# ATLAS OF FLEXIBLE BRONCHOFIBERSCOPY

SHIGETO IKEDA, M. D.

*Chief of Broncho-esophagological Division,*
*Chief of Chest Diagnosis,*
*National Cancer Center Hospital, Tokyo*

UNIVERSITY PARK PRESS BALTIMORE AND LONDON
IGAKU SHOIN LTD. TOKYO

**Library of Congress Cataloging in Publication Data**
Ikeda, Shigeto.
Atlas of flexible bronchofiberscopy.

Bibliography: p.
1. Bronchoscope and bronchoscopy. I. Title.
[DNLM: 1. Bronchoscopy—Atlases. WF 17 126a 1974 (P)]
RC 778. I 37 616.2′3′0754 74-4277
ISBN 0-8391-0686-6

PUBLISHERS

Sole distribution rights for USA and Canada granted to
UNIVERSITY PARK PRESS, Chamber of Commerce Building, Baltimore, Maryland 21202


Printed and bound in Japan

*This book is dedicated*

TO MY COLLEAGUES

*and*

TO MY WIFE, TAEKO

*Without whose help, this book would not have been possible*

# Foreword

When Dr. SHIGETO IKEDA attended the Ninth International Congress on Diseases of the Chest in Copenhagen in August 1966, he demonstrated the prototype of the present day bronchofiberscope. He brought a motion picture with him which showed that the instrument could be used for bronchoscopic cinematography. We were greatly impressed by Dr. IKEDA's presentation.

When he visited the Mayo Clinic some time later, he brought an improved version of the bronchofiberscope, which we had the opportunity to use in our endoscopic clinic. We were convinced that a tremendous advance had been made in the art and science of bronchoscopy. We were now able to probe the depths of the bronchial tree to a much greater extent than heretofore had been possible. The branches of the upper lobe were now accessible to direct vision. Even if lesions in the distal portions of the bronchial tree could not be visualized, material for histologic or microbiologic study could be obtained by brush, curette, or flexible biopsy forceps. In this regard, the bronchofiberscope was a significant advance over transbronchial brushing by catheter, a technique that also had been pioneered by Dr. IKEDA and his colleagues Drs. TSUBOI and ISHIKAWA and by Dr. HATTORI and his group in Japan.

In July 1969, I had the privilege of visiting the National Cancer Center Hospital in Tokyo. By this time, Dr. IKEDA was using the bronchofiberscope routinely in all cases of suspected bronchogenic carcinoma but especially the early and peripheral lesions. I marvelled at his dexterity and his skill in exploring the bronchial tree and his intimate knowledge of bronchial anatomy. Truly a new era in bronchology had begun.

Dr. IKEDA has reported his work with the bronchofiberscope at medical meetings in many parts of the world. The presentation, including a motion picture that he gave at the meeting of the American Bronchoesophagologic Association in April 1970, was particularly impressive. The bronchofiberscope has become an indispensable part of the armamentarium of the bronchologist. The instrument is now widely used in all thoracic centers and especially in clinics concerned with the early diagnosis of lung cancer.

Dr. IKEDA has presented us with a monumental treatise on the instrument that he had such a great role in developing. It would be impossible in this short foreword to emphasize more than a few of the important contributions that are made in this book. In Part I, Dr. IKEDA traces the development of the instruments that are currently available and makes it clear that further improvements can be expected. He does a good job of placing fiberbronchoscopy in its proper perspective. Bronchoscopy should be done in a specially equipped room by adequately trained personnel. Although the author prefers to use the fiberscope, he points out that the rigid bronchoscope is the instrument of choice for tracheal lesions and many lesions of the major bronchi, especially foreign bodies.

The new technique of fiberbronchoscopy necessitates knowledge of the detailed anatomy of the bronchial tree and requires a revision of present nomenclature. No longer is it sufficient to recognize the 18 segments described by JACKSON and HUBER or even the more detailed designations of BOYDEN and the Japanese Committee on Nomenclature for Bronchial Branching. Dr. IKEDA has devised a system that describes the bronchial tree up to the fifth generation of branching. Reports of bronchoscopic findings are best recorded on charts of the bronchial tree. In addition, a classification of bronchoscopic findings is advocated.

Considerable attention is devoted in this book to the usefulness of fiberoptic bronchoscopy in the early detection of cancer. Certainly the new instrument has proved to be most valuable in this area, and Dr. IKEDA describes his experience in considerable detail. In patients with positive cytology but negative chest roentgenograms, the examination of the bronchial tree may be very time-consuming. An orderly and meticulous exploration of the bronchial tree is essential if the neoplasm is to be localized. Experience in the Mayo Lung Project for early cancer detection has verified Dr. IKEDA's observations.

Part II is devoted to many case reports that reflect the author's experience. As might be expected, most of the cases are concerned with lung cancer. Certainly, the cases illustrate his success in utilizing all available endoscopic techniques. In addition to direct vision of the lesion, biopsy, brushing, irrigation, and aspiration, he often employs bronchography to aid in the localization of peripheral lesions. These case reports emphasize that the endoscopist is dependent on the cooperative efforts of expert radiologists and cytopathologists.

The role of the bronchofiberscope in therapy is obviously more limited. Nevertheless, the instrument may be useful in some circumstances. In the critically ill postoperative patient, secretions may be aspirated through the fiberscope. The author outlines the possible usefulness of the instrument in therapy and describes a case of foreign body removal. Undoubtedly, further improvements in the bronchofiberscope and flexible endoscopic forceps will lead to greater use of the instrument for therapeutic purposes.

As the reader will soon note, the volume is profusely illustrated and includes many magnificent color photos of the bronchial tree. In every respect, the volume lives up to the high standards of the publisher, Igaku Shoin Ltd. This volume certainly is an authoritative work on the newest and most impressive contribution to bronchology, the bronchofiberscope.

ARTHUR M. OLSEN, M. D.

*Professor of Medicine*
*Mayo Graduate School of Medicine*
*(University of Minnesota)*
*Rochester, Minnesota, U.S.A.*

# Foreword

Bronchoscopy was first introduced into Japan by Professor Inokichi Kubo who studied under Gustav Killian in 1903. As in other countries the utilization of a bronchoscope in those days was limited largely to the removal of foreign bodies in the air passages. Then the Chevalier Jackson system was introduced into this country in 1934 at the time when the bronchoscope had just become recognized as a useful instrument in the diagnosis and treatment of pulmonary tuberculosis.

After World War II, with the increasing incidence of tuberculosis, bronchoscopy became an indispensable armamentarium in dealing with chest diseases. Under the general acceptance of the role which bronchoscopy played, there emerged the Japan Broncho-esophagological Society in 1949 The Society, among others, was instrumental in creating closer bonds of mutual cooperation not only between broncho-esophagologists with otolaryngologists but also with thoracic surgeons, chest physicians, pediatricians, anaesthesiologists and roentgenologists in the study of their common interests in the bronchial trees. While the main objective was initially directed towards the solution of problems in tuberculosis, the rising incidence of lung cancer made the clinicians switch their interest to early diagnosis of bronchogenic carcinomas.

It was at this transitional period of decreasing pulmonary tuberculosis to increasing lung cancers that a flexible bronchofiberscope came to be recognized. The credit for the first to report on the subject must go to Dr. Shigeto Ikeda. He demonstrated it with motion pictures at the 9th International Congress on Diseases of the Chest held in Copenhagen in 1966. Also, Dr. Ikeda was the first to publish an article on the use of the flexible bronchofiberscope which appeared in the Journal of Japan Broncho-esophagological Society and Keio Journal of Medicine in 1968.

Dr. Ikeda was graduated from Keio University School of Medicine in 1952. Immediately, he joined the Department of Thoracic Surgery of his alma mater and studied under Visiting Prof Yasuyuki Kano, a renown surgeon in collapse therapy for tuberculosis. While under training on thoracic surgery centering on the treatment of pulmonary tuberculosis, Dr Ikeda showed special interest in diagnostics and pathology of bronchi through bronchography and bronchoscopy. His paper entitled "Patho-physiological Studies of Bronchi using Bronchographic Motion Pictures" presented at the 7th International Congress of Broncho-esophagology was acclaimed by those familiar with this problem as an outstanding contribution. Dr. Ikeda's research was aimed at grasping and analyzing in a clear and dynamic manner the organic structures of the human body. To achieve this end he had already been richly endowed with talents in technology and electrical engineering as well as in the practical skills of cinematography such as cinebronchography and endoscopic motion pictures.

In 1962, Dr. Ikeda was appointed Chief of the Division of Broncho-esophagology at the then newly created National Cancer Center Hospital, the first institute of its kind in Japan Incidentally, there seems to be two factors involved in his being named to this position. The first was that Dr. Shichiro Ishikawa, Director of the Hospital, had a keen sense of detecting the special talent and abilities possessed by Dr Ikeda The other factor was that Dr. Ikeda himself had the confidence that he was equal to the task of contributing to medicine by developing useful instruments.

While applying to practice his knowledge of bronchology acquired during his training, he realized that he was not satisfied with only a 40 per cent of accuracy in the diagnosis of lung cancer which was attainable with a rigid bronchoscope. Encouraged by the development of the gastrofiberscope, then of the glassfiber optics, he began to develop a bronchofiberscope in 1964 with which he succeeded in 1966 as the world's first model capable of practical use. Through further improvements, it has become increasingly popular. At present 2,000 fiberscopes are being used by medical men throughout the world. Thus, bronchofiberscopy has established itself on a firm basis as an important clinical armamentarium.

The concern that Dr. Ikeda shows in bronchology, however, is not limited to developing fiberscopes. As noted in this book, his studies cover a wide range of anatomical and pathological researches. To mention only a few: they include the new nomenclature of bronchi, classification of bronchoscopic findings, and endoscopic classification of lung cancers. Recently, he has launched a formidable project for the early diagnosis of cancer of the hilum of the lung. He has also designed and perfected various endoscopic cameras and endoscopic color television devices. The results of these investigations have frequently been reported at international meetings.

Bronchoscopy first brought to practical use by Dr. Killian and Dr. Jackson has been improved and streamlined to keep abreast of modern bronchology with the ingenuity of Dr. Ikeda. His flexible bronchofiberscopy, science-aided, is making rapid strides as a standard orthodox method. The progress, indeed, is short of a meteoric feat.

This Atlas of Flexible Bronchofiberscopy is the first authoritative monograph devoted to exploring hitherto unfathomed areas in bronchology. It is my fervent hope that the work will do much to evoke interest and stimulate further study for clinicians throughout the world.

*"He that does good to another man, does also good to himself;*
*not only in the consequence, but in the very act of doing;*
*for the consciousness of well-doing is an ample reward."*
——*Seneca*

JO ONO, M. D., Sc. D.
*Visiting Professor,*
*Keio University School of Medicine, Tokyo*
*President, Japan Broncho-esophagological Society*

# Foreword

I regard it a great credit to the National Cancer Center in Tokyo to have Dr. SHIGETO IKEDA, a prominent clinical physician on our medical staff.

Dr. S. IKEDA is one of the most outstanding contributors in the field of science in Japan, whose devoted efforts toward the development and improvement of the flexible bronchofiberscope, that have been made since the time of his appointment at the National Cancer Center 11 years ago, raised the standard of this instrument up to its present level.

Today, in Japan, the flexible bronchofiberscope is indispensable for the diagnosis of various diseases of the lung, especially the early detection of bronchial cancers admitted to our hospital. The applications of this instrument in practice proved very successful; and at the same time the results of these application brought forth many valuable suggestions for further improvements, which are now being studied.

Dr. IKEDA's atlas shows, with many beautifully and vividly illustrated colored pictures, the useful applications in practice and the facts of various forms of diseases discovered by the instrument. They are explained along with the history of the bronchoscope as its background.

It is my fervent desire that this atlas be made available to the specialists in European countries and the U. S. A. where the frequencies of male bronchogenic carcinomas were as predominent as 78, 70 and 40 per 100,000 population in Scotland, England and the U. S. A. respectively, during 1966–1967 rather than in Japan where the frequency was low (14 per 100,000 population although this type of cancer has increased rapidly in recent years). For this reason the Igaku Shoin Ltd. has consented to publish this book in English.

It is firmly believed that this atlas would not only bring credit to Dr. IKEDA personally, but would also become one of the great contributions that our National Cancer Center could make to the world in related fields. If this book would be widely utilized by scholars in this field and thus serve for the early detection and progress in the treatment of lung cancer, I will be gratefully pleased with the publication.

KEMPO TSUKAMOTO, M. D.

*President*
*National Cancer Center, Tokyo*

# Preface

In the summer of 1966, I had the opportunity of introducing the first flexible broncho fiberscope in the world to the IX International Congress on Diseases of the Chest held at Copenhagen. Since then the bronchofiberscope has been rapidly accepted and welcomed by bronchoscopists everywhere. Now that approximately 2,000 bronchofiberscopes are in world-wide use, they are replacing the conventional rigid bronchoscopes which have been in use for over 70 years.

In the past, many types of medical apparatus or instruments long utilized have been gradually supplanted by others newly developed; however, the flexible bronchofiberscope is unique in that it has seen world-wide diffusion in a very short period of time. This radical change in the field of examination of the tracheo-bronchial tree, extending the clinical indications for diagnosis and treatment carries with it potential dangers of complications as well as damage to the bronchofiberscope itself, unless the instrument is utilized with meticulous care and technique which comes only with proper training and practice. In order to perform the procedure with the highest degree of safety and efficiency, bronchofiberscopists must have a thorough knowledge of the anatomy and physiology of the tracheo-bronchial tree. At the same time, they should know the potentialities as well as limitations of the bronchofiberscope.

This Atlas is divided into two parts: Part I, General Information, describes the various models of the bronchofiberscopes, technique of performing orthodox examinations with these instruments, care and sterilization, recording of findings, and the bronchoscopic anatomy of the tracheo-bronchial tree. The second division, Part II, Case Presentations, includes clinical reports of 58 representative cases.

The theme and significance of each subdivision will be briefly mentioned here:

1) By presenting the evolution and development of the bronchofiberscope from its inception to the present form, the trainee is able to thoroughly understand the structure of the apparatus.

2) By learning the proper manipulation of the bronchofiberscope, the trainee will be able to minimize the potential dangers of damage to the instrument as well as avoiding any accident that may be inflicted upon the patient.

3) The three dimensional stereo-photograph of the bronchial tree which was especially prepared for this book will help the reader to acquire the anatomic nomenclature of the various branches out to the fourth order of branching. We are proud to present the first three dimensional stereo-photograph ever to appear in a medical book.

4) In order to enable the student to learn thoroughly the normal appearance of the bronchial tree as seen through the bronchofiberscope, these findings have been presented as a color Atlas. The photographs were taken with the 5 mm bronchofiberscope in common use.

5) Abnormalities have been classified according to types, and have been presented with colored photographs, diagrams, statements as to significance, and discussions.

6) More recently, the flexible bronchofiberscope is being utilized not only for diagnosis but also for therapeutic purposes. These therapeutic usages have been outlined

7) A large number of pages in the Atlas has been devoted to case presentations.

The main concern has been lung cancer. Detailed descriptions of each case with cytological diagnosis and pathological findings are presented. The following has been emphasized in this section:

Firstly, in the process of arriving at a diagnosis, one should thoroughly review the X-ray films. In this regard, tomograms and/or bronchograms are extremely helpful, as they often reflect the bronchoscopic findings accurately.

Secondly, bronchial findings are depicted by schematized diagrams in order to aid in interpreting the pathology; also, by a diagram of the bronchial tree accurately pinpointing the exact location of the lesion.

Thirdly, bronchoscopic diagnosis depends upon the endoscopic findings plus cytological examination of specimens obtained by bronchoscopic biopsy. For this reason, photographs of cytologic or biopsy findings are included in some cases.

Fourthly, bronchoscopic findings are verified by examination of the resected specimens. Thus, in as possible, the resected specimen with gross and microscopic findings have been included.

Finally, comments have been added giving the summary and impressions that we have gained.

About four years have been spent in the preparation and completion of this book. I had hoped that this publication would have been completed before the brochofiberscope became so popular, creating a demand for such an Atlas. The delay was due primarily to the fact that I wished to present a thorough and complete book on the subject. I apologize from the heart for this delay.

A final word: A video-cassette in color entitled "Technique of the Flexible Bronchofiberscope" is available as a supplement to this book. This will compensate for some of the shortcomings of a book in respect to actual techniques as they are presented audiovisually, including endoscopic colored movies. It is hoped that you use the cassette tape as an integral part of the book.


## ACKNOWLEDGEMENTS

In preparing this publication, the following persons have contributed a great deal, directly or indirectly, to the author No amount of words of appreciation would suffice for the gratitude I feel towards these persons.

Dr. Arthur M. Olsen, Professor of Medicine, Mayo Graduate School of Medicine, (Univ. of Minnesota), Rochester, Minnesota, U.S A.

For his invaluable Foreword to this book and his efforts expended in the worldwide diffusion of the flexible bronchofiberscope.

Dr. Jo Ono, Visiting Professor, School of Medicine, Keio Univ., Tokyo.

Also for his invaluable Foreword to this book and his effort given to the domestic diffusion of the same bronchofiberscope.

Dr. Kempo Tsukamoto, President, National Cancer Center, Tokyo.

For his taking the trouble to write a invaluable Foreword to this book.

Dr. Yoshihiko Fred Fujikawa, Consulting Bronchoscopist, Long Beach (California) Veterans Administration Hospital and Univ. of California at Los Angeles Medical Center, U.S.A

For his painstaking and correction of the English version of the manuscript and his highly important suggestions for the book, from the standpoint of an American chest surgeon and bronchoscopist.

Dr. Yasuyuki Kano, Visiting Professor, School of Medicine, Keio Univ., Tokyo, and Director of the National Kasumigaura Hospital, Tsuchiura.

For his early instructions in chest surgery and as a teacher.

Dr. SHICHIRO ISHIKAWA, Visiting Professor, School of Medicine, Keio Univ., Tokyo, and Director of the National Cancer Center Hospital, Tokyo.
For his instruction which directed the author's attention to the diagnosis of lung cancer, and his generosity in allowing me a free hand in research along this line.

Dr. YUZIRO DOTAI, Formerly Assistant Professor, School of Medicine, Keio Univ., Tokyo.
For his early guidance in providing the author with the theme of research of bronchology.

Dr. YUKIO SHIMOZATO, Chief Pathologist, National Cancer Center Hospital, Tokyo.
For his valued advice as one of the leading pathologists on lung cancer in Japan, and for his kindness in supplying the valuable photographs of gross and microscopic specimens which are contained herein as plates.

Dr. RYOSUKE ONO, National Cancer Center Hospital, Tokyo.
One of the most indispensable cooperators in bronchofiberscopy who worked in the field of cytology for the preparation of this book.

Dr. NAOTO MIYAZAWA, National Cancer Center Hospital, Tokyo.
Also one of the most important cooperators in this field, devoting his attention mainly in the field of pathology in this book.

Dr. KOJI NAMBA, National Cancer Center Hospital, Tokyo.
A third most highly valued cooperator, who produced the replicas of bronchographic schemata in this book.

Dr. AKI KOETSU, National Cancer Center Hospital, Tokyo.
For his ample cooperation in the field of cytopathology.

Dr. KIICHI FURUYA, Tokyo Medical and Dental Univ., School of Medicine, Tokyo.
For his laborious work in producing bronchofiberscopic replicas.

Prof. HAJIME ORIYA, Professor of English, Japan Defense Academy, Yokosuka.
For his cooperation in turning out the English version of this book.

Mr. TSUNEO MACHIDA, President of Machida Endoscope Company, Ltd., Tokyo.
Mr. HARUHIKO MACHIDA, Vice President of Machida Eodoscope Company, Ltd., Tokyo.
For their generosity in listening to the author's original idea of newly costructing the flexible bronchofiberscope and incorporating all of the author's demands accurately in the actual manufacturing of the apparatus.

Mr. NAGASHIGE TAKAHASHI, Olympus Optical Co., Ltd., Tokyo, now retired.
For his effort in the manufacturing of the flexible bronchofiberscope as a person in exclusive charge of this work.

Mr. HIROYUKI FURIHATA, Olympus Optical Co., Ltd., Tokyo.
For his earnest efforts in manufacturing the recently developed type of bronchofiberscope.

Mr. SENTARO SHIMIZU, Mr. KAZUO ODA and Mr. TSUNETAKA KURODA, respectively of the Machida Endoscope Co., Ltd., Tokyo.
For their assistance in proof-reading.

Mr. RINSHI KOBAYASHI, Toppan Printing Co., Ltd., Tokyo
For his efforts in producing 3-dimensional printing of the bronchial tree.

November, 1973

SHIGETO IKEDA, M. D.
*National Cancer Center Hospital*
*Tokyo, Japan*

# Contents

## Part two : CASE PRESENTATION

# Case Index

# Part 1
# GENERAL

# I. The Development of the Bronchoscope

## HISTORICAL BACKGROUND OF THE RIGID BRONCHOSCOPE

Bronchoscopy, a method for directly visualizing pathologic changes in the trachea and bronchi, is an extremely useful procedure for the diagnosis of pulmonary disease. It would not be too much to say that the effectiveness of bronchoscopy is solely dependent on the efficiency of the apparatus used.

The rigid bronchoscope originated from GUSTAV KILLIAN (1860–1921), Freiburg, who has been called the father of bronchoscopy. Much of his achievement in this field, however, was dependent on the work of other pioneers. JOSEPH P. O'DWYER (1841–1894), famous for his intubation in diphtheria, contrived a tube of thin metal for the purpose of removing foreign bodies from the trachea or bronchus. This tubular contrivance, motivated later by the electric bulb invented by THOMAS EDISON in 1878, established the foundation for endoscopic examination of the lower air way including the larynx. In 1895, KIRSTEIN of Berlin examined the interior of a patient's larynx directly with O'DWYER's tube, aided by CASPER's prismatic electric bulb, by depressing the tongue and epiglottis. These pioneering attempts by physicians in other countries preceeded the work of G. KILLIAN. KILLIAN employed an esophagoscope for the direct inspection of the esophagus and an endoscope for the direct examination of the bronchus. KILLIAN's endoscope was illuminated by an external light source and a head mirror; while BRUNNING, his disciple, designed another type of endoscope equipped with an ocular illumination. This contributed greatly to the diffusion of direct inspection technique.

In the United States, in 1897, MAX EINHORN (1865–1928) published his first essay on esophagoscopy; and in 1902, he succeeded in developing an esophagoscope illuminated at the distal tip. CHEVALIER JACKSON, Philadelphia, produced a bronchoscope incorporating a suction tube as well as tip-illumination in 1904. Since then, bronchoscopists all over the world have been utilizing the KILLIAN or the JACKSON type, or a modification of one of these instruments (Fig. 1).

In the meantime, a demand arose for a magnified field of vision for observing the interior of the bronchus. The demand created two types of accessories. One was a telescope which could be inserted into a bronchoscope for magnification. The other invention consisted of attaching a telephoto-lens to the distal end of the open tube rigid bronchoscope, the end of which was obliquely

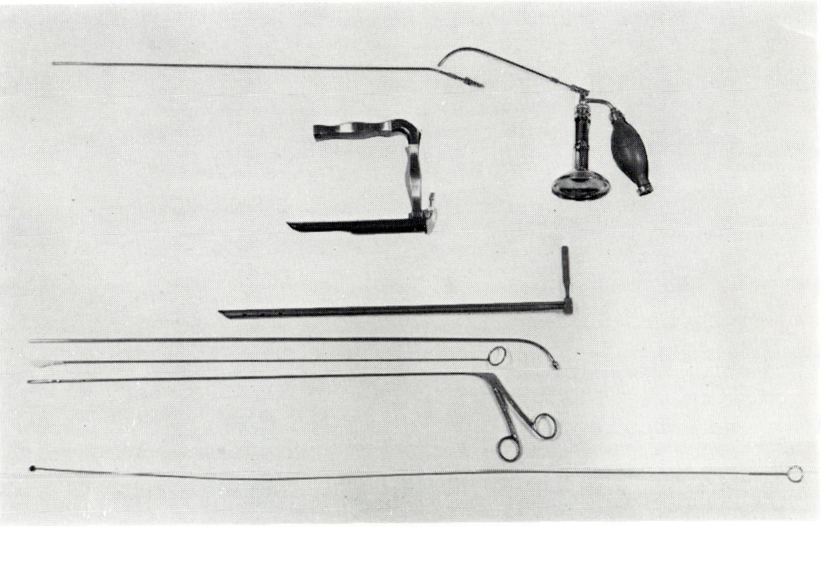

**Fig. 1** A set of rigid bronchoscopy.

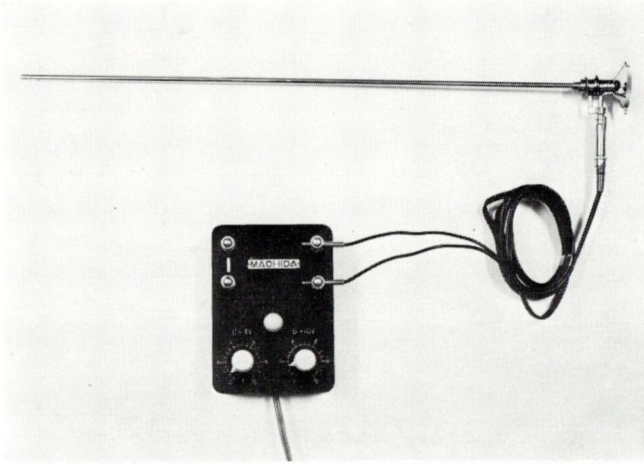


**Fig. 2** A telescope with an electric bulb attached.

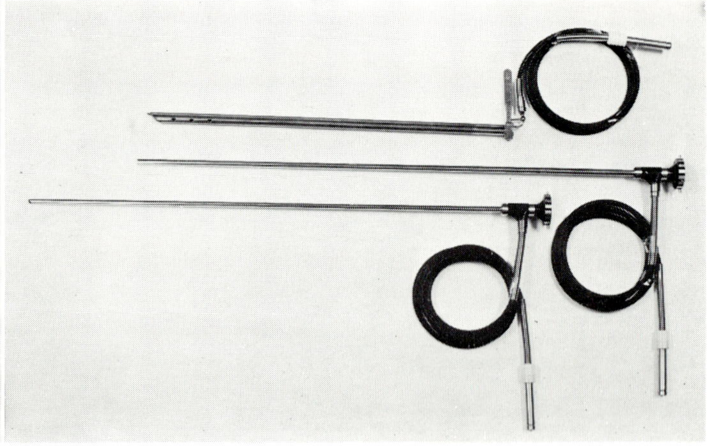

**Fig. 3** A rigid bronchoscope with optic glass fiber and optic glass fiber telescopes (one is a lateral viewing and the other is direct viewing).

angled. The bronchoscopic telescopes were illuminated at the tip by a small electric bulb with foroblique view or lateral-view lenses. This modification greatly increased the range of visibility (Fig. 2).

In recent years an attempt was made to further increase illumination by employing a quartz rod instead of the small electric bulb. With the recent development of the optic glass fiber, a new telescope made of glass fiber as light-guide was manufactured (Fig. 3). The illumination obtained was several times brighter than the older system. It has several other features : completely unobstructed, well illuminated and larger visual field without parallax, as the fixed bulb at the tip has been eliminated ; and most importantly, a reduction in the diameter of the tip. This improved the range of visibility, extending it from the subsegmental to the sub-subsegmental bronchi in the middle and the lower lobes. Thus, the range of visibility for the diagnosis of lung cancer was extended to these areas.

## EVALUATION OF A RIGID BRONCHOSCOPE

In spite of ceaseless efforts to improve the rigid bronchoscope, many problems were left unsolved as a bronchoscope for diagnosing lung cancer. Admittedly, if tumors are found within the visible range of this instrument, the diagnosis will be definitive, the location and aspects of the tumors will be well observed, and histologic examination may be performed. But the detection range of lung cancer, even aided by a telescope (Fig. 4) is limited to the hilar type or those located in the lobar, segmental, or subsegmental bronchi of the middle and the lower lobes. Most importantly, the segmental and subsegmental bronchi in both upper lobes cannot be visualized : $B^1$, $B^2$, $B^3$ on the right and $B^{1+2}$ and $B^3$ on the left. Cytologic and histologic examinations are often extremely difficult in these areas because of their inaccessibility.

Among 217 cases of lung cancer resected at the National Cancer Center Hospital in Tokyo in the past 5 years, 48 cases were classified as "early lung cancer" that is, the size of the tumor in these cases was less than 30 mm in diameter. Pathologic tracing was done on these resected lung specimens, and the locations of lesions exposing themselves or infiltrating the bronchi are plotted on a diagram of the bronchial tree (Fig. 5). Many of these early small tumors are located in the upper lobes and are probably visible in only 10 out of 48 cases (20.8%) based on the visible range of the conventional rigid bronchoscope. Thus, it is apparent that the rigid bronchoscope loses its effectiveness for smaller tumors, when early diagnosis is imperative. Since a majority of early small cancerous lesions are located in the branch bronchi of the upper lobes, that is the segmental bronchi (II order of branching), subsegmental bronchi (III order) and sub-subsegmental (IV order), extension of the visible range over these areas could conceivably have made another 30 cases (62.4%) visible. Extension as far as the bronchi of V order of branching would possibly raise the detection rate even further. The locations of these resected lesions in relation to pathologic histology was studied. The examination revealed that many of the small tumors at the hilum were squamous cell carcinoma, and that many of the peripheral small tumors were adenocarcinoma. The small tumors found between the subseg-

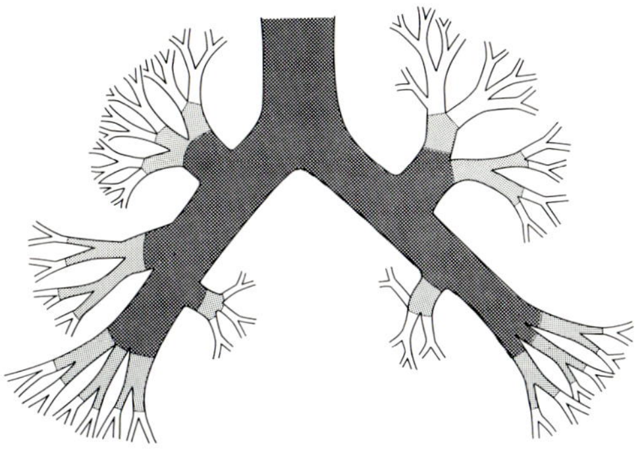


**Fig. 4** Visible range with a rigid bronchoscope.

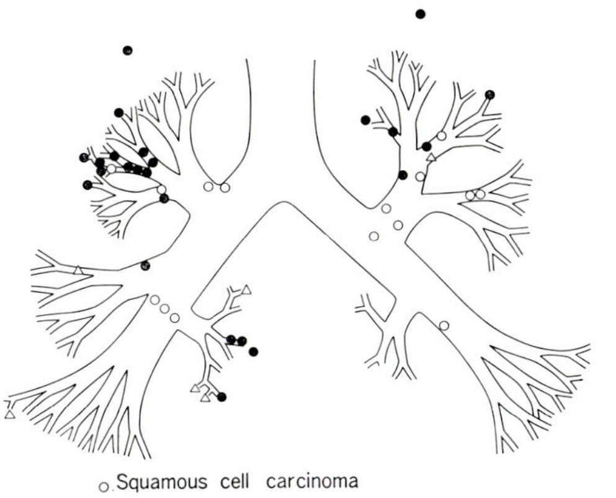


**Fig. 5** Types of carcinoma and locations in 48 resected tumors less than 30 mm in diameter (1963–1965).

mental bronchi (III order) and V order of bronchi were designated intermediate tumors. Of 48 cases of small early tumors, 25 cases (52%) were intermediate, *i. e.*, 13 of 14 cases of squamous cell carcinoma, 9 of 27 cases of adenocarcinoma, and 3 of 7 cases of undifferentiated cell carcinoma. Thus, another type of bronchoscope was required, which would permit inspection deeper into the upper lobes extending to at least IV to V order of branching and allow brushing or biopsy during observation for the definitive diagnosis of early lung cancer.

Another shortcoming of the rigid bronchoscope is that it requires special skill in insertion (Figs. 6 and 7) and is uncomfortable to the patient during examination. Difficulties often occur during prolonged examination under local anesthesia. This is another reason that spurred the development of a flexible bronchoscope.

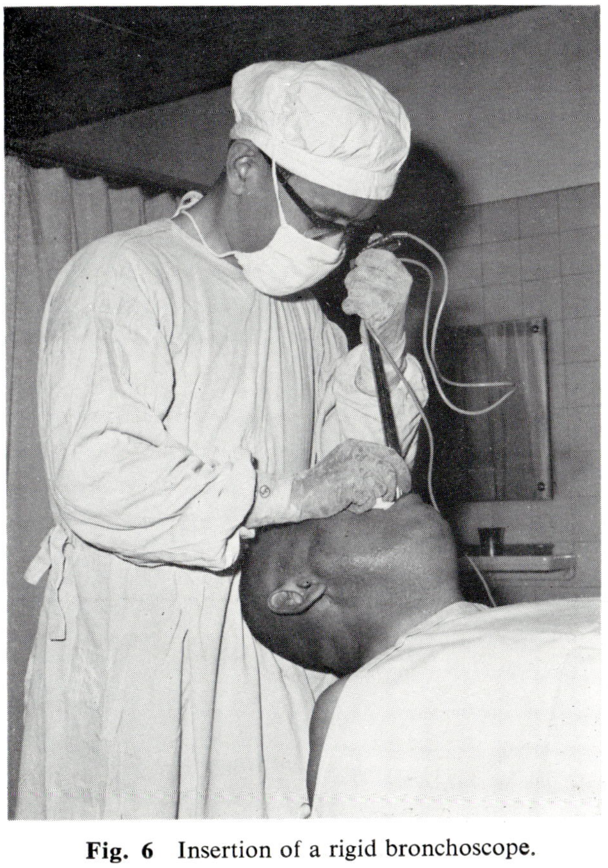

**Fig. 6** Insertion of a rigid bronchoscope.

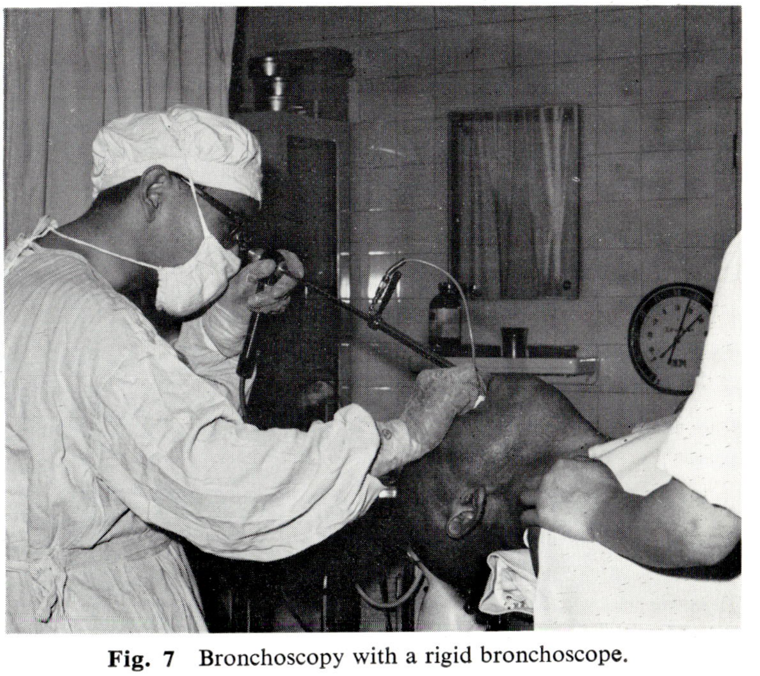

**Fig. 7** Bronchoscopy with a rigid bronchoscope.

# GLASS FIBER AND A FIBERSCOPE

**1. Glass fiber** (Figs. 8 and 9)

When a glass stick is melted by heat and is rapidly pulled apart, the melted portion forms a long fine silk-like thread. If this piece of thread is 10 $\mu$ or less in diameter, it will possess a property similar to that of a fiber, quite different from the ordinary conception of glass. Thus, flexible glass fibers were created. John Tyndall, an Englishman, 1870, described the optical properties of such fibers. But it was not until J. L. Baird (1927), an Englishman and C. W. Hansell (1930), an American put forth the proposal that this property could be utilized. In 1930, H. Lamm, a German, advocated the application of the glass fibers to a flexible gastroscope. It was not until the 1950s, however, that real progress was made on research into the optical properties of the glass fiber. In most cases fibers are utilized in the form of bundles in fiberoptic systems. One of the essentials for such an application is the complete optical insulation of each fiber in the bundle.

The present method of accomplishing this insulation is to coat the exterior of the core of each light-transmitting fiber with a transparent material (actually melted glass) of lower refractive index than the core glass, a cladding method. The principle of light transmission through the fiber is that the light, entering at a certain angle of incidence from the cut-end surface of a fiber, travels through the fiber, striking the cladding glass and repeatedly reflects internally even though the fiber is bent or twisted on the way (Fig. 10).

Cladding glass, an indispensable component of currently used glass fibers, is an invention by V. Heel, a

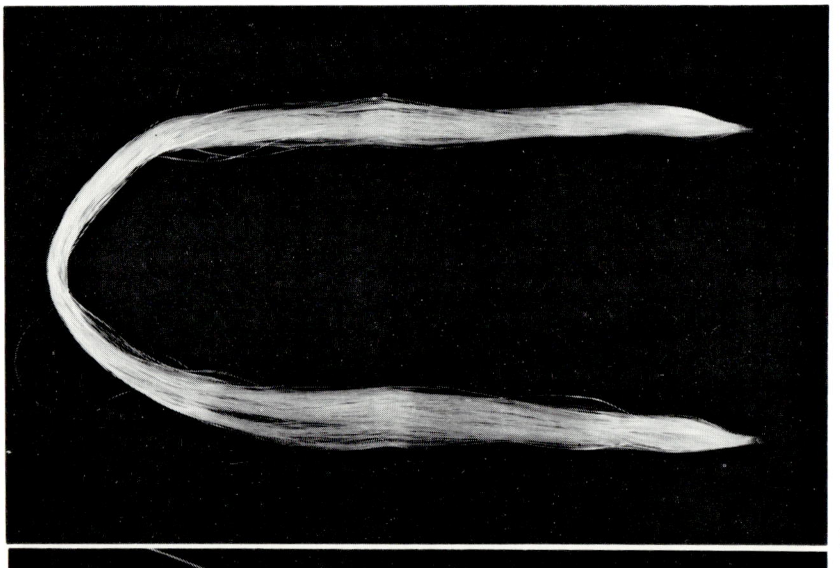

**Fig. 8** A glass fiber bundle.

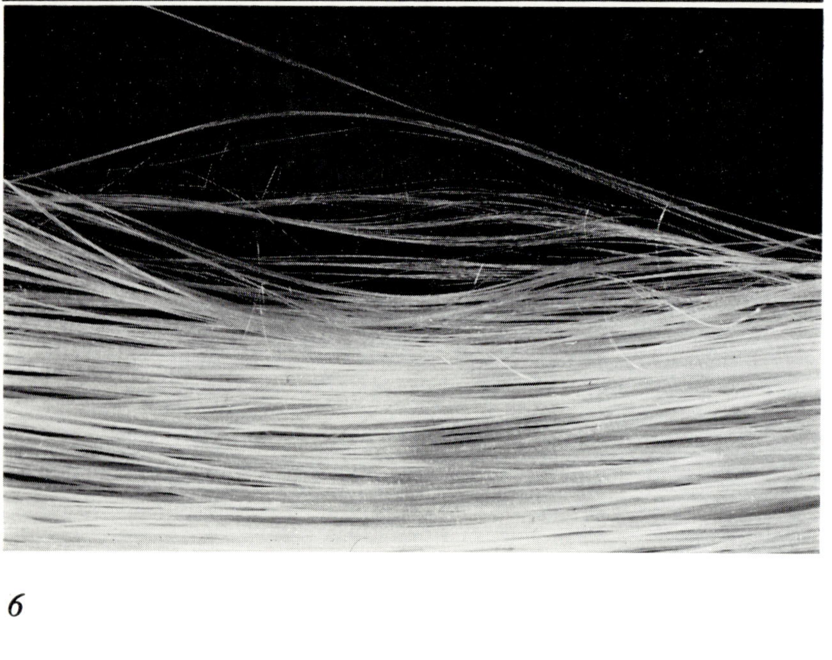

**Fig. 9** Part of a glass fiber bundle, magnified.

Dutchman and B. O'Brien, an American. Later H. H. Hopkins and N. S. Kapany, both Englishmen, developed the optically-arranged fiber bundle and named it the fiberscope.

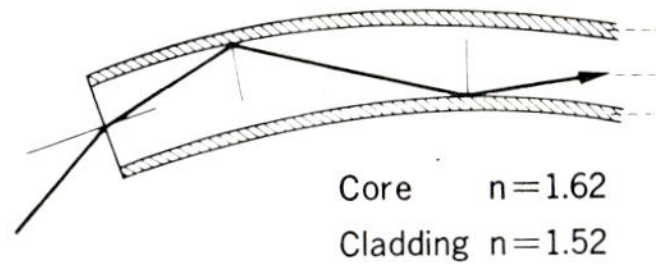


**Fig. 10** Principle of glass fiber : Reflection and guide of light within the coated glass fiber.

## 2. Fiberscope

A large number of optical fibers fastened together with both ends tightly fixed makes a flexible bundle. When an optical image enters one end of the bundle, the image is transmitted to the other end. To accomplish this, it is essential that the regular arrangement compactness of fibers at one end of the bundle are precisely the same as at the other end. If so, each fiber will convey its own light volume to the other end in strict accordance with the light and shade of the image focused (Fig. 11). This is the principle of a fiberscope. The resolution of a fiberscope is solely dependent on the regularity, density and compactness of fibers at both ends. The smaller the fiber size, the better the resolution ; but if the fiber is too thin it loses its mechanical strength and light transmission capacity. It has generally been assumed that about 5 $\mu$ is the limit.

There are varieties of technical methods in the manufacture of a fiberscope, especially in the relationship of fibers to each other. The pattern of fiber arrangement in each manufacturer is a closely guarded secret. This is evidence of the high precision and accuracy required for the arrangement of fibers. When both cut-ends of bundled fibers have been polished, a set of objectives and oculars are set in the ends. A fiberscope is thus completed (Figs. 12 and 13).

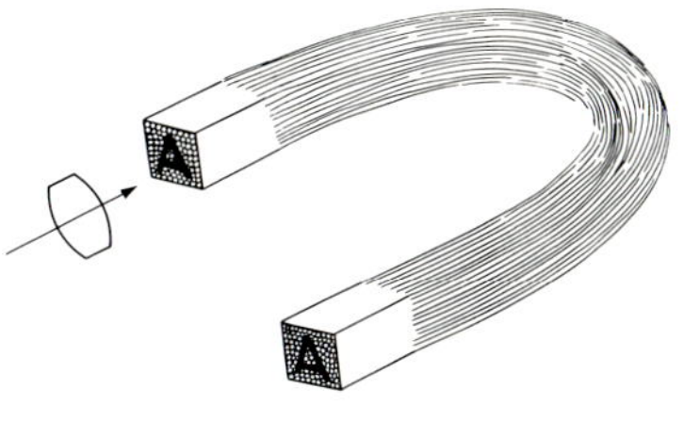

**Fig. 11** Principle of glass fiber : Transmission of an image through a glass fiber bundle from the distal end to the proximal end.

## 3. Development of the fiberscope

An early type of fiberscope was invented and so named by H. H. Hopkins and N. S. Kapany who brought it to the United States. There, investigational work was carried on by the University of Rochester and Bausch and Lomb, Optical Technology Inc. At the University of Michigan, work on the gastrofiberscope was conducted separately by B. Hirschowitz and his group. In 1957, a type of fiberscope was demonstrated at the Gastroscopic Society of America, and the appratus was named the gastroduodenal fiberscope.

In Japan, a test gastrofiberscope of modified type (F. G. S.) was manufactured in October, 1962, at Machida Endoscope Co., Ltd., under the supervision of T. Kondo, T. Takemoto and K. Tsuneoka. The modified gastrofiberscope retained the advantages and improved the deficiencies of Hirschowitz's gastrofiberscope. In the following year, 1964, a gastrocamera equipped fiberscope was manufactured at Olympus Optical Co., Ltd. In 1966, an esophagofiberscope was produced by Machida under the guidance of T. Takemoto, T. Kogure and T. Kondo, and another of similar structure was made by Olympus. At the 1st. Congress of International Society of Endoscopy held

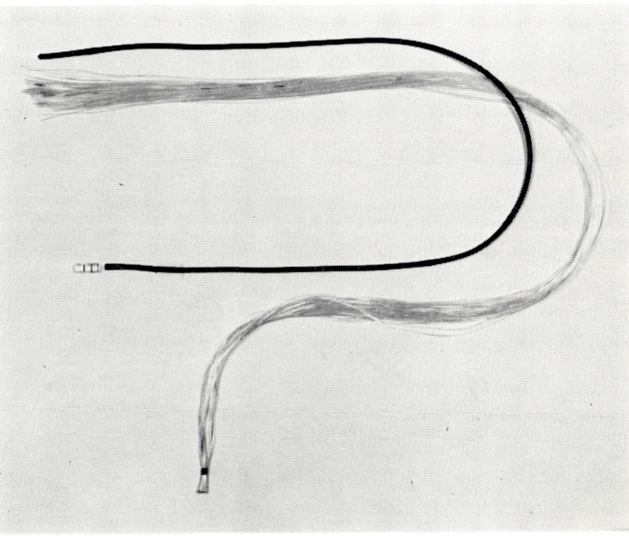

**Fig. 12** Glass fiber bundle taken out.

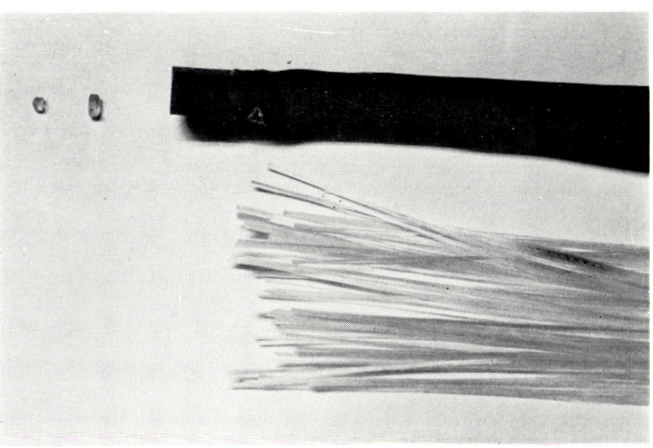

**Fig. 13** Disjointed glass fiber and distal tip, magnified.

in Tokyo in September, 1966, both Japanese and foreign makes were exhibited and demonstrated. Among them, those of Japanese make were very highly regarded internationally.

## DEVELOPMENT OF THE FLEXIBLE BRONCHOFIBERSCOPE

### a. Initial ideas

The specifications and characteristics of our initial proposal for a bronchofiberscope (1964) were as follows:

1. Outer diameter : less than 6 mm
2. Image-guide fiber : 15 μ, more than 15,000 in a bundle
3. Light-guide fiber : 15–20 μ, more than 10,000
4. Length of the distal rigid tip : less than 10 mm
5. Focal distance, fixed focus visible 5–30 mm
6. Angle : flexible by about 60 degrees at 30 mm from the distal end
7. Direct vision be provided
8. Total length : 1 m
9. Angle of vision : 80 degrees

The trial production of the above outlined apparatus was entrusted to Machida Endoscope Co., Ltd. Toward the end of 1965 similar specifications were given to Olympus Optical Co., Ltd. for production.

### b. Trial products by Machida Endoscope Co., Ltd.

In July, 1966, the first apparatus for test use was completed at Machida Endoscope Co., Ltd., satisfying most of our specifications and demands (Fig. 14). It was an excellent flexible fiberscope, with a 5 mm outer diameter, high flexibility, 90 degrees field of vision, and clear image resolution. Contrary to our original expectations, however, controlled angular bending of the distal tip was not achieved, so that free insertion into the targeted bronchus was not possible. It had other essential advantage however. It made possible visualization of the inside of a bronchus due to its flexibility, provided there had previously been inserted in the trachea another tube for anesthetizing that part. This is a memorable advantage : the patient was allowed to be examined in a natural supine position. Thus Machida No. 1 bronchofiberscope was the first ever utilized in the medical field in the world, together with Olympus No. 1 bronchofiberscope which will be discussed later. Both of these were reported and demonstrated at the 9th International Congress of Diseases of the Chest in Copenhagen, 1967, and were named Flexible Bronchofiberscopes.

Trials with the first two models of the bronchofiberscope disclosed various deficiencies. These can be summarized as follows : first, the distal end could not be flexed at will; second, there was no means by which anesthetic could be infused into the bronchus. Machida No. 2 instrument, made in September of the same year, improved upon these shortcomings. Its tip was flexible by 100 degrees in one direction and 10 degrees in the opposite direction at 15 mm from the distal end. Machida No. 3 (Fig. 15–2), produced in October of the same year, was equipped with a channel

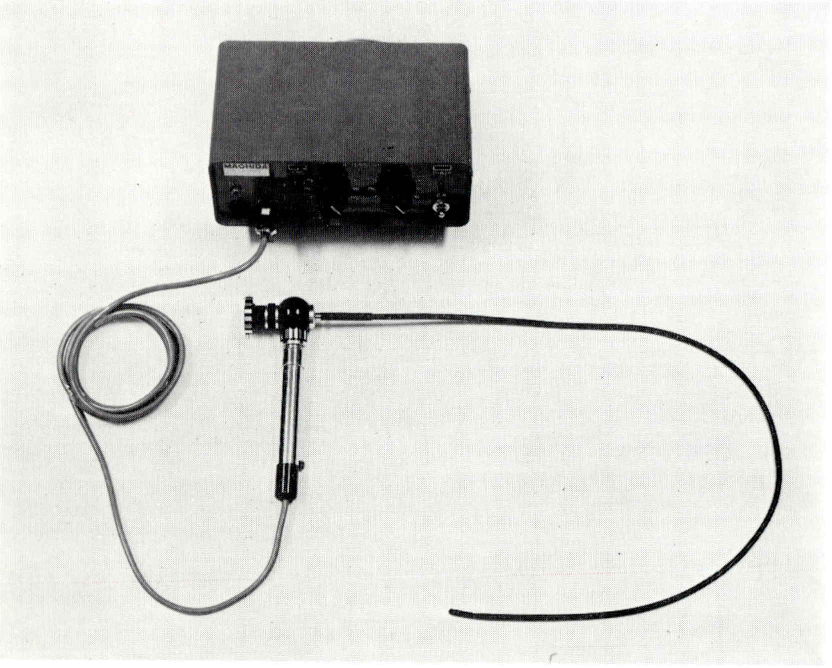


**Fig. 14** Flexible bronchofiberscope of Machida make, prototype fiberscope No. 1 (1966).

for infusing anesthetic solutions into the bronchus, and had a 5 mm outer diameter as in Machida No. 1. The No. 3 instrument not only satisfied the above mentioned items specified for the No. 1 bronchofiberscope but exceeded the original specifications as to the outer diameter and the angular flexibility. With this scope, the instrument could be introduced into III–IV order of branching in the middle and lower lobes, allowing visualization of bronchi of IV-V order. In the upper division bronchi of the upper lobes, however, visualization did not extend beyond the orifices of the subsegmental bronchi, due to limited angulation of the distal tip to only 100 degrees.

To overcome this deficiency, Machida No. 4 was completed in December of the same year (Fig. 15–3). This new model could be flexed to more than 150 degrees at the tip and its flexible tip was extended to 50 mm. The angulation of this tip was manipulated with two handles. A channel for the instillation of anesthetic preparation and another channel 1.0 mm in diameter for biopsy instruments was added to facilitate obtaining specimens for cytological examination. A small pin-head shaped curette could be introduced through the channel, with which one could scrape off tumor cells under direct vision. This was a distinct improvement. Insertion into the upper lobes was extended to segmental bronchi of $B^1$ (apical segmental bronchus), $B^2$ (posterior segmental bronchus), $B^{1+2}$ (apical-posterior segmental bronchus) and $B^3$ (anterior segmental bronchus); and, if necessary, to subsegmental bronchi. Visualization was possible as far as the bronchi of IV-V order of branching. With this instrument practically all the bronchi up to IV order were visualized, except for $B^6$a right and left, right $B^3$ and left $B^5$b.

In order to overcome these shortcomings in Machida No. 4 apparatus, further improvements were made. Thus in 1967, Machida No. 5 was born (Fig. 15–4). The following specifications for further improvements were submitted: 1) Angulation be manipulated by one handle and the bending angle of the tip increased to a perfect U-turn of 180 degrees. 2) The co-ordinate movement of the basal and apical parts be further improved so that any turn made at the basal part will be precisely transmitted to the apical end making it possible to aim the tip in any desired direction. 3) In addition to the co-ordinated movements of the eyepiece and tip, 30 degrees rotation of the tip to the right or left by a revolving ring on the base of the eyepiece be provided. 4) The inner surface of the biopsy forceps be hollowed out like a spoon to increase the amount of biopsy material obtainable. 5) The channel for the biopsy forceps be also used for instilling anesthetic solutions. These were great advancements but still two other items were added. One was to increase durability and the other to make the light-guide glass fiber longer so that it could be connected to an outside light source. Thus, Machida No. 6 was produced in July, 1967.

In September of the same year, the diameter of image-guide glass fiber was reduced from 15 μ to 12 μ for better image resolution, and a special treatment was given to the light-guide glass fiber to strengthen it physically. For the external light source, a 500W Xenon lamp was developed to increase the brightness of the visualized field. As a result, endoscopic photography and cinematography became possible. Thus Machida No. 7 bronchofiberscope was manufactured and it was the model finally marketed.

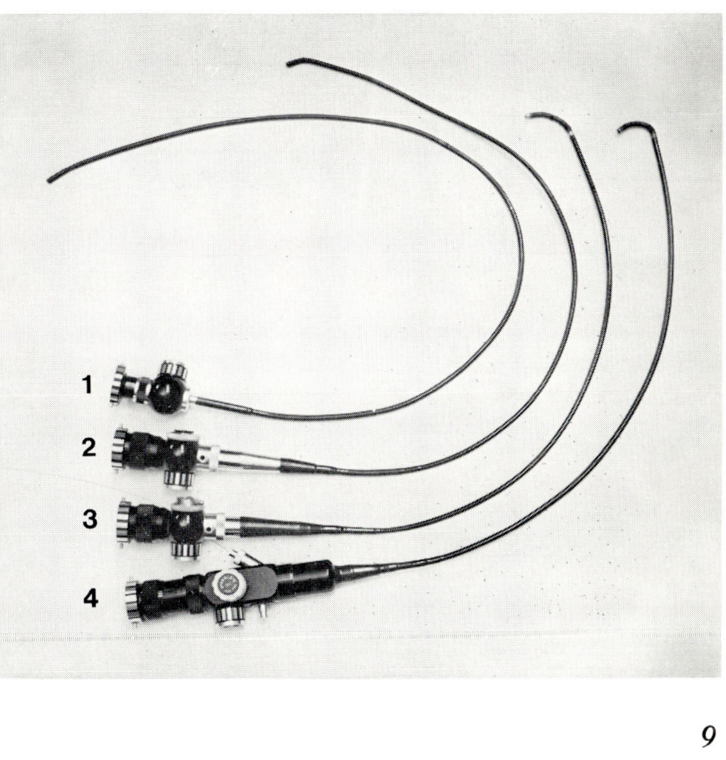


**Fig. 15** Transitional history of the bronchofiberscope of Machida make:
1. Trial fiberscope No. 1
2. Trial fiberscope No. 3
3. Trial fiberscope No. 4
4. Trial fiberscope No. 5

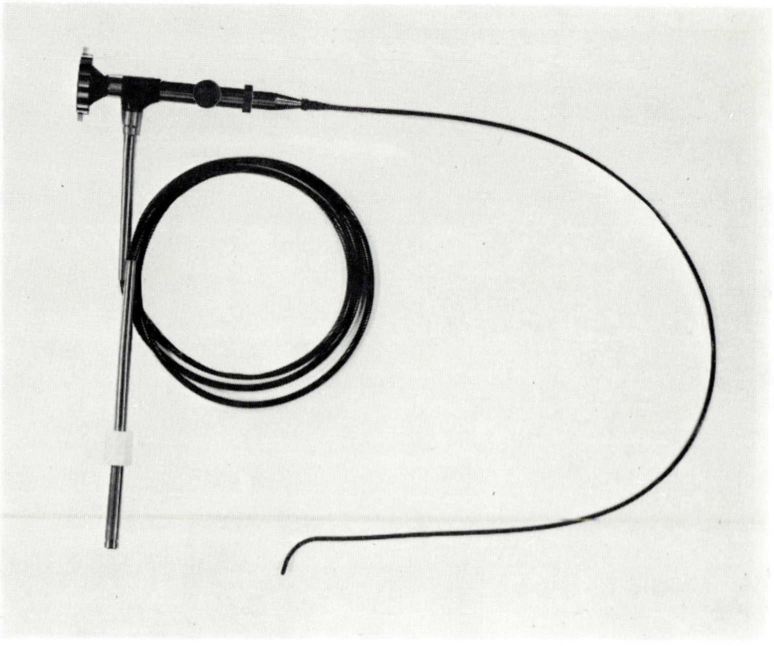

**Fig. 16** Bronchofiberscope of Machida make, 2.5 mm in diameter.

Following the above, Machida No. 8 was produced in August, 1969. In this model the diameter of the channel was increased from 1.0 mm to 1.4 mm making it possible to aspirate more easily viscous sputum. In order to accomplish this, the outer diameter of the sheath was increased slightly, from 5.0 mm to 5.2 mm.

Concurrently with the above improvements, another series of instruments was developed. A flexible bronchofiberscope with an outer diameter of 4 mm was developed in August, 1969, for the purpose of extending the visible range. In this model, the flexible tip was lengthened by 25 mm to 75 mm in order to make it possible to enter into the more peripheral bronchi. Both the diameter and number of image-guide fibers remained unchanged. The anesthetic infusion channel was narrowed to 0.8 mm, making it more difficult to aspirate sputum. Another development was a flexible bronchofiberscope with the outer diameter of 2.5 mm at the tip, manufactured in September, 1968 (Fig. 16). This is the smallest bronchofiberscope ever employed for clinical purposes. The tip is capable of bending by 60 degrees but lateral panning is not possible. The instrument has no hole for the infusion of anesthetic. The primary advantage of the flexible bronchofiberscope is improved visibility throughout the bronchial tree, making possible the earlier diagnosis of lung cancer.

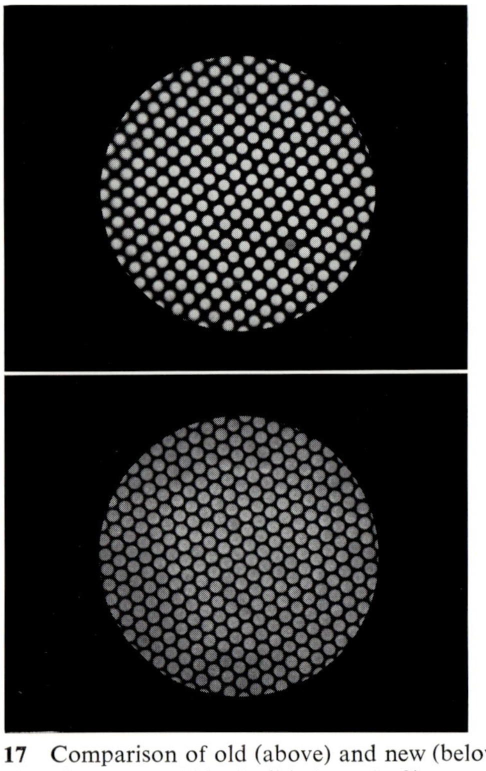

**Fig. 17** Comparison of old (above) and new (below) image bundles of Machida flexible bronchofiberscope.

In 1971, the 6 mm bronchofiberscope was manufactured for the purpose of aspirating viscous sputum and introducing larger biopsy forceps and curettes, by enlarging the diameter of the channel that is now in the present 5 mm bronchofiberscope. In addition to enlarging the diameter of the channel to 2.2 mm, the number of light-guide fibers was increased. The size and total number of the image fibers are the same as in the 5 mm scope. This new 6 mm instrument can also be used as a diagnostic instrument in the relatively larger bronchi.

In June 1972, Machida Endoscope Co., Ltd. devised and improved the image obtained with the 6 mm bronchofiberscope by making the individual glass fibers more uniform in size and by arranging the bundles in a honeycomb fashion (Fig. 17). This, together with a 20% increase in the number of light-guide fibers, improved not only the image but its brightness.

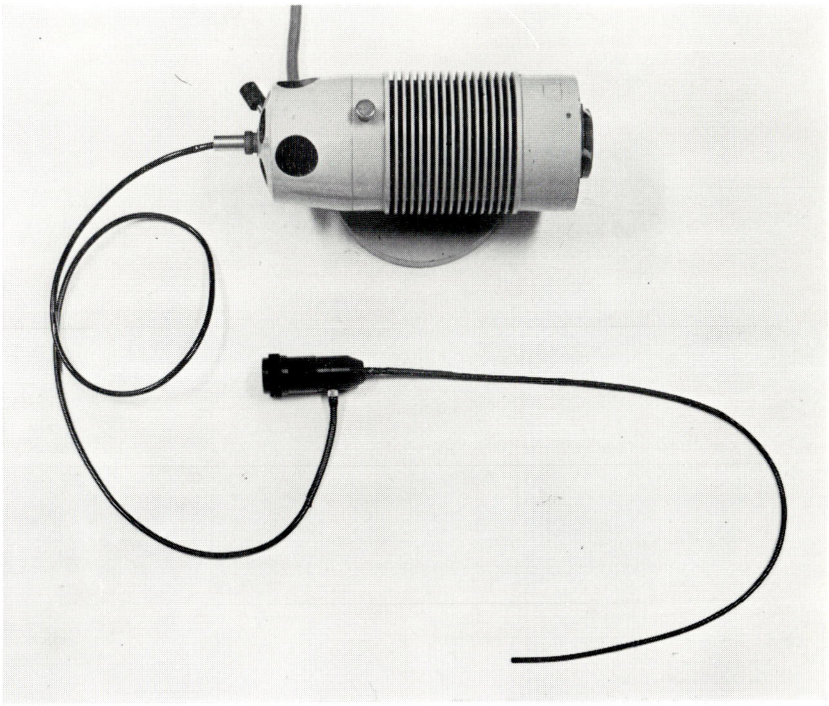

**Fig. 18** Bronchofiberscope of Olympus make, prototype fiberscope No. 1 (1966).

### c. Trial products by Olympus Optical Co., Ltd.

Olympus Optical Co., Ltd. has had extensive experience in the field of the gastrocamera and other types of flexible fiberoptic scopes. Olympus No. 1 flexible bronchofiberscope was completed in August, 1966, under our supervision (Fig. 18).

The outer diameter of the main body was 3.3mm but the distal end did not bend. Olympus No. 1 was thinner than Machida No. 1, so that it could be inserted into narrower bronchi ; but the field of vision, 45 degrees, was too narrow. These shortcomings precluded the use of this instrument for clinical practice.

Because Olympus Optical Co., Ltd. put so much effort and energy into the pattern of the image-guide glass fiber, Olympus No. 2 was not completed until September, 1967. The tip of this scope could be bent about 120 degrees by two handles and its diameter was 5.5 mm. This instrument was subject to frequent prob lems, but it served as a model for Olympus No. 3 and No. 4, which were developed in rapid succession. These two were quite similar mechanically except for their diameters ; No. 3 being 5 mm and No. 4 being 4 mm.

Olympus technicians directed their efforts to develop an instrument with unique characteristics, differing from the Machida scopes which were already being marketed. Thus, Olympus No. 3 (BF-5B) was an instrument which could be manipulated by one hand. The lever for controlling the flexible tip could be maneuvered by the fingers of the left hand which also supported the eyepiece, freeing the right hand for supporting the body of the scope, suctioning, handling accessory instruments, etc. The second improvement was the greater flexibility of the entire main body, instead of just the flexible distal part. However, if the portion near the tip is angled too sharply, it is liable to be damaged because of the characteristics of the Olympus fiber bundle. With the high flexibility of its entire body, the bronchofiberscope could be inserted as far as $B^1$ and $B^{1+2}$ (similar to introducing Metra's catheter into the upper lobe) when the scope-tip is bent and the entire scope is pushed in gently. The third is better co-ordinated rotation of the proximal basal part with the tip. Instead of panning, the tip can be turned in any direction by rotating the proximal eyepiece. The fourth is a notch in the field of vision denoting the axis of the flexible tip of the instrument. Improvement in the arrangement of fibers in the bundle is one of the best characteristics of Olympus fiberscope. All of these laid the foundation for Olympus No. 4. In the No. 3 the channel for anesthetic infusion, suction, and brush was wide enough (1.4 mm in inner diameter) so that aspiration of sputum under direct vision was extremely easy and even thick sputum could be aspirated with ease. A brush could be inserted through the channel from the proximal part.

Olympus No. 4 (BF-4B) has a 4 mm outer diameter at the tip so that it can be inserted into the sub-subsegmental bronchi. In June, 1968, the bronchofiberscope was modified into a cardiofiberscope ; the tip was covered with silicone rubber. At first a cardiofiberscope with 5.5 mm outer diameter was tested experimentally. Then another with 4 mm outer diameter treated overall with silicone rubber resulting in diameter of 4.4 mm was used clinically. The length of this instrument was elongated to 800 mm.

A test fiberscope, Olympus No. 5 (Fig. 19) was pro-

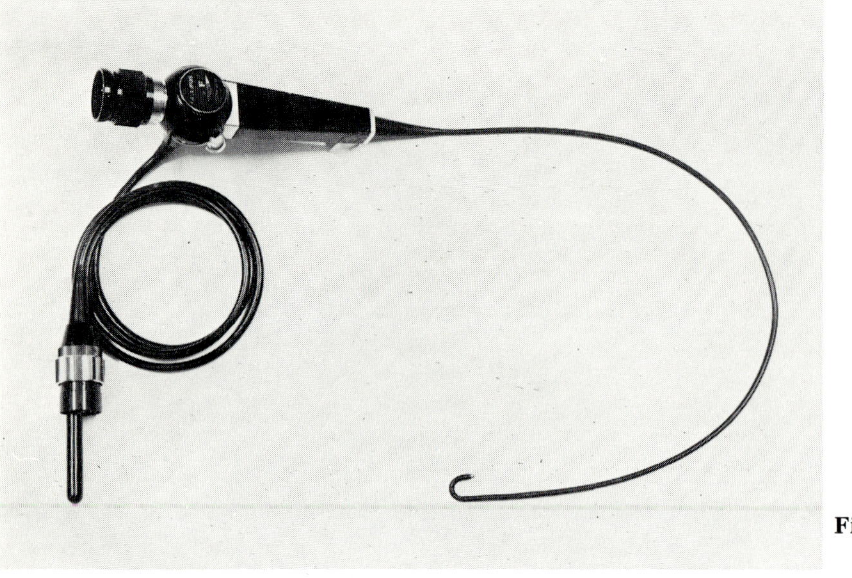

**Fig. 19** Bronchofiberscope of Olympus make No. 5 (1968).

duced in August, 1968, to expand the visible range beyond that of Olympus No. 3 or No. 4. The new instrument featured the following: the outer diameter was 3.2 mm, the field of vision was 53 degrees in the diagonal direction, and the angle flexible by 180 degrees. These, combined with the softness of the fiberscope itself, allowed insertion into bronchi of IV-V order of branching. The small diameter of bronchofiberscope precluded incorporating a channel for infusing, suctioning or obtaining biopsy specimens. However, spiral ridges at the tip may be utilized as a curette.

Olympus BF-5B bronchofiberscope was improved in the latter part of 1971. The new model BF-B (or BF-5B-2 as it was formerly called, but revised recently to BF-B) is 5 mm in diameter at the tip and 5.8 mm in the main body. The most important feature of this new model is the increase in diameter of the channel from 1.4 mm to 1.9 mm. This improvement enables the BF-B to be utilized for therapeutic bronchofiberscopy because of its added capability of aspirating viscous sputum in addition to accomodating larger biopsy forceps.

## DEVELOPMENT OF A TRACHEAL TUBE

A tracheal tube is indispensable for bronchofiberscopy. Prior to the insertion of flexible bronchofiberscope, a tracheal tube must be introduced. The bronchofiberscope is then passed through the tracheal tube which has already been placed in the upper air way. This is necessary for three reasons; maintenance of an adequate air way, suctioning of sputum and occasional cleansing of the tip of the scope.

Although a conventional bronchoscope may be used as a tracheal tube, a flexible intratracheal tube such as that used for general anesthesia is much more comfortable as the patient's head need not be kept unnaturally hyperextended. With the usual type endotracheal tube the insertion of a flexible bronchoscope is difficult because of increased friction between the tube and the scope, due to difference in materials composing the

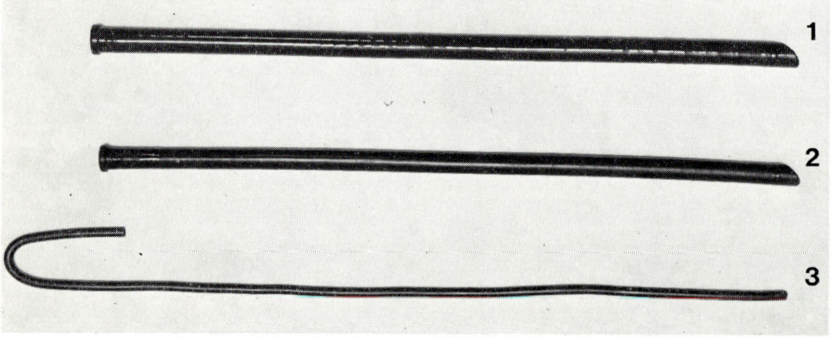


**Fig. 20** Flexible tracheal tube:
1. Large (11.5 mm in outer diameter, 9.0 mm in inner diameter)
2. Small (10.0 mm in outer diameter, 8.5 mm in inner diameter)
3. Stylet

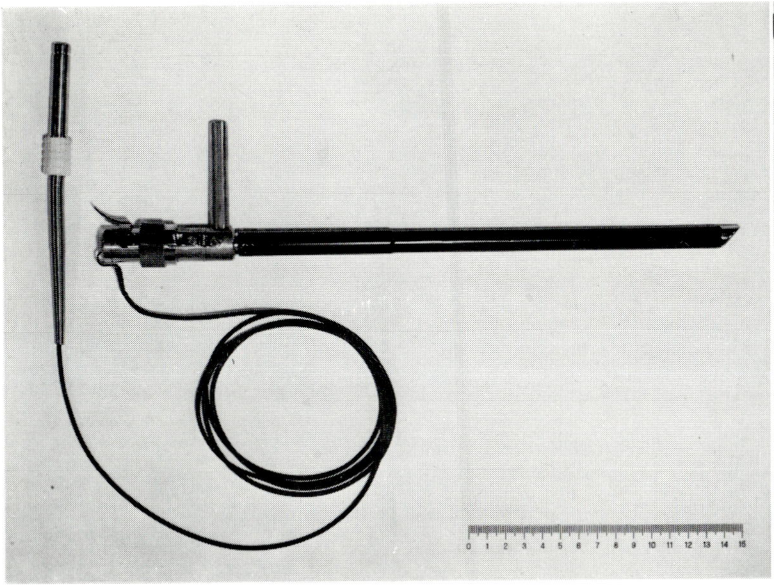


**Fig. 21** Rigid-or-flexible tracheal tube (prototype).

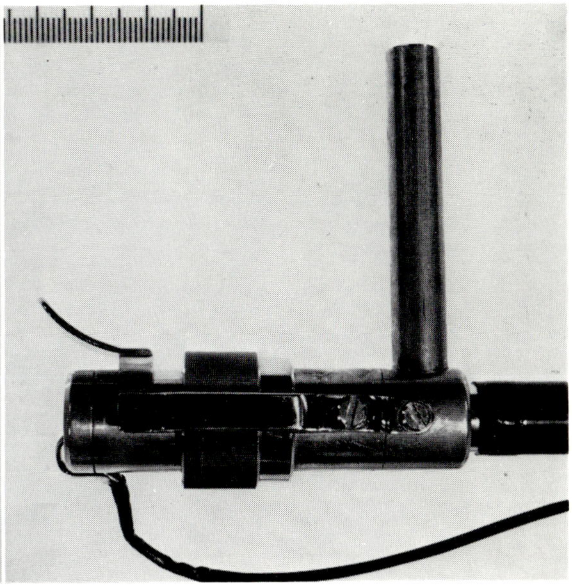

**Fig. 22** Handle part of the tube in Fig. 21, magnified.

two instruments. Therefore a flexible tracheal tube (Fig. 20) made of the same material as the outer covering of the bronchofiberscope was developed. With this improvement local anesthesia was entirely sufficient when properly applied to the larynx, trachea and bronchi.

In the process of introducing the intratracheal tube, the possibility of overlooking pathologic changes, in the upper air way was realized. This urged us to design another type of a tube. This new tube (Fig. 21) had an outer diameter of 11 mm, inner diameter of 8.5 mm, 20 cm in length, and the body was made of a spiral metal tape covered with vinyl chloride, with a handle at the proximal end. The tube can be rigid or flexible: when the knob (Fig. 22) connected to the handle is turned clockwise the intratracheal tube becomes straight and rigid, and when counterclockwise, it becomes flexible and curved. A light-guide glass fiber rod connected to a light source can be inserted through a channel for illumination. The tracheal tube thus equipped with tip illumination has two clinical applications. One is its utility as a rigid bronchoscope by holding the tube in a straight line with the knob tightened. The other is its use for insertion of the flexible bronchofiberscope in a natural supine position, minimizing the discomfort of the patient (Fig. 23). Minimum discomfort to the patient facilitates performing a thorough examination and obtaining adequate biopsy specimens.

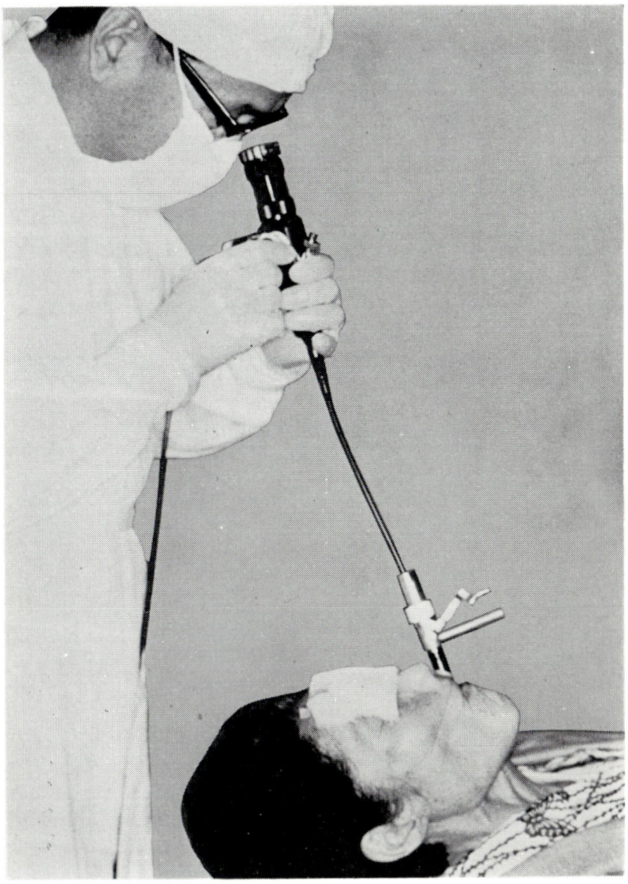

**Fig. 23** Rigid-or-flexible tracheal tube in the flexible position.

## DEVELOPMENT OF INSTRUMENTS FOR HISTOLOGY AND CYTOLOGY

Bronchoscopy comprises two clinical functions. The first is visualizing pathologic changes in the tracheobronchial tree. The second is the definitive diagnosis by obtaining cytologic and histologic specimens under direct visualization. The flexible bronchofiberscope has conspicuously broadened the range of cytology by direct visualization.

For the collection of cytologic material, several different types of instruments have been tested (Fig. 24). In the initial stage a needle with a small head (Fig. 24-1) was tried. With this instrument the biopsy specimens obtained often fell off the needle head as it was withdrawn. The second implements, brushes, (Fig. 24-2 and 3) interrupted the field of vision since they overlapped the optic lenses at the tip-end of the fiberscope. A small curette was next tried (Fig. 24-4). A curette had already been developed by E. Tsuboi and had been used through a Metra's catheter. This curette was further reduced in size, so that it could be passed through the channel of a bronchofiberscope. This implement can be flexed 40 degrees by a handle at the proximal part and guided to the target. Another type of small curette is one in which distal part is double hinged (Fig. 25-4). A recent development is a small biopsy forceps (Fig. 25-5), like the miniature one commonly used for gastrofiberscopy. This is suitable for sampling histologic material rather than just cytologic specimens.

The disadvantages of the small curettes and biopsy forceps used with the 5 mm bronchofiberscope are that sometimes an adequate biopsy specimen cannot be obtained and that the instruments are quite fragile.

The newer 6 mm Machida FBS-6 and Olympus BF-6 bronchofiberscopes, with their larger channels, permit the use of a curette as large as that used in Metra's catheter (Fig. 25–7), and larger, more durable biopsy forceps with which more adequate biopsy specimens can be obtained (Fig. 25–6).

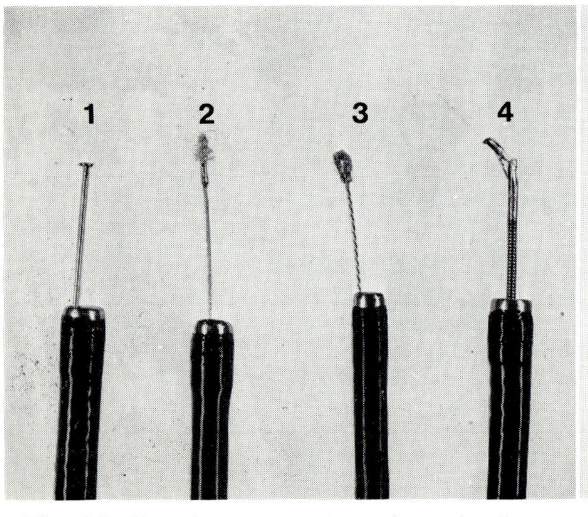


**Fig. 24** Development of various implements for curettage and brushing in bronchofiberscopy:
1. Drill 2. Brush 3. Brush
4. Small curette

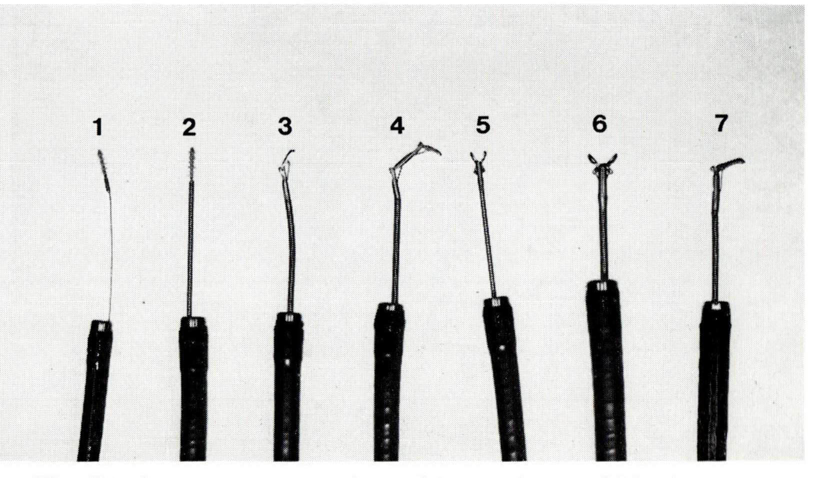


**Fig. 25** Apparatuses currently used for cytology and histology:
1. Small brush (for 4 mm bronchofiberscope)
2. Small brush (for 5 mm)
3. Single small curette (for 5 mm)
4. Double small curette (for 5 mm)
5. Small biopsy forceps (for 5 mm)
6. Biopsy forceps (for 6 mm)
7. Single curette (for 6 mm)

# BRONCHOFIBERSCOPES IN CURRENT USE

A variety of flexible bronchofiberscopes manufactured by either Machida Endoscope Co., Ltd. or Olympus Optical Co., Ltd. are commercially available in Japan. Some of them are experimental models used for research while others are for general purposes. Machida 4 mm (FBS-4), 5 mm (FBS-5), 6 mm (FBS-6) and Olympus 4 mm (BF-4B), 5 mm (BF 5B) and 5.8 mm (BF-B) are commercially available at the present time.

Proper examination with a bronchofiberscope requires an adequate topical anesthesia and aspiration of secretions. A channel for performing these functions, particularly aspiration of moderately thick secretions, is incorporated in the 5 mm or larger instruments; since the small channel in the 4 mm bronchofiberscope permits aspiration of only thin, watery secretions. Thus, it is obvious that the 4 mm instrument is used interchangeably with the larger bronchofiberscopes for examining the smaller peripheral bronchi, and should not be used alone.

**a. Machida bronchofiberscopes and accessories** (Table 1)

1. Commercially available bronchofiberscopes (Figs. 27–29)
2. Tracheal tube; its structure
3. Light source (Fig. 30)
4. Camera (Figs. 31–33)
5. Cytological sampling instruments

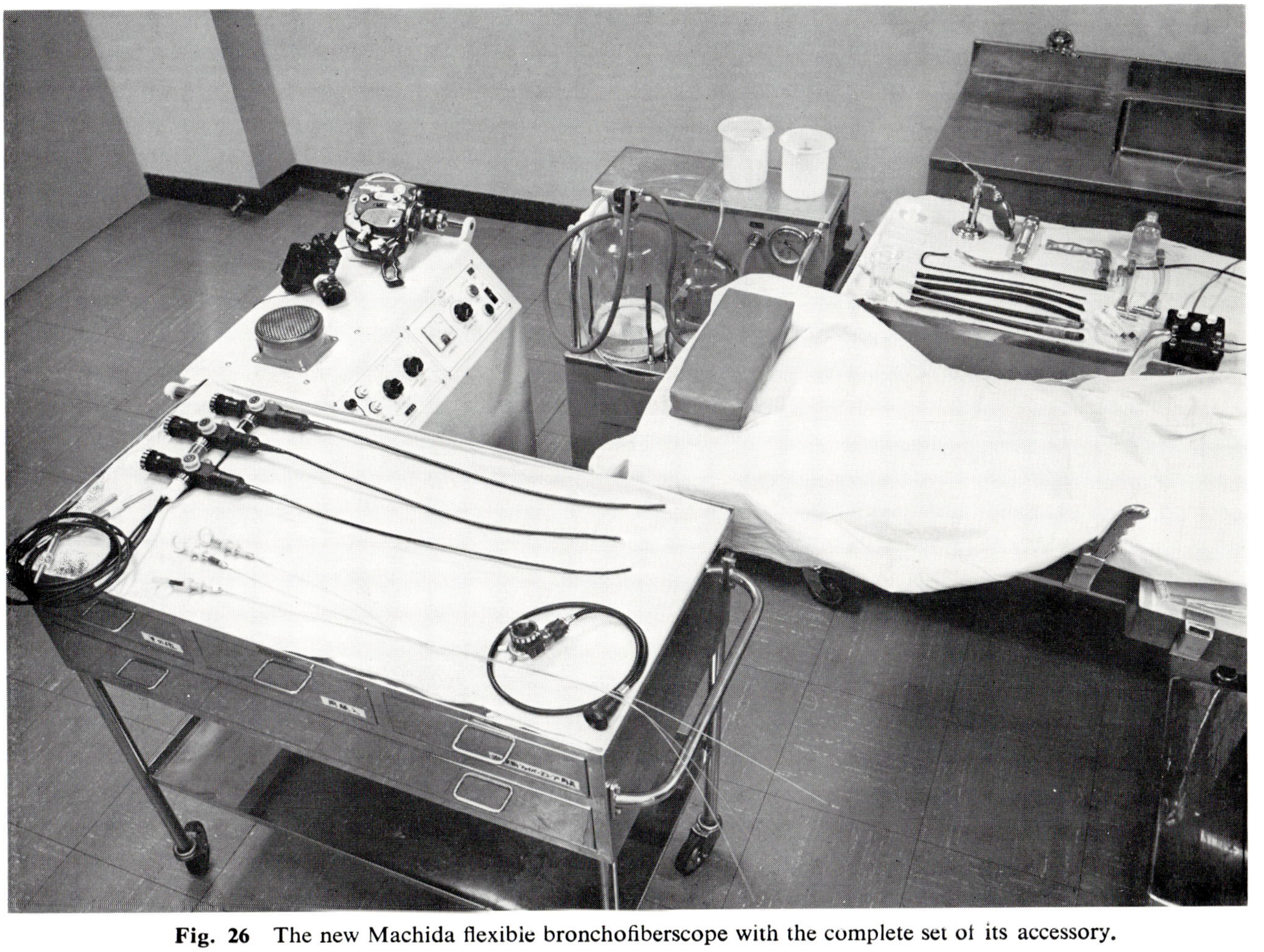

**Fig. 26** The new Machida flexible bronchofiberscope with the complete set of its accessory.

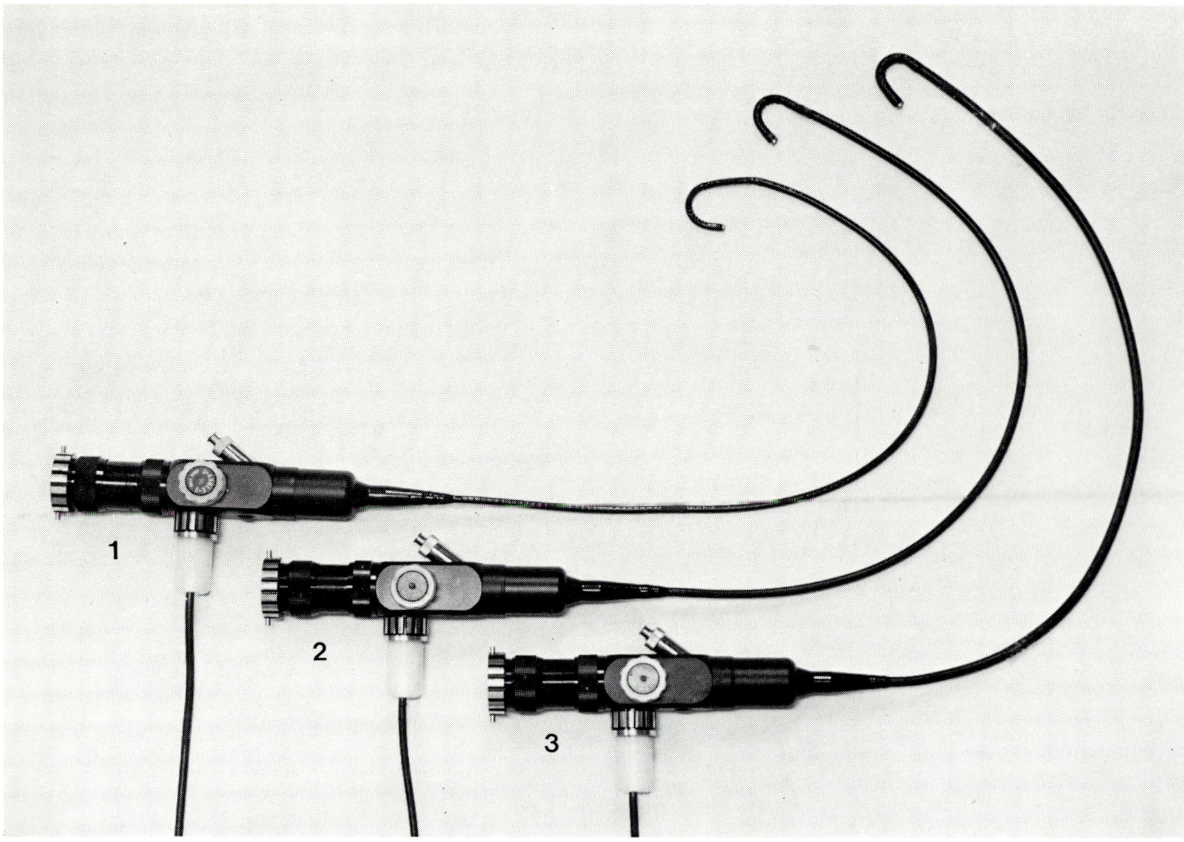


**Fig. 27** Bronchofiberscopes in current use, Machida make:
1. Model FBS-4 (diameter of the distal tip: 4 mm) 2. Model FBS-5 (5.2 mm)
3. Model FBS-6 (6 mm)

*Characteristic features of a Machida flexible bronchofiberscope*

1) Angulation of the distal tip is 180 degrees in one direction, forming a perfect U-turn, and 10 degrees in the opposite direction.

2) The distal tip may be rotated 30 degrees to the right or left.

3) The visible range is wider than with the Olympus.

4) Maneuvering the instrument for endobronchial visualization is rather simple.

5) Endoscopic picture is larger than with the Olympus.

6) A variety of instruments for cytological sampling are provided: a small curette, a small biopsy forceps and a brush for the 5mm bronchofiberscope; a small brush for the 4 mm scope; a biopsy forceps and a curette for the 6 mm one. All of these may be utilized in accordance with the location of lesions and the indications present.

**Table 1** Specifications, Machida Flexible Bronchofiberscope in Current Use

| | 4 mm | 5 mm | 6 mm |
|---|---|---|---|
| Commercial name | FBS-4 | FBS-5 | FBS-6 |
| Total length | 770 mm | 770 mm | 770 mm |
| Effective length | 600 mm | 600 mm | 600 mm |
| Distal rigid part: | | | |
| length | 8 mm | 8 mm | 8 mm |
| Diameter | 4.2 mm $\phi$ | 5.2 mm $\phi$ | 6.2 mm $\phi$ |
| Angle of vision | 70° (circular) | 70° (circular) | 70° (circular) |
| Visible range | 5–50 mm | 5–50 mm | 5–50 mm |
| Angle: | | | |
| Up | 180° | 180° | 180° |
| Down | 10° | 10° | 10° |
| Rotation of the distal part: | | | |
| Right | 90° | 30° | 30° |
| Left | 90° | 30° | 30° |
| Focusing | Fixed | Fixed | Fixed |
| Diameter of glass fiber: | | | |
| Image | 12 $\mu$ | 12 $\mu$ | 12 $\mu$ |
| Light | 20 $\mu$ | 20 $\mu$ | 20 $\mu$ |
| Inside channel diameter | 0.8 mm | 1.4 mm | 2.2 mm |
| Cytologic and histologic sampling implements | Small brush | Brush or single small curette, double small curette, small biopsy forceps | Biopsy forceps, or single curette, double curette |

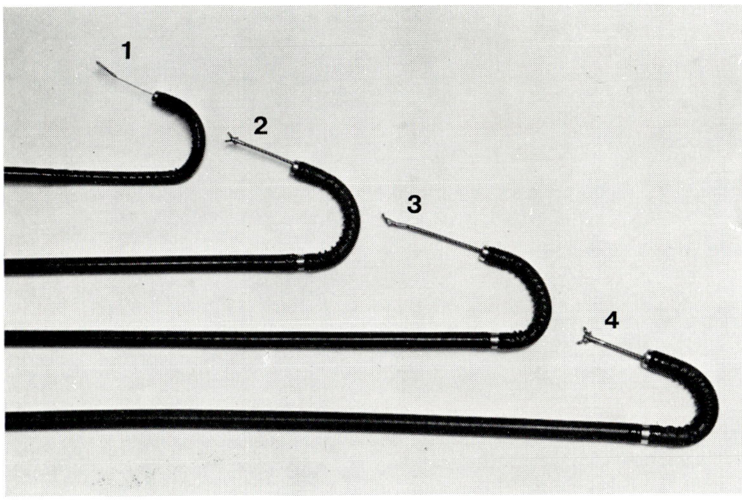


**Fig. 28** Sampling instruments intubated into bronchofiberscopes and the distal tip, Machida make : 1. Small brush intubated into a 4 mm bronchofiberscope 2. Small biopsy forceps intubated into a 5 mm brochofiberscope 3. Single small curette intubated into a 5 mm brochofiberscope 4. Biopsy forceps intubated into a 6 mm bronchofiberscope

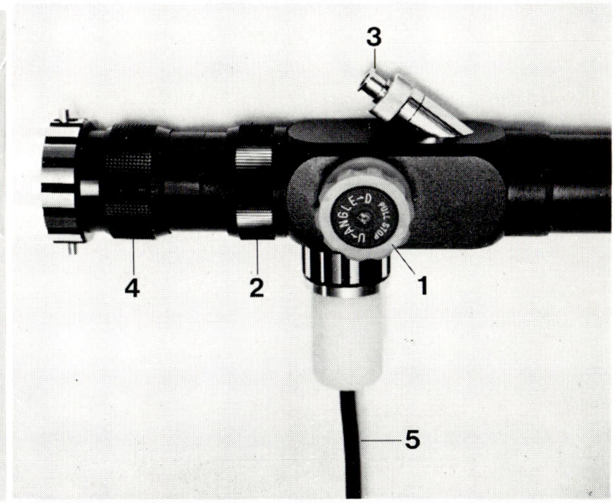


**Fig. 29** The proximal part of a bronchofiberscope, Machida make : 1. Angulation knob 2. Rotation ring (panning rim) 3. Channel for suction and injection. 4. Eyepiece focus (diopto-adjustor ring) 5. Light guide glass fiber bundle

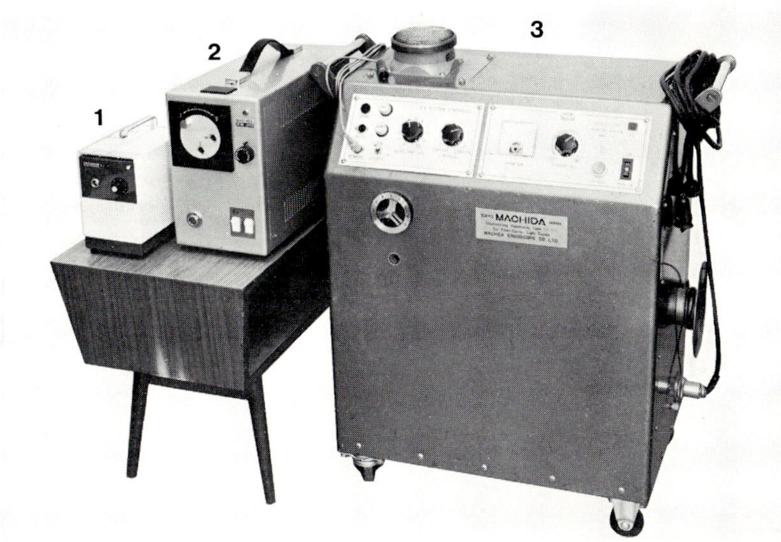


**Fig. 30** Light source :
1. 150 W Halogen lamp, light source (Model RH-150)
2. 300 W Mercury lamp, light source (Model RM-300)
3. 500 W Xenon lamp, light source (Model RX-500)

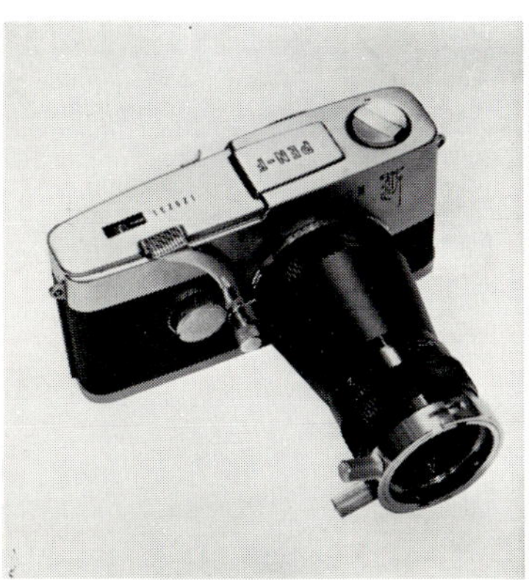

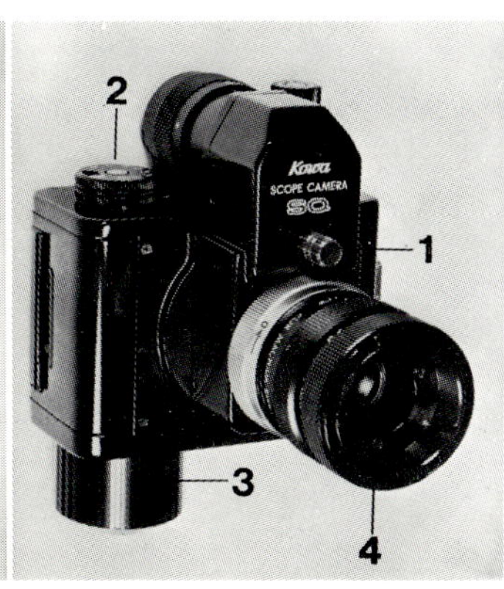


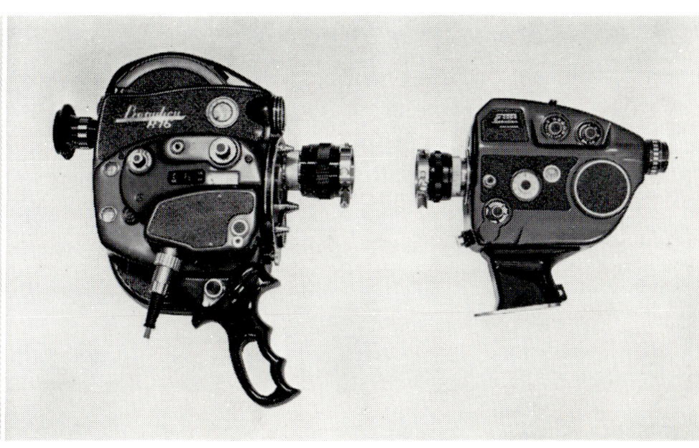

31 32 33

**Fig. 31** Olympus Pen Camera with the lens for the exclusive use with Machida f-75 mm adapter lens.
**Fig. 32** New type, Kowa Scope Camera SQ : 1. Shutter button 2. Timer shutter speed dial 3. Automatic film winder 4. Lens with the exclusive automatic joint device.
**Fig. 33** Movie cameras. Left : For 16 mm (Beaulieu R 16), Right : For 8 mm (Beaulieu S 2008).

**b. Olympus bronchofiberscopes and accessories** (Table 2)

1. Commercially available bronchofiberscopes (Figs. 35–37)
2. Light source (Fig. 38)
3. Camera (Fig. 39)
4. Cytological sampling instruments

*Characteristic features of an Olympus flexible bronchofiberscope*

1) Angulation of the distal tip may be controlled by one hand.
2) Although it has no specific rotating mechanism, this maneuver can be performed by rotating the entire instrument at the eyepiece.
3) The image glass fibers used are 9 $\mu$ in diameter and are well arranged so that resolution is clear and definite.
4) Visible field is rectangular. The angle of vision is 80 degrees diagonally ; narrower than Machida scope.
5) For cytological sampling, a brush can be passed through the channel from the proximal part in the 5 mm (BF-5) instrument.

**Table 2** Specifications, Olympus Flexible Bronchofiberscope in Current Use.

| | 4 mm | 5 mm | 6 mm |
|---|---|---|---|
| Commercial name | BF-4B | BF-5B | BF-B(BF-5B-2)* |
| Total length | 775 mm | 775 mm | 775 mm |
| Effective length | 560 mm | 560 mm | 560 mm |
| Distal rigid part: length | 8 mm | 8 mm | 8 mm |
| Diameter of body | 4 mm $\phi$ | 5.5 mm $\phi$ | 5.8 mm $\phi$ |
| Angle of vision | 82° (Diagonal angle) | 83° (Diagonal angle) | 83° (Diagonal angle) |
| Visible range | 4–40 mm | 5–45 mm | 5–45 mm |
| Angle: | | | |
| Up | 160° | 130° | 100° |
| Down | 30° | 30° | 10° |
| Rotation of the distal part | (−) | (−) | (−) |
| Focusing | Fixed | Fixed | Fixed |
| Diameter of glass fiber: | | | |
| Image | 9 $\mu$ | 9 $\mu$ | 9 $\mu$ |
| Light | 20 $\mu$ | 20 $\mu$ | 20 $\mu$ |
| Inside channel diameter | 0.8 mm | 1.4 mm | 1.9 mm |
| Cytologic and histologic sampling implements | Small brush | Brush or single small curette | Biopsy forceps |

* The name "BF-5B-2" has recently been revised to "BF-B".

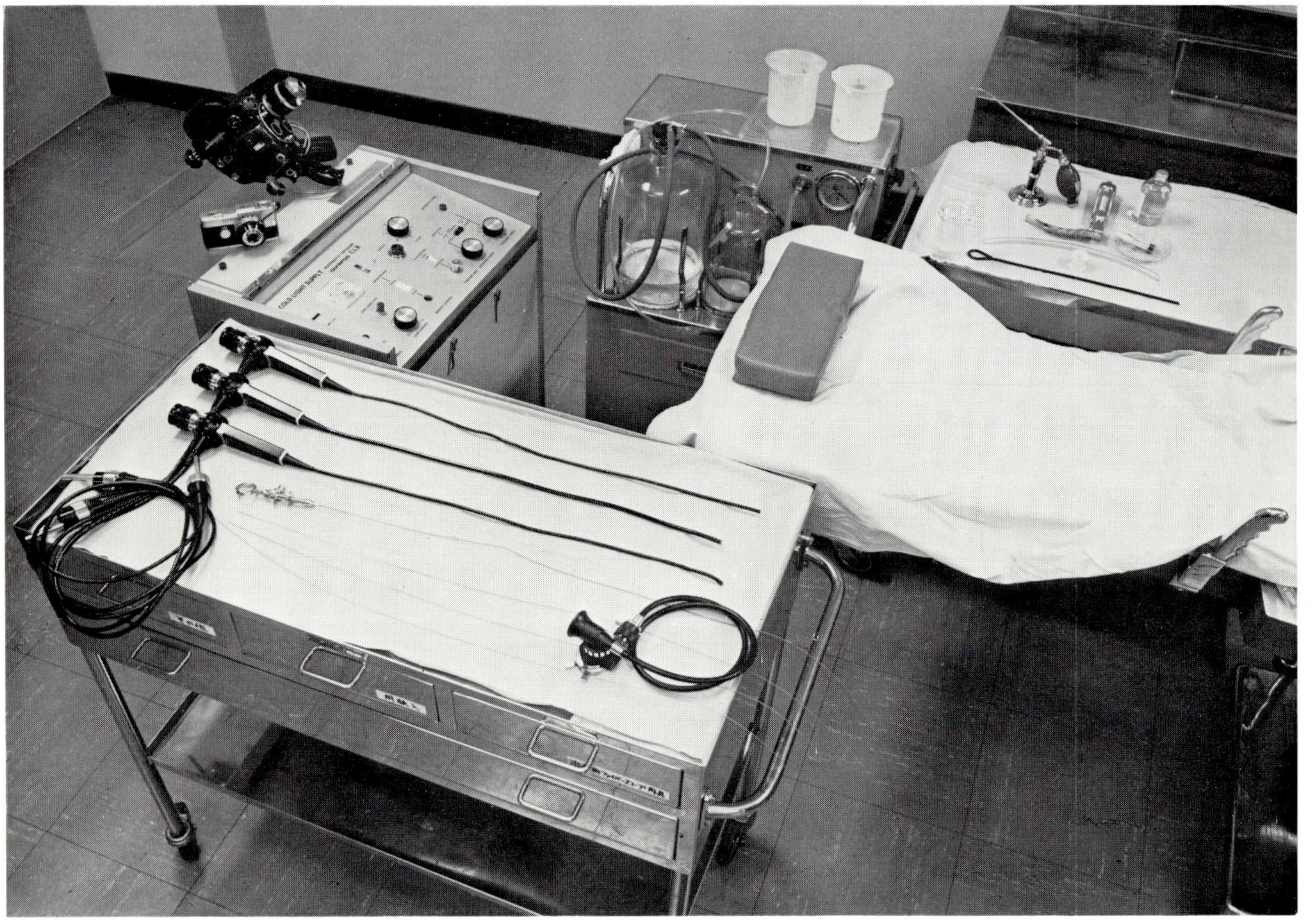

**Fig. 34** The new Olympus flexible bronchofiberscope with the complete set of its accessories.

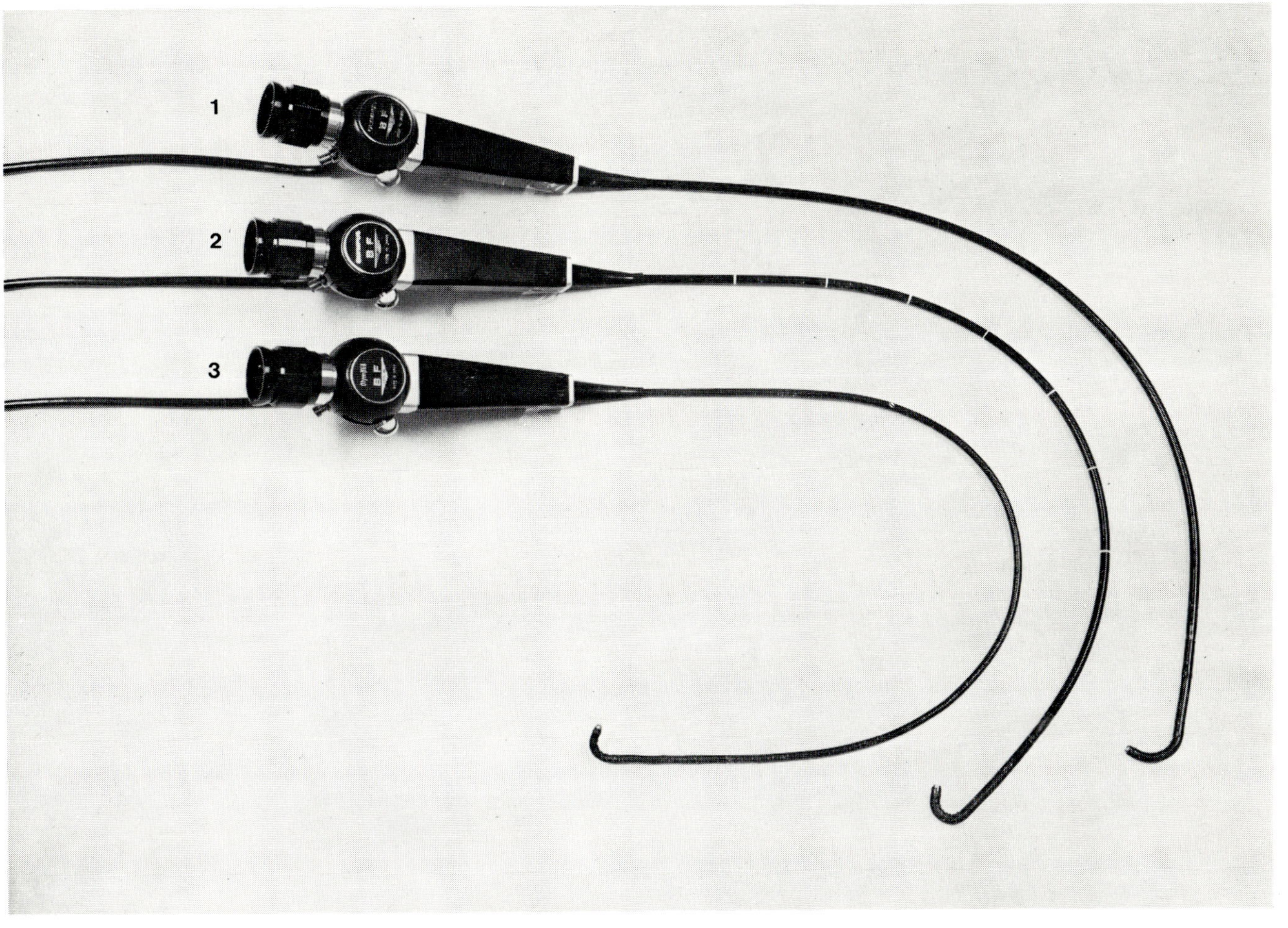


**Fig. 35** Flexible bronchofiberscopes in current use, Olympus make:
1. Model BF-B (diameter of distal tip: 5.8mm) 2. Model BF-5B (5.5mm) 3. Model BF-4B (4.0mm)

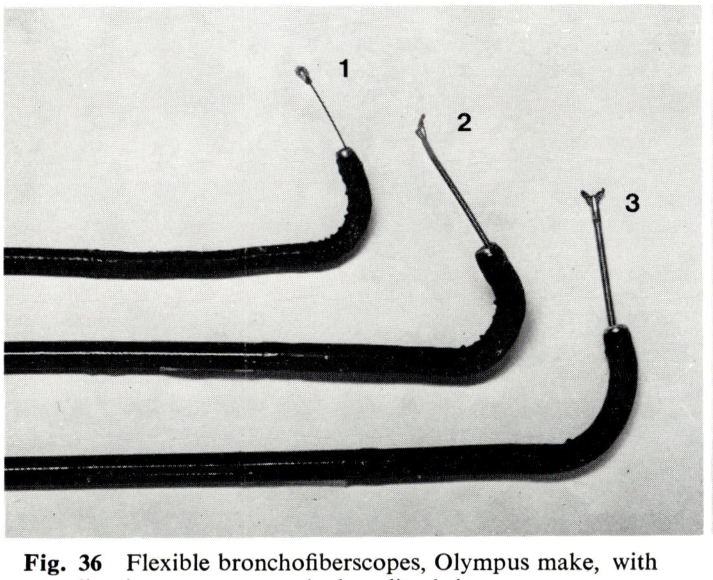


**Fig. 36** Flexible bronchofiberscopes, Olympus make, with sampling instruments attached to distal tips:
1. Model BF-4B with a small brush intubated
2. Model BF-5B with a single curette intubated
3. Model BF-B with a biopsy forceps intubated

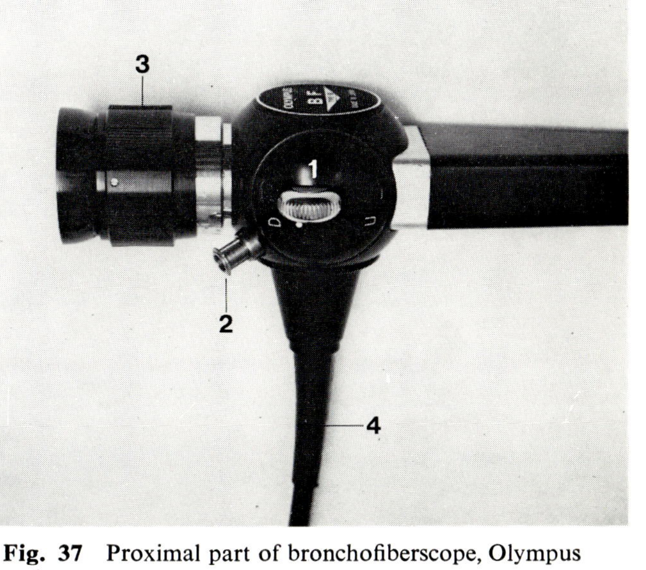


**Fig. 37** Proximal part of bronchofiberscope, Olympus make:
1. Angle bar
2. Channel for suction and injection
3. Eyepiece focus (diopto-adjustor ring)
4. Light-guide glass fiber bundle

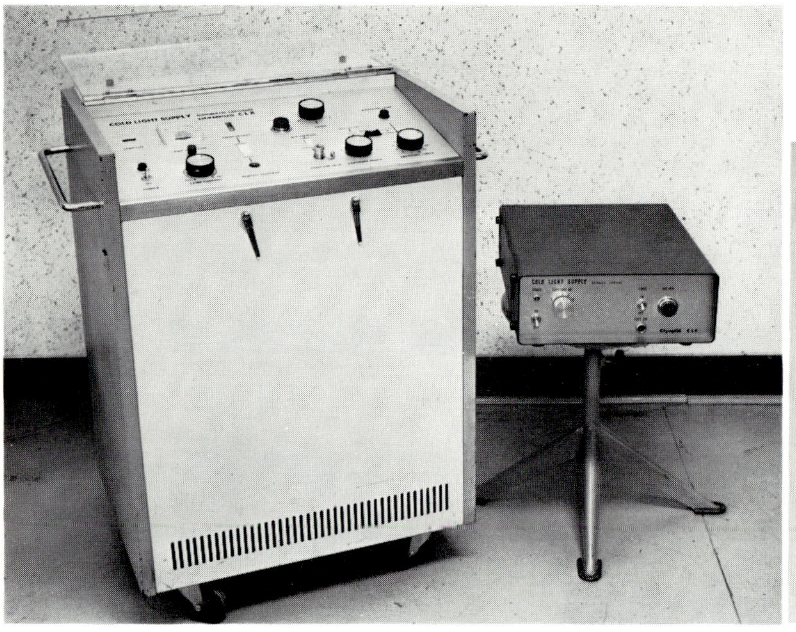

**Fig. 38** Light source :
Left : 300 W Xenon lamp, light source, Model CLX
Right : 150 W Halogen lamp, light source, Model CLE

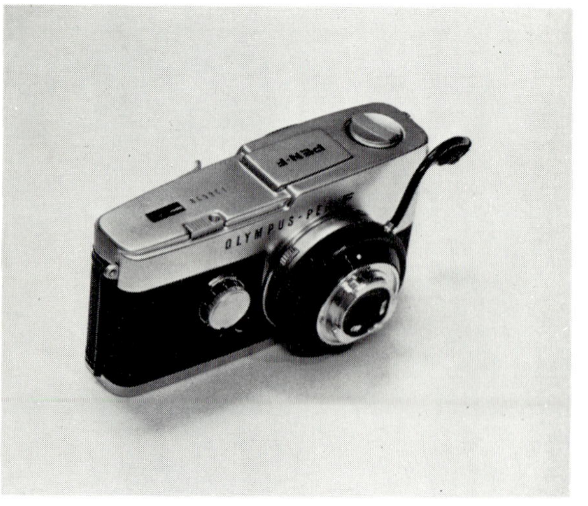

**Fig. 39** Olympus camera for the bronchoscopic use.

**c. General characteristics of the two makes**

| | MACHIDA | OLYMPUS |
|---|---|---|
| Image | Fairly good (fiber bundle arrangement: good) | Good (fiber bundle arrangement: very good) |
| Light volume | Slightly inadequate | Adequate |
| General handling capacity | Extremely good | Good |
| Feasibility in insertion into apical part | Good | Moderately good |
| Visible field | Wide | Slightly narrow |
| Picture for recording | Large | Small |
| Instruments for cytological and histological sampling | All types available | Brush and biopsy forceps |

**d. The latest flexible bronchofiberscope**

Since 1972 quite a number of flexible bronchofiberscopes have been exported to various foreign countries, especially to the United States. With the wide use of this apparatus, the medical terms such as therapeutic bronchofiberscopy and bedside bronchofiberscopy were newly coined and are now popularly used. Side by side with the popularity there have arisen demand for varied improvements to be made on the flexible bronchofiberscope itself.

In the following the new designs and improvements will be described. Of course, some of them are not finished but on the way to completion in the very near future.

*The new Machida flexible bronchofiberscope*

(a) Type T (Fig. 40) : The body of the present Machida flexible bronchofiberscope is slightly stiff. This is the reason why it is somewhat difficult to insert transnasally and impossible to intubate directly through the tracheotomy tube. In order to overcome this deficiency, the body of the newest type has been made more flexible. It is 5.2mm in the outer diameter (same as that of FBS-5) and can be bent approximately 200 degrees at the distal part, but cannot be rotated to the right and left.

(b) The laryngeal fiberscope for inserting the tracheal tube (Fig. 41) : As has often been mentioned, there is necessity for the tracheal tube to be inserted into the trachea. This insertion is difficult at times and has motivated the development of the laryngofiberscope.

This fiberscope is clad with the spirally shaped Anaconda tube, which is flexible and, once bent, maintains its shape until changed manually into another shape. In flexible bronchofiberscopy, the laryngeal fiberscope is intubated through the tracheal tube which can be fixed by the stopper equipped at the root. Thus the whole thing can be introduced orally or nasally into the larynx through the vocal chords under direct vision. When the intubation is finished, the laryngeal fiberscope is removed, leaving the tracheal tube behind.

The laryngeal fiberscope can be utilized for intubating an anesthetic tube. Another type of a laryngofiberscope larger in diameter is now under manufacture.

(c) The adaptor for suction : In order to avoid the repeated insertion and removal of the suction tip for aspiration of secretions through the channel, an adaptor (Fig 40-1) has been made by Machida Endoscope Co., Ltd. for use with any of their bronchofiberscopes. The adaptor has a hole in its body (Fig. 40-2).

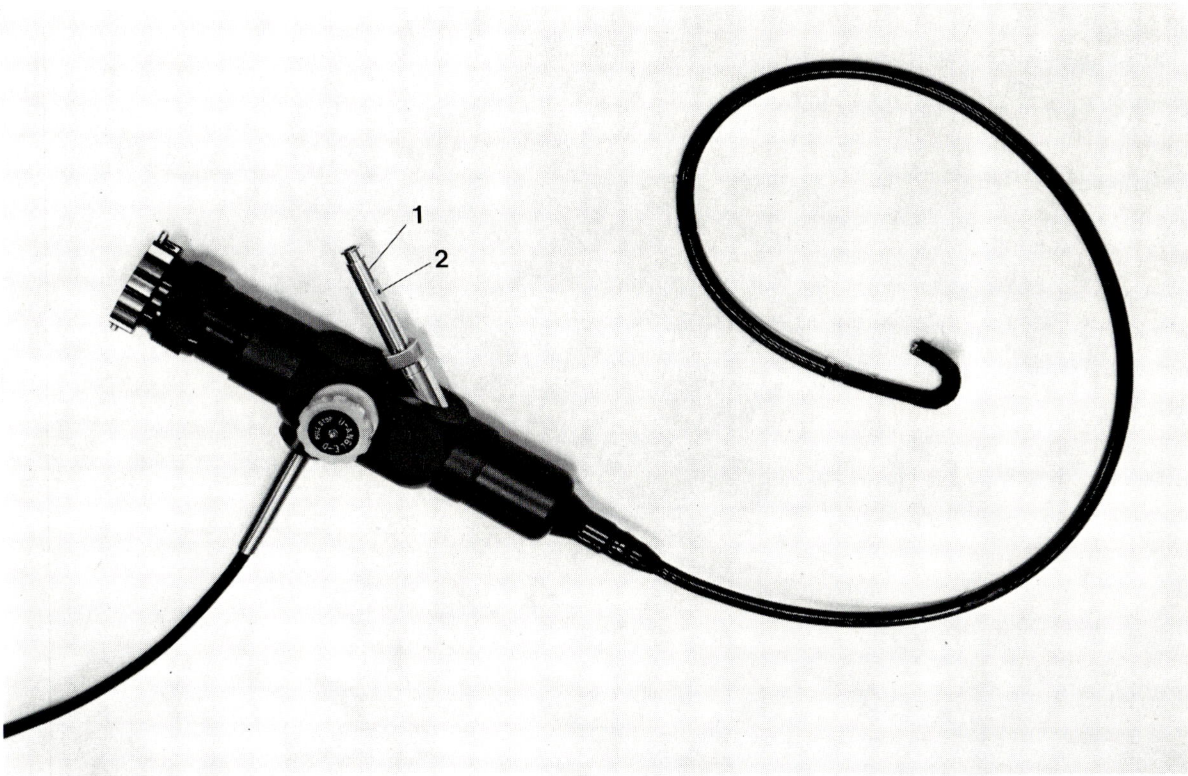


**Fig. 40** Machida flexible bronchofiberscope, type T. The arrow 1 is the connector of the newly made suction pipe. When the suction pipe has been connected with this part and the hole indicated by the arrow 2 is closed with a finger-tip, the suction starts, and when the finger-tip is removed the suction ceases. When instilling anesthetics, the hole (2) is closed with the finger-tip. The connector can be attached to any kind of Machida flexible bronchofiberscope.

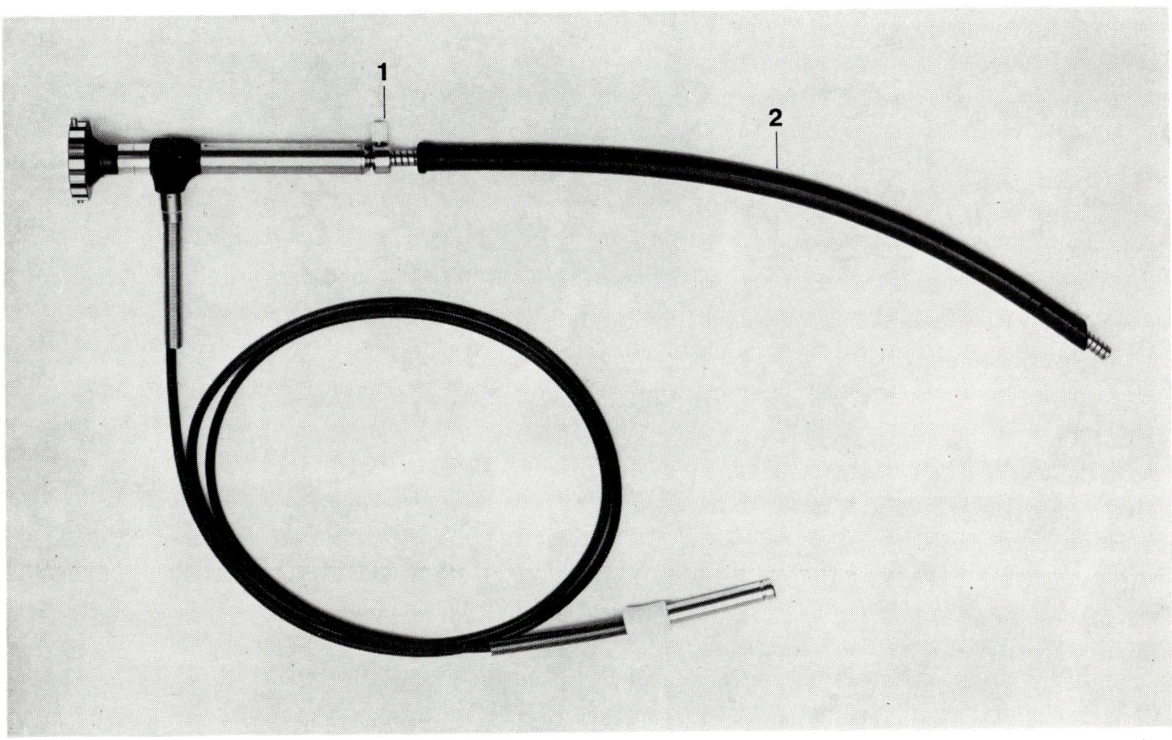


**Fig. 41** Laryngofiberscope for the insertion of the flexible bronchofiberscope (The tracheal tube is seen with the laryngeal fiberscope inserted through it)
1. The stopper 2. The tracheal tube

The adaptor is connected to a suction tube. When the hole is closed with a finger, the suction is activated.

*The latest Olympus flexible bronchofiberscope* (Fig. 42)

In the early part of 1973, Olympus Optical Co., Ltd. set out to modify its flexible bronchofiberscope. Part of the model changes have been accomplished but the new type models will not be available until early in 1974.

First, the proximal part was revamped. In this model, the lever for manipulating the tip was replaced by a round knob with two wings. However, this model is difficult to manipulate with one hand and furthermore, it cannot be manipulated at all with only the right hand.

The second improved model is similar to the old type with a lever control; however, manipulation of this instrument has been made easier and smoother by relocating the lever in a more accessible position (Fig 45). Also, one of the best features of this improved model is that, by capping the eyepiece with a specially designed water proof cover, the entire instrument can now be immersed in liquid. This is a great advance in the area of sterilizing the instrument.

The third is also a significant improvement. The suctioning of sputum can be accomplished just by covering a small opening on the upper part of the proximal end (Fig. 43). Through this opening, anesthetic or irrigating solution can be instilled with a syringe.

The fourth improvement is related to photography. First, a 16 mm compact camera for still pictures has been completed, and second, the setting and removing of its attachments has been much facilitated (Fig. 44). The photography will be done easily as the film winding and exposure are both automatically performed. For example, when 20 frames are used up, the film is automatically wound up.

Furthermore, exposure time is 1/15 to 1/60, if a 300 W Xenon lamp is used, and if a flash is utilized, 1/100 exposure is sufficient. Endobronchial photography can be achieved with two times longer intensifying development than the standard process. The film to be used is 16 mm Ektachrome, Kodak, so that the image obtained is a bit small, 5 × 5 mm.

The improvements mentioned above are mainly concerned with the capability of the apparatus, and its function including flexibility of the body or the bending of the tip remains unchanged.

As this Atlas goes to press, the improved model of the new Olympus bronchofiberscopes mentioned above are not yet available.

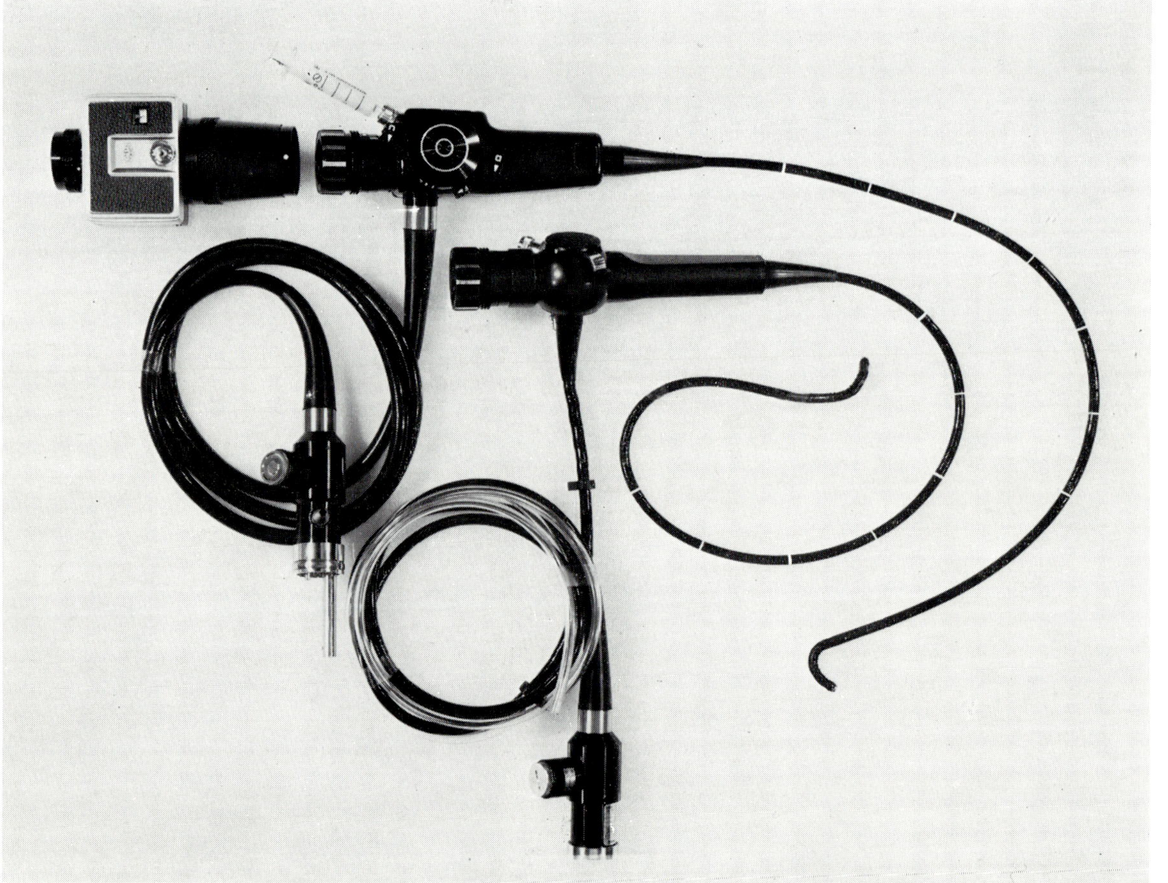

**Fig. 42** Olympus flexible bronchofiberscope, new model: No. 1 (upper) and No. 2 (lower).

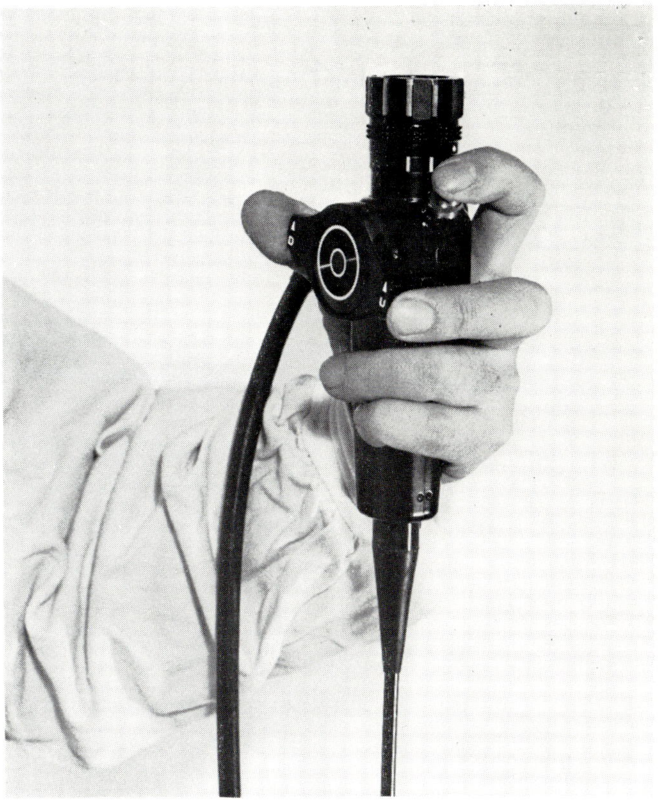

**Fig. 43** How to hold the new Olympus flexible bronchofiberscope, No. 1 and use the suction button.

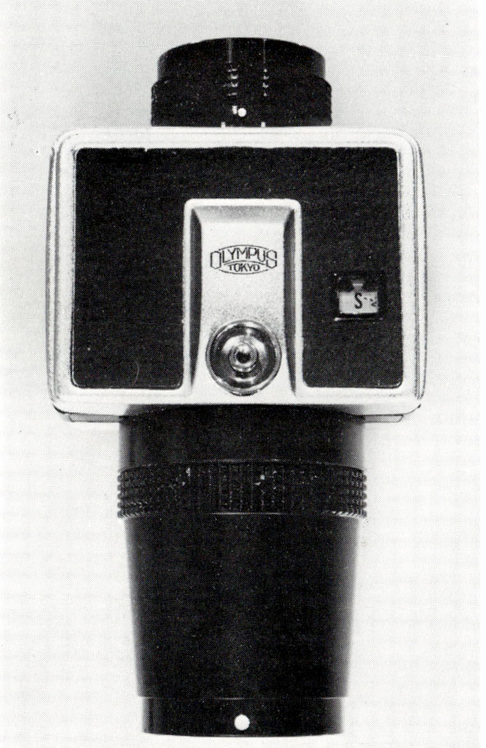


**Fig. 44** New 16 mm camera.

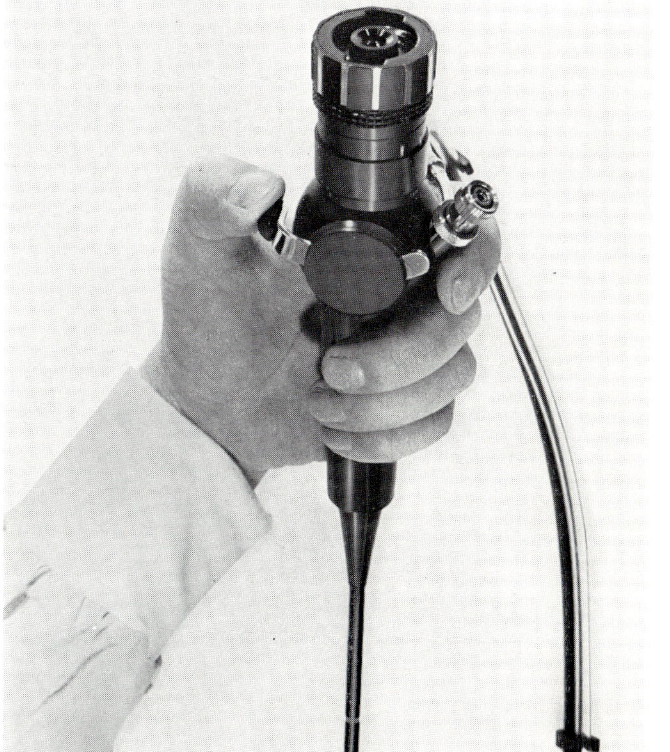

**Fig. 45** How to hold the new Olympus flexible bronchofiberscope, No. 2.

**e. Flexible bronchofiberscope in the United States** (Figs. 46 and 47)

In the United States, American Cystoscope Makers, Inc. (ACMI) has been developing a flexible bronchofiberscope since 1968 under the guidance of Dr. F. N. Marici. This bronchofiberscope, ACMI-MARICI instrument, is expected to be marketed in the near future (personal communication, August 1972).

The general outline of the specifications are: The diameter of the body is 6.5 mm and the short distal tip can be deflected to more than 120° in opposite directions. It has an 1.8 mm channel which will allow the use of a 5 Fr. biopsy forceps. There are two other channels: one for oxygen insufflation and the other for washing the distal optics. The distal tip cannot be rotated as in Machida scope.

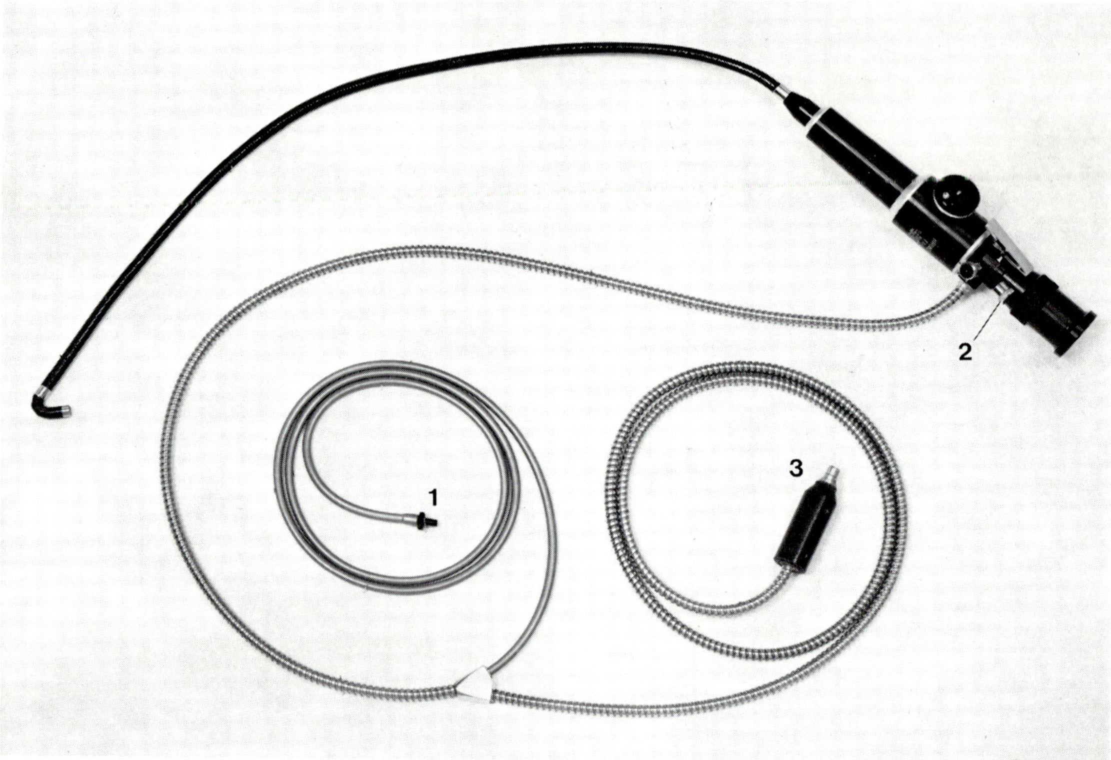


**Fig. 46** Flexible bronchoscope of ACMI-MARICI make.
1. Channel for oxygen insufflation 2. Channel for washing and biopsy forceps
3. Light-guide glass fiber bundle

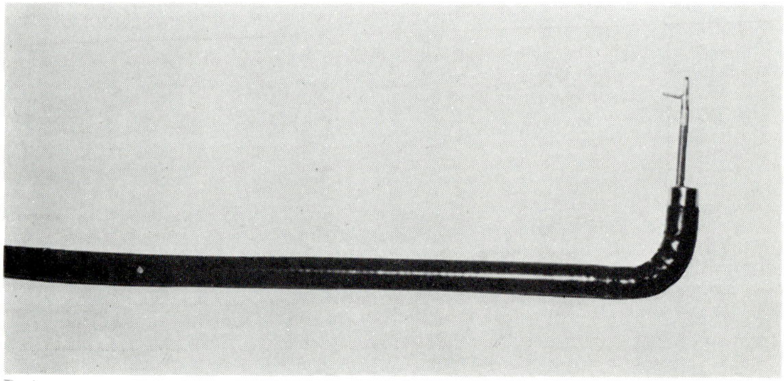

**Fig. 47** Distal tip of ACMI-MARICI make.

# II. Significance of the Flexible Bronchofiberscope

Rigid bronchoscopy has a history of seventy years. The newly developed bronchoscope with great flexibility has opened a new era for effective bronchoscopy. Its advantages may be summarized as follows :

**a. Extension of visible range** (Fig. 48)

The 5 mm bronchofiberscope now commercially available is capable of being inserted into any subsegmental bronchus of an adult male, and visualizing sub-subsegmental bronchi up to IV order of branching. With the 4 mm flexible bronchofiberscope, bronchi of V-VI order of branching may be visualized. Such an extension of visual range in the bronchus has been unprecedented in its history.

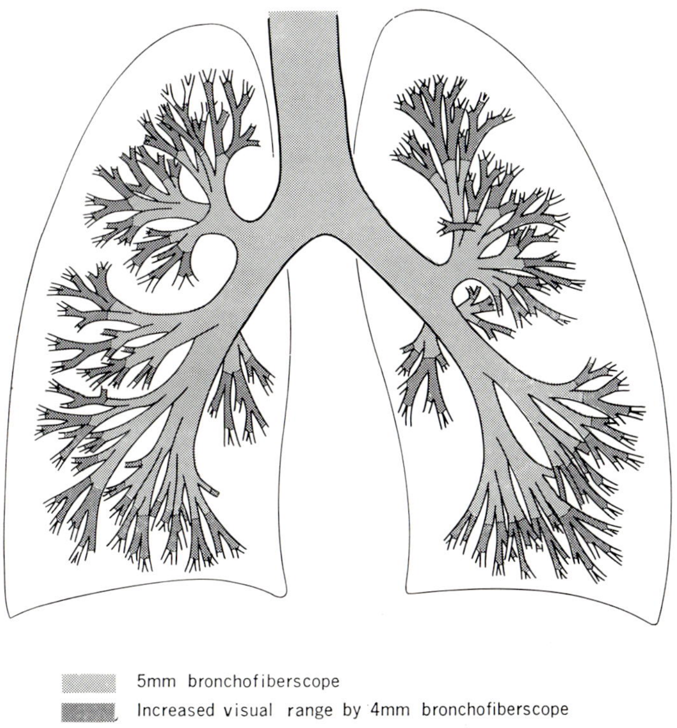


**Fig. 48** Comparison of visual range by 5 mm and 4 mm bronchofiberscopes.

**b. Patient's discomfort minimized** (Fig. 49)

A bronchofiberscope introduced through a flexible tracheal tube has made it possible to examine a patient in a natural supine position. This has diminished the patient's discomfort remarkably. Consequently, it is now possible to make longer and more precise inspection of the lesion, obtain cytological specimens, and perform endoscopic photography or cinematography for the record.

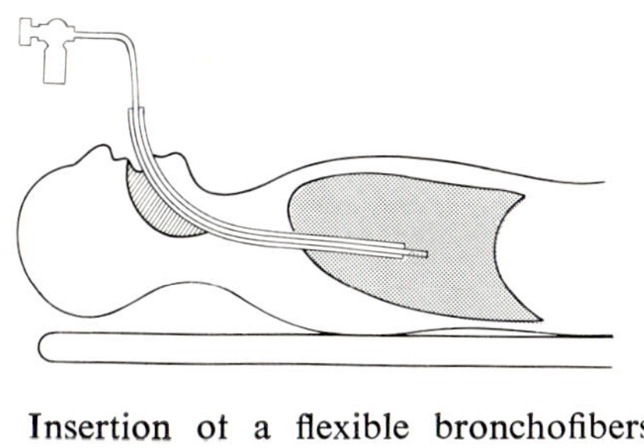

**Fig. 49** Insertion of a flexible bronchofiberscope.

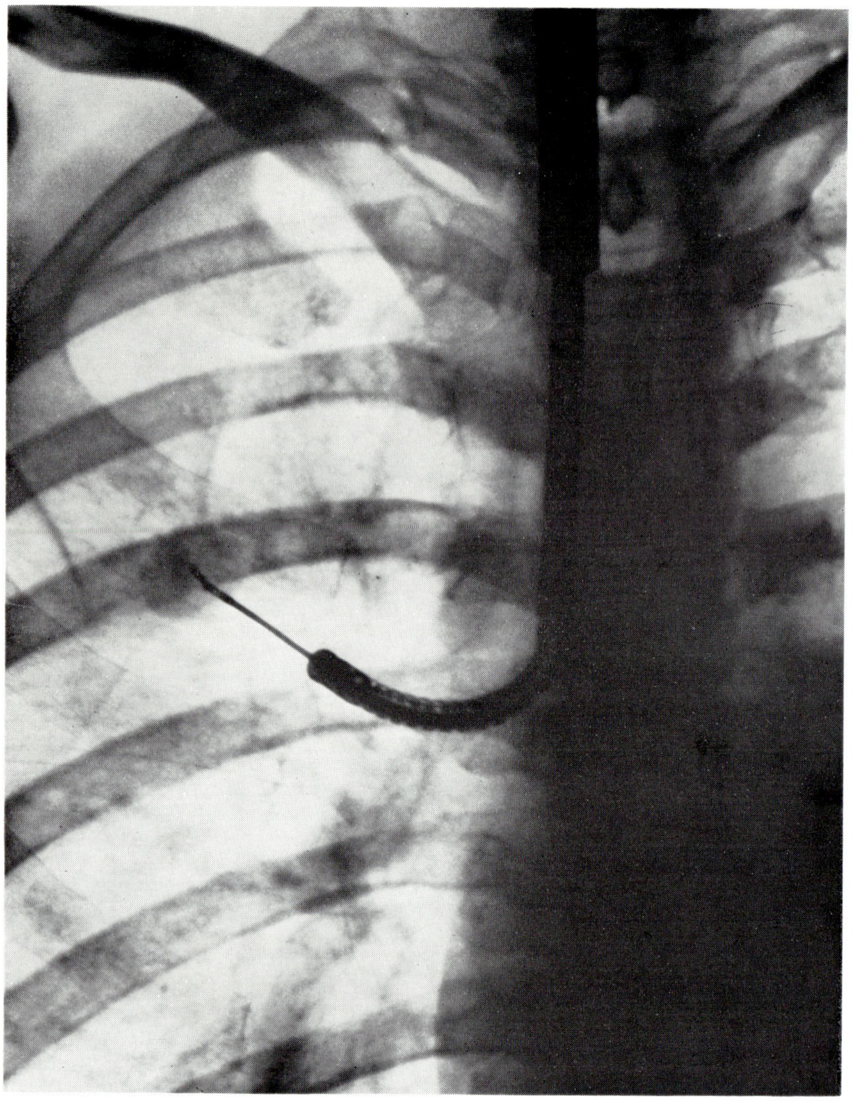

**Fig. 50** X-ray photo showing the confirmation of a bronchofiberscope hitting the lesion.

**c. Precision in cytologic and histologic diagnoses** (Fig. 50)

The increase in the visible range has naturally expanded the area that can be diagnosed cytologically and histologically under direct vision. If a lesion is located in the periphery beyond bronchofiberscopic visualization, a small curette projected from the tip of the fiber scope can be introduced into the lesion by identifying and locating the involved bronchus based on the study of a bronchogram prepared several days previously (usually 4–7 days). In other words, when the orifice of the lesional bronchus is visualized the curette can be directly inserted into the bronchus. When the lesion in the bronchus is more peripheral, the curette can be guided into the target bronchus under X-ray TV fluoroscopy. Thus, the collection of cytologic specimens can be accurately performed with perfect precision.

# III. Indications and Contraindications for Bronchofiberscopic Examination

## INDICATIONS FOR BRONCHOFIBERSCOPIC EXAMINATION

First is pulmonary hemorrhage or hemoptysis. Most common causes of hemoptysis are; bronchogenic carcinoma, bronchial adenoma, metastatic tumors, pulmonary tuberculosis and other granulomas, bronchiectasis and lung abscess. When the hemorrhage is excessive, the bronchofiberscope with its small aspirating channel obviously should not be used. After the gross hemoptysis has subsided, then the bronchofiberscope is invaluable in detecting the source in the lesion and for making the definitive diagnosis in the bronchi.

Second is chronic, severe, unexplained cough. A chronic cough may be due to a chronic bronchitis, bronchial tuberculosis, foreign bodies in a bronchus, bronchogenic carcinoma, or bronchial adenoma.

Third is wheezing, which may be due to a partial stenosis or obstruction in the trachea or bronchus. The wheezing may be due to a foreign body, neoplasm, tuberculous bronchitis, bronchospasm due to bronchial asthma, bronchitis or emphysema, or to cicatricial stenosis. Other causes may be due to extrinsic pressure on the trachea or bronchus from tumors of the thyroid, esophagus, thymomas, enlarged paratracheal glands due to granulomas, lymphomas, or malignant metastases.

Fourth, indications based on roentgenographic findings including atelectasis, and shadows suggesting neoplasia.

As mentioned previously, persons over the age of 40 who have such symptoms and no findings in the chest X-ray films must be examined with the flexible bronchofiberscope to make an early diagnosis of lung cancer.

## CONTRAINDICATIONS FOR BRONCHOFIBERSCOPIC EXAMINATION

The extent of indications and contraindications in bronchoscopy largely depends on the skill of the physician and his choice of technique. It may be affirmed, however, that there are no contraindications to this method of examination if bronchoscopy is imperative. The relative contraindications to the use of the bronchofiberscope are the same as those with a rigid bronchoscope, except that in many cases where a rigid bronchoscopy is not possible because of the poor condition of a patient, it is occasionally possible to perform flexible bronchofiberscopy under either general or local anesthesia.

Contraindications in bronchoscopy:

1) Extreme depression of cardiac or pulmonary function

2) Physical condition immediately after heavy hemoptysis. In a patient with blood-stained sputum, bronchoscopic examination is essential.

3) Abnormal emaciation due to fever.

4) General debilitation of the patient due to other causes.

## CHOICE OF TECHNIQUES

With the development of the flexible bronchofiberscope, the bronchoscopist now has a choice of either the rigid or flexible instruments, depending on the indication, the objective of the examination, and the location of the lesion.

Confirmation of the precise location of a peripheral lesion is very important. First prerequisite is a careful study of the frontal and lateral X-rays of the chest. If the lesion is near the hilum in a segmental or a subsegmental bronchus, tomograms are especially helpful. If the lesion is located peripherally, bronchograms are essential in confirming the specific branch bronchus leading to the lesion. This is especially important in lesions in IV to VI order of branching, which are accessible for viewing with the 4 mm bronchofiberscope.

After locating the lesion precisely, the following technique is utilized (Fig. 51):

1. For tracheal lesions, the rigid bronchoscope is preferred.

2. For lesions in any of the major bronchi, either the rigid or flexible instruments can be utilized. If a flexible bronchofiberscope is used, the larger instruments such as Machida FBS-6 or Olympus BF-B are recommended because of their large channels enabling good suction and introduction of larger instruments for biopsy specimens. For foreign bodies at this level, the rigid bronchoscope is recommended.

3. For lesions in the segmental or subsegmental level, the bronchofiberscope is advised.

4. For lesions in the more peripheral bronchi such as in IV to VI order of branching, the examination can only be performed with a bronchofiberscope. In such cases, both the 5 mm and 4 mm instruments are used to supplement each other.

1) The 4 mm bronchofiberscope can be introduced into bronchi of IV to VI order of branching. However, because of the small caliber of the channel, only thin secretions can be aspirated. Furthermore, neither a curette nor a biopsy forceps can be used with the 4 mm instrument.
2) The 5 mm bronchofiberscope can be passed through a segmental bronchus into a subsegmental branch, and visualization beyond this level is limited. The channel, as mentioned before, is quite adequate for aspiration, curettage or biopsy.

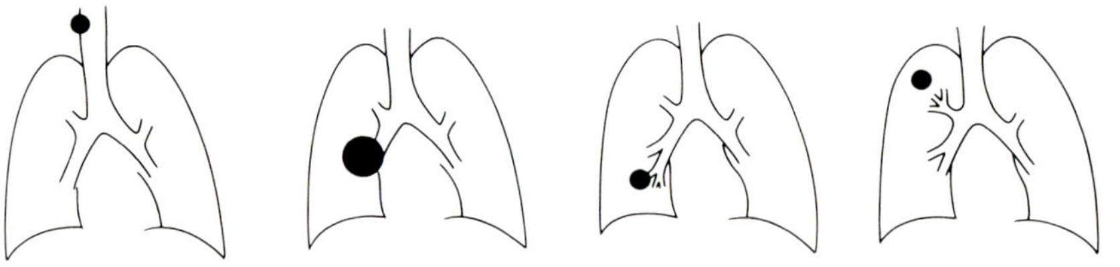


**Fig. 51** Choice of apparatus in bronchoscopic examination—bronchoscopic analysis is requested in the case of a peripheral lesion.

Bearing in mind the advantages of each model, the following procedure utilizing both instruments is suggested:

a) First the 5mm bronchofiberscope is introduced for observation and examination as far as possible. If necessary, additional instillation of anesthetic solution and/or aspiration of secretions can be accomplished at this time. The fiberscope is removed.
b) Next, the 4 mm bronchofiberscope is introduced for more detailed examination and deeper insertion. Again, the fiberscope is removed.
c) Following this, the 5 mm bronchofiberscope is reintroduced into the target bronchus for obtaining curettage or biopsy specimens of the lesion in question. This should be performed under X-ray TV fluoroscopy.

On many occasions X-ray television is a most important supplement in obtaining a proper biopsy specimen, even in cases where the target bronchus has been confirmed previously by bronchograms. This is particularly true when the lesion is large, involving several segmental or subsegmental bronchi, and accompanied by stenoses or obstructions. In such cases, the curette or biopsy forceps can be guided into the final target bronchus under X ray TV fluoroscopy.

5 In cases with negative chest X-ray but blood-streaked sputa, examination with the 5 mm broncho-fiberscope is the proper instrument of choice. If the source of bleeding is more peripheral than the subsegmental level, abnormalities are usually reflected on the chest X-ray; while lesions in the larger bronchi without obstruction usually do not reveal abnormal X-ray findings.

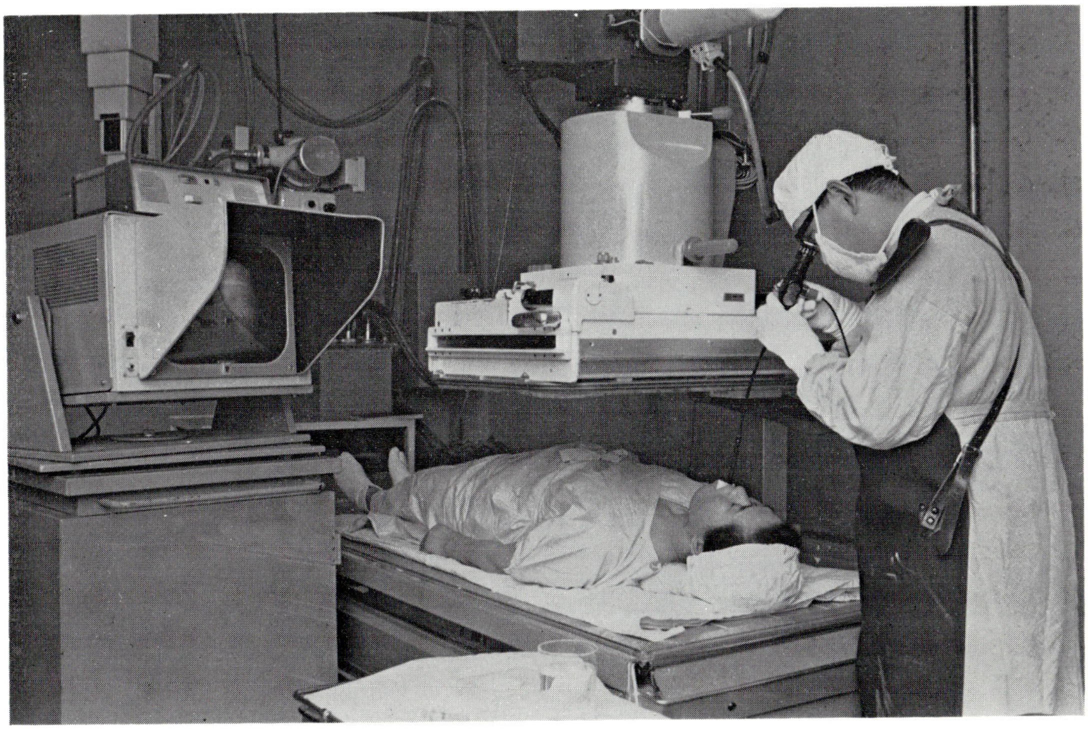

**Fig. 52** TV fluoroscopy.

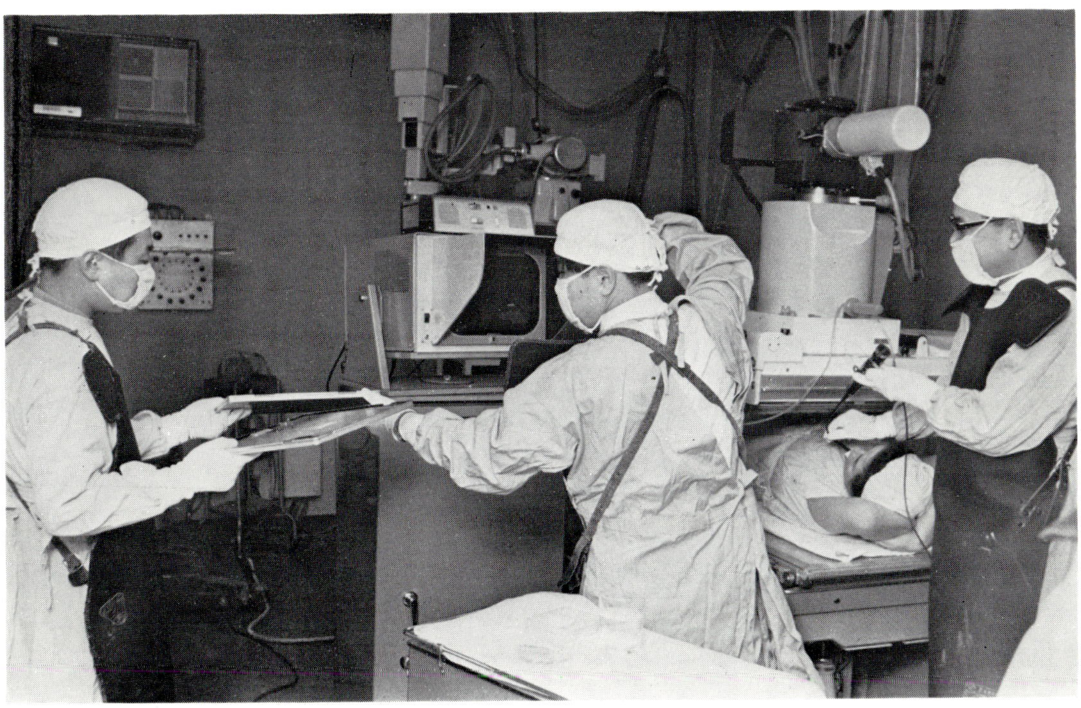

**Fig. 53** TV photofluoroscopy.

## COMPLICATIONS AND THEIR TREATMENT

Cautions and precautions when using a flexible bronchofiberscope are the same as those with an ordinary rigid bronchoscope. The incidence of complications is much less with the flexible bronchofiberscope.

Complications may be caused by the following:

### a. Local anesthesia of mucosa

In the past when cocaine or Cocaine T® was used for local anesthesia, toxic reactions were frequent; but at the present time with lidocaine, toxic reactions are rare. Caution must be exercised, however; overdose must be avoided. About 4–8 ml of 4 % lidocaine is a safe dose. In an ordinary adult the maximum dosage of 4 % lidocaine is 12 ml (200–400 mg). Intoxication due to lidocaine is manifested by marked weakness or loss of consciousness; rarely convulsion may occur. Treatment is to secure the air way and supply a sufficient amount of oxygen. Fortunately these side effects are of very brief duration.

### b. Insertion of a bronchofiberscope

Avoid rough insertion of the bronchoscope which may injure the mucosa of the throat. Forcible introduction through the larynx may injure the arytenoid cartilages or cause dyskinesia of the vocal chords. Spasmodic stricture of vocal chords is treated with local anesthetic in the larynx. Laryngospasm rarely leads to asphyxia and death.

### c. Post-insertion handling of the instrument

The sharp tip of the tracheal tube should not be allowed to injure the membranous part of the trachea. This can easily be prevented if the tube is inserted with the tip upturned. In patients whose pulmonary function is low prolonged inspection with the bronchofiberscope may cause dyspnea. It is preferable to supply oxygen through the bronchofiberscope in patients with reduced cardiac and/or pulmonary function, and the examining time limited to 10 or 15 minutes. General anesthesia may be preferable in such cases.

### d. Intrabronchial maneuvering of attachments for cytology, biopsy or removal of foreign bodies

Hemorrhage is the most frequent complication resulting from operation for cytology, biopsy or removal of foreign bodies. Hemostasis by compression can be accomplished with a forceps with a cotton ball fastened at the tip since the site of bleeding is clearly seen in many cases. If the hemorrhage is profuse it is essential that the blood not be allowed to overflow into the contralateral bronchus.

Presence of mind is the rule for a physician when bleeding occurs. Instruct the patient to suppress coughing as much as possible. Sudden and abrupt change of patient's posture must be avoided.

### e. Withdrawal of bronchofiberscopic instruments

Coughing or fever after the extraction of the tracheal tube and bronchofiberscope may be treated by administration of an ordinary antibiotic agent.

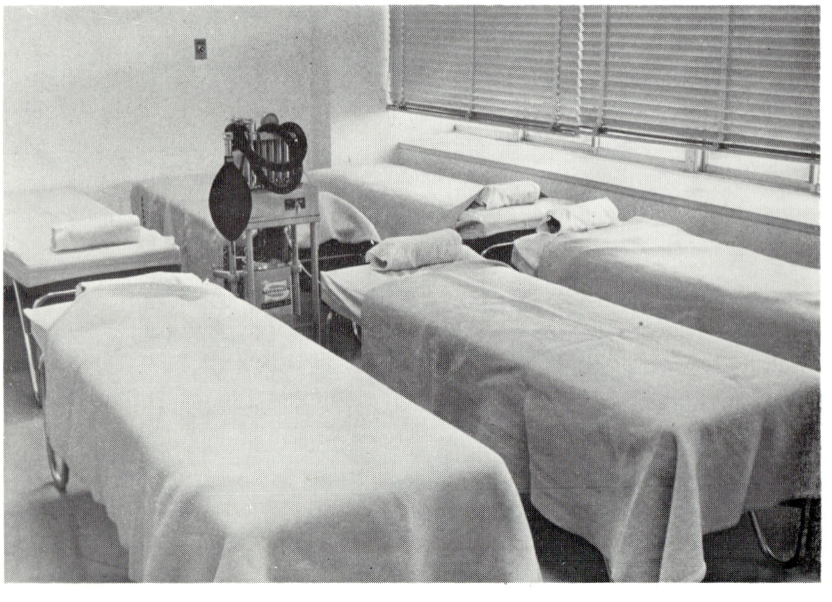

**Fig. 54** Unit for general anesthesia in case of emergency equipped in the endoscopic recovery room.

# IV. Manipulation of a Flexible Bronchofiberscope

## EQUIPMENT

The room for performing flexible bronchofiberscopy should be equipped with an X-ray television for two reasons: 1) for confirming the position of the tip of the bronchofiberscope and 2) for guiding the brush or curette into a peripheral lesion to obtain specimens for accurate cytological diagnosis. Needless to say, the lack of such equipment would greatly reduce the accuracy of diagnosis.

A room especially designed for the above purpose is illustrated in Fig. 55. The TV set connected to a 9-inch image intensifier includes a C-shaped arm which encircles the patient. The table is made of wood and plastic in order to permit X-ray fluoroscopy.

A suction set and an oxygen inhalation set are also essential (Fig. 56). The latter must always be available for a dyspneic patient or one likely to develop dyspnea during bronchoscopy.

Various instruments utilized for rigid bronchoscopy are prepared for flexible bronchoscopy as well. Apparatus for cytologic diagnosis, smear preparation, fixation and so forth are indispensable.

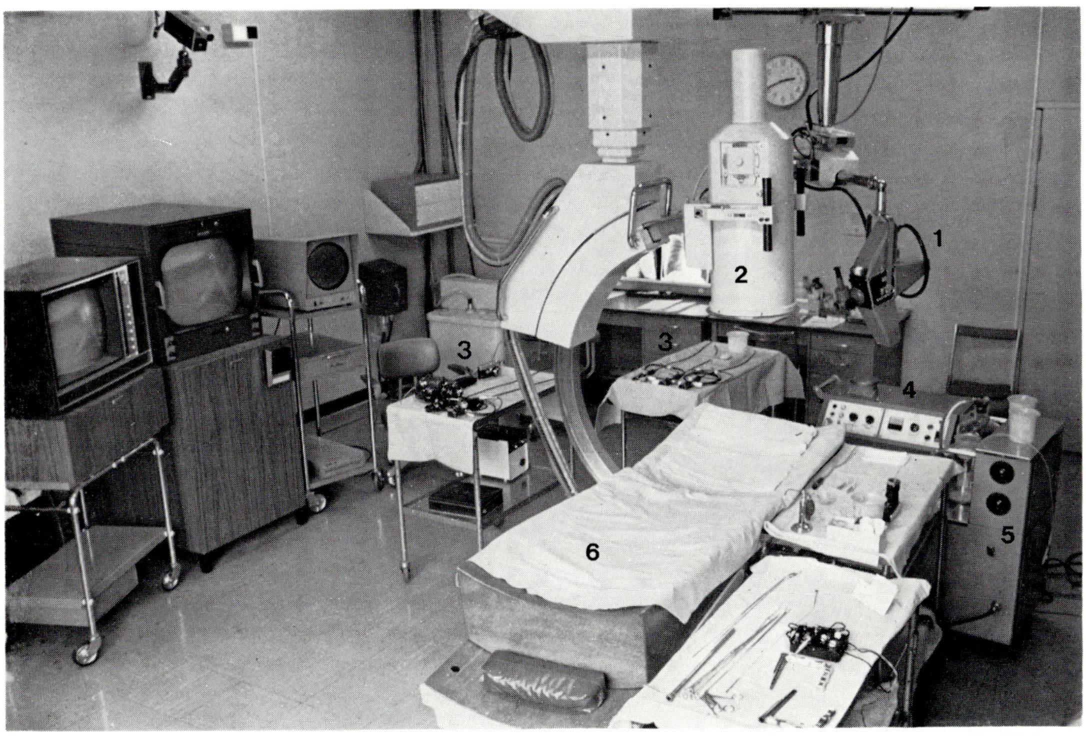


**Fig. 55** Bronchoscopic examination room.

1. Set of color TV for bronchoscopy
2. Set of X-ray TV for bronchoscopy
3. Various bronchofiberscopes
4. Light source
5. Suction instruments
6. Table for bronchoscopy (usable with fluoroscopy)

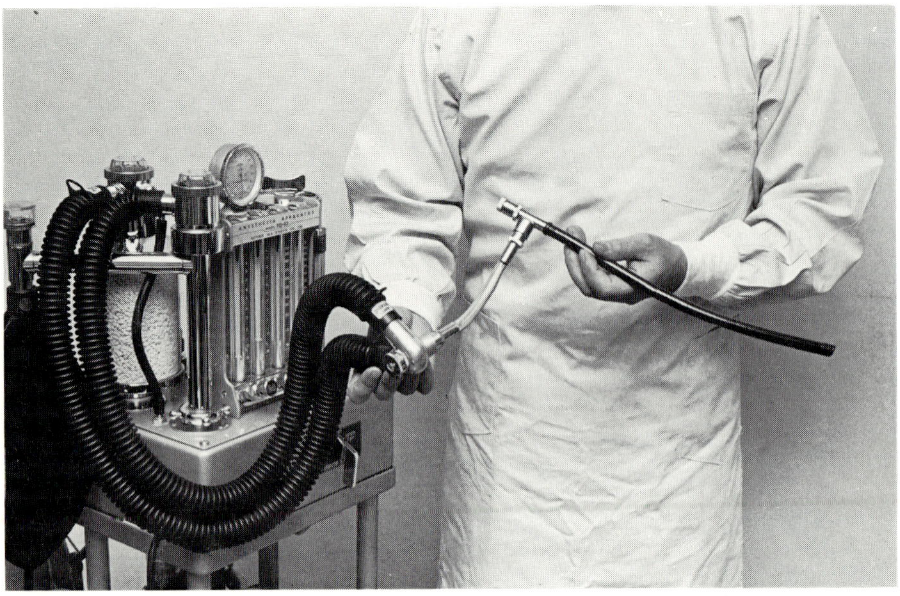

**Fig. 56** The oxygen inhalator of general anesthetic unit connected to the tracheal tube with a two-way adaptor may be utilized in the low pulmonary function cases.

## CAUTION IN HANDLING

A flexible bronchofiberscope is an extremely delicate apparatus. The body contains tens of thousands of glass fibers and its distal end contains special mechanisms for bending and twisting. Rough handling cannot be allowed under any circumstances. The instruments must be manipulated with the utmost care. Mishandling distal end or the tip may damage the glass fibers.

## PREPARATION OF THE PATIENT

The patient should not take any food or drink for at least three hours prior to bronchoscopy.

Cooperation of the patient and confidence in his physician are indispensable. For this purpose, the patient should be :

1) Given a thorough explanation of the objective of the procedure.
2) Instructed that there is no danger involved in the operation.
3) Assured that his cooperation facilitates the examination.
4) Relieved of any feeling of oppression or pain during bronchoscopy by appropriate medication.
5) Convinced that he should try to breathe as normally as possible during the examination, instead of holding his breath.

Usually 30 minutes before bronchoscopy, the adult patient should have 5–10 mg morphine injected intramuscularly. If salivation is excessive, 0.5 mg atropine sulfate is recommended for intramuscular injection.

## ANESTHESIA

The choice of anesthetic varies depending upon the technique the doctor employs, his preference, and the hospital system. Unlike rigid bronchoscopy general anesthesia is rarely necessary, because the patient experiences minimal discomfort.

For local anesthesia 2–4 % lidocaine (Xylocaine®) is recommended.

1) Prior to the insertion of a flexible bronchofiberscope 2 ml of 2 % lidocaine is sprayed into the pharynx and the larynx with a nebulizer (Fig. 58).

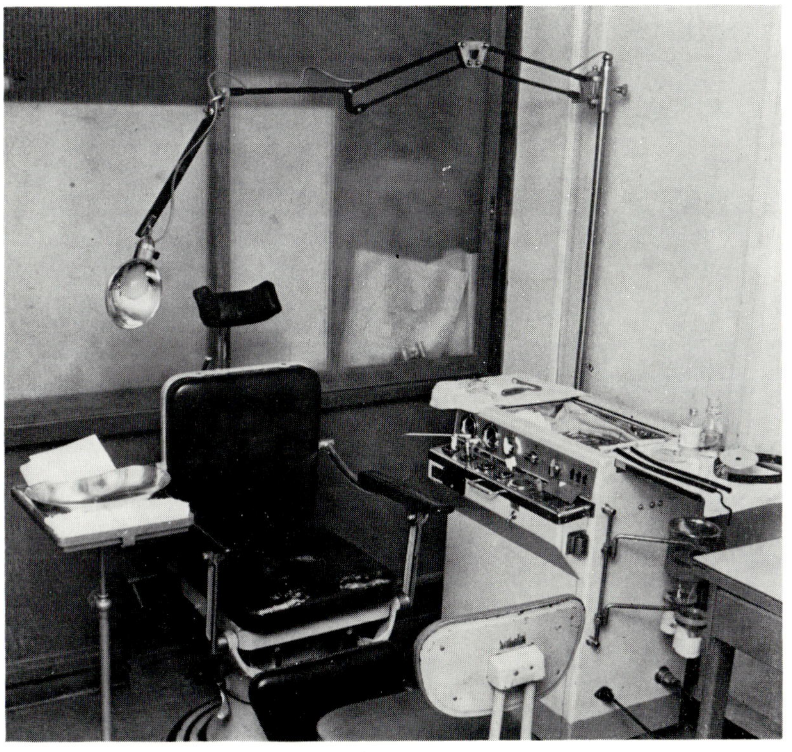

Fig. 57 Room for larynx-pharynx anesthesia.

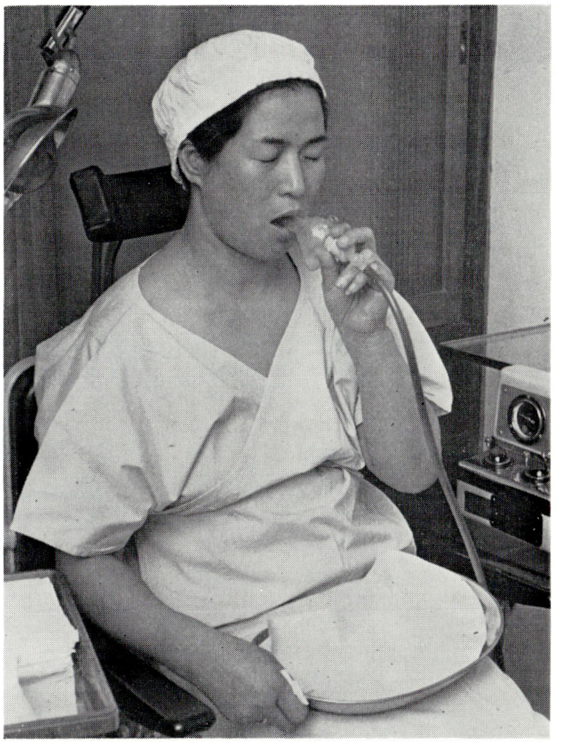

Fig. 58 Nebulizer for larynx anesthesia.

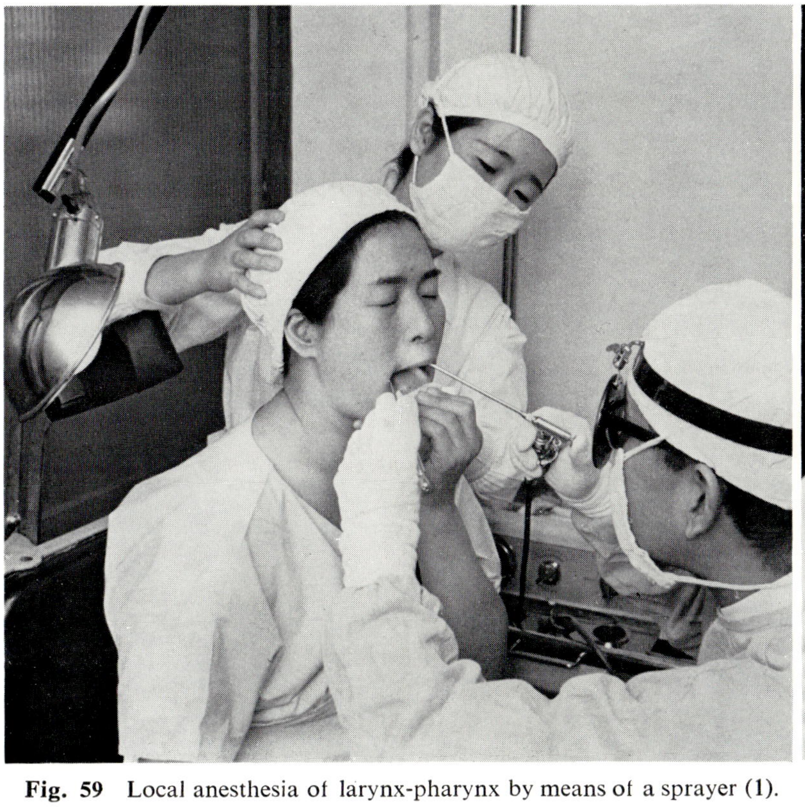

Fig. 59 Local anesthesia of larynx-pharynx by means of a sprayer (1).

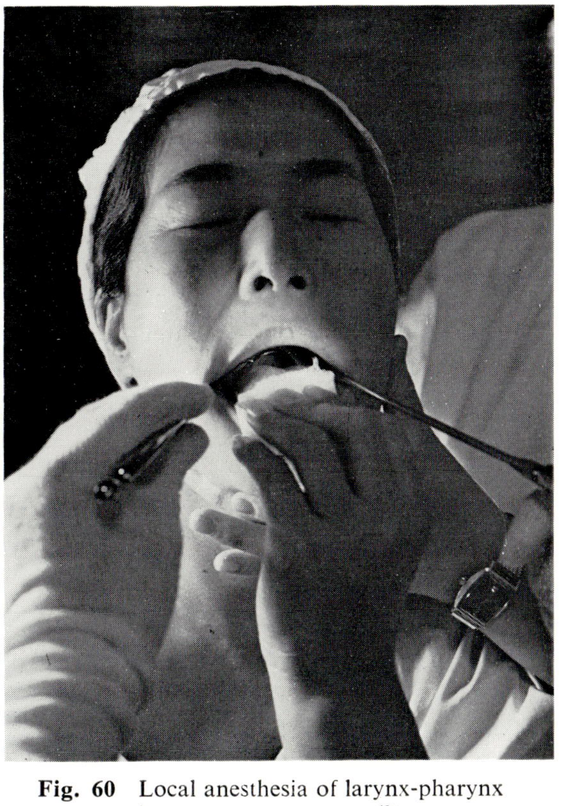

Fig. 60 Local anesthesia of larynx-pharynx by means of a sprayer (2).

2) After nebulization, 2–4 ml of 4 % lidocaine is again sprayed into the larynx (Figs. 59 and 60).
3) After the insertion of the flexible bronchofiberscope, 4 % lidocaine solution is instilled through the channel.
4) The total amount of 4 % lidocaine should not exceed 5–10 ml, otherwise lidocaine toxicity may occur.

# TECHNICAL PROCEDURE

### a. Tracheal intubation—Variations in techniques of introducing the bronchofiberscope

There are roughly two techniques of bronchofiberscopy. The first is the method in which a tracheal tube is employed for the insertion of the fiberscope (1, 2). In the second, no intratracheal intubation is employed and the fiberscope is inserted transorally (3) or transnasally (4).

1. After local anesthesia is accomplished by nebulizing lidocaine into the pharynx and larynx, the next process is to insert a tube into the trachea. This step is necessary because of the reasons given later.

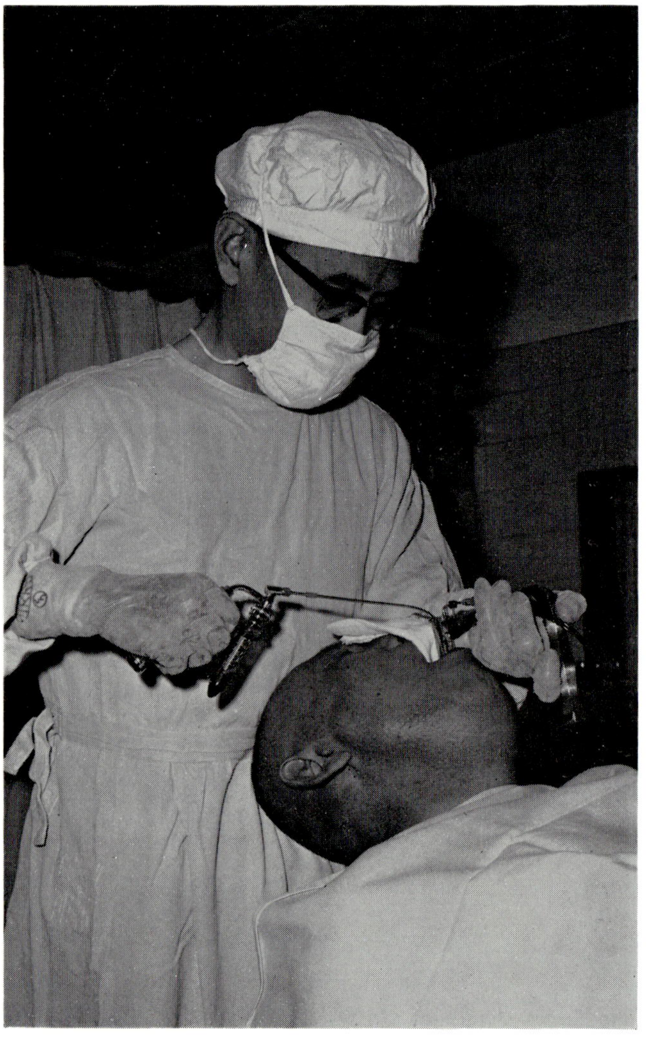

**Fig. 61** Local anesthesia in the supine position by a sprayer.

The tracheal tube, either a soft or combination flexible-rigid one, is introduced into the trachea with the patient in the supine position using a laryngoscope to keep the larynx in view. Any of the laryngoscopes will do, such as the Jackson, the Wis Foregger (L-shaped), or the Macintosh type.

With a flexible intratracheal tube, a malleable stylet is inserted in order to maintain the curve (Figs. 61–66). The stylet is lubricated with some types of lubricant such as olive oil to reduce friction between it and the intratracheal tube. Viscous lidocaine is used as a lubricant for the tube for smoother introduction.

The tracheal tube may be introduced directly with the patient sitting ; much in the same manner as when introducing a Metra's catheter for performing bronchograms (Figs. 69–72).

The combination flexible-rigid tracheal tube is inserted into the trachea in the rigid state in the same manner as when using a rigid bronchoscope.

Once the tracheal tube is inserted, a cylindrical bite-block is placed about the tube and fixed between the upper and the lower teeth of the patient in order to prevent him from biting the tube (Fig. 67) The bite block and the tracheal tube are firmly fixed in place with adhesive tape (Fig. 68).

The insertion of the tracheal tube must be accomplished with the utmost gentleness and care , particularly so as the patient is conscious and fully aware of the proceedings. Patient's cooperation is essential. The operator should strive to develop a skillful technique.

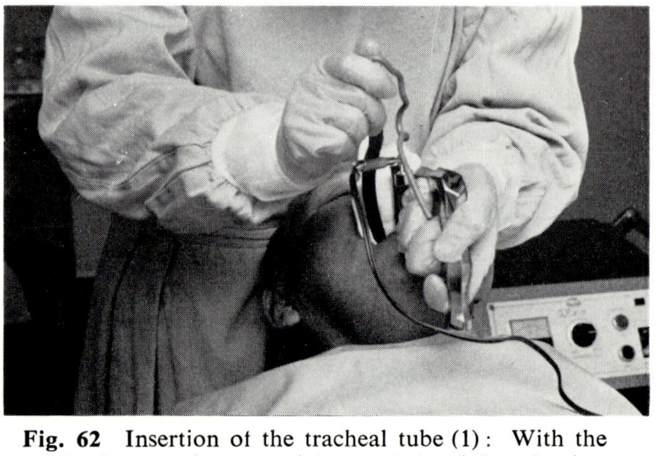

**Fig. 62** Insertion of the tracheal tube (1) : With the epiglottis pressed away and the vocal chords kept in view aided by the laryngoscope, the tracheal tube with a stylet intubated is inserted into the trachea, the distal tip upturned.

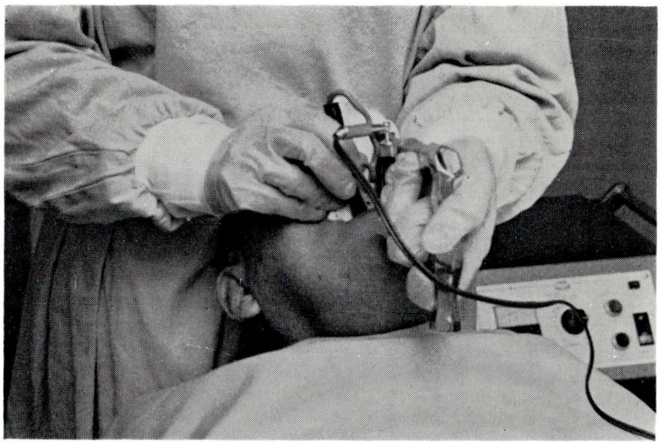

**Fig. 63** Insertion of the tracheal tube (2) : The tracheal tube is farther advanced toward the depth of the trachea.

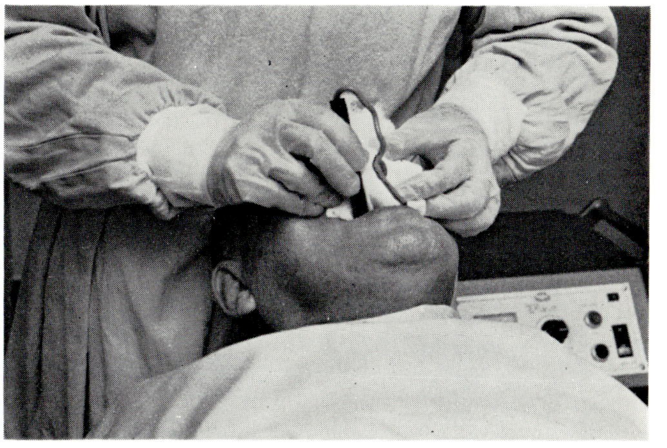

**Fig. 64** Insertion of the tracheal tube (3) : The laryngoscope is removed.

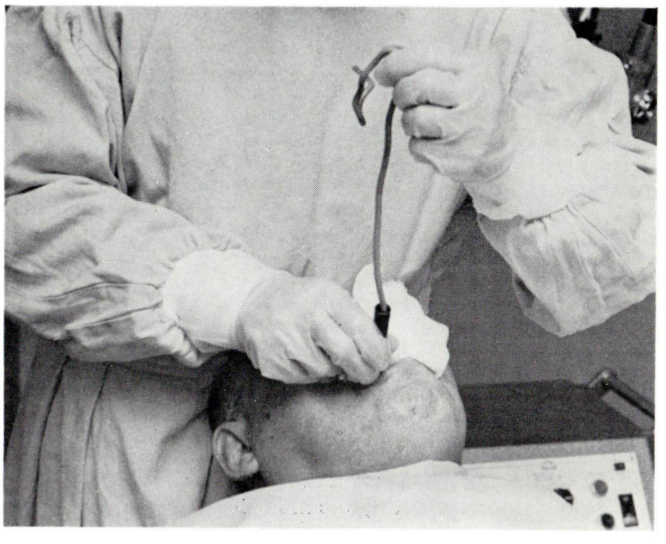

**Fig. 65** Insertion of the tracheal tube (4) : The stylet is withdrawn.

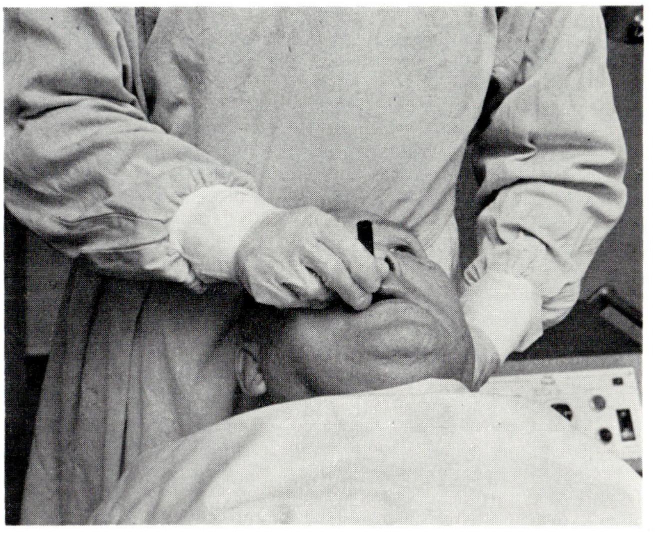

**Fig. 66** Insertion of the tracheal tube (4) : The tracheal tube is so fixed that about 50 to 70 mm of the tube remains out of the mouth. It is desirable that the distal end of the tube be situated about 20 mm from the tracheal bifurcation.

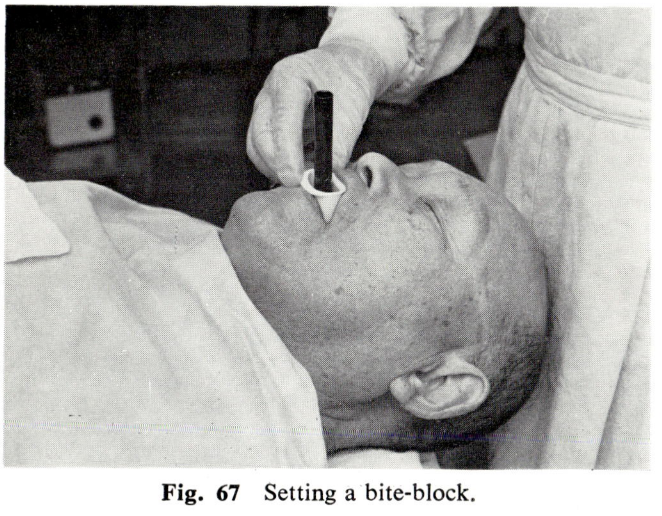

**Fig. 67** Setting a bite-block.

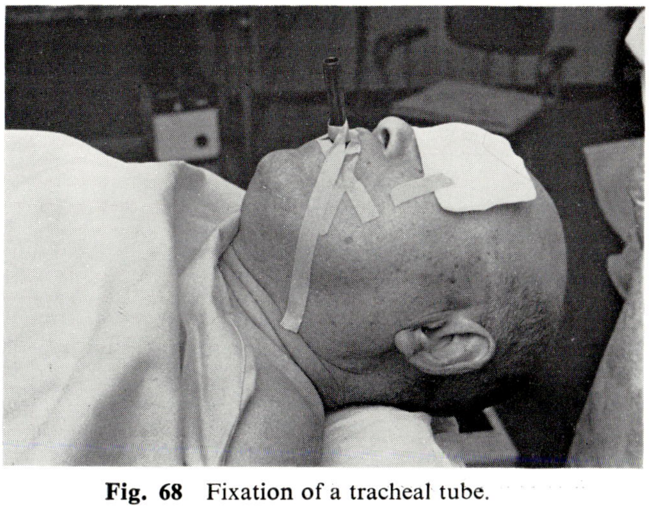

**Fig. 68** Fixation of a tracheal tube.

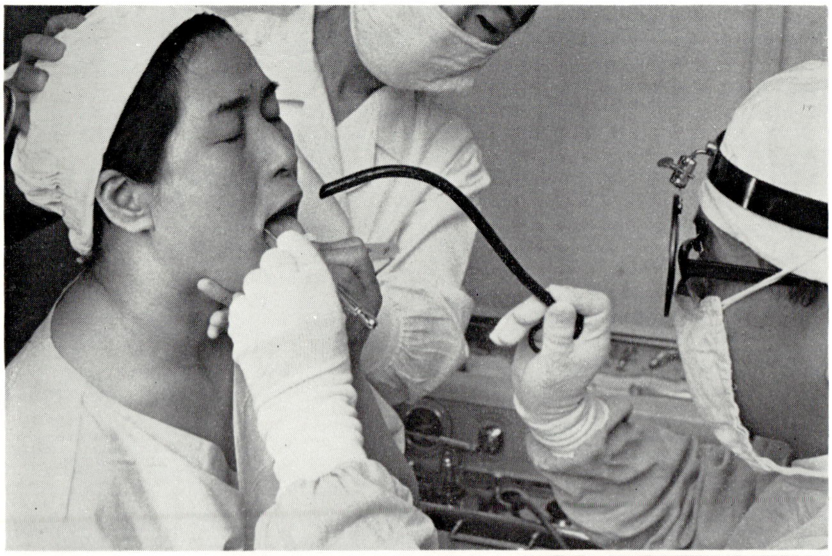

**Fig. 69** Insertion of the tracheal tube in the sitting position(1) Aided by an indirect laryngoscope (mirror) introduced just in front of the uvula, the tracheal tube with a stylet intubated is inserted into the mouth. Essential is to hold the distal end upturned (basal downward). Position of the patient's body enabling the insertion easy The patient sits deep in the chair, a bit leaning forward, both shoulders kept relaxed, the head tilting backward only slightly, and jaws held in a protruding manner.

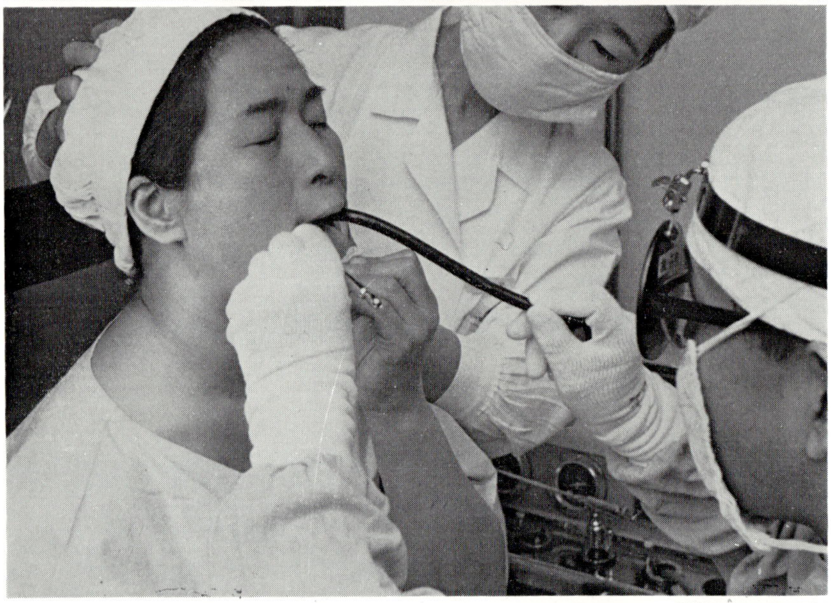

**Fig. 70** Insertion of the tracheal tube in the sitting position (2): The tracheal tube is inserted into the glottis, with the larynx in full view aided by the indirect laryngoscope.

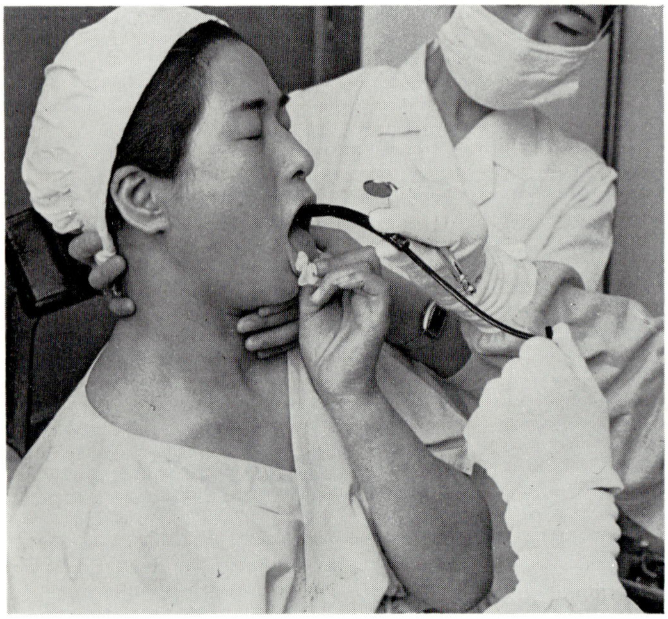

**Fig. 71** Insertion of the tracheal tube in the sitting position (3) When the tracheal tube has been well inserted, the stylet is slowly removed.

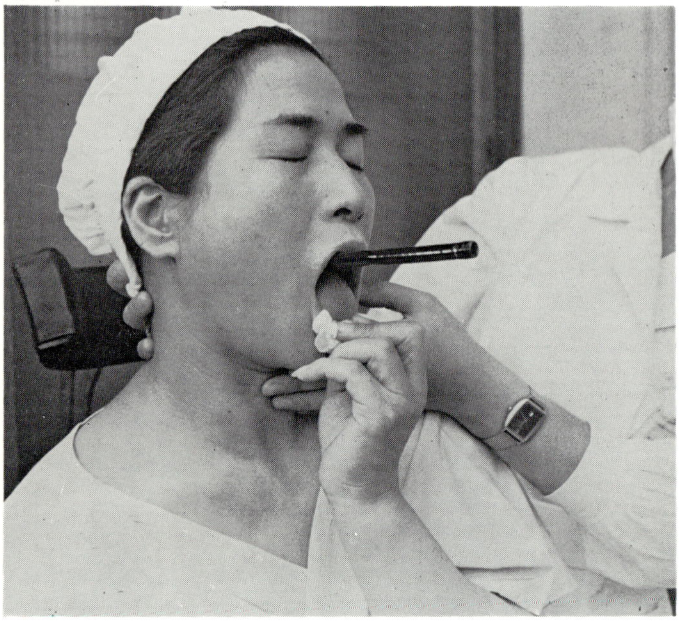

**Fig. 72** Inserted tracheal tube. As has been stated, it is desirable for the proximal part of the tracheal tube to protrude about 50 mm to 70 mm.

2. In some circumstances when the intratracheal tube cannot be introduced in the usual manner described earlier (*e. g.* if the patient is not able to open his mouth adequately or if the operator is inexperienced), the intratracheal tube may be introduced by utilizing the bronchofiberscope itself as a guide (Figs. 73–77).

First, the body of the bronchofiberscope is inserted through the intratracheal tube which is then held proximally close to the eyepiece. Next, the bronchofiber scope is introduced gently under direct vision through the mouth, between the vocal chords, and advanced gently down the trachea. When the tip of the bronchofiberscope reaches the level of the carina, the intratracheal tube is gently pushed into the trachea guided by the body of the bronchofiberscope.

The advantages of this technique are that the vocal chords as well as the upper trachea can be examined, and the technique itself may be easier for the beginner. The disadvantage is that the flexible tip of the instrument may be damaged. However, this danger can be minimized by making certain that the tip of the instrument is at or near the level of the carina before the tracheal tube is inserted into the trachea.

3. Another technique is the transoral method without the intratracheal tube (Figs. 78–81). The pharynx and larynx are anesthetized by spraying as described above. The patient will be laid supine. He is instructed to hold the tip of his tongue out while the bronchofiberscope is inserted. The fiberscope must be advanced gently directly in the median line. The operator's free fingers should be placed within the patient's mouth to protect the fiberscope and prevent its being bitten as occasionally happens with an extremely nervous patient. Thus the fiberscope is gently advanced into the trachea, as has already been mentioned before.

When the insertion has nearly reached the tracheal carina, a bite-block is applied around the body of the fiberscope. The rest of the operation follows the above description.

This is a handy method but not suitable for cases producing large amounts of sputum or requiring biopsy or curettage, as the lack of a tracheal tube precludes repeated extraction and reintroduction of the fiberscope.

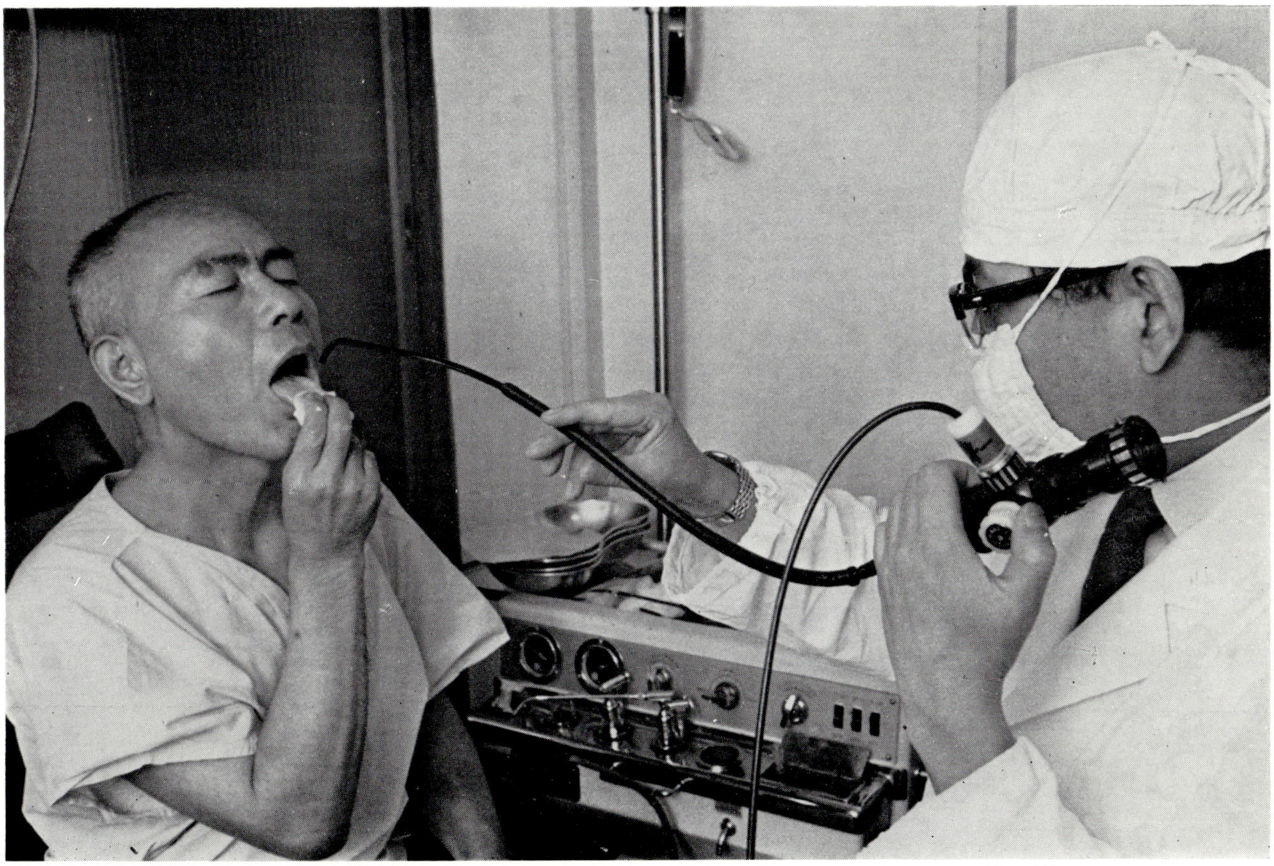

**Fig. 73** Insertion of the tracheal tube making use of the bronchofiberscope (1) : The tracheal tube is held thus near the proximal part of the bronchofiberscope. The fiberscope is put into the patient's mouth.

Fig. 74 Insertion of the tracheal tube (2) : The fiberscope, with its tip bent, is inserted into the trachea through the glottis which is under direct vision.

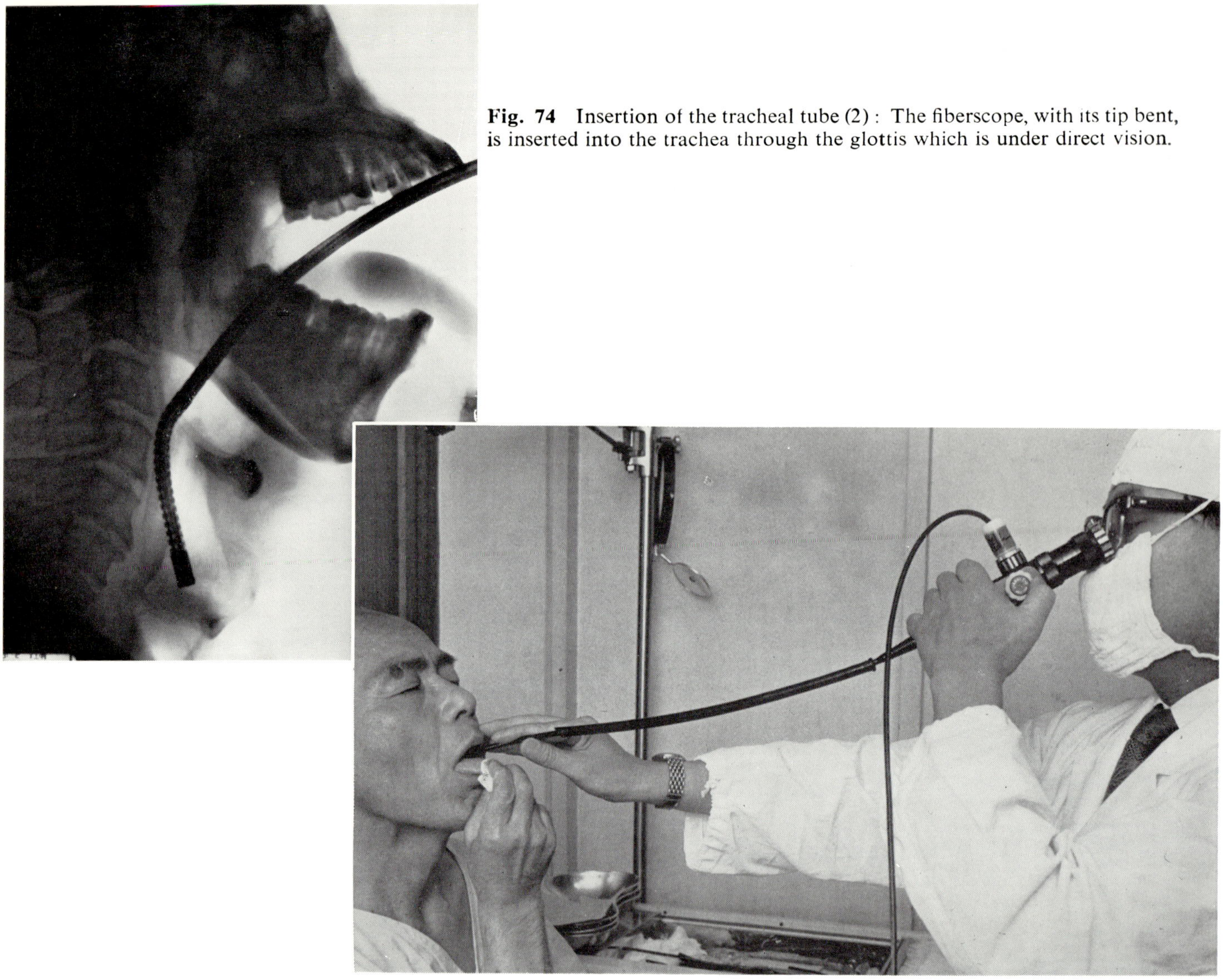

Fig. 75 Insertion of the tracheal tube (3): When the distal part of the fiberscope is at the level of the tracheal bifurcation, the tracheal tube is then introduced, guided by the body of the fiberscope. Caution here is that the bevel of the tracheal tube be directed posteriorly.

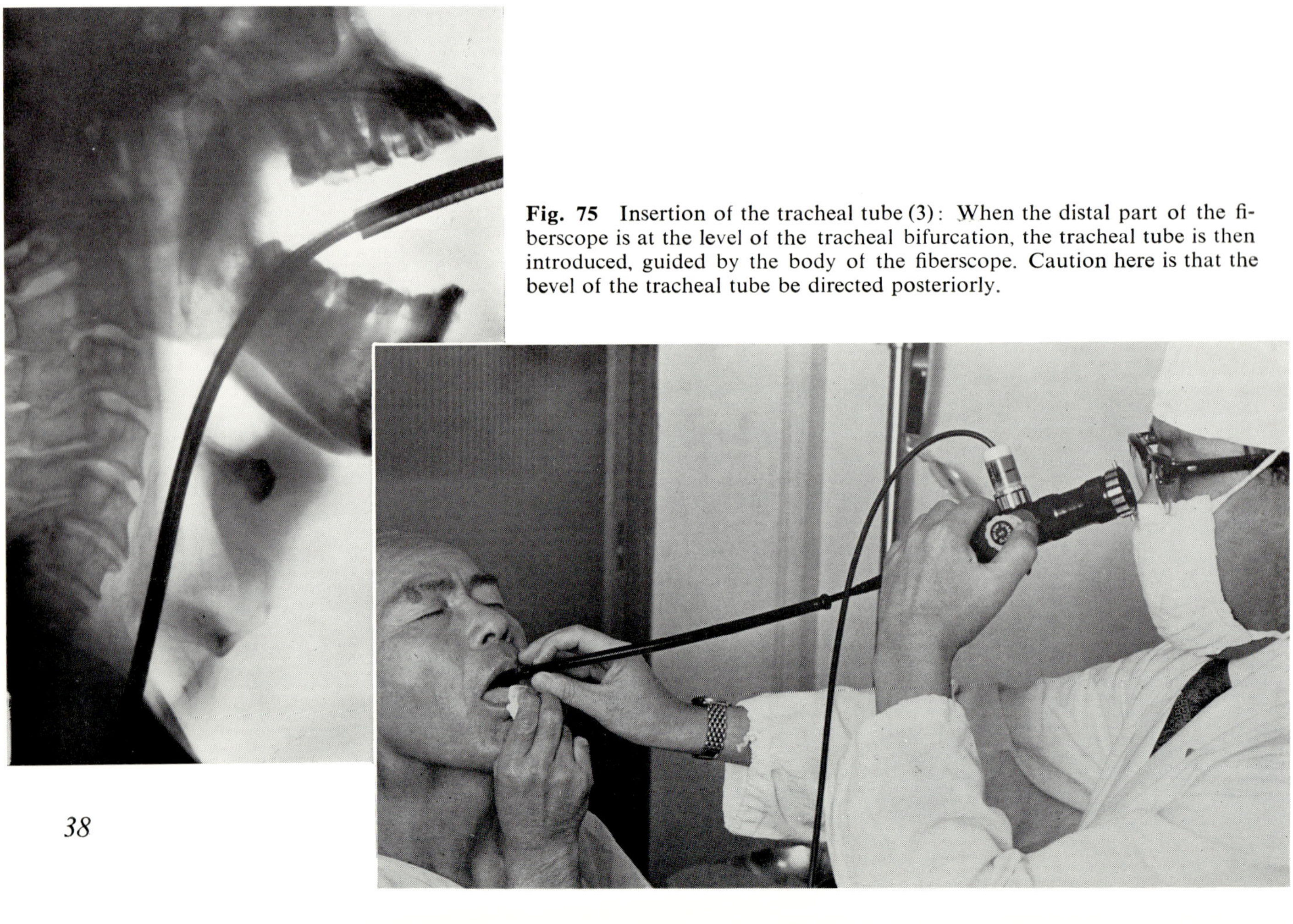

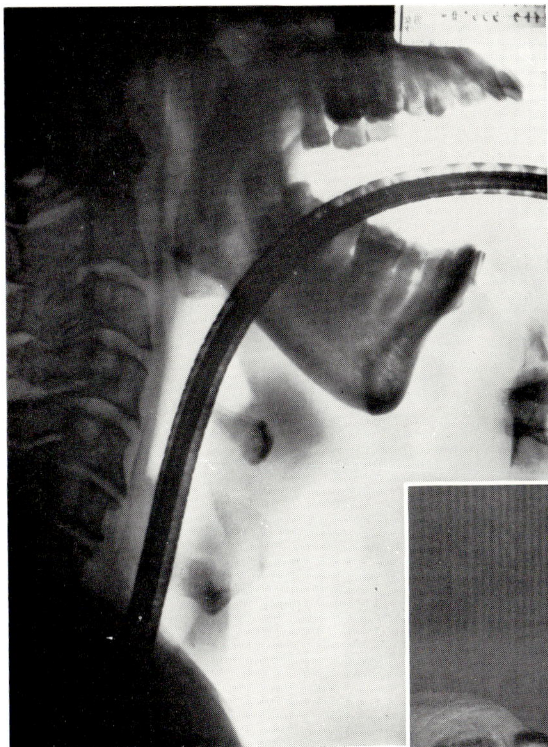

Fig. 76 Insertion of the tracheal tube (4): When the insertion of the tracheal tube is finished the fiberscope is slowly removed.

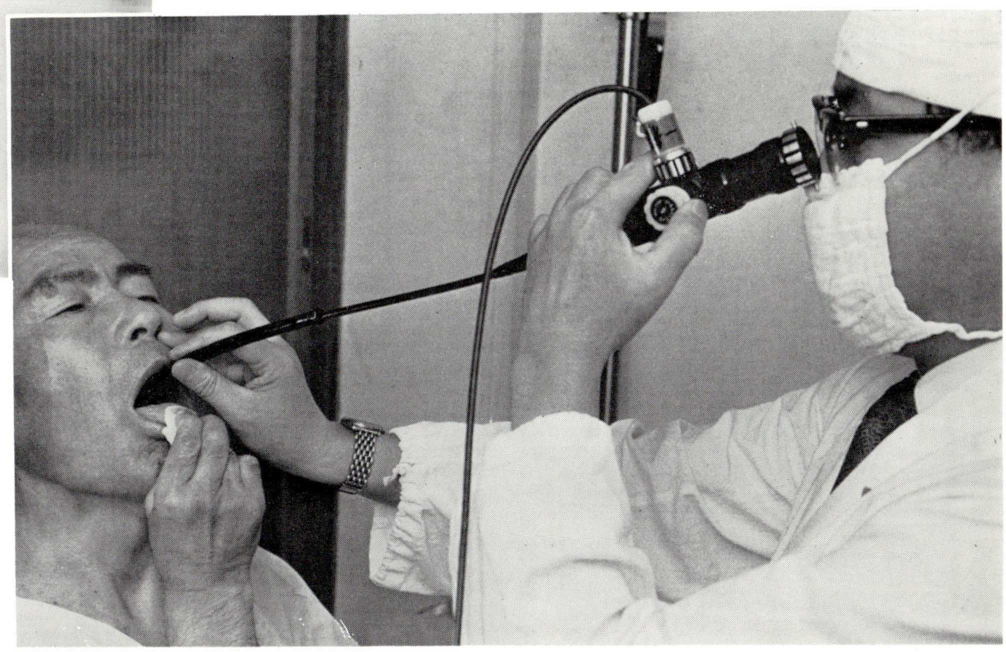

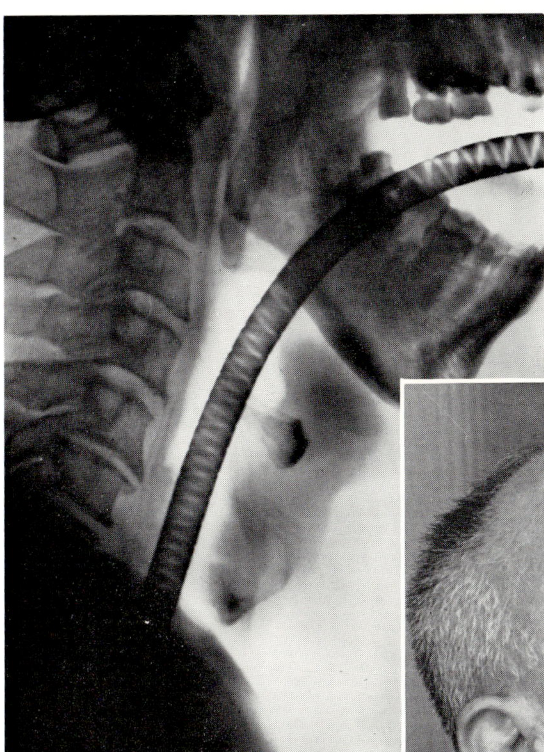

Fig. 77 Insertion of the tracheal tube (5): After the insertion, the tracheal tube is so fixed that it may not be bitten by the patient.

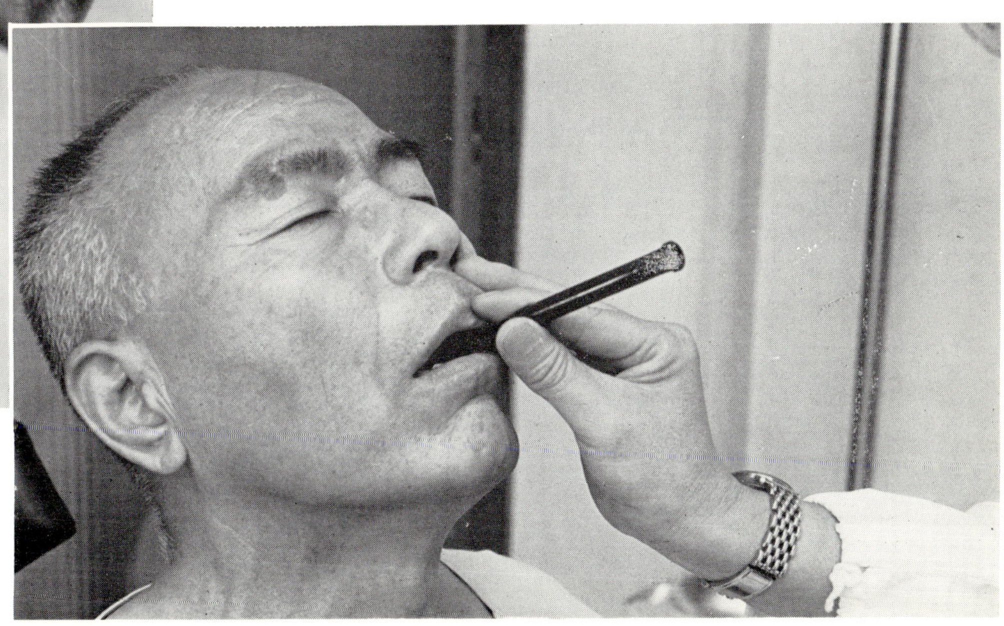

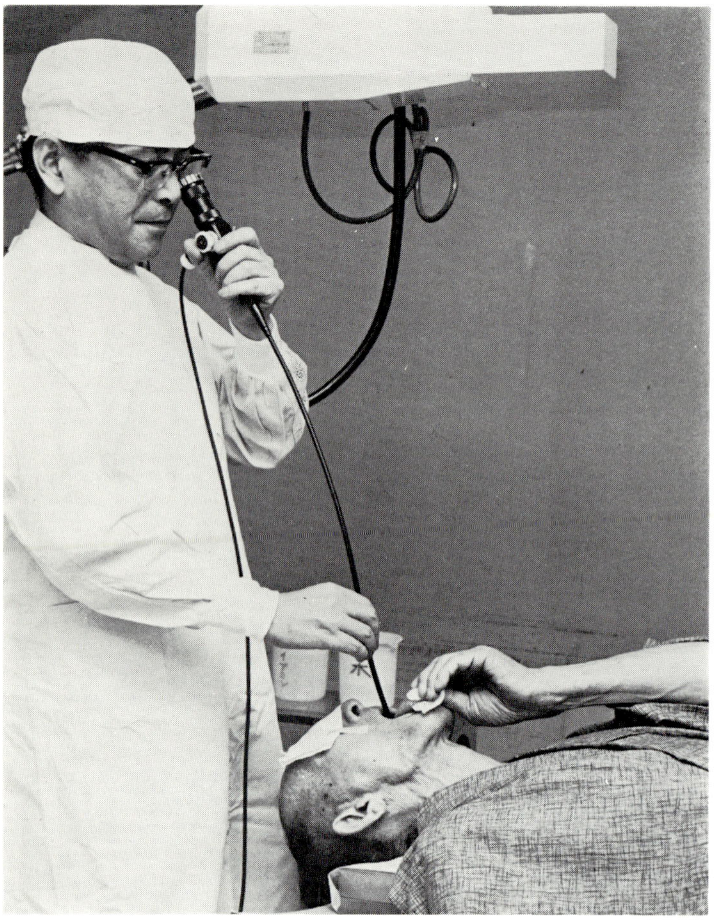

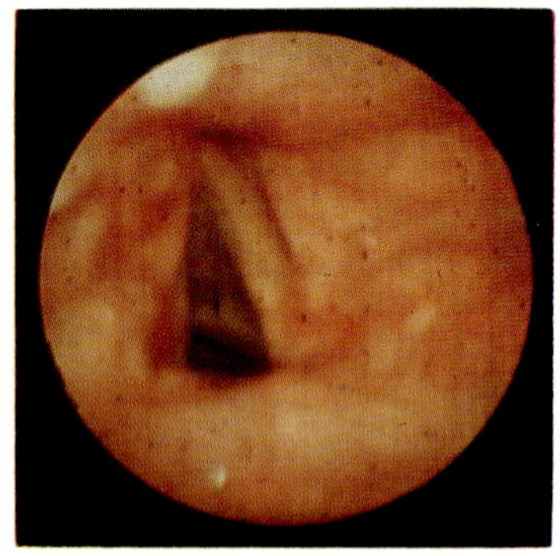

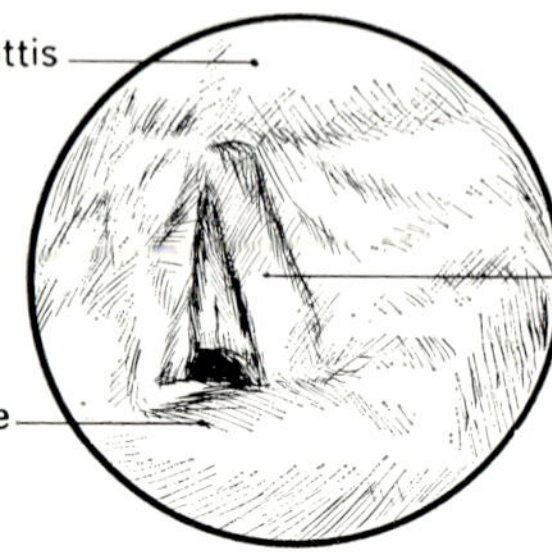


**Fig. 78** The bronchofiberscope is put into the mouth, with the pharynx and larynx in full view of the operator while the patient keeps his tongue pulled out. When the posterior wall of the pharynx comes into view, the tip of the fiberscope is given an upward angulation. The operator holds the fiberscope body with his right hand in order for the fiberscope to enter into the mouth in the median line. The epiglottis, vocal chords and arytenoid cartilages are well seen.

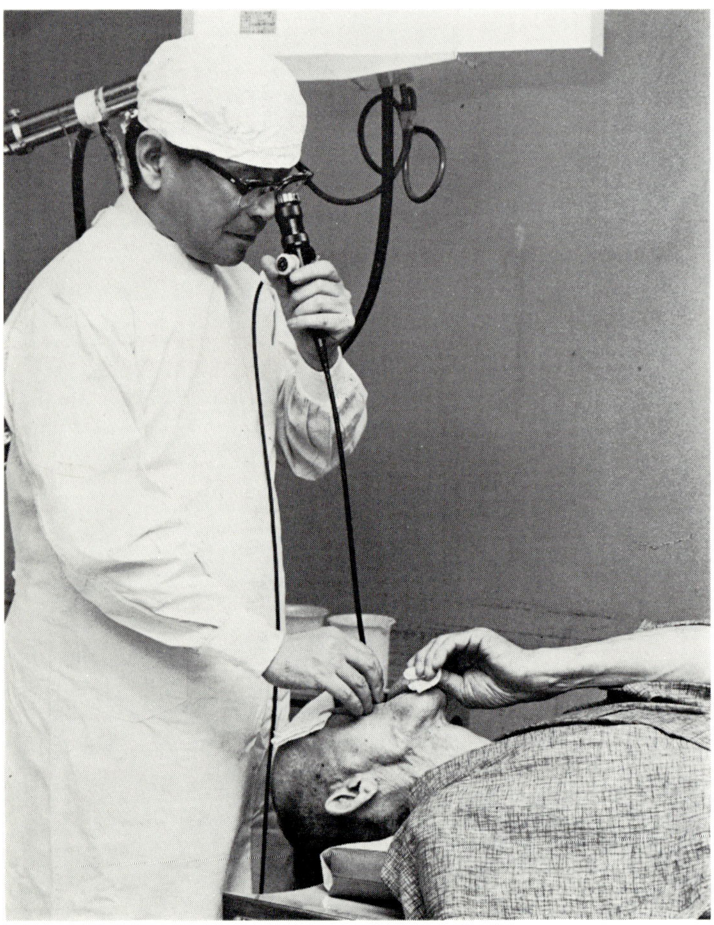

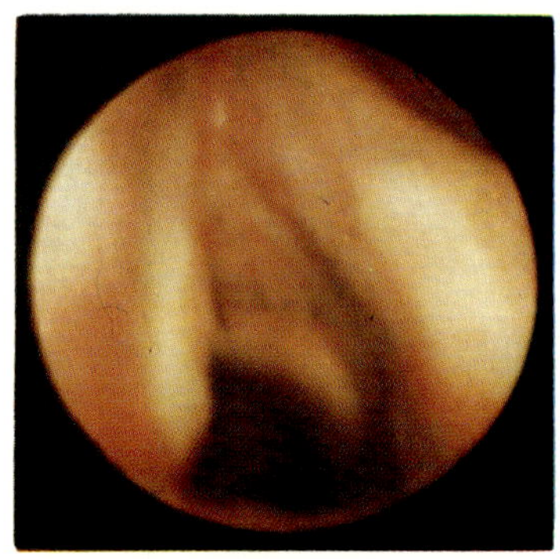

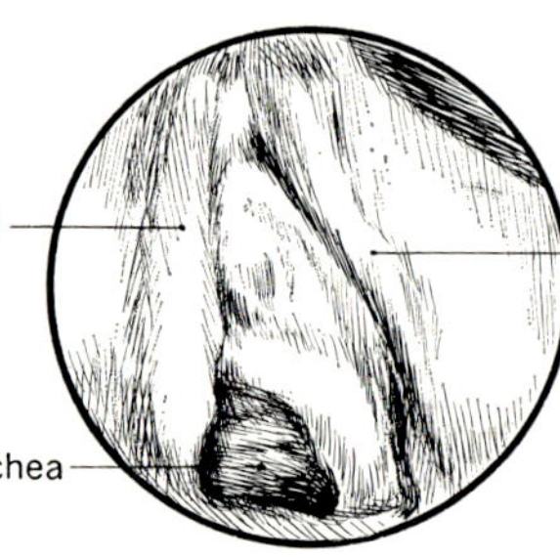


**Fig. 79** A little additional angulation is given to the tip, which holds up the epiglottis, then the fiberscope is advanced into the entrance of the larynx. At this stage, also, the midline; otherwise it may deviate into the pyriform recess and may not get into the trachea. The vocal folds are well viewed in the endoscopic picture.

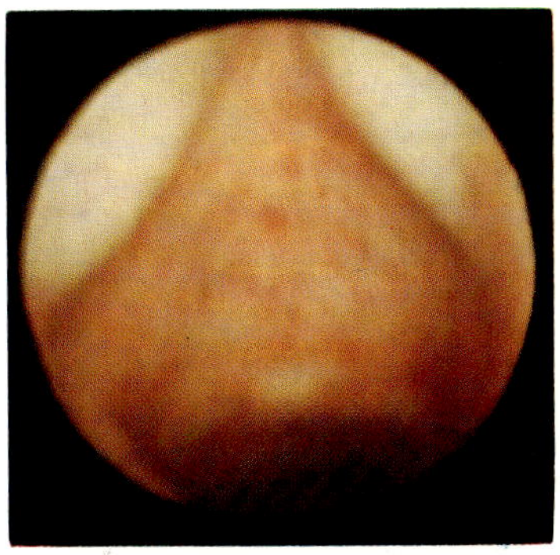

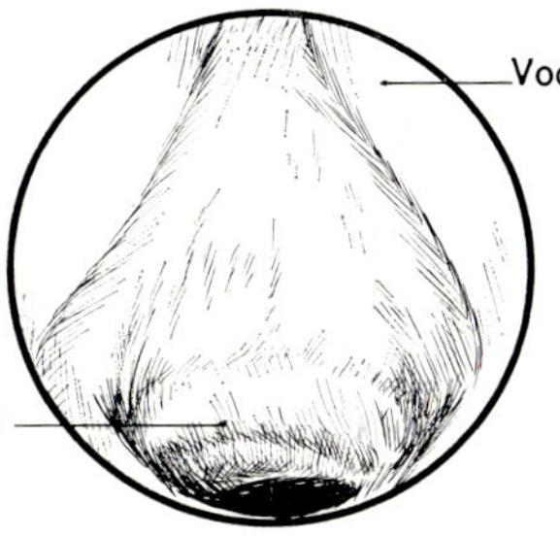


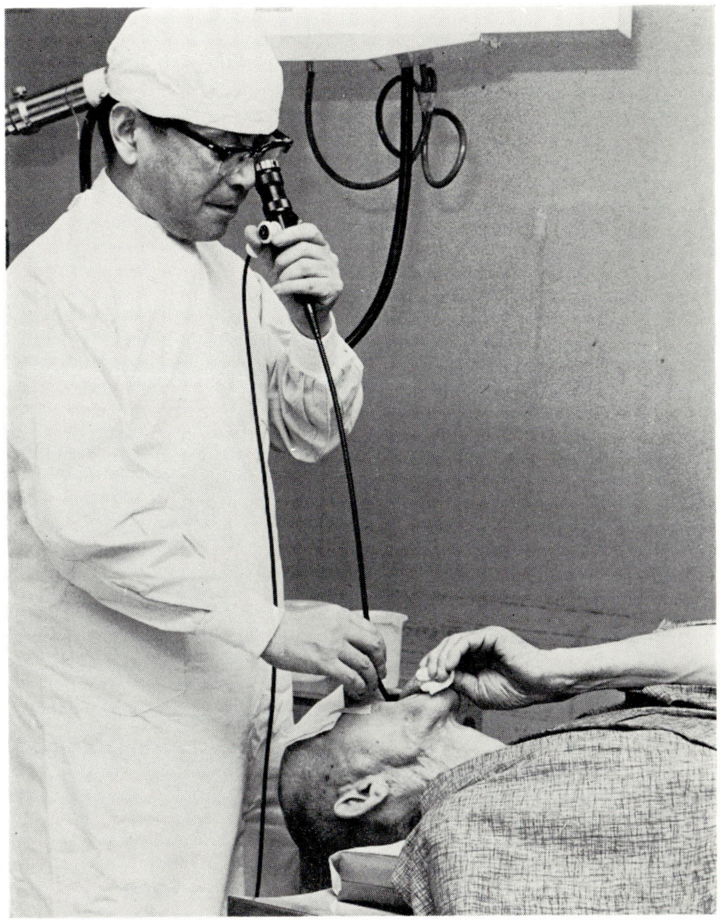

**Fig. 80** When the tip is inserted farther into the larynx, the anterior wall of the trachea comes in view ahead of the vocal chords. If the advancement is continued without any adjustment the tip hits the anterior wall of the trachea; so therefore, a slight angulation is given to direct the tip downward. Thus it is inserted into the trachea in a straight line.

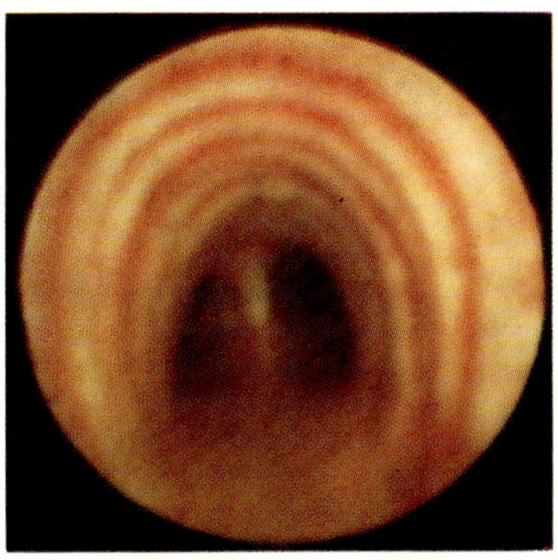

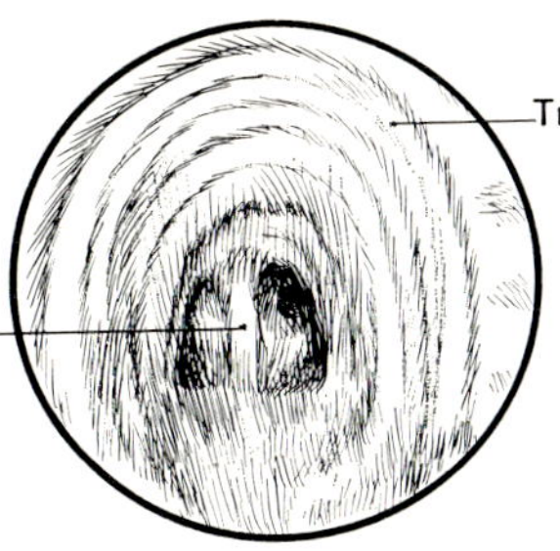


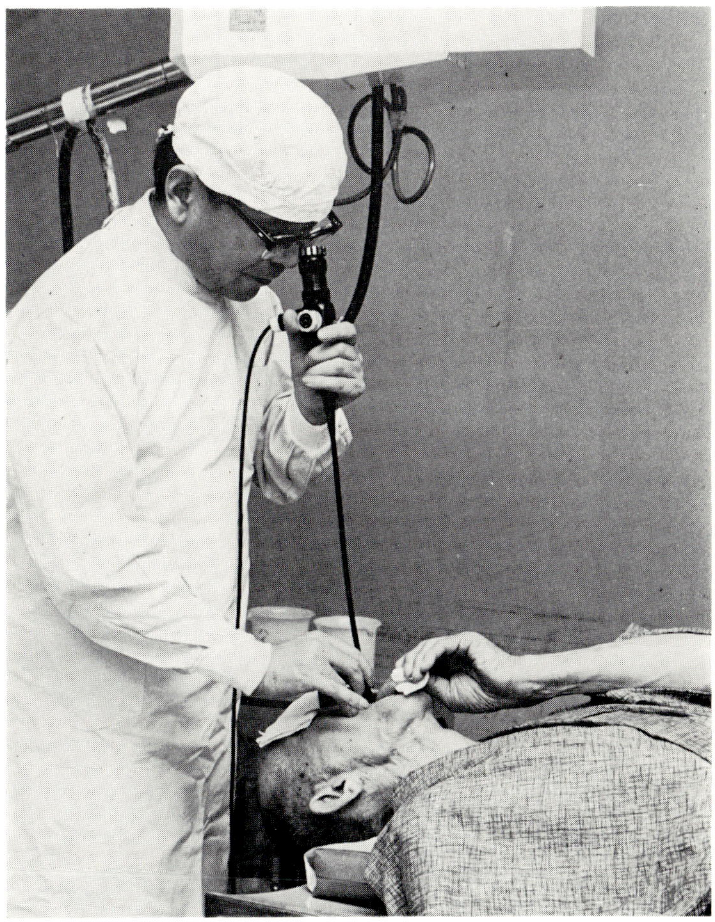

**Fig. 81** The fiberscope is advanced down the trachea. The tracheal bifurcation is seen far ahead of the tracheal rings.

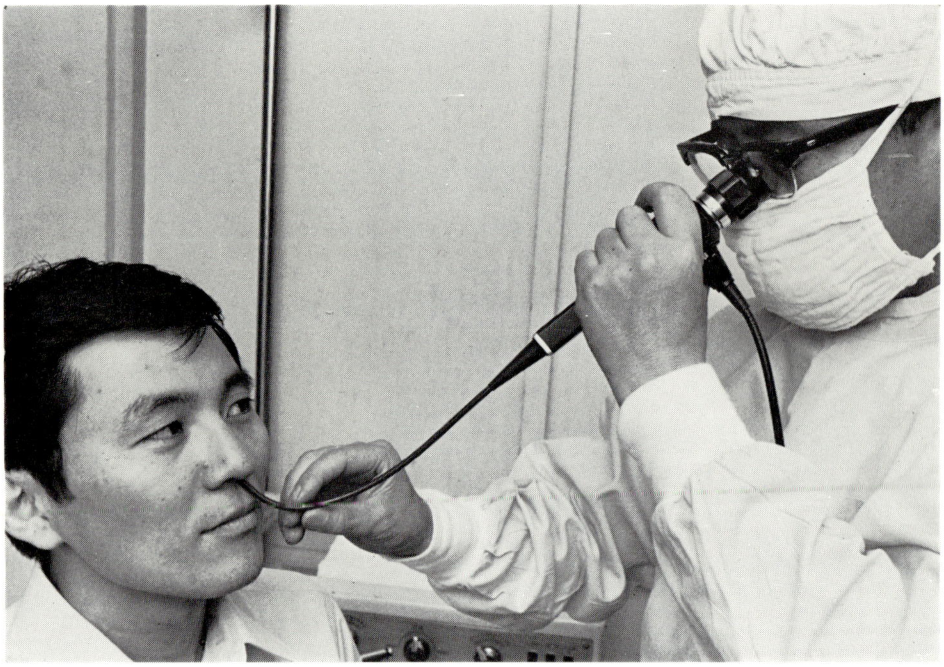

**Fig. 82** Transnasal bronchofiberscopy. Handy bronchofiberscopy at the sitting position.

4. Transnasal technique initiated by SMIDDY, SACKNER and others in the United States is to insert the bronchofiberscope directly through either of the nares without the auxiliary intratracheal tube. The nasal mucosa is anesthetized by injection and/or spraying, then the bronchofiberscope is introduced through the naris, larynx, glottis and trachea under direct vision (Fig. 82).

Another modification, also initiated by SMIDDY, is to introduce a catheter into the nasal cavity down to the region of the larynx, through which the bronchofiberscope is then introduced. The advantages of this method are: 1) Facility in inserting the bronchofiberscope into the trachea because of the direct passage from the posterior naso-pharynx into the trachea; 2) Feasibility of conducting the examination with the patient in the sitting position, and 3) Expediency in handling the instrument. The disadvantages are: 1) Unsuited for most Asian people whose nares are not as large as those of Americans or Europeans; 2) Contamination of the instrument when introduced through the nasal cavity without a protective sleeve; 3) Potential damage to the nasal septum with possibility of subsequent bleeding; 4) Inadequate air way might become a cause of bronchospasm; 5) Difficult in cleansing the lens at the tip when necessary; 6) Cumbersome and unwieldy when a different sized bronchofiberscope is indicated, and 7) Difficulty controlling hemorrhage should it arise.

Under the circumstances, transnasal bronchofiberscopy may be adequate for gross examination of the major bronchi but not for minute diagnostic or therapeutic bronchofiberscopy.

**b. Insertion of the bronchofiberscope**

Prior to introduction of the bronchofiberscope into the tracheal tube, the following preliminary procedures are performed:

1. The small lens at the distal end of the bronchofiberscope is wiped with silicone or soapy water to prevent fogging.

2. To reduce friction between the bronchofiberscope and the tracheal tube, a lubricant such as olive oil or Xylocaine Jelly® applied on the outer surface of the instrument. When the contacting surfaces of the bronchofiberscope and the tracheal tube are of different materials, considerable friction may be encountered. This may be overcome by a more liberal application of lubricant.

3. The panning angle of the bronchofiberscope should be adjusted to neutral position before insertion into the tracheal tube. This is to assure that the instrument will be in the correct visual plane.

4. When the intubation is finished, on introducing the bronchofiberscope, 1–2 ml of 4 % lidocaine is usually injected through the channel of the instrument. Sputum in the trachea and bronchi is aspirated as necessary.

When the tip of the fiberscope is advanced into a narrow bronchus and sputum is observed, it should be aspirated very gently and carefully in order to avoid bronchial spasm or bleeding from the mucosa. The bronchoscope may be removed at will for cleaning the tip or clearing the channel. The latter is especially important prior to instilling anesthetic solutions, as otherwise the secretions will be reintroduced into the bronchial tree.

### c. Caution for insertion training

There are two essentials in achieving the most effective bronchofiberscopy in the shortest possible time for the patient. One is the thorough proficiency and skill in handling the flexible bronchofiberscopy ; the other is the perfect knowledge of the anatomy of the bronchus and bronchial tree.

A bronchial tree made of ordinary hard glass is available for training the bronchofiberscopist to attain the above objectives. The glass model (see Fig. 101) is ideal in many ways, but it is not soft nor flexible as the human bronchial tree and the tip of the bronochofiberscope is sensitive and delicate. The trainee should never force the tip of the fiberscope into the deeper parts of the bronchus, attempting to see more clearly by forcible twisting the proximal part of the instrument, when the tip has been fixed in the bronchus. This can not be overemphasized in any case.

### d. Holding the flexible bronchofiberscope

The technique of holding a flexible bronchofiberscope differs depending on the type, whether it is Machida or Olympus type.

*a) Machida type.* The proximal eyepiece part of Machida bronchofiberscope is usually held in the left hand (Fig. 83), reserving the right hand for minor yet delicate manipulations such as maneuvering the various handles at the proximal end, including insertion of the scope into the tracheal tube by supporting both the end of the tube and the fiberscope (Fig. 84).

If the proximal eyepiece of the fiberscope is rotated clockwise, the distal tip of the scope is twisted to the right and orientated in that direction. This is called the coordination of a flexible bronchofiberscope (Fig. 85). When a bronchus in the right lung is the target, the proximal basal part of the fiberscope is slowly and gently rotated to the right. If the target bronchus is on the left, it is gently turned counterclockwise, and advanced into it.

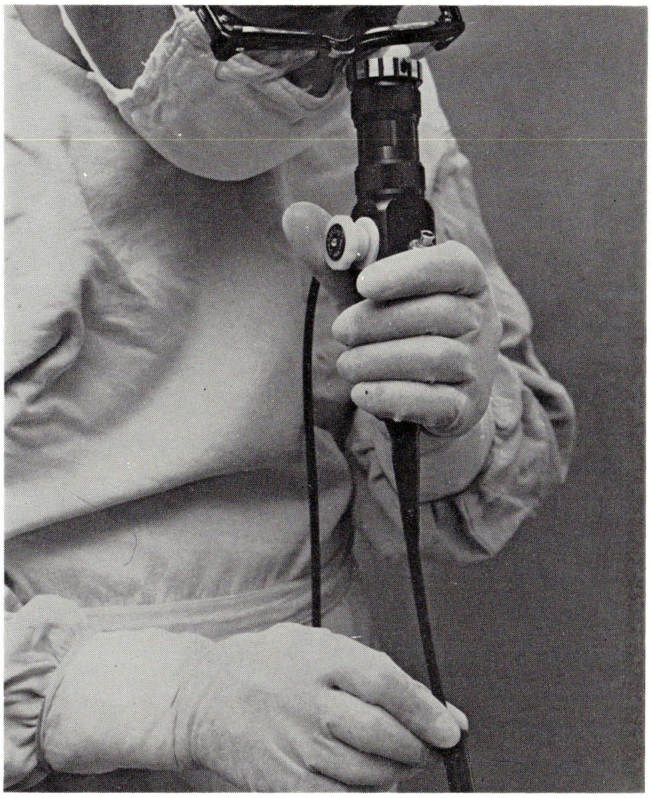

**Fig. 83** How to hold a Machida bronchofiberscope correctly.

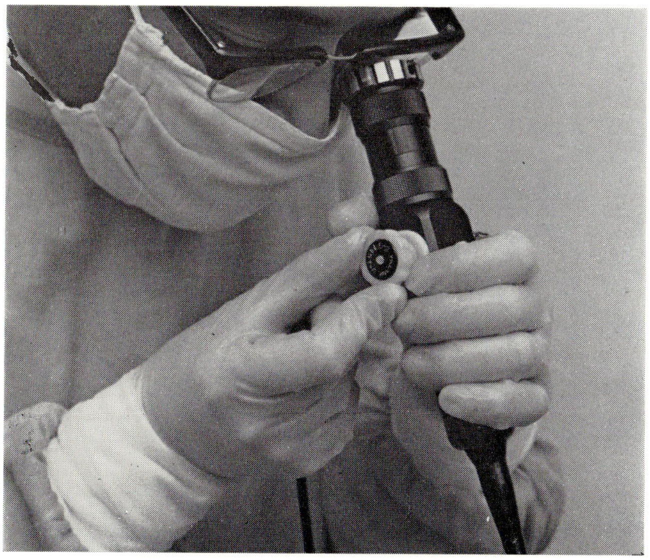

**Fig. 84** Right hand is used if a large angulation is required.

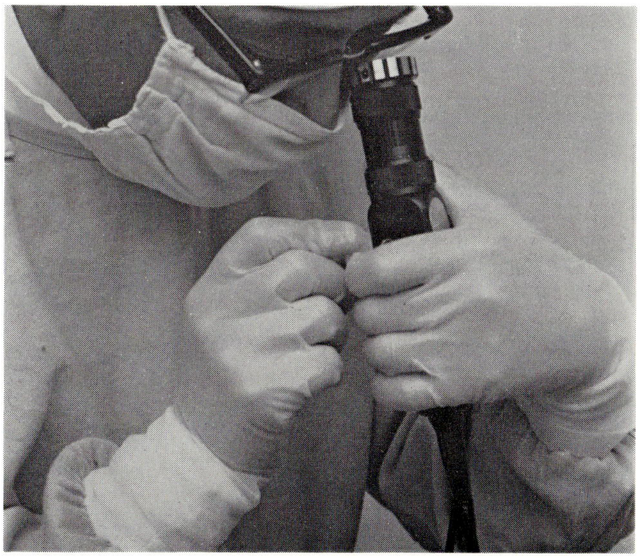

**Fig. 85** In directing the distal tip to the large target bronchus, the coordinating function between the proximal and distal parts should be utilized by twisting the proximal grip of the scope. If the target is the small bronchus with the tip already in it, the twisting must be avoided.

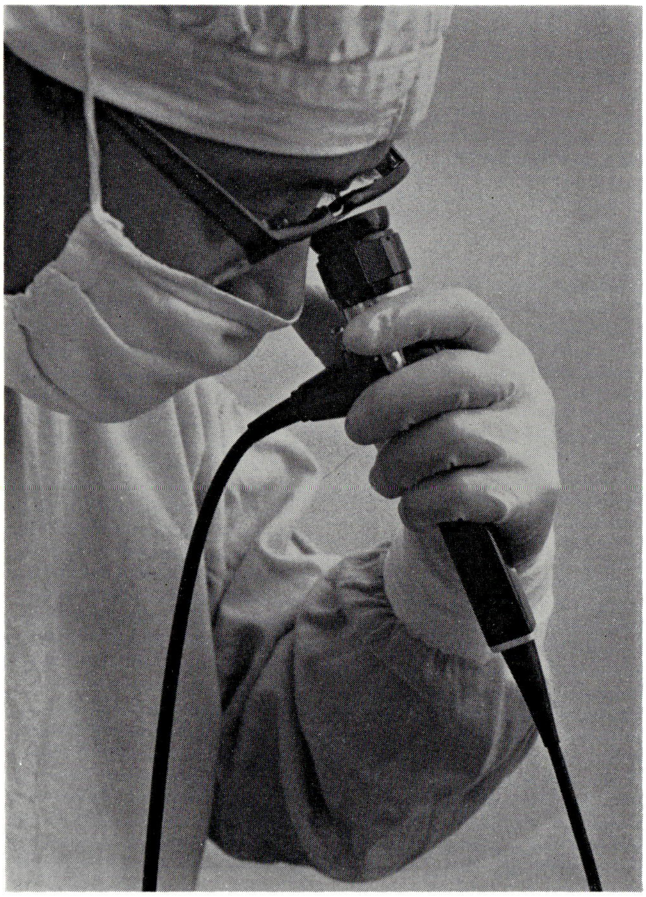

**Fig. 86** How to hold an Olympus bronchofiberscope. For the fiberscope to be inserted into the right bronchus, it is to be held by the left hand.

*b) Olympus type.* One of the distinctive features of Olympus type of bronchofiberscope lies in the advantage that both the proximal eyepiece of the fiberscope and the angle lever, which controls the angulation of the tip, can be held and controlled by one hand; either the right hand or the left (Figs. 86–88). Because of the flexibility of the body of the bronchofiberscope, the free hand may be engaged in guiding it into the tracheal tube. As the tip cannot be rotated independently, this is accomplished by rotating the entire fiberscope.

### e. Insertion of the flexible bronchofiberscope into a lobar bronchus, a segmental bronchus and a subsegmental bronchus

In advancing a bronchofiberscope its relative position in a bronchus must be correct. That is, the entire circumference of the bronchus of any size through which the fiberscope is advancing should be seen straight ahead. If not, the tip may impinge on the bronchial wall or abrade the bifurcation of a bronchus, causing cough or bleeding.

*a) Insertion into major bronchi : the trachea, main bronchus and lobar bronchus.* If the fiberscope is to be inserted into a relatively large bronchus, the eyepiece is rotated so as to orientate the tip correctly to that bronchus. If for instance, the target is the right main bronchus, the eyepiece is rotated clockwise and at the

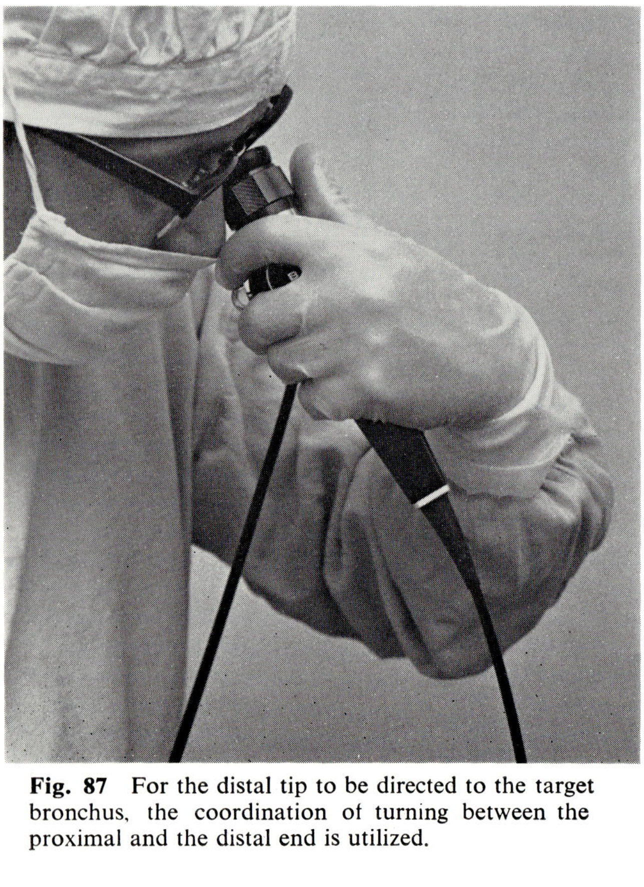

**Fig. 87** For the distal tip to be directed to the target bronchus, the coordination of turning between the proximal and the distal end is utilized.

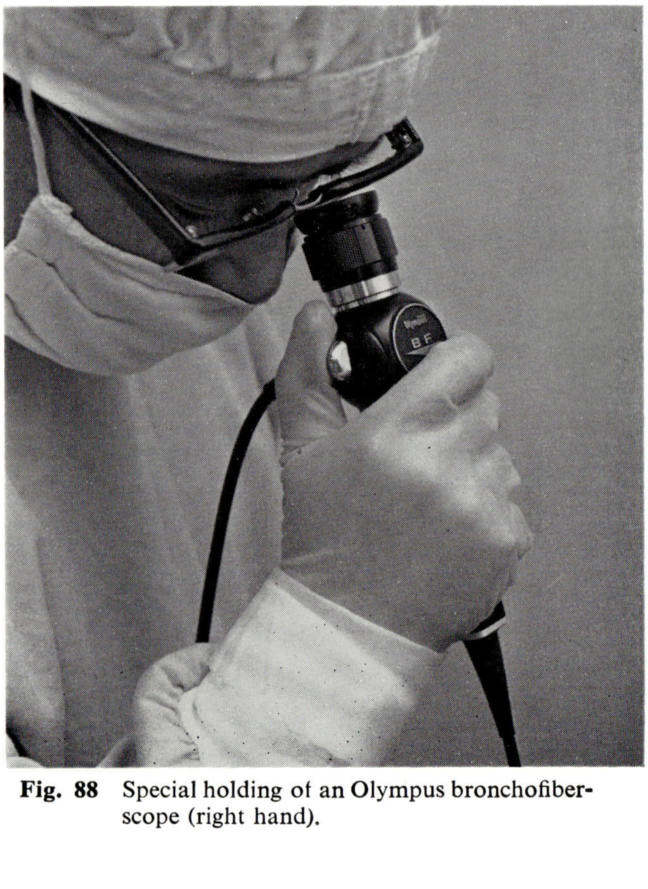

**Fig. 88** Special holding of an Olympus bronchofiberscope (right hand).

same time, the handle is maneuvered to bend the tip slightly to the proper angle so that the inside of that bronchus is visible in its entirety In order for the tip to enter the right upper lobe bronchus, the tip is angulated more and advanced gently. This general principle may be applied to any type of a flexible bronchofiberscope. If Machida type is selected for use, the proximal part itself is rotated to maneuver it into a major bronchus. The use of the rotation ring should be reserved for insertion into a narrower, smaller order bronchus branching from a segmental bronchus. This rotation ring is one of the main advantages of Machida type.

If Olympus type is used, it is advanced into the target bronchus, either main bronchus or narrower one, by rotation of the proximal part. Olympus type has no rotation ring. Lack of this ring is supplemented by flexible coordination of the tip.

*b) Insertion into $B^6$ (the superior segmental bronchi of the lower lobes).* The tip of a bronchofiberscope can be bent 150 to 180 degrees upward and 10 degrees downward. When the target is $B^6$, either right or left, the eyepiece of the fiberscope must be rotated 180 degrees immediately in front of the bronchial entrance (Figs. 89–91).

When the orifice of $B^6$ becomes visible directly ahead, the tip is slowly advanced and inserted into $B^6$ by rotating the angulation handle.

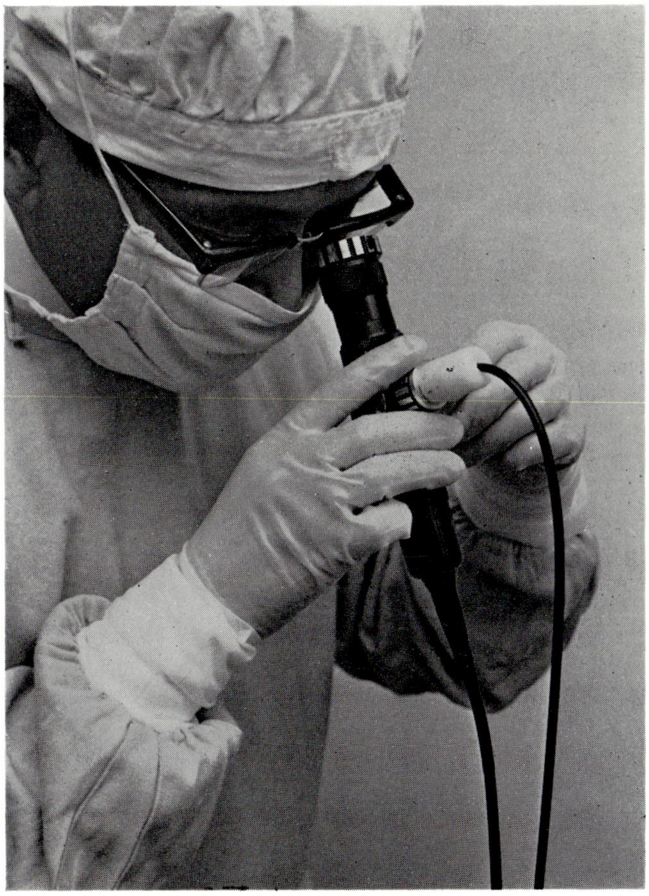

**Fig. 89** Holding of Machida bronchofiberscope in inserting into the superior bronchus of the lower lobe ($B^6$).

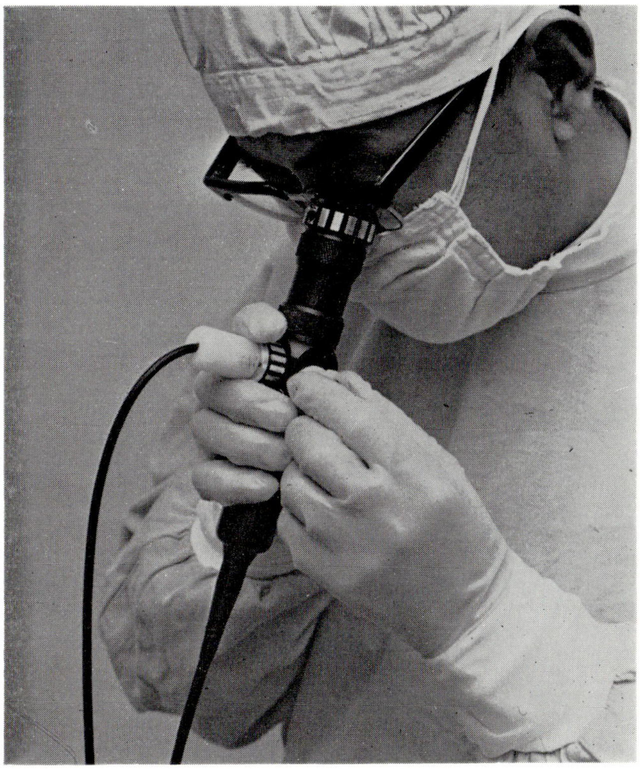

**Fig. 90** Same as Fig. 89.

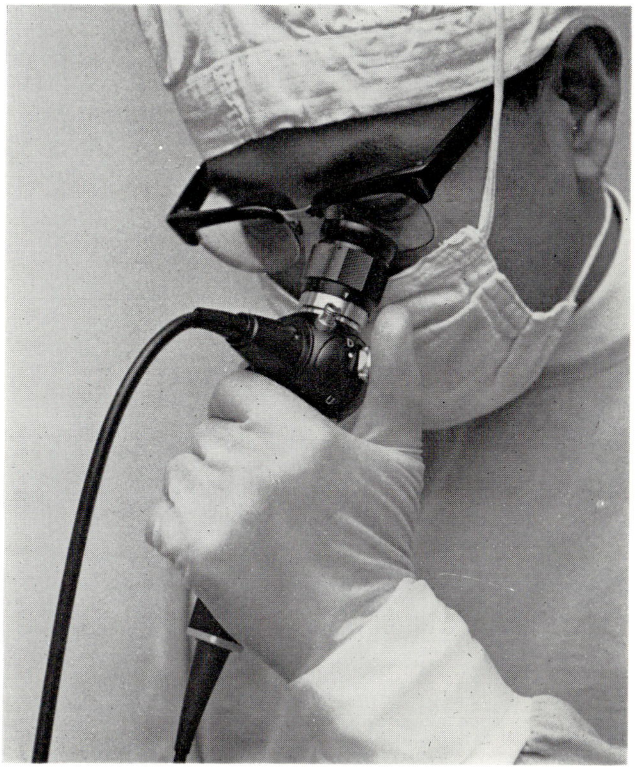

**Fig. 91** How to hold an Olympus bronchofiberscope correctly, in order to insert it into the left bronchus.

*c) Insertion into other bronchi.* The technique of inserting the fiberscope into a middle or lower lobe bronchus is the same as that described for the upper lobe.

*d) Insertion into the segmental or subsegmental bronchus from the lobar bronchus.* After the tip has been inserted into the lobar bronchus, it is advanced to a segmental bronchus. In an ordinary male adult a 5 mm bronchofiberscope may reach the segmental bronchi, and a 4 mm bronchofiberscope is capable of entering IV order of branching from a subsegmental bronchus. The technique of inserting the instrument into a segmental bronchus also depends on the type of the bronchoscope used. Of course, the coordinating function of the tip can be utilized in such cases, but, if forcibly utilized, there is a danger of damaging the tip when it has already been inserted into a narrower bronchus. If Machida scope is used, the rotation ring at the proximal part should be utilized at this stage.

Lack of the rotation ring in Olympus type, when this is employed, makes it necessary to advance the tip by twisting the eyepiece and making full use of the coordination of the tip.

The tip of a 5 mm fiberscope may hardly be inserted into a subsegmental bronchus of a normal adult male, but the entrance may be reached with it.

Occasionally, abnormal location of a bronchus will not permit the instrument to be introduced even into a segmental bronchus. One of the alternatives in such a case is to advance the fiberscope by taking advantage of the respiratory movements of the bronchus. Caution must be taken, however, of never forcing the tip into the target bronchus, as this may damage the fiberscope. The following will clarify this situation.

When the instrument is inserted into a peripheral bronchus, the bronchus distal to this is magnified more than the actual size, since the field of vision of the bronchofiberscope is 65–80 degrees. Accordingly, an examiner might get the impression that there is enough space for the tip to be advanced further. In trying to push the instrument forwards, the tip seems to be drawn out backwards, and the adjacent part remains in sigmoid-like shape in the bronchus (Fig. 92). In such a case, the forcible insertion must not be continued, as the angling part of instrument may be broken.

As has been mentioned above, sputum, if any, in the bronchus must be removed. However, if it is in a nar-

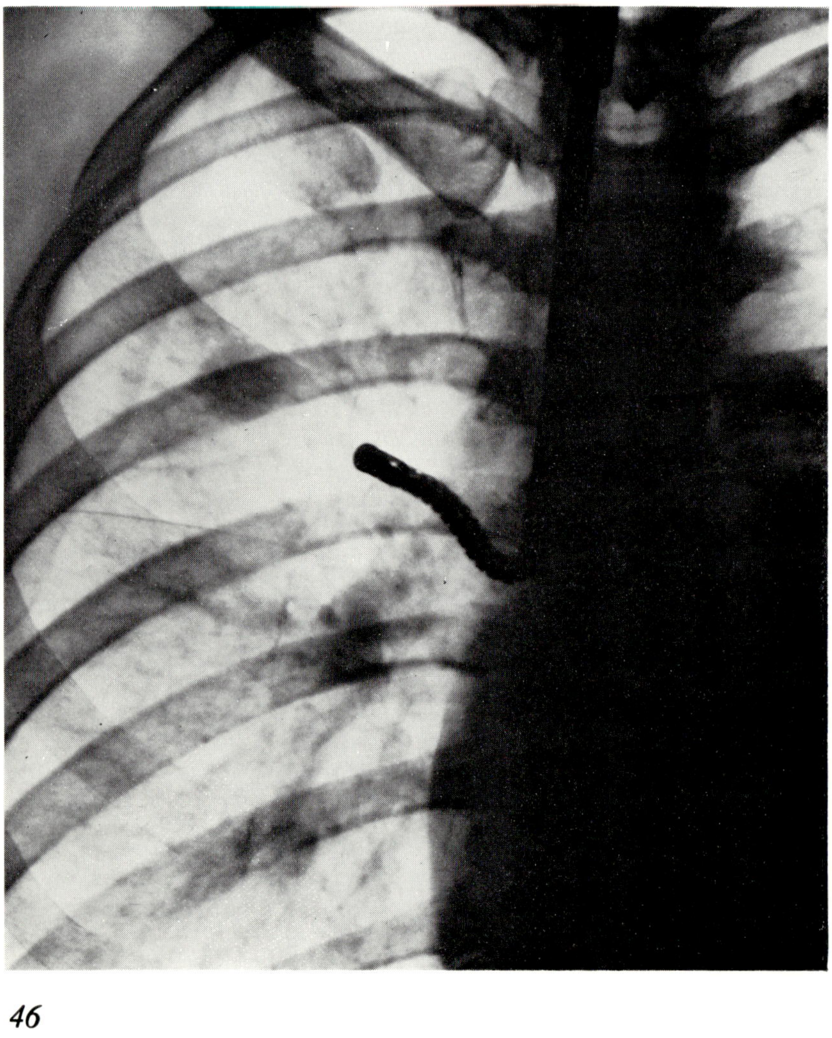

**Fig. 92** X-ray picture showing the tip of Machida bronchofiberscope in a sigmoid-like shape.

row bronchus, spasm is liable to occur. In order to prevent this, it is recommended that the suction tube be applied gently and lightly to the channel mouth for aspiration (Figs. 93 and 94). The suction channel in a 5 mm bronchofiberscope functions better because its inner diameter is 1.4 mm, while that for a 4 mm fiberscope is capable of aspirating only watery sputum because its inner diameter is only 0.8 mm. Another shortcoming of the latter is that sputum stuck to the lens at the tip causes the field of vision to be blurred since the suction power is weaker. When this happens, the fiberscope should be removed from the tracheal tube for cleansing the tip.

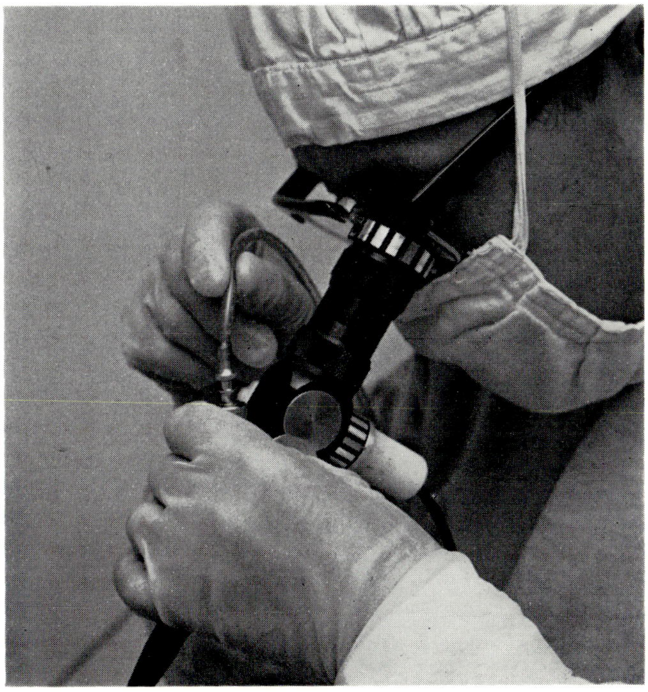

**Fig. 93** Suction of the sputum by a bronchofiberscope, Machida make.

### f. Cytology and biopsy

*a) Technique of inserting accessory instruments.* Cytology and biopsy are essential for bronchoscopy. A brush or a curette fo cytologic purpose can be inserted into the small channel used for aspiration of sputum or injection of anesthetics. A small curette, a small biopsy forceps or a very small brush can be inserted through the channel at the proximal part of the fiberscope. This is possible in the 5 mm or larger fiberscope, but not in the 4 mm. Whenever one of these implements is inserted into the channel, the fiberscope should be removed from the tracheal tube. The reason is that if either a curette or a biopsy forceps is inserted into a bronchofiberscope while its tip is bent in a bronchus, it may damage the fiber bundles at the tip. Also, if the insertion is done immediately after the sputum is aspirated, the backed-up secretions may fog the lens at the tip.

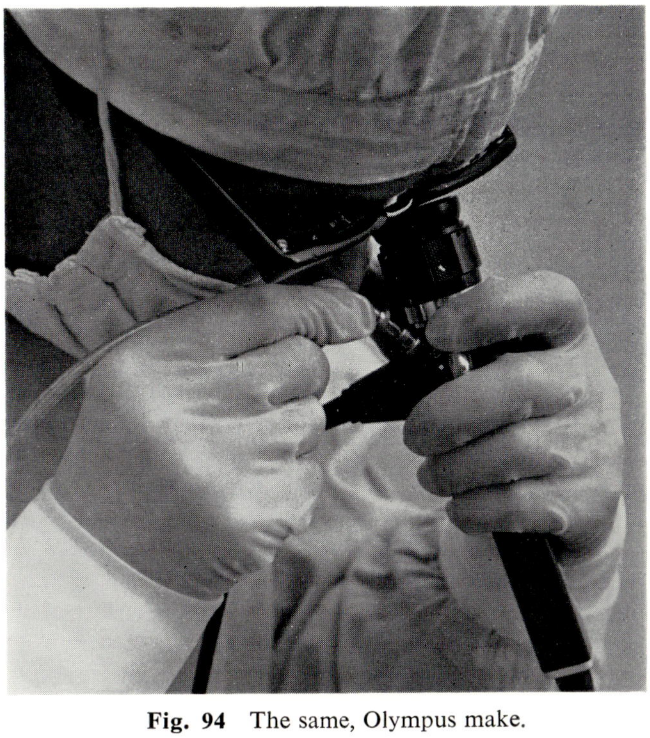

**Fig. 94** The same, Olympus make.

In inserting a biopsy forceps or a curette, it occasionally may not pass smoothly, as if it were caught in the fiberscope To overcome this difficulty, insertion should be made by rotating it. When the head of a forceps or a curette has emerged from the tip after insertion, the extruding part should be kept at 3 mm (Fig. 95) When a larger brush is utilized it is inserted through the channel from the tip of the fiberscope in a retrograde fashion.

In performing cytologic or histologic examination, first the physician must recall the endoscopic anatomy of the target bronchus so that he may be able to reach that bronchus without error. This forms an essential part of his preparation The second is to remove any sputum in the pathway completely and to anesthetize the part sufficiently in order to inhibit cough. Coughing is often induced when the brush head carries along sputum or touches and irritates the bronchial wall.

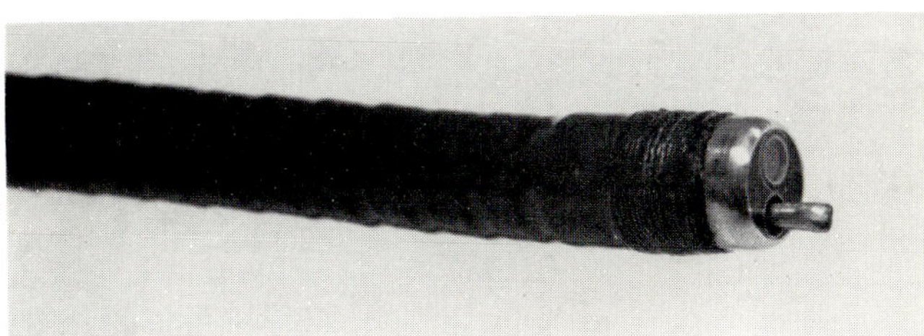

**Fig. 95** The distal tip with a sampling instrument protruding from the end.

*b) Indications and choice of instruments.* If a tumor is located in the trachea or major bronchus, such as the main bronchus, truncus intermedius or lobar bronchus, biopsy forceps should be used. This is easily accomplished under direct visualization.

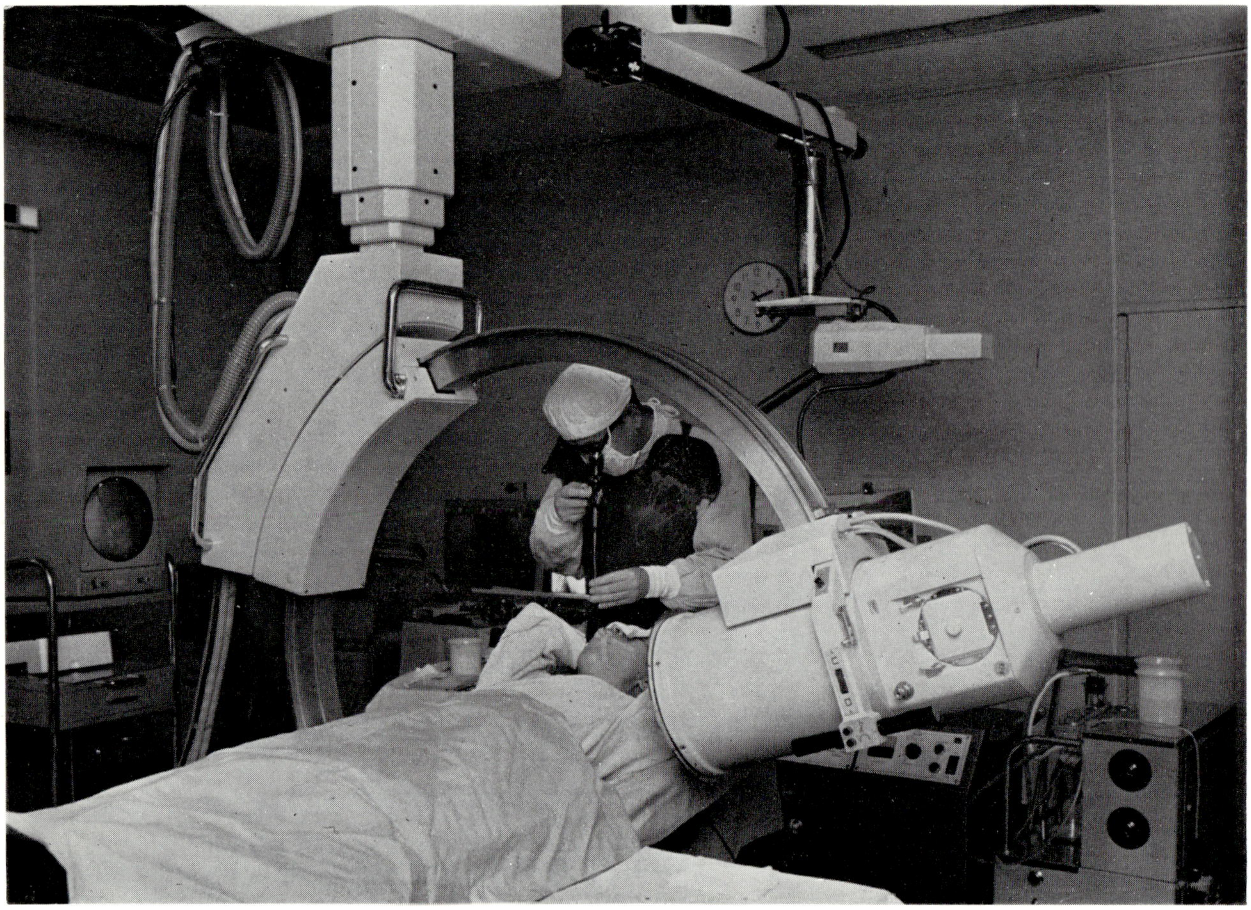

**Fig. 96** Bronchofiberscopy with the assistance of X-ray TV designed exclusively for bronchoscopic examination.

The tumor in a segmental or a more peripherally located bronchus, if visible, is better biopsied for cytology with a small curette. It is in such a tumor located in an obstructed bronchus that a small curette displays its great utility. The small head can pass through the obstruction. It can be advanced under direct vision into a bronchus which does not permit a 4 mm bronchofiberscope to pass. The curette head can be bent about 40 degrees by maneuvering the handle of the instrument. Under fluoroscopy (Fig. 96) the curette can be advanced to an extremely peripherally located lesion.

The instrument should be held in the manner shown in Fig. 97 for it to be bent smoothly and avoid sharp angulation which may damage the glass fibers. Obtaining biopsy specimens is greatly facilitated by having an assistant hold the proximal part so that the operator can work with both hands. The biopsy instrument should not be held with the operator's finger or thumb in the ring of the instrument, as this may cause the tip of the instrument to be angulated too sharply

A brush is rarely used. This is due to the fact that a brush is liable to catch and carry along sputum or unnecessarily stimulate the bronchial wall. However, it is used to abrade the bronchial wall and obtain a specimen when the tumor is not visible, when there is redness or edema in the bronchus, or when some irregularity prevents the usual biopsy forceps or small curette from obtaining the desired tissue.

*c) Smearing and fixing.* When the desired material has been collected, the biopsy instrument is taken out of the patient's tracheobronchial tree together with the fiberscope as soon as possible. After the instruments are withdrawn, the collected material is immediately smeared on a glass slide without removing the biopsy instrument from the fiberscope (Fig 98) The material at the tip of a curette should be removed with a needle.

After smearing the material on a slide, it is quickly dipped into a fixative of 95% alcohol. Speed is essential. The reason is that cells collected with a curette are so small in number that they dry quickly, and, when dried, they are hardly usable for cytological diagnosis.

The specimen obtained with a small biopsy forceps may either be smeared on a glass slide or fixed, if the specimen is fairly large, in the 10 % formalin solution.

*d) Bleeding after curettage or biopsy.* Curettage or biopsy of a tumor often causes bleeding. If the bleeding is mild, the blood is aspirated in order to prevent coughing. In many cases bleeding from the lesions of cancer can be controlled if the bronchial tree is not stimulated However, on some occasions, excessive bleeding results in outpouring of blood into the trachea. In such cases, the patient is instructed to lie recumbent with the operated side down to prevent aspiration of blood into the contralateral side, and the physician suctions out the overflowing blood from the trachea. The other alternative is to control bleeding by tamponading with a small cotton ball fastened with a piece of thread at the tip of a brush under direct vision of the fiberscope

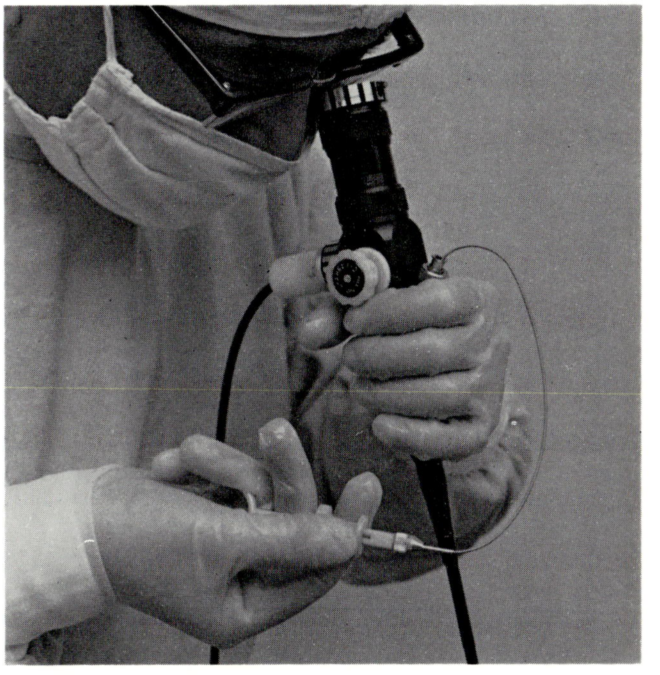

**Fig. 97** Manipulation of a sampling instrument.

### g. Summary on the usage of a flexible bronchofiberscope

1) Prepare all the necessary apparatus and implements and be sure that they function satisfactorily.
2) Remember that a flexible bronchofiberscope is an extremely delicate and precise apparatus. Be cautious in handling it, avoiding any roughness.
3) Skill in inserting the fiberscope can be gained step by step Do not try to introduce the scope with any force in any case.
4) Do not leave the bronchofiberscope within a bronchus more than 10 minutes at the longest. If necessary, remove the scope from the tracheal tube to give ample airway to the patient. This is essential
5) Fix the material obtained for cytology as quickly as possible.
6) Caution is requested in handling the apparatus for cytological diagnosis in bronchofiberscopy.

In biopsy repeated sampling is frequently necessary. Efforts to obtain satisfactory sampling result in greater percentage of definitive diagnoses.

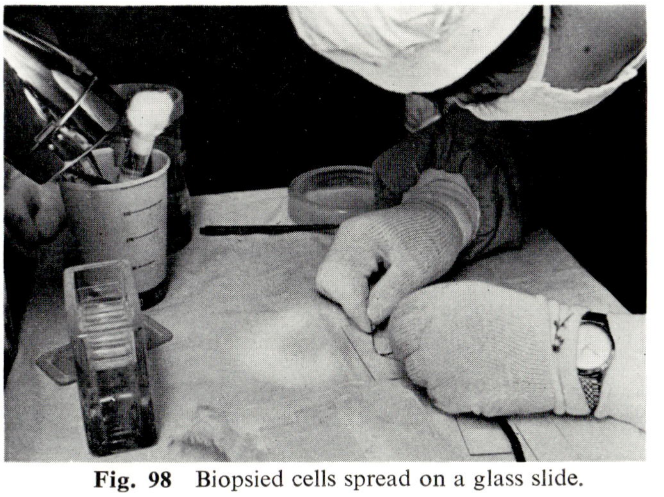

**Fig. 98** Biopsied cells spread on a glass slide.

## CLEANING OF THE INSTRUMENT

Careful cleaning of the instrument after each use to maintain the life of the bronchofiberscope :

### a. The body of a bronchofiberscope

The main body is cleaned and wiped with gauze soaked in 70 % alcohol. The proximal part of the instrument may also be wiped with a moist gauze, but excessive amount of alcohol must be avoided as the sterilizing solution might invade the instrument through the narrow spaces or apertures. Do not dip the whole body and the proximal part of the instrument into the sterilizing solution.

### b. The channel for insufflation and suction

Sputum clogged in the suction channel is cleaned and washed by irrigating the channel with water. A good method is to connect the mouth of the channel to a suction source and immerse the tip in water Then a cleaning brush or a cytologic brush is passed through the channel, followed by irrigation with water. The inside of the channel is sterilized by aspirating 1 % Hyamin T® or Betadine® so solution followed by sterile water. Lastly, the channel is completely dried by compressed air blown through it.

**c. The channel of 4 mm flexible fiberscope**

The channel of the 4 mm fiberscope is often clogged with sputum since the diameter of the channel is narrower than the larger scope. The best method of removing the sputum is to irrigate with water using a 10 ml syringe fitted into the entrance of the suction channel at the proximal part.

**d. Tracheal tube**

The same cleaning method as in the suction channel of a bronchofiberscope may be applied to this instrument. Special care must be taken to remove sputum or other secretions which may be sticking to the inside of the tube.

**e. Brush, curette and biopsy forceps**

These small instruments are cleaned with a soft tooth brush in running water. Since they are made of thin metal, brushing should be done lightly and gently.

## STORAGE AND STERILIZATION OF BRONCHOFIBERSCOPE

1. Prior to storing a flexible bronchofiberscope, its tip, main body and proximal part must be completely dried.
2. After drying, the bronchoscope is best stored in a hanging position with the tip down. This prevents the main body or the tip from bending in an unnatural way.

Ideally, as has been described above, the best method of sterilizing a bronchofiberscope is by means of ethylene oxide gas. However, if the temperature is over 40°C and the inside pressure over 1.5 kg/cm$^2$ (as is the case when sterilizing other surgical instruments), the tip may be damaged. Accordingly, an ethylene oxide gas sterilizer specifically for bronchofiberscopes was designed (Fig. 99), which accomplished perfect sterilization in about 4 hours keeping the temperature under 40°C and inside atmospheric pressure under 1.5 kg/cm$^2$. If these two conditions are satisfied, the ordinary ethylene oxide gas sterilizer can be utilized in hospitals which do not have the special sterilizer.

The disadvantages of gas sterilization are the time required (4 hrs.) and the several days the instrument must be shelved to allow the ethylen oxide gas to dissipate. This is extremely inconvenient for the doctor who must daily perform several bronchoscopies. Therefore, 70 % alcohol, 1 % benzethonium chloride (Hyamin T®) or Betadine® can usually be substituted as has been described before (p. 49).

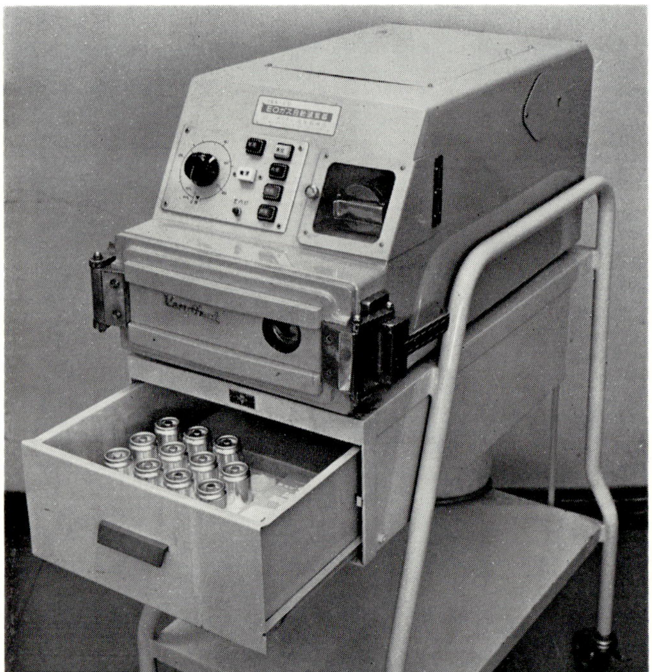

99

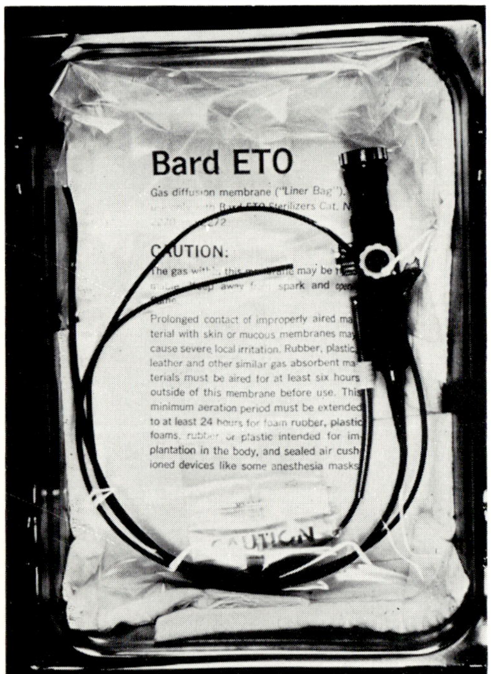


100

**Fig. 99** Automatic sterilizer for exclusive use of the endoscope, utilizing ethylene oxide gas.

**Fig. 100** Handy sterilizer by ethylene oxide gas. The fiberscopes are sterilized in 24 hours when left to stand overnight (by the courtesy of B. Marsh, M. D., Johns Hopkins University, U.S.A.).

# BRONCHOFIBERSCOPIC TRAINING

For bronchofiberscopy to be performed efficiently, training is indispensable until the bronchofiberscope literally becomes an extension of the operator's hand.

For training purposes, a bronchial tree made of hard glass has been manufactured. This glass model, Fig.101, is life-sized and is complete from the trachea down to the subsegmental bronchi. The inside diameters approximate that of an adult male, and the branching is representative of the average man or woman.

Of course, the model differs from living human in moisture, flexibility and texture ; so, in using the model, the following factors should be considered :

1) A moderate amount of olive oil should be applied to the inside surface of each bronchus of the model before use.

2) The same oil must be applied to the tip of the bronchofiberscope to minimize friction.

3) Unncessary force should never be used in advancing the tip into a more distal bronchus. As often happens, forcible twisting of the proximal part will damage the tip of the instrument.

4) A 5 mm fiberscope can be inserted readily into a segmental bronchus directed toward the entrance of the subsegmental bronchus. When further insertion is required, the instrument must be replaced by the 4 mm model.

5) Since the glass model is hand-made, unavoidable minor differences in the caliber of the smaller bronchi may occur. For example, a segmental bronchus in the model may not admit the tips of a fiberscope, whereas the corresponding bronchus of a living human may readily admit the same instrument.

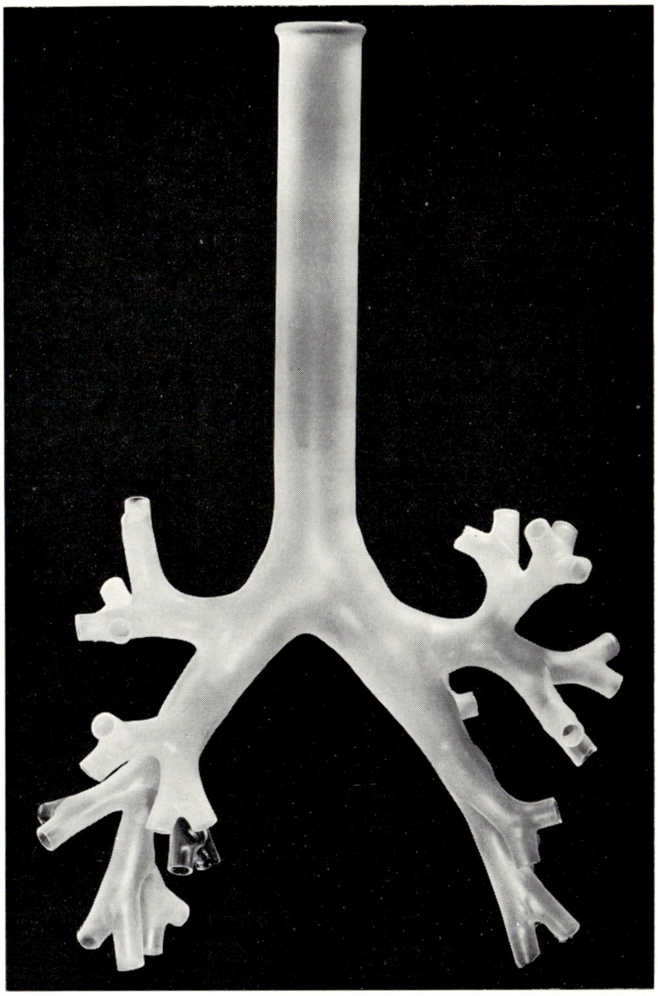

**Fig. 101** Glass bronchial tree for bronchofiberscopic training.

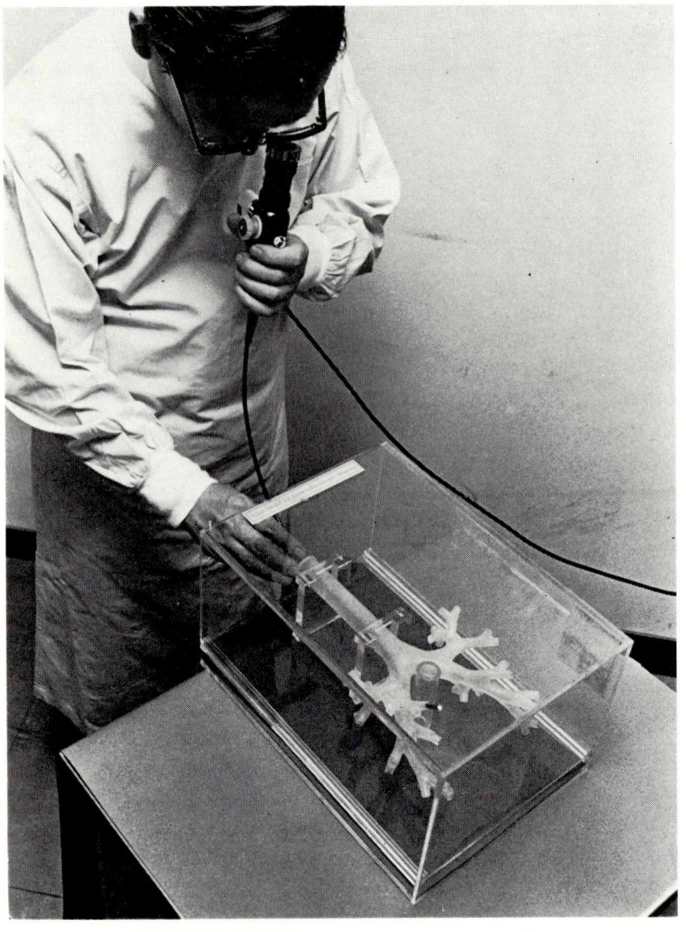

**Fig. 102** Initial training should start with the bare glass model. This makes it easy for the trainee bronchofiberscopist to maneuver the tip of the fiberscope under direct vision.

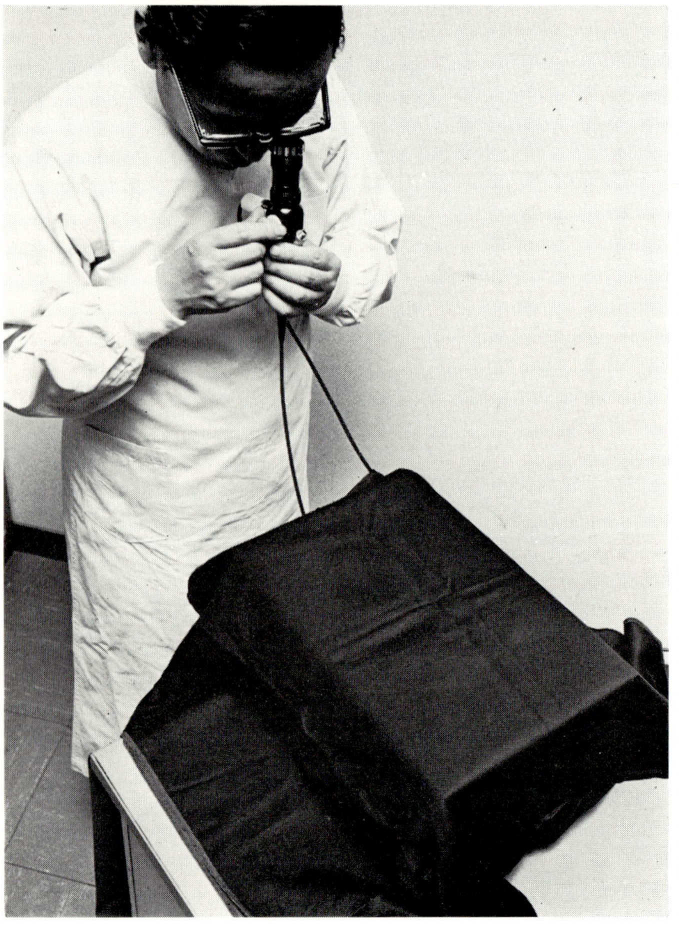

**Fig. 103** Later training, after he has achieved satisfactory skill in insertion, should be done with the model covered with an opaque, sheet of black cloth. In this step, the fiberscope is connected with the light source, as in the practical use of the scope. The trainee should concentrate his mind on the orientation.

# V. Recording of Bronchoscopic Pictures

In reporting bronchoscopic findings, it is essential that the records be as objective, accurate and detailed as possible, excluding any subjective judgement of a physician. Records in the form of drawings or writing alone are not satisfactory for later reference, since they lack accuracy and objectivity. The flexible bronchofiberscope of today can visualize peripheral bronchi beyond III order of branching which may not have characteristic bifurcations. This also demands objectivity in the recorded findings.

Previously, it was difficult to deliver sufficient light into a bronchus due to the slenderness of a bronchofiberscope. But with improvements in the field of light source, it is now possible to obtain permanent, objective records. There are three methods for recording: photography, cinematography and television.

## PHOTOGRAPHY

**a. Camera** (Figs. 104 and 105)

Olympus Pen F camera is the one most commonly used at the present time. This is a single lens reflex camera using 35 mm film for half-size pictures. It may be used with either Machida or Olympus bronchofiberscope, using their respective adaptors which are different.

**b. Time of exposure**

Time of exposure depends on the brightness of the light source and the size of the fiberscope. It is also variable in accordance with the focal length of the lens used in the case of Machida bronchofiberscope. Furthermore, the condition of the object to be photographed also is a factor in determining the time of ex-

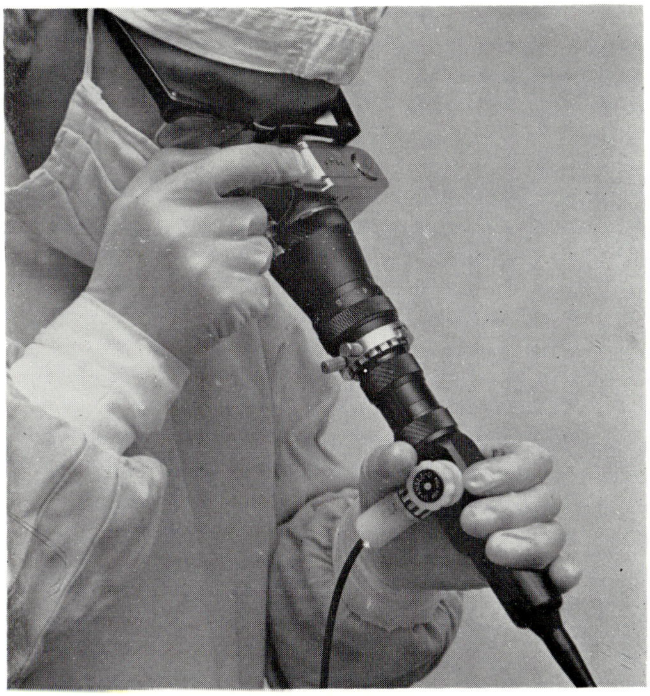

**Fig. 104** Endoscopic photography employing a bronchofiberscope of Machida make.

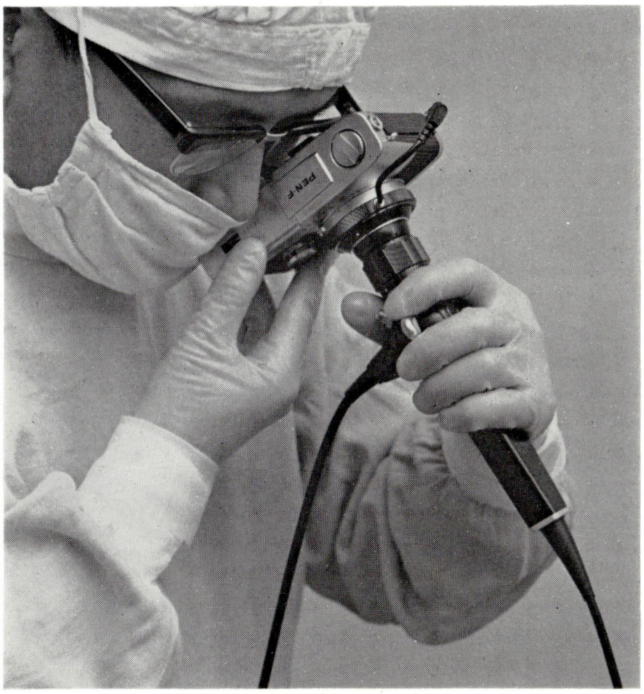

**Fig. 105** Endoscopic photography using a bronchofiberscope of Olympus make.

posure: in taking a picture of a bronchial bifurcation, for instance, the exposure time is twice as long as in the segmental bronchus.

The size of the picture to be obtained on a film also determines the time of exposure. When Olympus 5mm flexible bronchofiberscope is employed, the picture obtained is 5 mm in diameter; while, when Machida type is used with a 51.6 mm lens, the picture produced on a film is 6 mm in diameter. The exposure time in these instances are essentially the same. If a 75 mm lens is used with a Machida bronchoscope, the picture is enlarged to 9 mm. That is, in the latter case the exposure time must be twice as much as in with the 51.6 mm lens. This is partly due to the magnified image and also because of a longer-focus lens.

The following are the data obtained under the condition of maximum brightness with a Xenon lamp as light source. They may be applied to either the Machida or Olympus bronchofiberscopes.

*a) Bronchial bifurcation*:

Machida 5 mm bronchofiberscope (75 mm lens)
1/8 second,
Machida 5 mm bronchofiberscope (51.6 mm lens)
1/5 second,
Olympus 5 mm bronchofiberscope (no lens)
1/15 second.

*b) Entrance of the segmental bronchus*:

Half of exposure time of each item in (a) is enough.

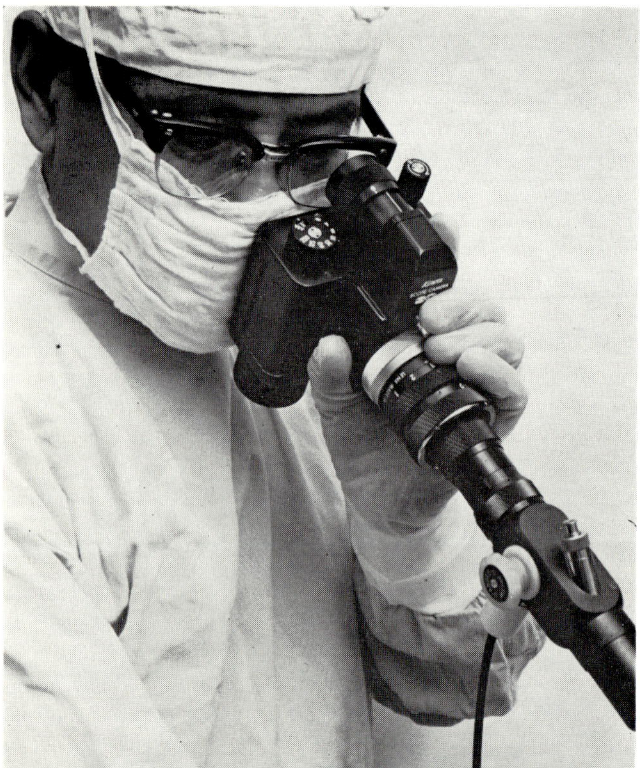

**Fig. 106** How to hold a bronchofiberscope of Machida make for endoscopic photography utilizing the new Kowa camera.

**c. New type of endoscopic camera**

*a) Kowa scope camera SQ* (Fig. 106). In a newly developed camera for exclusive bronchofiberscopic use, the following is different from Olympus Pen F.

1. Pictures obtained with Olympus Pen F camera, being only 5 mm in diameter, require magnification because of their small sizes. The newly developed camera for use with Machida scope has a 125 mm lens system. The resultant pictures are markedly enlarged to 14 mm in diameter, permitting examination with the naked eye. The exposure time, however, is double that of the 75 mm lens under similar conditions of light and location within the bronchial tree.

2. The new bronchofiberscope camera possesses another great advantage over Olympus type. The latter requires both hands for holding and picture taking. With the new camera, the camera and the proximal part of the fiberscope can be held by one hand and the shutter operated simultaneously, making photography much easier.

3. An automatic film winder is incorporated in the new camera, so that serial photography can be accomplished with ease.

The present model is being modified incorporating an automatic exposure meter.

*b) Olympus new camera.* A new miniature 16 mm camera has been developed by Olympus Optical Co., Ltd. (Fig. 107). At the present time, it is used exclusively with the gastrofiberscope by attaching it to the eyepiece. This camera is being modified for use with the flexible bronchofiberscope.

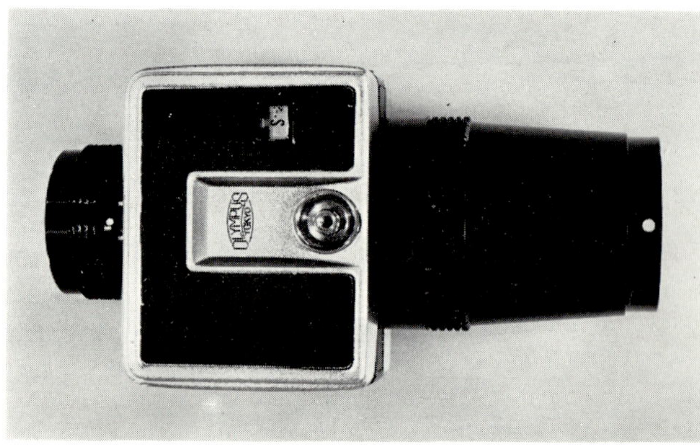

**Fig. 107** A new endoscopic camera of Olympus make.

**d. Film**

High speed EKTACHROME®, Kodak (daylight, ASA 160, DIN 23) is recommended.

If the light source is a 500 W, 300 W or 150 W Xenon lamp, the usual processing technique as with any color film is satisfactory. However, of necessity, if the exposure time is shortened, then the film must be developed by a special processing method whereby the sensitivity of the film is increased to the equivalent of

ASA 400, DIN 57. 5. This special processing process does not alter the grain of the film.

**e. Cautions for bronchoscopic photography**

The extremely peripheral bronchi into which a flexible bronchofiberscope can be advanced, do not have distinct characteristics of their own. Also, because of their small size, the mucosa is easily injured by aspiration of sputum or other manipulative procedures, and, caution must be exercised.

1. Pictures should be taken not only of the lesion but also of the bronchus leading up to the area in serial fashion. This will put the pictures in their relative order for reviewing at a later time.

2. The sites of photographed areas should be recorded accurately in a memorandum. This is also very helpful for later review of films.

3. Pictures should be taken prior to any possible injuries which may occur on bronchial walls.

4. Photographing is occasionally easier when withdrawing the bronchofiberscope than when inserting it into a bronchus.

## CINEMATOGRAPHY

Although serial pictures may be taken with a hand camera, it is frequently difficult to grasp the exact location of a lesion when pictures are referred to later on. In this respect the endoscopic cine film is more convenient since, needless to say, the inside of a bronchus can be observed continuously as the bronchofiberscope is maneuvered, with much clearer understanding of the relative location of the lesion. The only shortcomings are that the cine camera is heavy and that the film is expensive.

In our hospital when some definite and convincing findings are seen, the cine camera is utilized in almost every case.

**a. Film**

The importance of the case at hand determines whether the 16 mm or 8 mm film is used. The reason is that 16 mm is suitable for public exhibition as in a general assembly but 8 mm is not.

Emphatically recommended is, if 16 mm is selected it is strongly recommended that EKTACHROME EF® (7241, daylight type), Kodak film be used. In developing this film, special processing is required increasing the sensitivity four times.

**b. Light source and time of exposure**

The light source should be set at its utmost intensity. In cinematography the recommended speed, using EKTACHROME EF® with special processing, is 12–16 frame/sec at the bronchial bifurcation and 16–24 frame/sec at the segmental bronchus, when a 16 mm cine camera is connected to a 5 mm bronchofiberscope of either Machida make or Olympus make. If an 8 mm cine camera is selected, the time of exposure may be 2/3 that of the 16 mm, using EKTACHROME EF®, with twice longer intensifying development. Recently an automatic exposure control (so-called electric eye system) has been attached to the light source unit.

**c. Cine camera** (Figs. 108 and 109)

One of the excellent endoscopic cine cameras available is the Beaulieu® of French make. They have two models, R-16 for the 16 mm and, S-2008 for 8 mm films. It can be connected to an electric eye system which automatically controls the light volume from the light source. Other advantages of this camera are its light weight and the speed-regulator, which is very convenient for bronchofiberscopic purposes. A lens specific for endoscopy must be used.

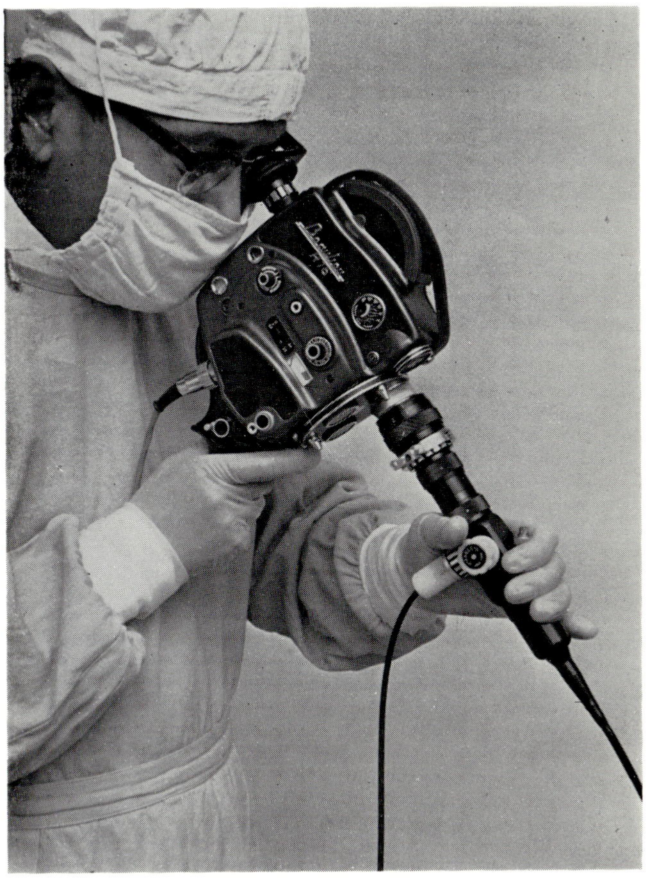

**Fig. 108** Endoscopic cinematography with a 16 mm camera.

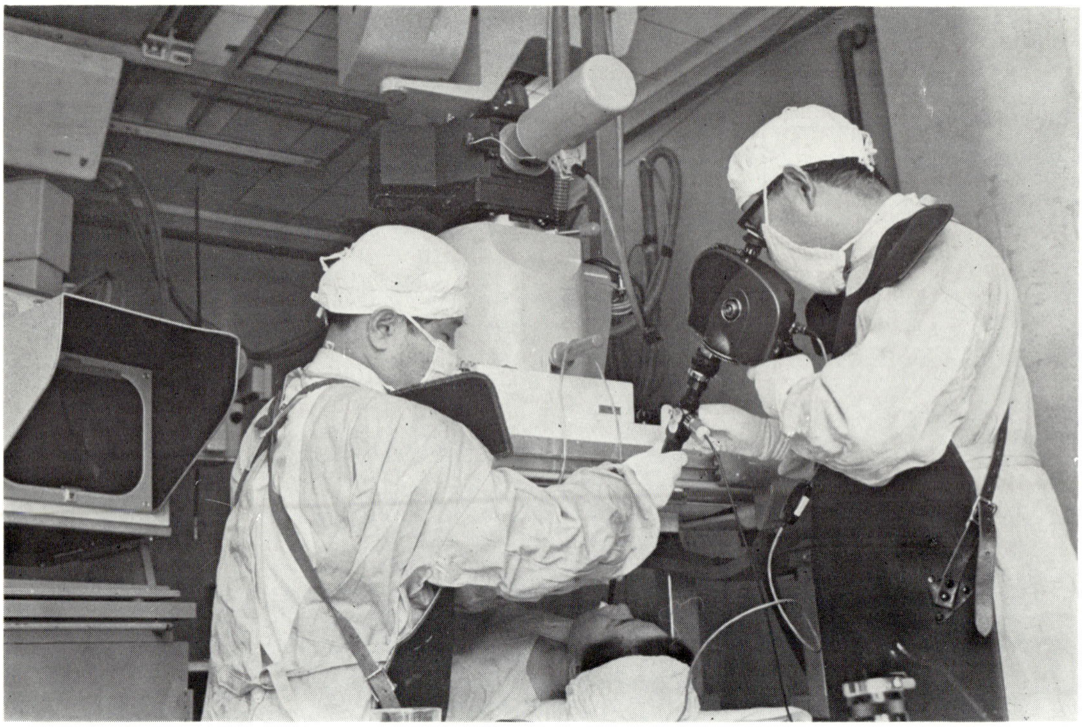

**Fig. 109** Endoscopic cinematography with a 16 mm camera under X-ray TV fluoroscopy.

**d. Analysis of exposed films** (Fig. 110)

Unlike ordinary commercial movies, the projected pictures are darker but are still of great value medically. They are frequently shown at a slower speed or even just one frame at a time for close analysis and study. For this purpose, a projector with special features accomplishing the above is necessary The projectors currently in common use and recommended are the Analector® for 16 mm manufactured by De Oude Delft Co. (Holland) or Ektagraphic MFS-8® for 8 mm by Kodak Co. (U.S.A.). The Analector, for example, has variable speeds from 1 frame/sec to 24 frame/sec and can hold one frame as a still picture for as long as two minutes without damaging the film. For these reasons, this projector is recommended as one of the most suitable for analysis of endoscopic pictures.

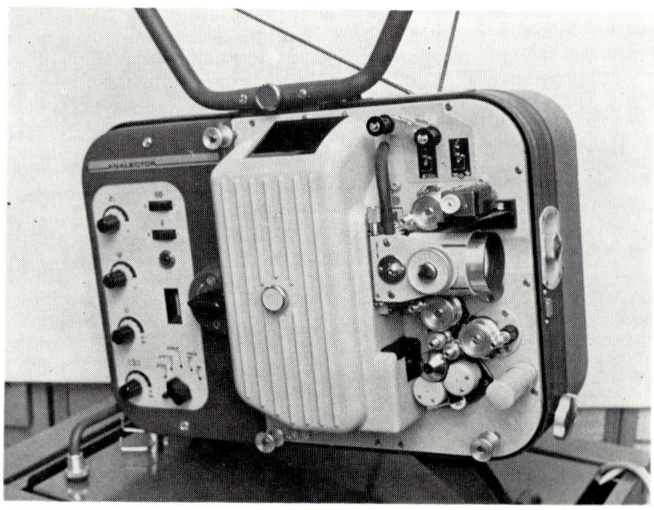

**Fig. 110** Analector ; Special 16 mm projector for analyzing endoscopic findings.

## TELEVISION

A color television camera has recently been developed, which can simultaneously televise endoscopic images as the lesions are visualized by a flexible bronchofiberscope. The light volume which a fiberscope can transmit into the bronchus is extremely small due to the narrowness of the scope body. This demands a TV camera which is small both in size and weight, has high sensitivity and excellent resolution. A camera which satisfies these requirements has been completed after several years' trials and investigations since 1968. This simultaneous color TV camera weighing 7.5 kg in its body alone, with three Plumbicons®* used in it, was developed by Matsushita Communication Co.Ltd.,Japan.

Very clear-cut pictures can be watched on TV, with the camera hung on a specially designed hanger and connected to a flexible bronchofiberscope. Furthermore, the pictures may be recorded in the color video tape recorder.

* Trade name for TV camera tube, Philips, Holland.

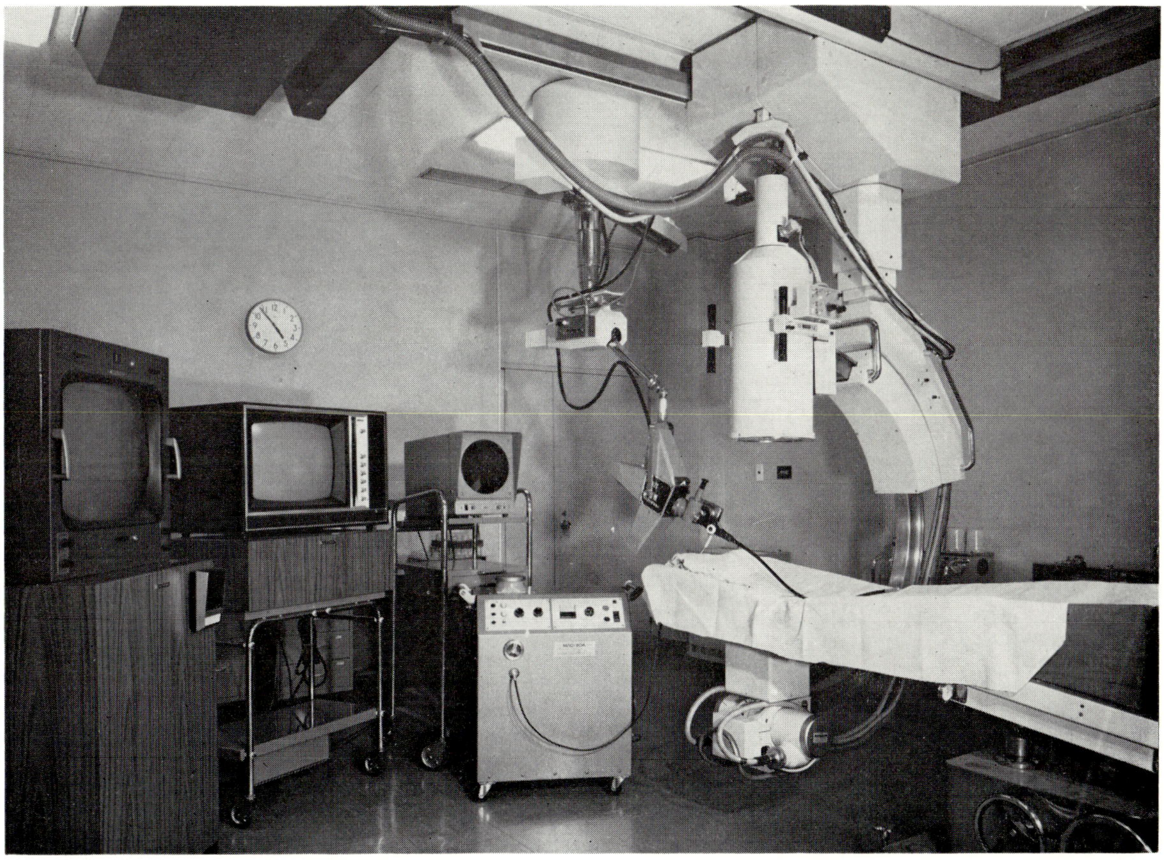

**Fig. 111** A color TV set for endoscopic purpose.

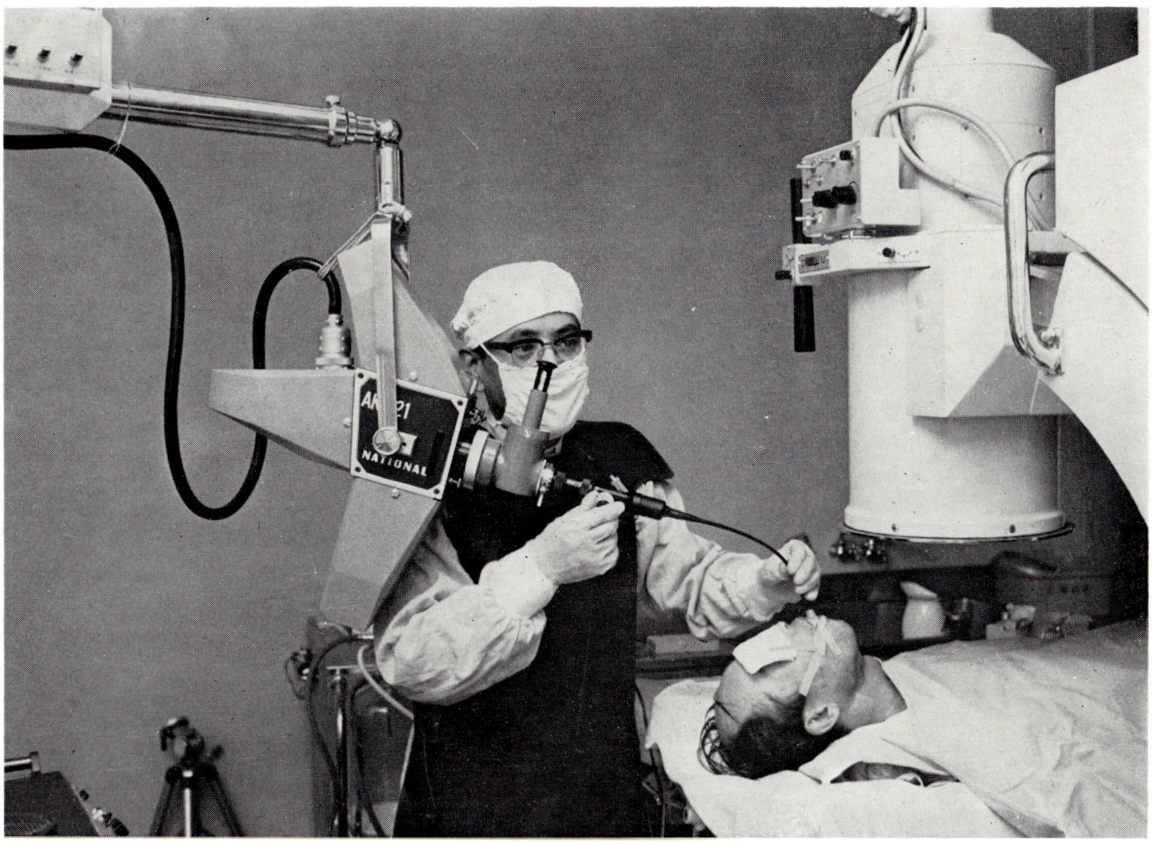


**Fig. 112** How to make use of color TV.

# VI. Normal and Abnormal Findings

## NOMENCLATURE FOR PERIPHERAL BRONCHI

The present names of the bronchi are based on the nomenclature of JACKSON-HUBER or BOYDEN abroad and in Japan, established by the Committee on the Nomenclature for Bronchial Branching (Fig. 113). None of these systems extends beyond the subsegmental bronchi. With the recent development of a flexible bronchofiberscope, the visual range encompasses the sub-subsegmental bronchi (IV order of branching) to the bronchi of VI order of division. With an improved bronchofiberscope of a smaller diameter now being developed, visualization would be extended further towards the more peripheral bronchi. There may be many

### RIGHT

A. Bronchus dexter
B. Truncus [bronchialis] superior
C. Truncus [bronchialis] intermedius
D. Truncus [bronchialis] inferior

- UPPER LOBE
  - $B^1$: R. apicalis
    - a. Rm. apicalis proprius
    - b. Rm. [subapicalis] ventralis
  - $B^2$: R. [lobi superioris] dorsalis
    - a. Rm. [subapicalis] dorsalis
    - b. Rm. [lobi sup.] horizontalis
  - $B^3$: R. [lobi superioris] ventralis
    - a. Rm. [lobi sup. ventr.] lateralis
    - b. Rm. [lobi sup. ventr.] medialis
- MIDDLE LOBE
  - $B^4$: R. medius lateralis
    - a. Rm. lateralis
    - b. Rm. medialis
  - $B^5$: R. medius medialis
    - a. Rm. superior
    - b. Rm. inferior
- LOWER LOBE
  - $B^6$: R. [lobi inferioris] superior
    - a. Rm. superior
    - b. Rm. lateralis
    - c. Rm. medialis
  - B*: R. [lobi inferioris] subsuperior
  - $B^7$: R. mediobasalis
    - a. Rm. ventralis
    - b. Rm. dorsalis
  - $B^8$: R. ventrobasalis
    - a. Rm. lateralis
    - b. Rm. basalis
  - $B^9$: R. laterobasalis
    - a. Rm. lateralis
    - b. Rm. basalis
  - $B^{10}$: R. dorsobasalis
    - a. Rm. dorsalis
    - b. Rm. lateralis
    - c. Rm. medialis

### LEFT

A. Bronchus sinister
B. Truncus [bronchialis] superior
D. Truncus [bronchialis] inferior

- UPPER LOBE
  - $B^{1+2}$: R. apicodorsalis
    - a. Rm. apicalis
    - b. Rm. [subapicalis] dorsalis
    - c. Rm. [lobi sup.] horizontalis
  - $B^3$: R. [lobi superioris] ventralis
    - a. Rm. [lobi sub. ventr.] lateralis
    - b. Rm. [lobi sub. ventr.] medialis
    - c Rm. [lobi sub. ventr.] superior
  - R. lingualis
    - $B^4$: R. lingualis superior
      - a. Rm. lateralis
      - b. Rm ventralis
    - $B^5$: R. lingualis inferior
      - a. Rm. superior
      - b. Rm. inferior
- LOWER LOBE
  - $B^6$: R. [lobi inferioris] superior
    - a. Rm. superior
    - b. Rm lateralis
    - c. Rm medialis
  - B*: R. [lobi inferioris] supsuperior
  - $B^8$: R. ventrobasalis
    - a. Rm. lateralis
    - b. Rm. basalis
  - $B^9$: R. laterobasalis
    - a. Rm. lateralis
    - b. Rm. basalis
  - $B^{10}$: R. dorsobasalis
    - a. Rm. dorsalis
    - b. Rm. lateralis
    - c. Rm. medialis

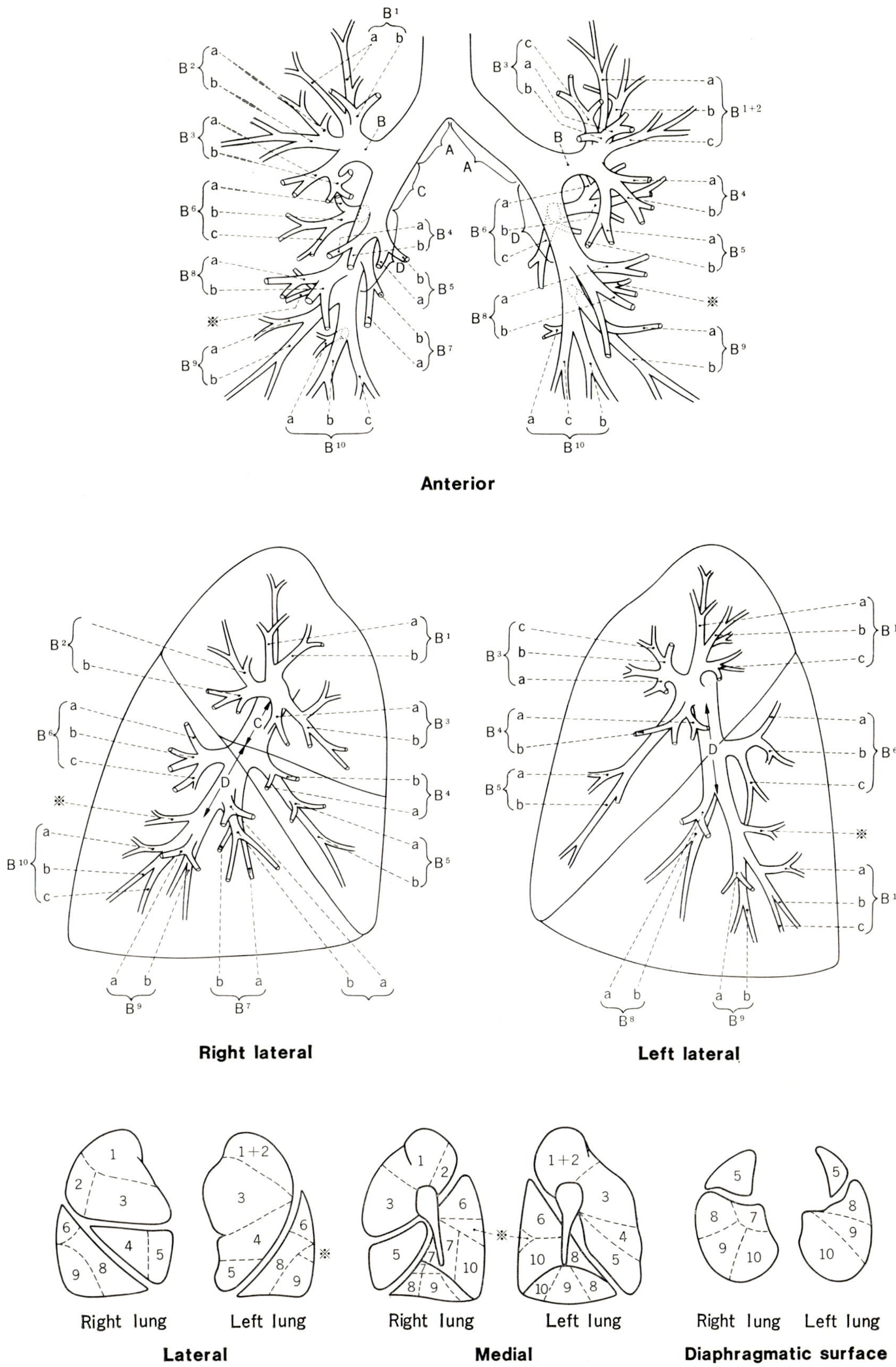


**Fig. 113** Nomenclature for the bronchi by the Japanese Committee on the Nomenclature for Bronchial Branching, 1950.

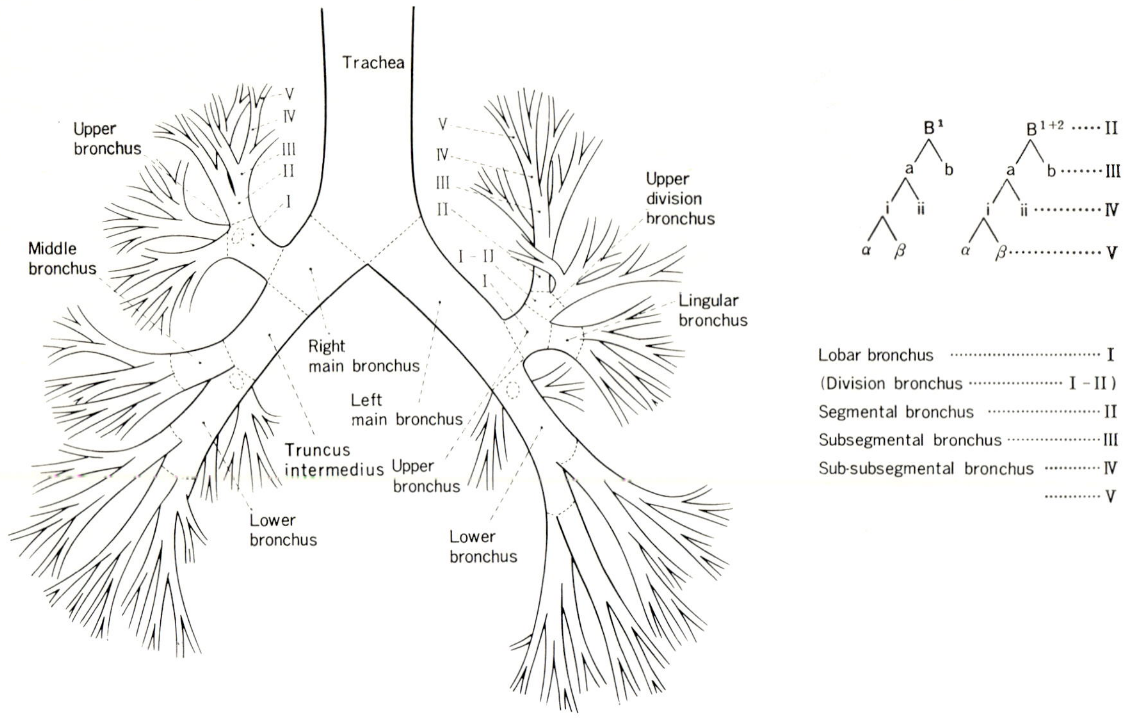


**Fig. 114** Establishment of the nomenclature for bronchi by Ikeda, 1969.

anomalies in branching in the periphery. Nomenclature for bronchi of IV to VI order has not been established, not to speak of the more peripheral ones.

In order to fill this gap in bronchial nomenclature, a system of symbols has been adopted in our clinic (Fig. 114). The system has two aspects: one is the names of branching order and the other is concerned with the names of peripheral bronchi.

### a. Designation of bronchi in accordance to the order of branching

All the lobe bronchi are generically called the bronchi of I order of branching; the segmental bronchi are all designated by the names of the bronchi of II order of branching; and so on up to IV and V branches. The large bronchi, such as the right main bronchus, need not be given a new name; traditional names will suffice.

### b. Nomenclature for the peripheral bronchi

Traditional names to the subsegmental bronchi raise no problems. Traditional nomenclature by Jackson-Huber or the Committee on the Nomenclature for Bronchial Branching are adequate. A subtle question however, arose here. Take an example of a subsegmental bronchus. It may be called "the posterior branch bronchus of the apical segmental bronchus of the right upper lobe" (which is long enough). In the same way, a more peripherally located bronchus of V order of branching will be "the anterior branch bronchus of the anterior branch bronchus of the posterior branch bronchus of the apical segmental bronchus of the right upper lobe". These names are too long and rather misleading for practical purposes. Of the two, the first may be expressed as $B^1a$ as Jackson does occasionally, but as we do routinely; and the second $B^1ai\alpha$ in our terms. The problem is the complete absence of names for the bronchi beyond the subsegments.

Our proposition is as follows. A bronchus of IV order of branching (subsegmental) is designated by "i" if it is located posteriorly, and "ii" if anteriorly, just as a bronchus of III order of branching (segmental) is differentiated by "a" (posterior) and "b" (anterior). The same criterion is applied to the bronchi of V order (sub-subsegmental): alpha ($\alpha$) if posterior and beta ($\beta$) if anterior. Further designation for VI order and beyond are reserved. They will be called by their respective names as in the preceding paragraph though extremely complicated. The above proposed nomenclature is, it must be admitted, for the sake of clinical conveniences and not based on anatomical structure.

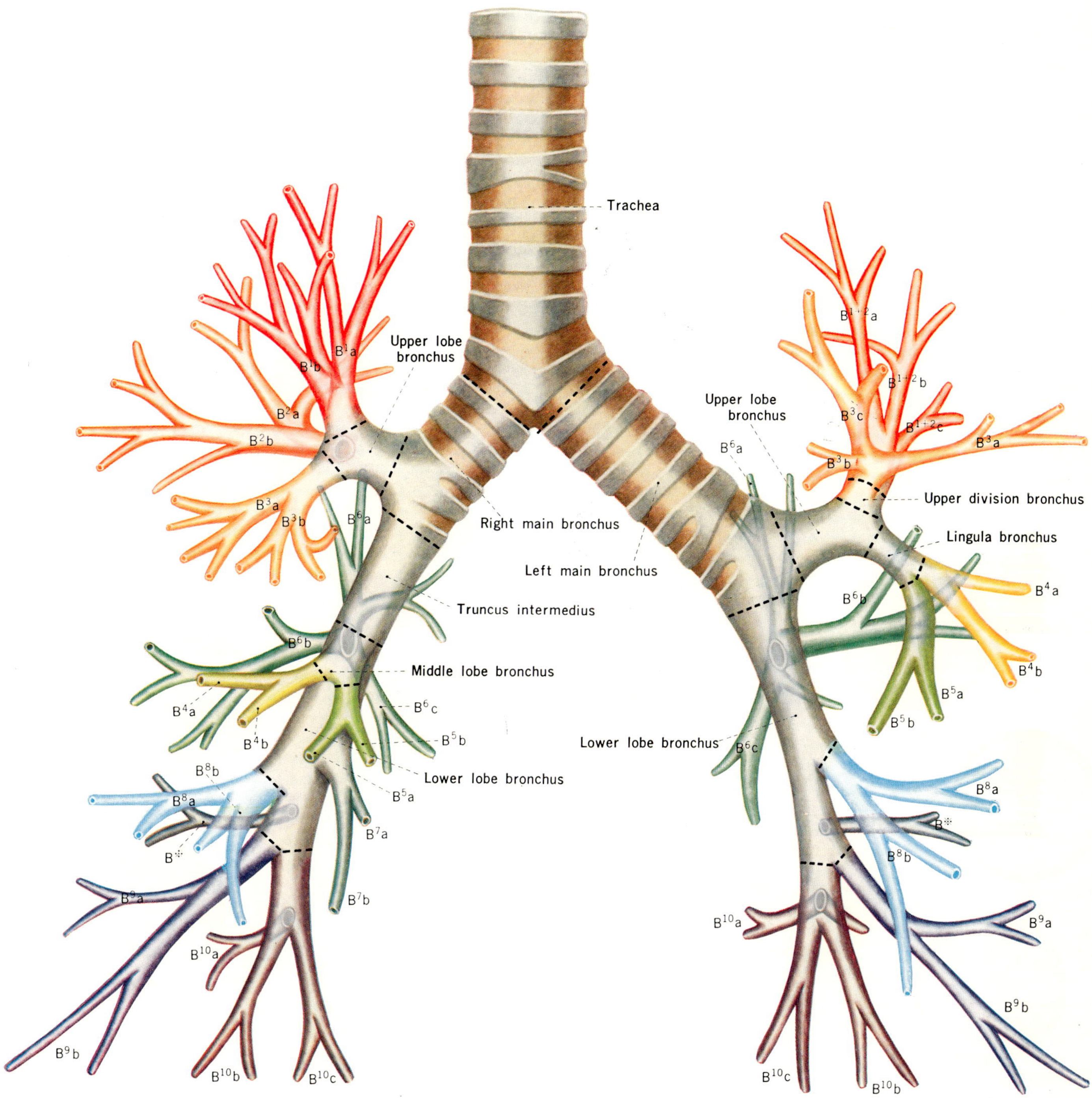


**Fig. 115** The bronchial tree.

## NORMAL FINDINGS OF BRONCHI

Following bronchofiberscopic photographs of normal bronchi (Japanese, male) are taken through the 5 mm flexible bronchofiberscope of Machida make (FBS-5) (Figs. 116–120).

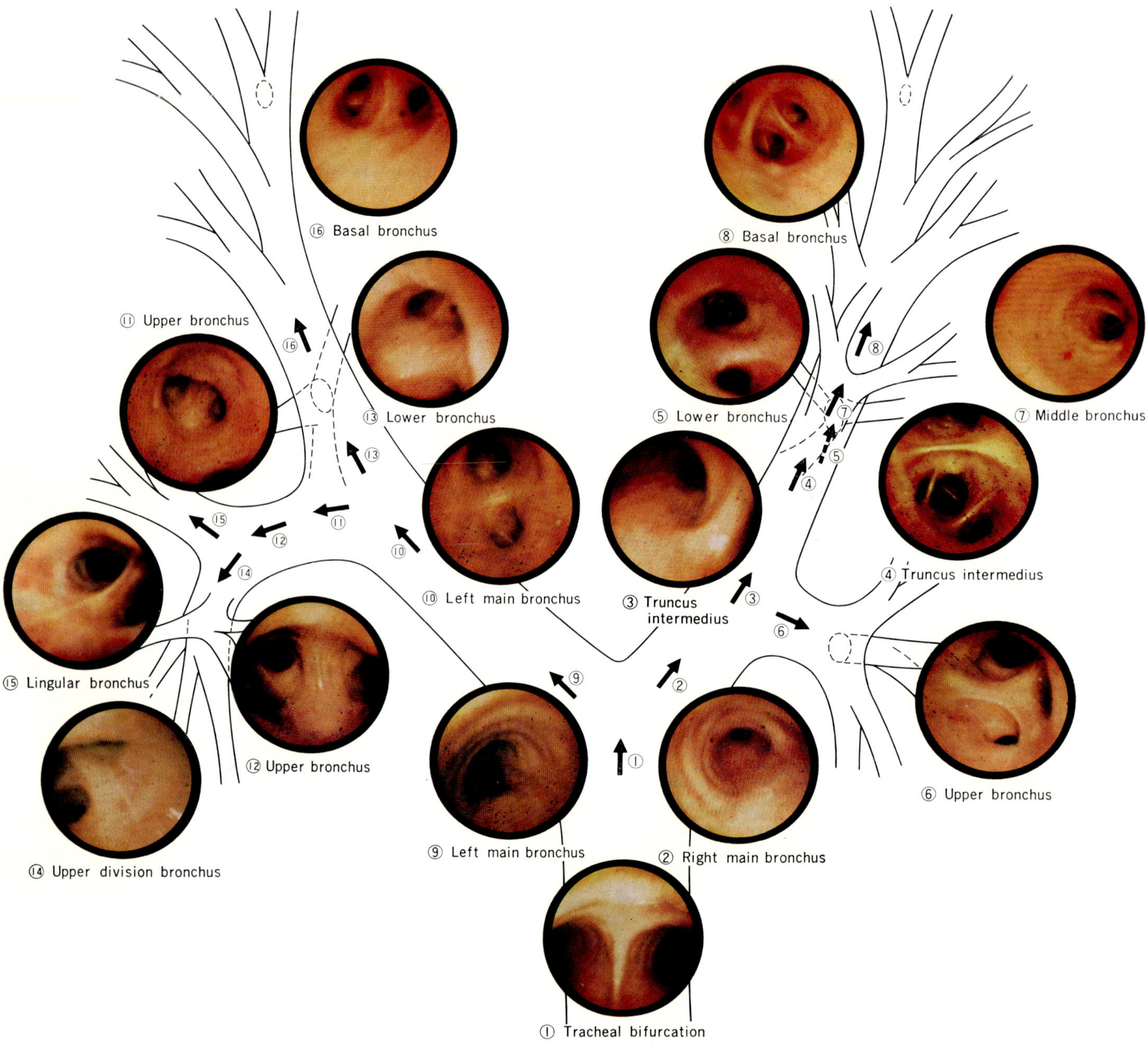


**Fig. 116** Main bronchi.

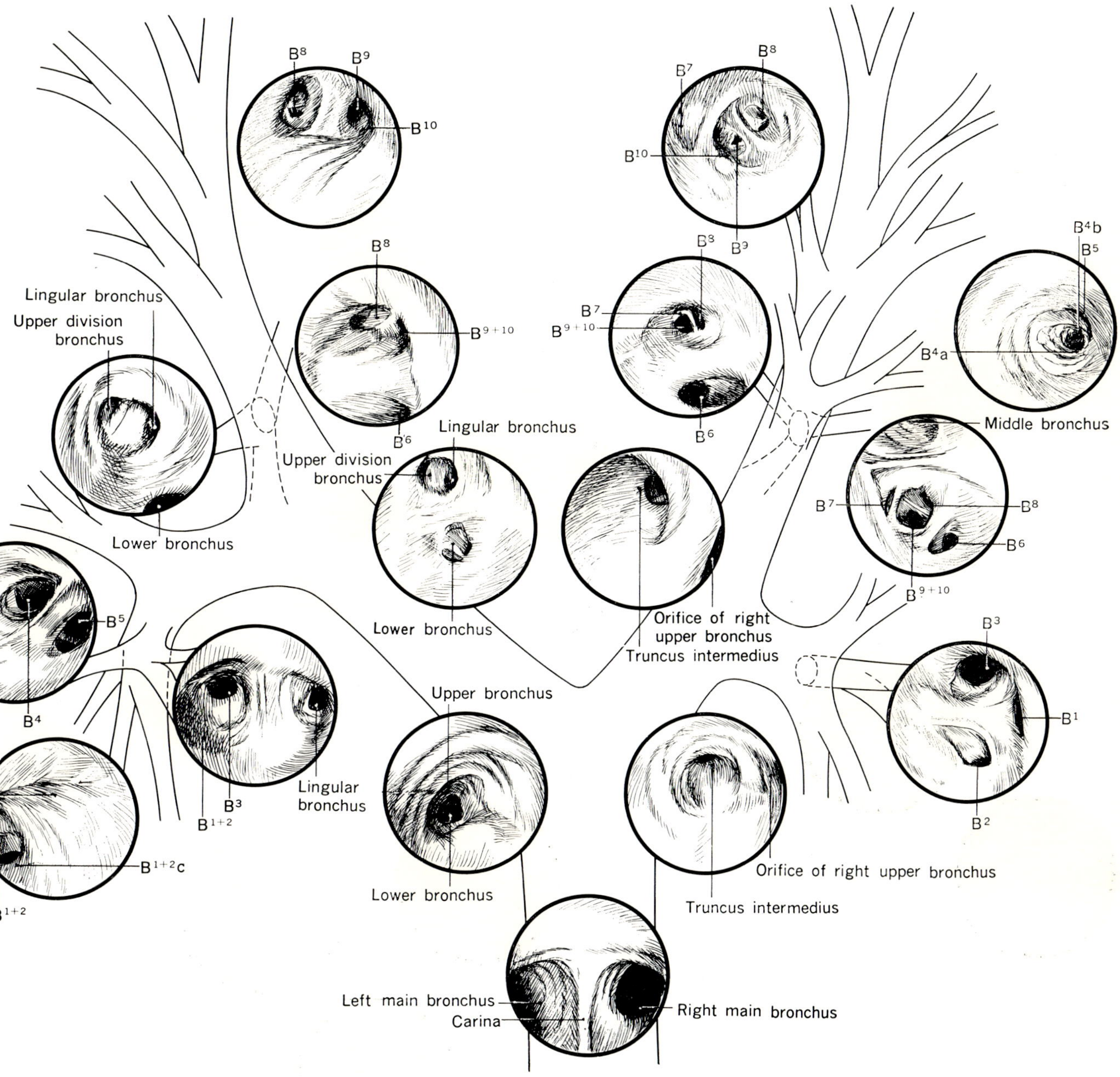

B8
B9
B10
B7
B8
B10
B9
B8
B9+10
B3
B7
B9+10
B9
B4b
B5
B4a
Lingular bronchus
Upper division bronchus
B6
B6
Lingular bronchus
Middle bronchus
Upper division bronchus
B7
B8
B6
Lower bronchus
B5
Lower bronchus
B9+10
Orifice of right upper bronchus
Truncus intermedius
B3
B4
Upper bronchus
B1
B3
B3
B1+2
Lingular bronchus
B2
B1+2c
B1+2
Lower bronchus
Orifice of right upper bronchus
Truncus intermedius
Left main bronchus
Carina
Right main bronchus

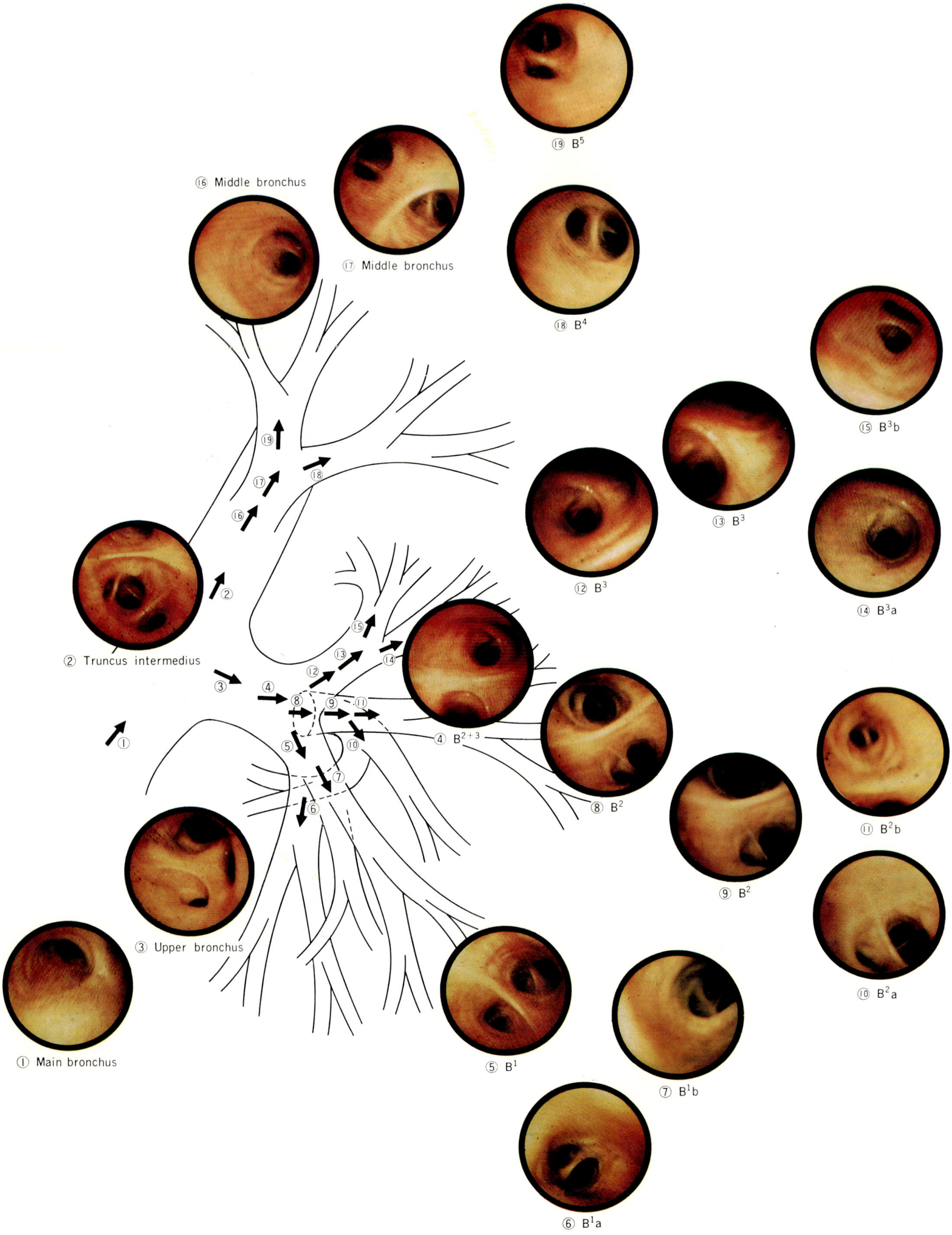


**Fig. 117** Right upper and middle lobe bronchi.

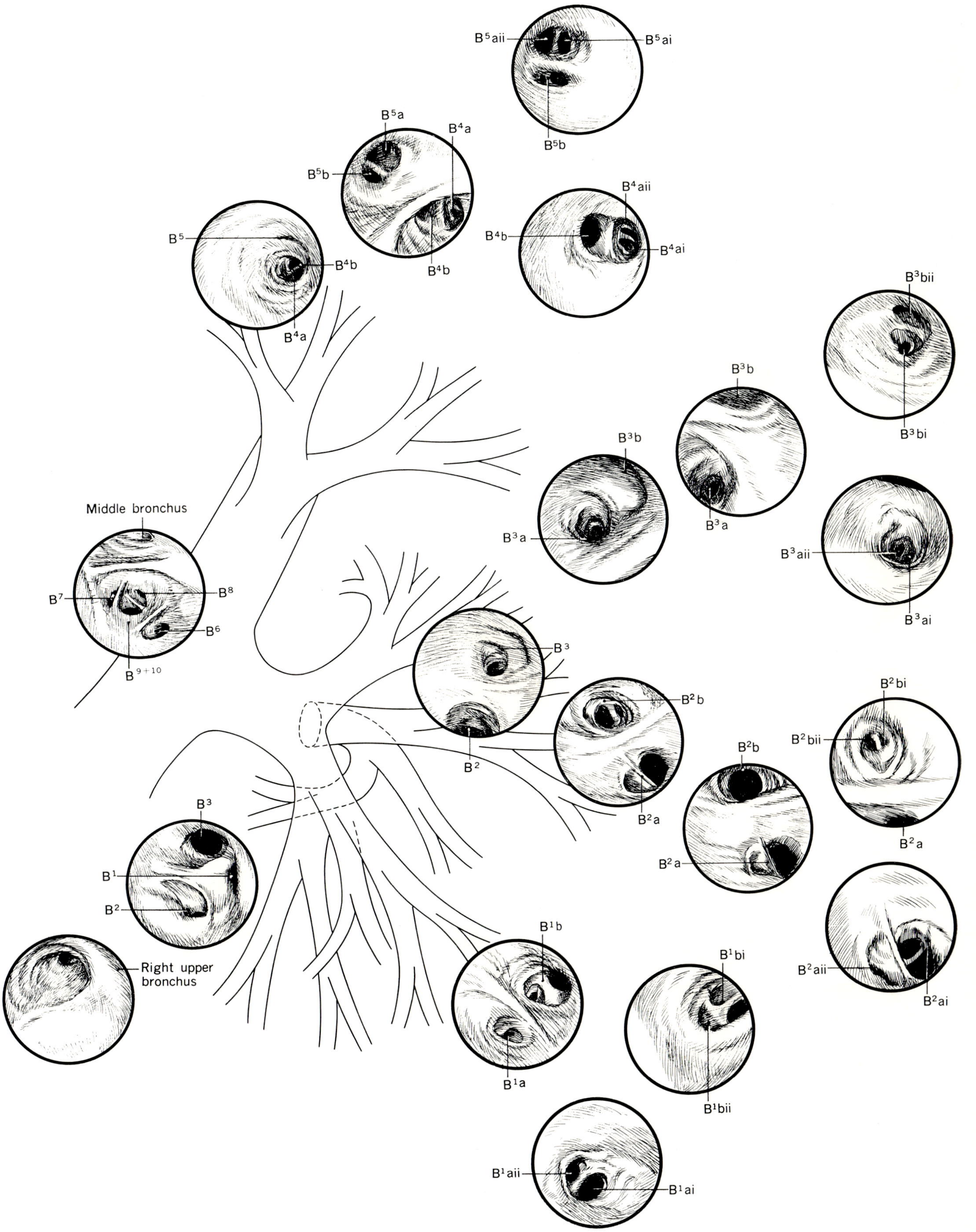
B⁵aii
B⁵ai
B⁵b
B⁵a
B⁴a
B⁵b
B⁴b
B⁴aii
B⁴b
B⁴ai
B⁵
B⁴b
B⁴a
B³bii
B³bi
B³b
B³b
B³a
B³a
B³aii
B³ai
Middle bronchus
B⁷
B⁸
B⁶
B⁹⁺¹⁰
B³
B²b
B²
B²bi
B²bii
B²b
B²a
B²a
B²a
B³
B¹
B²
Right upper bronchus
B¹b
B¹bi
B²aii
B²ai
B¹a
B¹bii
B¹aii
B¹ai

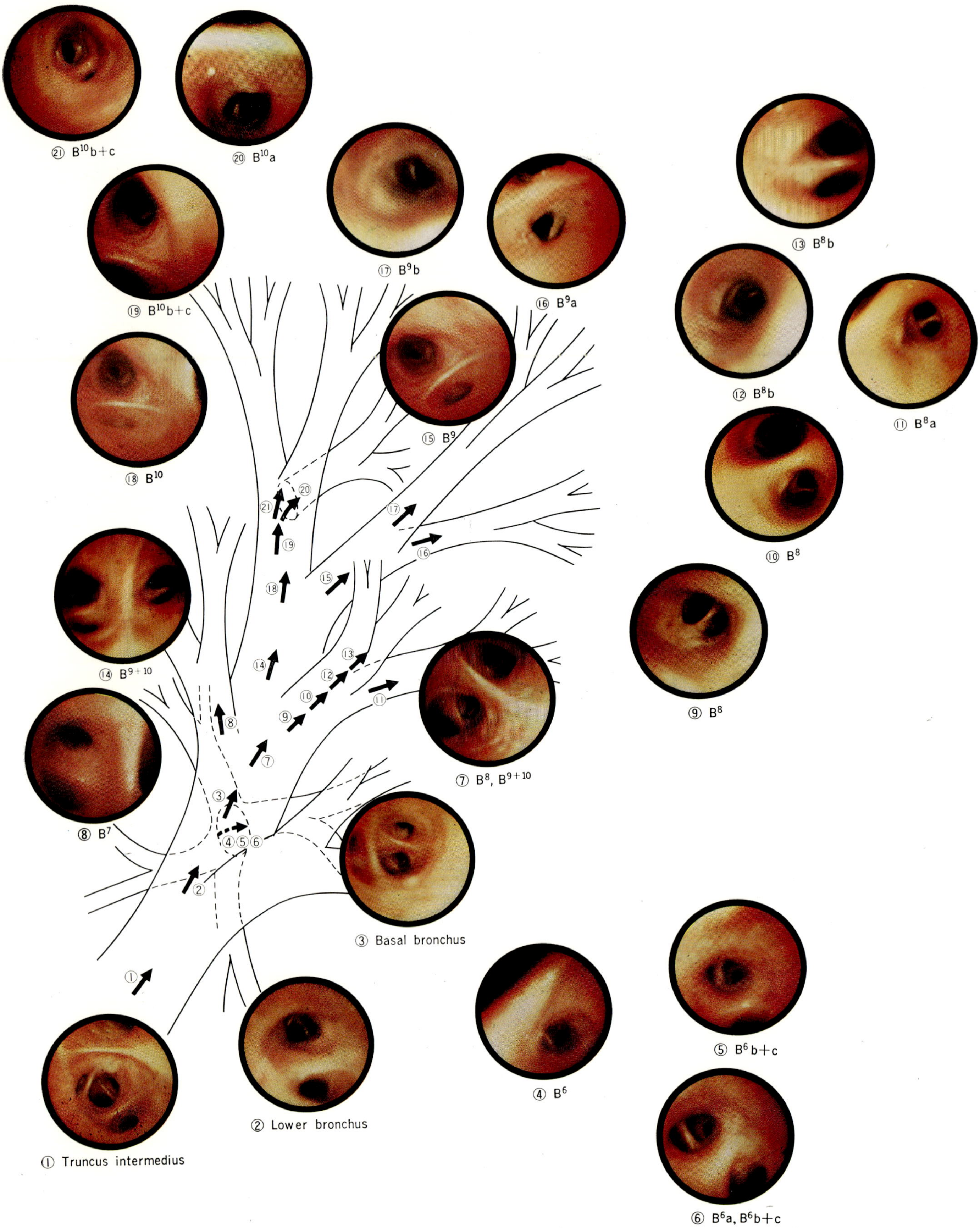


**Fig. 118** Right lower lobe bronchi.

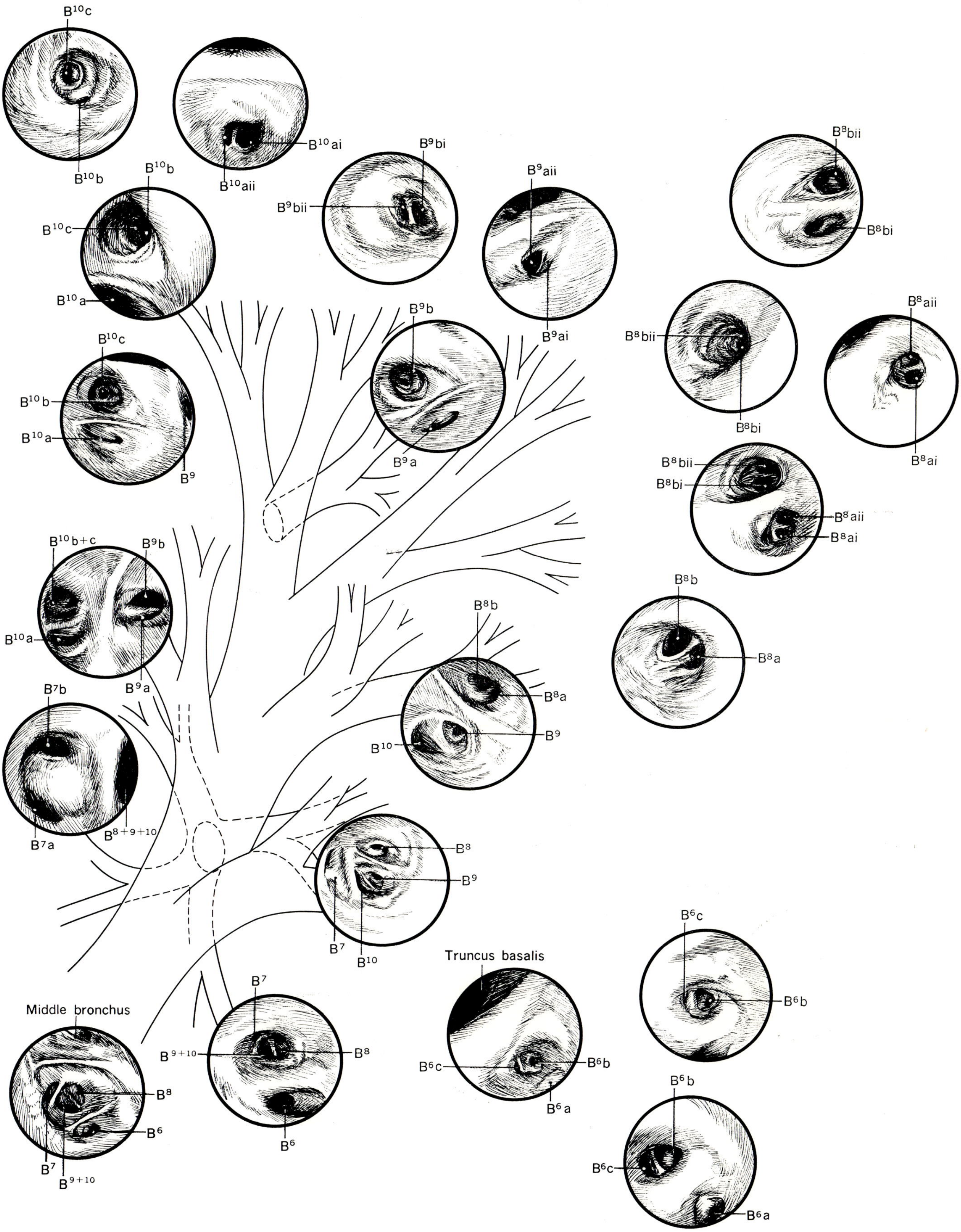
B10c
B10b
B10ai
B10aii
B9bi
B9bii
B9aii
B9ai
B8bii
B8bi
B10b
B10c
B10a
B9b
B9a
B8aii
B8ai
B10c
B10b
B10a
B9
B8bii
B8bi
B8aii
B8ai
B10b+c
B9b
B10a
B9a
B8b
B8a
B8b
B8a
B9
B10
B7b
B7a
B8+9+10
B8
B9
B7
B10
Truncus basalis
B6c
B6b
Middle bronchus
B7
B9+10
B8
B8
B6
B7
B9+10
B6
B6c
B6b
B6a
B6b
B6c
B6a

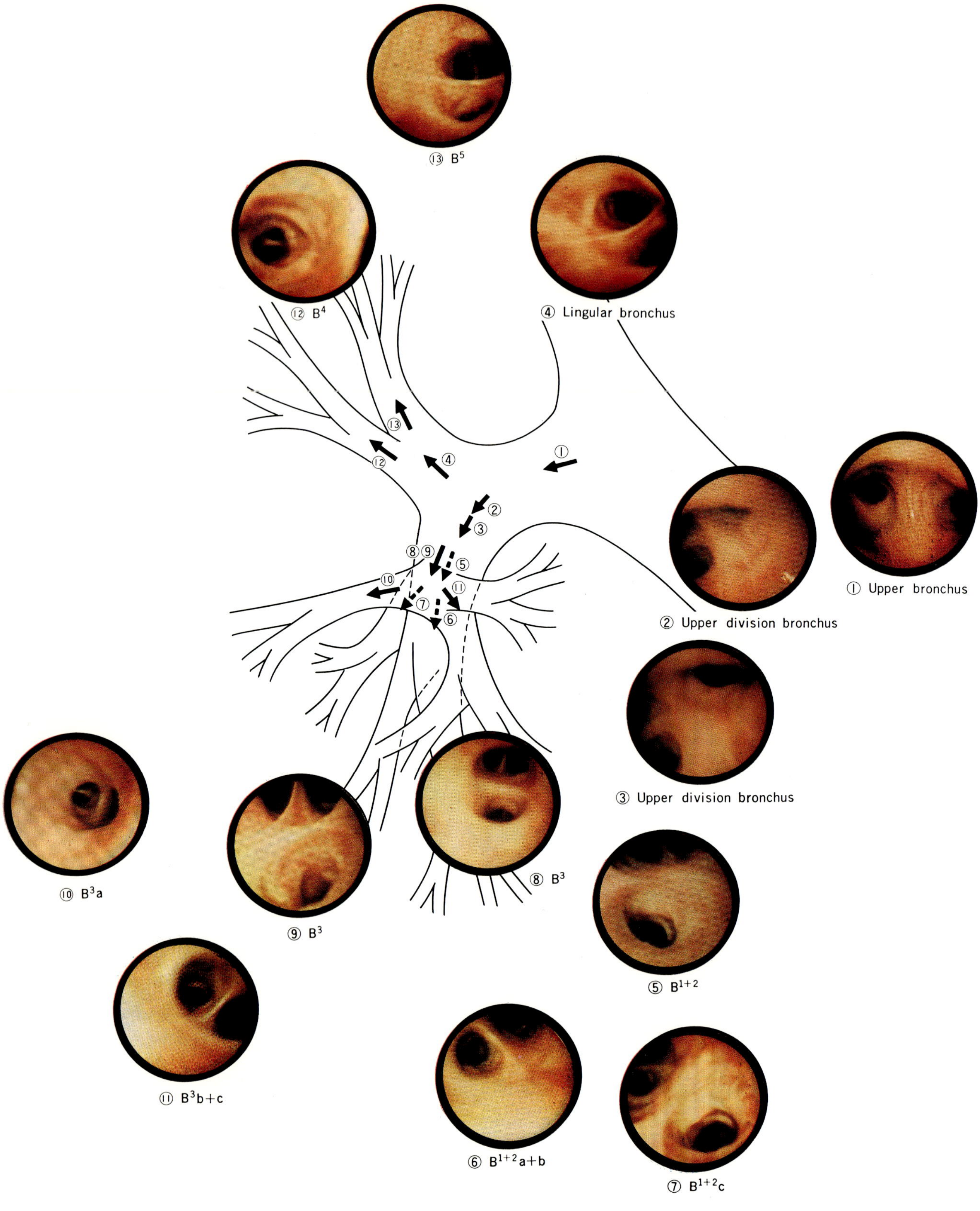


**Fig. 119** Left upper lobe bronchi.

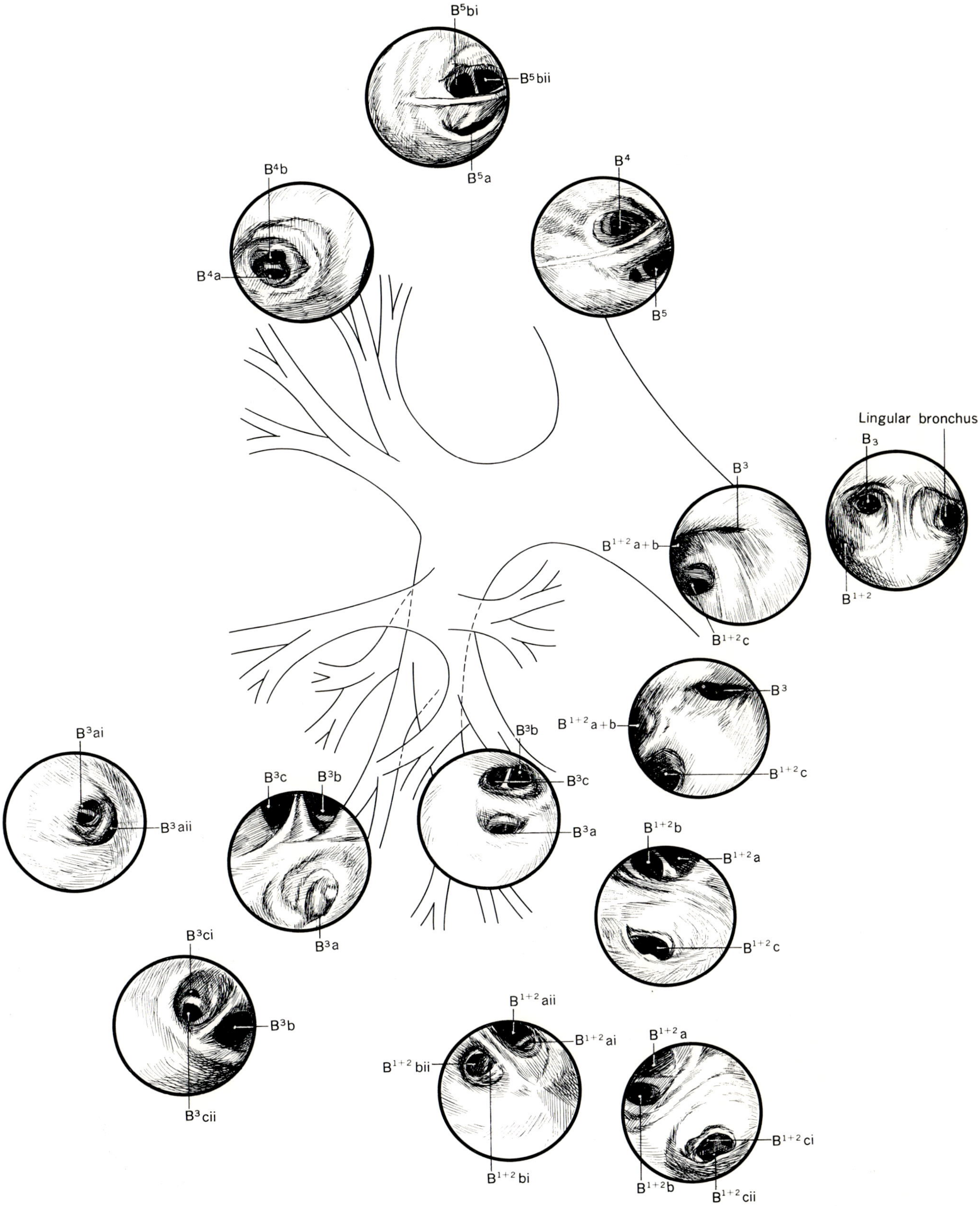
B$^{5}$bi
B$^{5}$bii
B$^{5}$a
B$^{4}$b
B$^{4}$a
B$^{4}$
B$^{5}$
Lingular bronchus
B$_{3}$
B$^{1+2}$
B$^{3}$
B$^{1+2}$a+b
B$^{1+2}$c
B$^{3}$
B$^{1+2}$a+b
B$^{1+2}$c
B$^{3}$ai
B$^{3}$aii
B$^{3}$c
B$^{3}$b
B$^{3}$a
B$^{3}$b
B$^{3}$c
B$^{3}$a
B$^{1+2}$b
B$^{1+2}$a
B$^{1+2}$c
B$^{3}$ci
B$^{3}$b
B$^{3}$cii
B$^{1+2}$aii
B$^{1+2}$ai
B$^{1+2}$bii
B$^{1+2}$bi
B$^{1+2}$a
B$^{1+2}$ci
B$^{1+2}$b
B$^{1+2}$cii

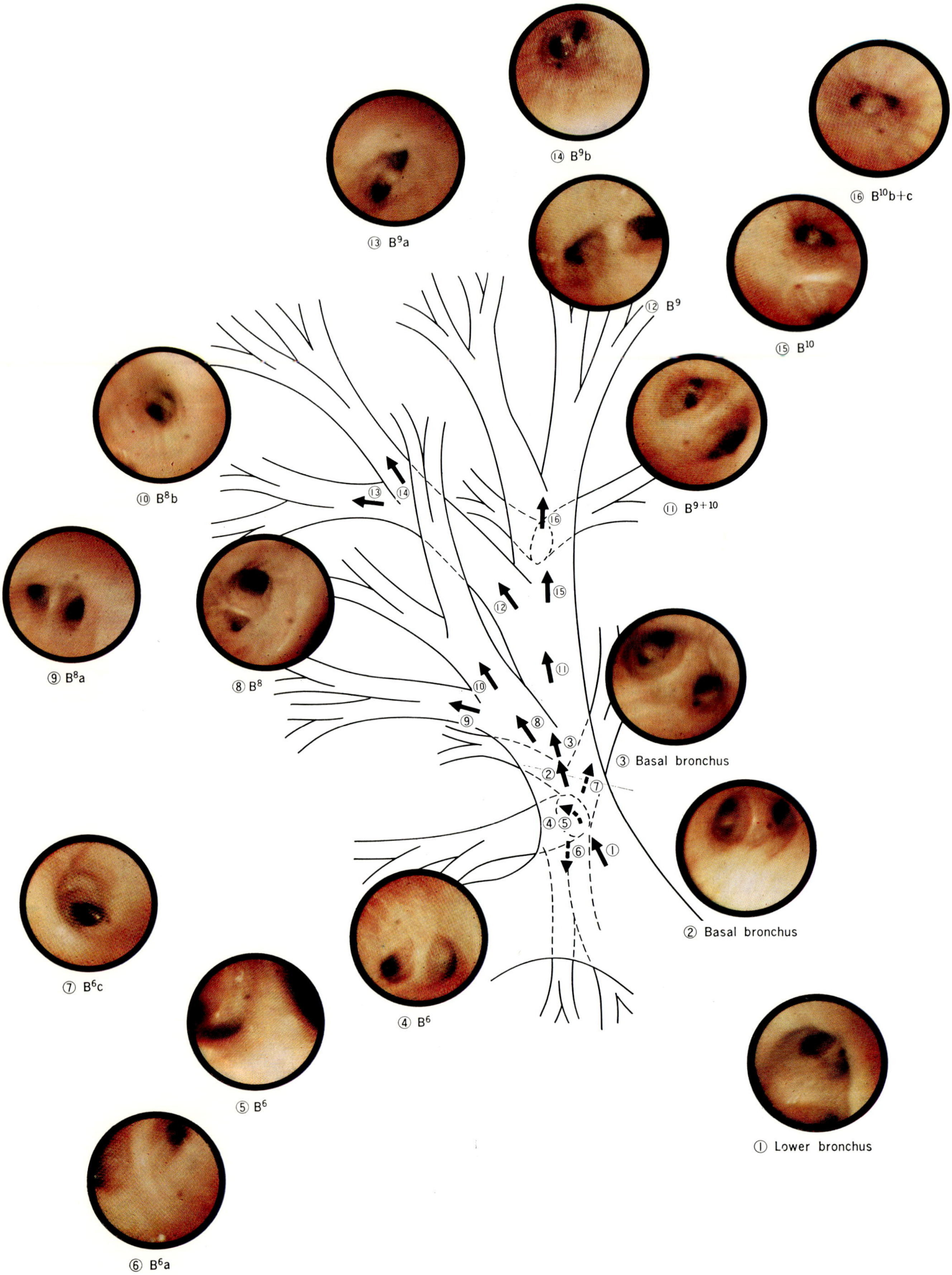


**Fig. 120** Left lower lobe bronchi.

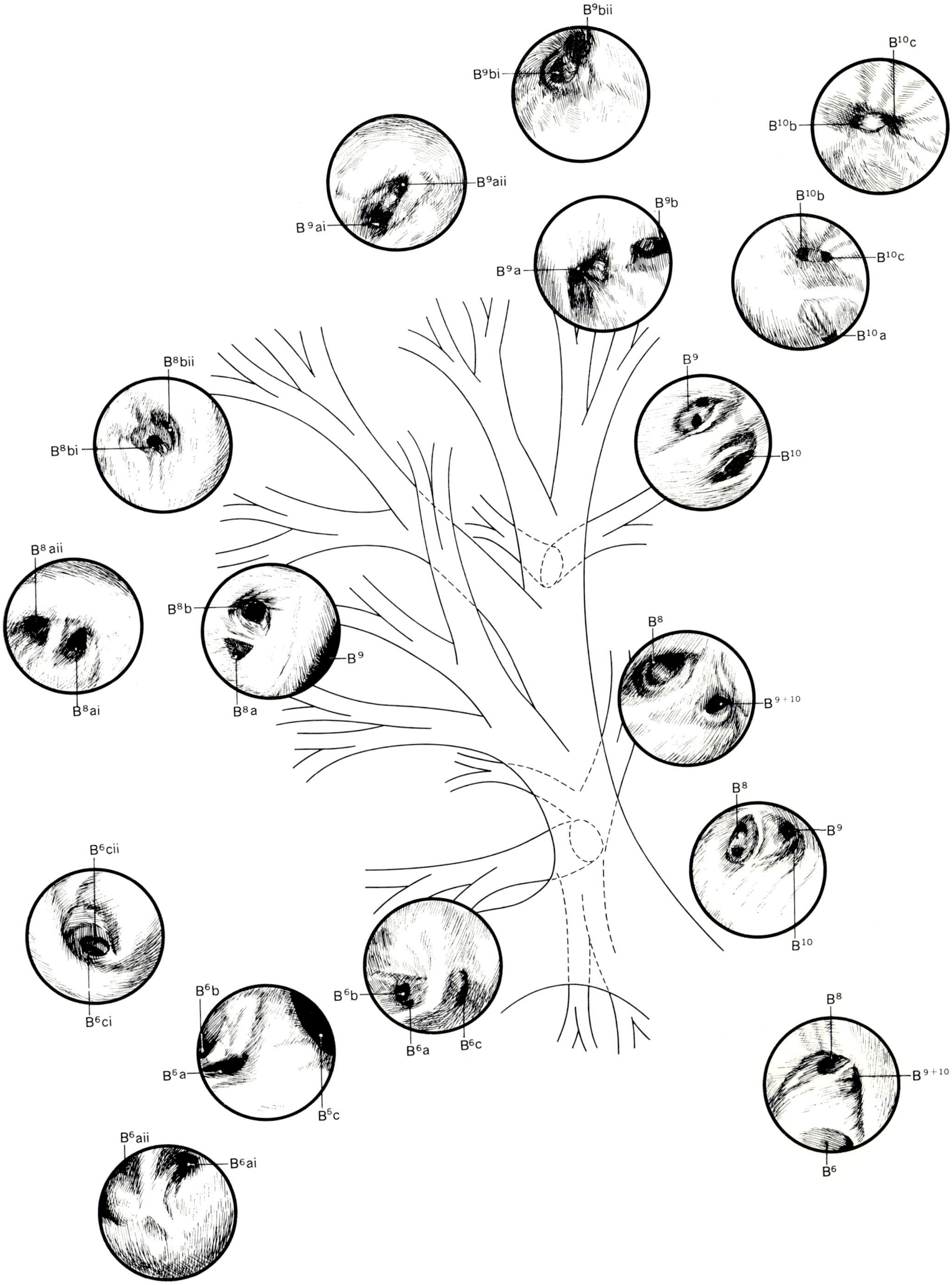
$B^{9}bii$
$B^{9}bi$
$B^{10}c$
$B^{10}b$
$B^{9}aii$
$B^{9}ai$
$B^{9}b$
$B^{9}a$
$B^{10}b$
$B^{10}c$
$B^{10}a$
$B^{8}bii$
$B^{8}bi$
$B^{9}$
$B^{10}$
$B^{8}aii$
$B^{8}ai$
$B^{8}b$
$B^{9}$
$B^{8}a$
$B^{8}$
$B^{9+10}$
$B^{8}$
$B^{9}$
$B^{10}$
$B^{6}cii$
$B^{6}ci$
$B^{6}b$
$B^{6}a$
$B^{6}c$
$B^{6}b$
$B^{6}a$
$B^{6}c$
$B^{8}$
$B^{9+10}$
$B^{6}$
$B^{6}aii$
$B^{6}ai$

# CLASSIFICATION OF BRONCHOSCOPIC FINDINGS

A standardized classification of bronchoscopic findings was discussed by HUZLY and STRADLING. This classification, however, is limited to findings obtained in the major bronchi and is not applicable to findings with the bronchofiberscope, especially when they involve the smaller bronchi of IV to VI order of branching.

The following Classification Standard of Bronchoscopic Findings, proposed by the Japan Society of Lung Cancer in October, 1970, would be acceptable for present purposes.

**a. Abnormal organic changes of the bronchial wall**

1. Redness
2. Swelling (edema)
3. Engorgement of blood vessels or vascular engorgement with tortuosity of the vessels
4. Irregularity of bronchial mucosa
5. Unclearness (indistinct) of bronchial cartilages
6. Protruding bronchial cartilages
7. Ulceration
8. Enlarged mucous gland orifices
9. Submucosal lymph nodes
10. Atrophy of the bronchial wall
11.* Hypertrophy
12. Tumor
13. Necrosis
14. Longitudinal infolding (corrugations ; striations)

**b. Endobronchial Abnormalities**

1. Narrowing
2. Stenosis
3. Ectasis
4. Compression (bulging)
5. Abnormal bifurcation due to a diverticulum
6. Anomalous bronchial branching

**c. Abnormal substances in the bronchial lumen**

1. Secretion
2. Blood
3.* Calculus
4. Foreign bodies

**d. Dynamic disorders**

1.* During respiration
2.* During cough

The asterisks indicate that the picture of the bronchoscopic findings of these items are ommited in this Atlas.

The findings of the "bronchial stumps" are added to the Classification Standard in the following pages.

**a. Abnormal organic changes of the bronchial wall**

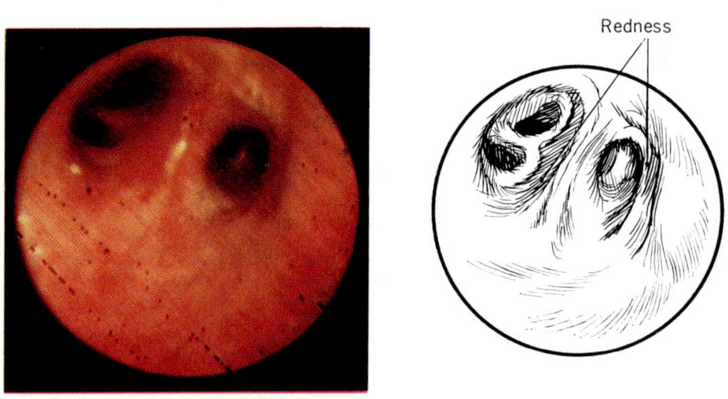


**Fig. 121 Redness** (or reddening) : The middle lobe bronchi are reddened. Bronchial cartilages are not clearly visualized. The reddening here is due to bronchiectatic secretions.

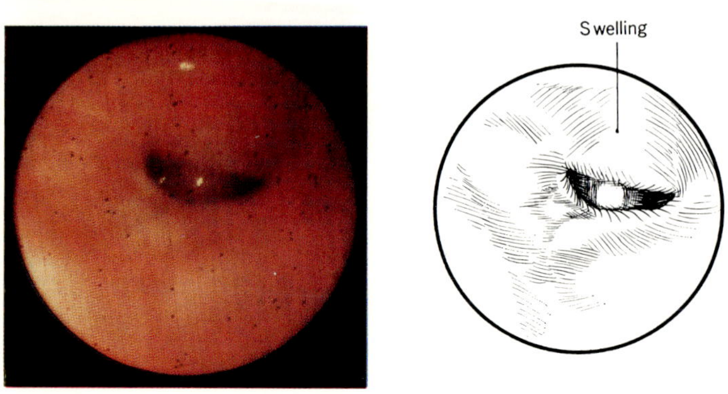


**Fig. 122 Swelling** (or tumescence) : The orifice of $B^6$ (superior segmental bronchus of the lower lobe) is swollen and compressed. The bifurcation of $B^6b$ and $B^6a+c$ is swollen and narrowed. This swelling is caused by bronchial inflammation.

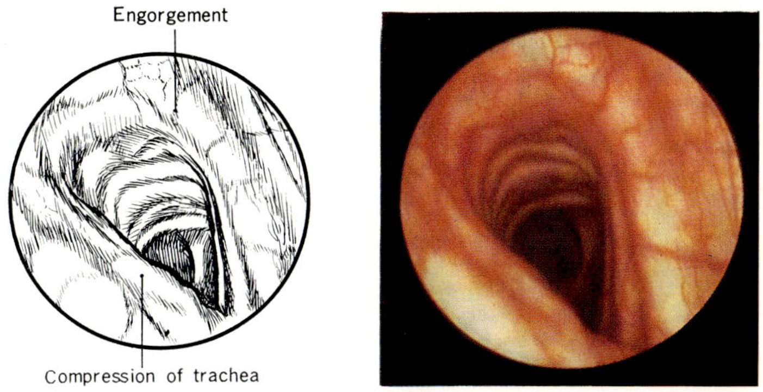


**Fig. 123 Engorgement of small blood vessels:** The trachea is compressed by a mediastinal tumor.

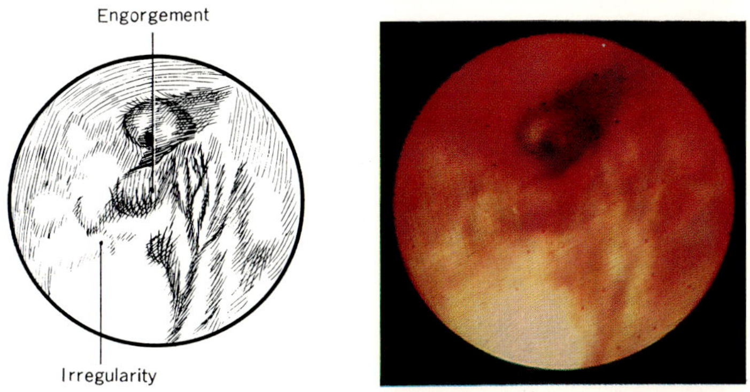


**Fig. 124 Engorgement:** The orifice of the lingular bronchus is irregular and accompanied by engorgement of small blood vessels. The intensive irregularity is seen on the posterior wall. The changes are due to infiltration by a carcinoma.

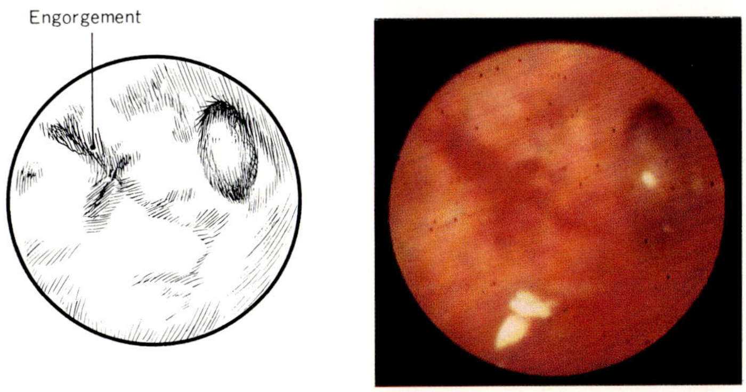


**Fig. 125 Engorgement:** The small blood vessels at the orifice of the left $B^6$ (superior segmental bronchus of the lower lobe) are engorged. This change is due to pulmonary tuberculosis.

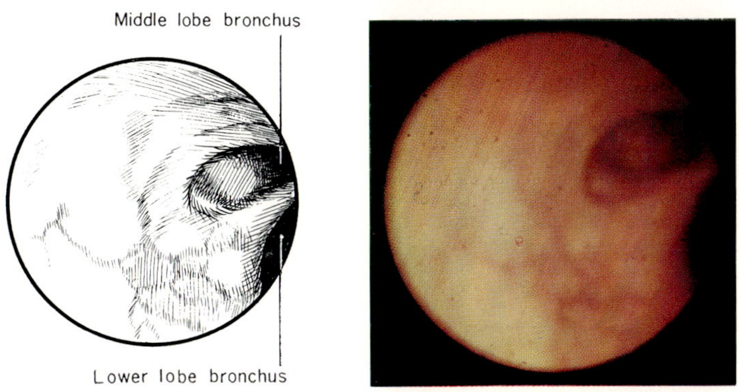


**Fig. 126 Engorgement:** On the left lateral wall near the bifurcation of the middle and lower lobe bronchi, at the lower part of the truncus intermedius, there is observed a cicatrization with tortuous engorgement of converging capillaries.

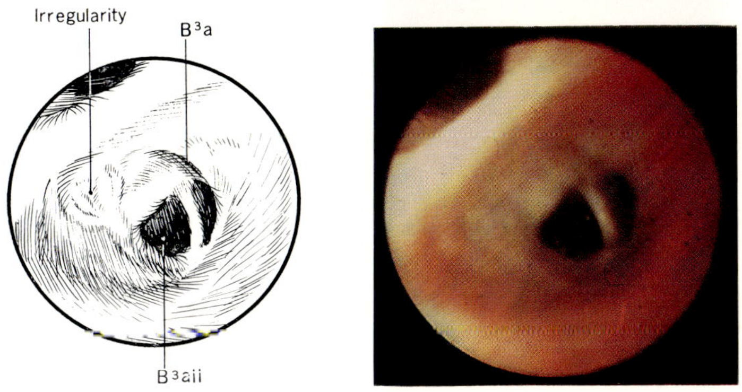


**Fig. 127 Irregularity of bronchial mucosa:** An example of irregularity with moderate stenosis of the right $B^3$a is seen. The septum between i and ii is normal. Further peripherally, an obstruction caused by adenocarcinoma was found in $B^3$aii.

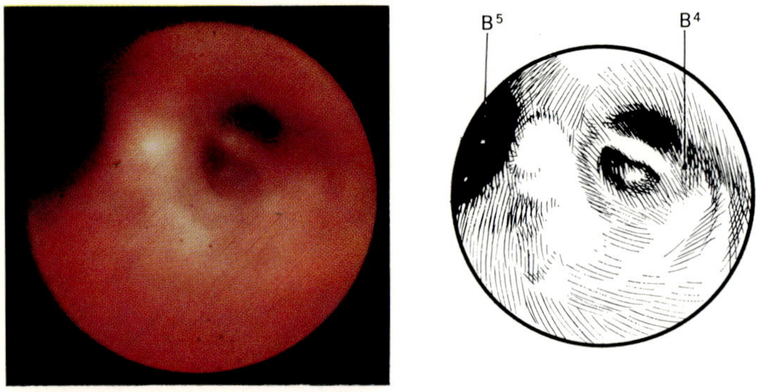


**Fig. 128 Unclearness of bronchial cartilages:** Normally, bronchial catilages are clearly seen; however, in the presence of certain changes such as mucosal thickening, the bronchial cartilages become obscured. The example here shows bronchitis within the middle lobe bronchus. This has caused unclearness of the bronchial cartilages, together with reddening and swelling.

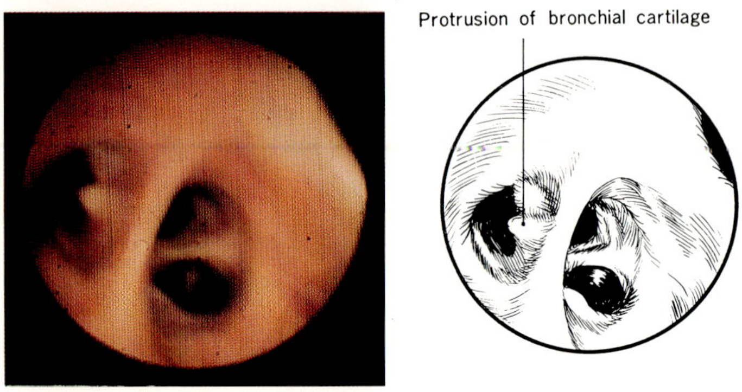


**Fig. 129 Protruding bronchial cartilages:** A protrusion is seen on the right lateral wall very near the orifice of right $B^{10}$. This proved to be an abnormal protrusion of a bronchial cartilage.

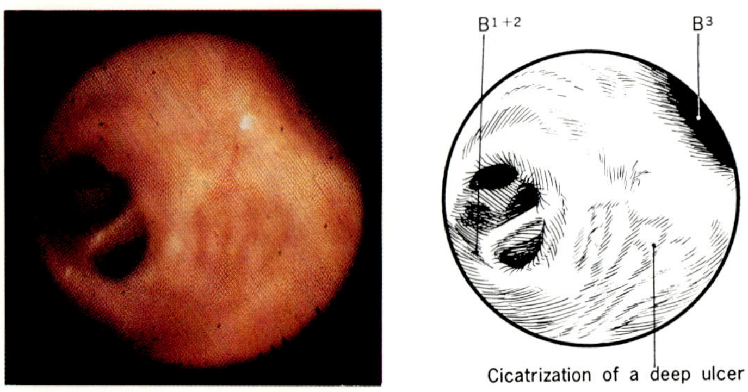


**Fig. 130 Ulcerations:** On the posterior wall near the orifice of the left upper division bronchus a cicatrization of a deep ulcer is present. Occasionally, an anthracotic lymph node may be seen through the bed of a healed ulcer.

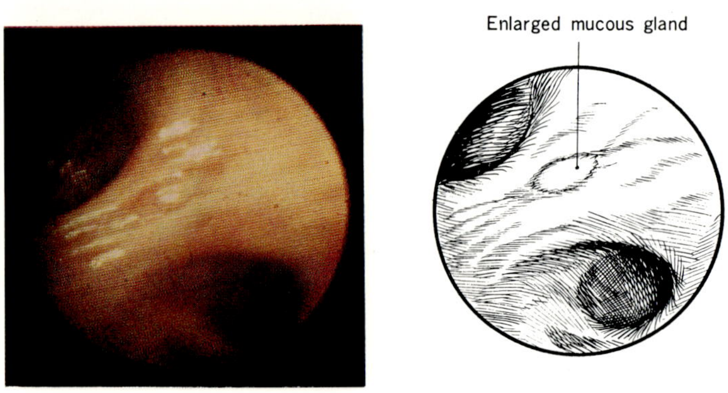


**Fig. 131 Enlarged mucous gland orifices:** This picture shows an enlarged bronchial gland extruding from the septum between the right upper and lower lobe bronchi. Long standing chronic bronchitis can present such a finding.

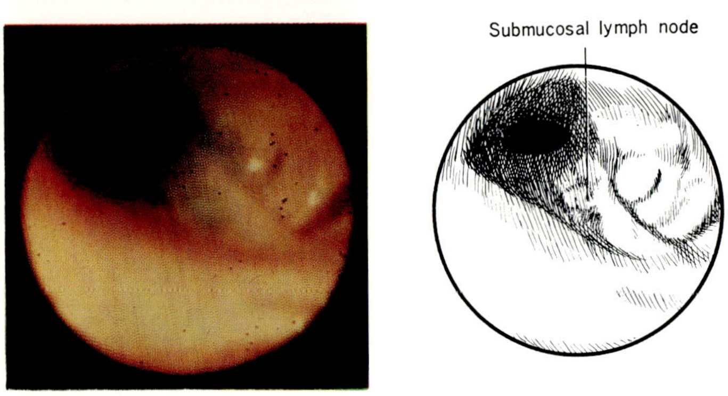


**Fig. 132 Submucosal lymph node:** Lymph node seen through the mucosa; A black lymph node is visible through the right $B^3$ mucosa. An enlarged bronchial gland is also noted just to the left and adjacent to the above. As in Fig. 131, this finding is a feature frequently obtained on patients with chronic bronchitis or chronic pulmonary tuberculosis.

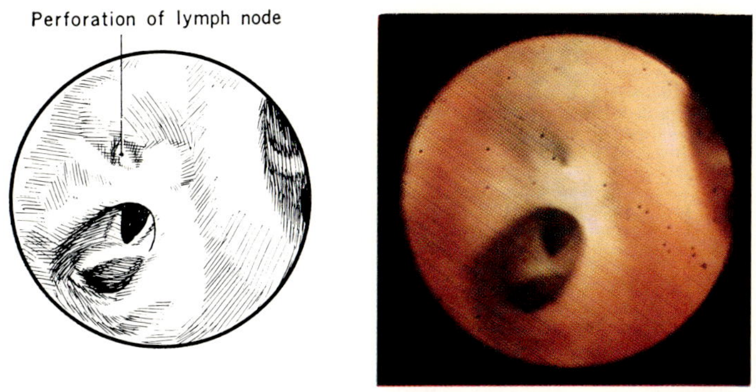


**Fig. 133 Submucosal lymph node :** Perforation of a lymph node; small blackish holes are visible near the orifice of $B^{1+2}$. This is an example of a healed perforated lymph node. Notice the cicatrization around the holes.

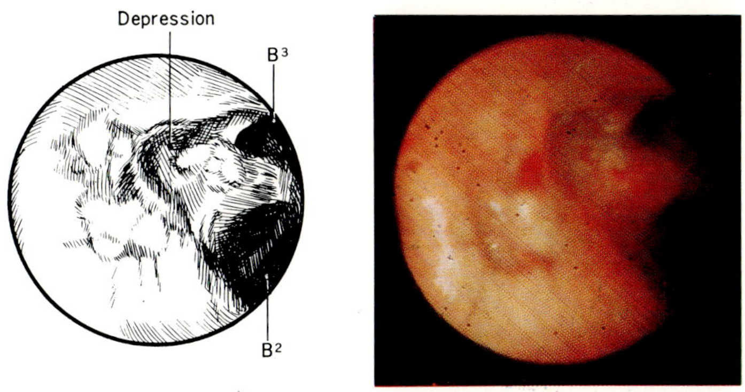


**Fig. 134 Atrophy of the bronchial wall :** Wrinkles are visualized at the entrance of the right upper lobe bronchus and at $B^3$. This is an example of bronchial atrophy.

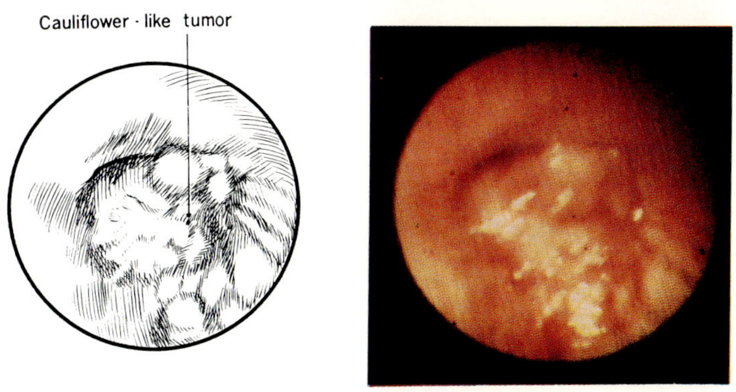


**Fig. 135 Tumor :** Squamous cell carcinoma. Note the irregular cauliflower-like tumor obstructing the right truncus intermedius.

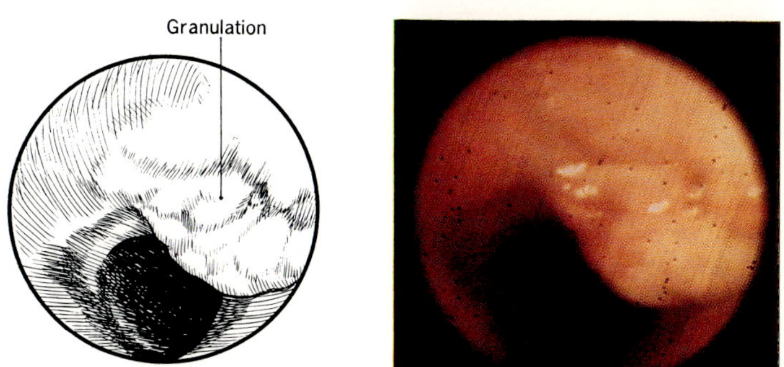


**Fig. 136 Tumor :** Granulation. On the anterior wall of the trachea is located a soft tumor, with a slightly rough, undulating surface. Scrutinize the difference in surface contour as compared with Fig. 135. This is a granuloma due to tracheostomy tube.

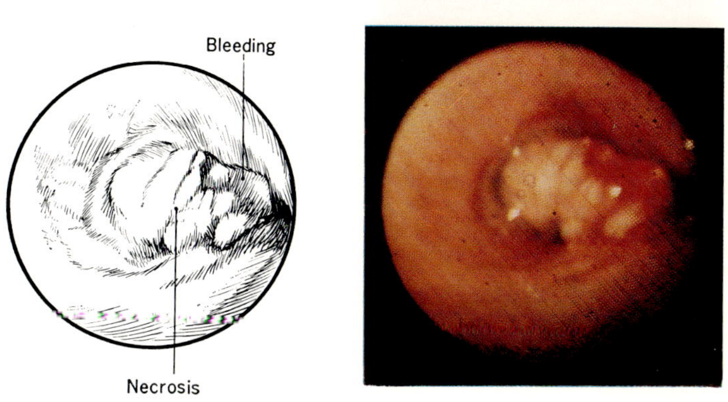


**Fig. 137 Necrosis :** Polyp-like tumor protruding from the truncus intermedius with necrosis on the surface. Pathologically, this was squamous cell carcinoma.

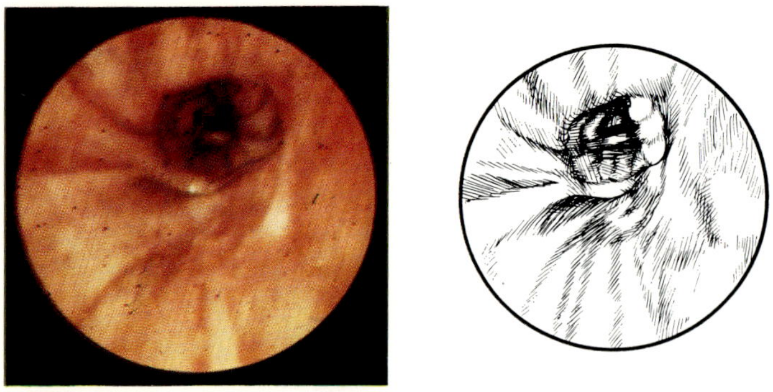

**Fig. 138 Longitudinal infolding:** Longitudinal corrugations are present around the orifice of the right main bronchus with funnel-shaped narrowing. This is one type of bronchial atrophy.

**b. Endobronchial abnormalities**

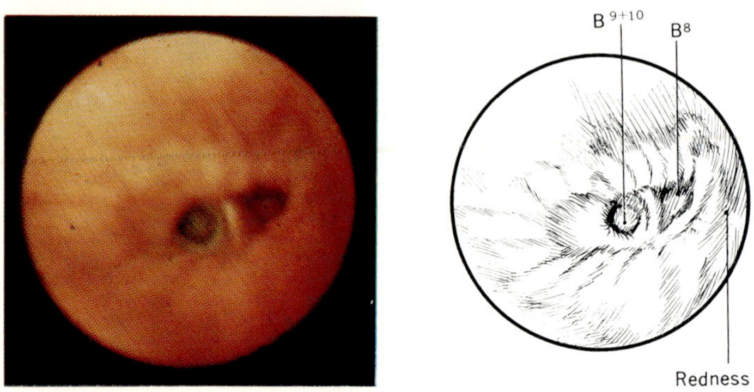


**Fig. 139 Narrowing:** The entire bronchus just proximal to the bifurcation of $B^{8}$ and $B^{9+10}$ is narrowed, forming a lily-like appearance. The narrowed part is slightly reddened.

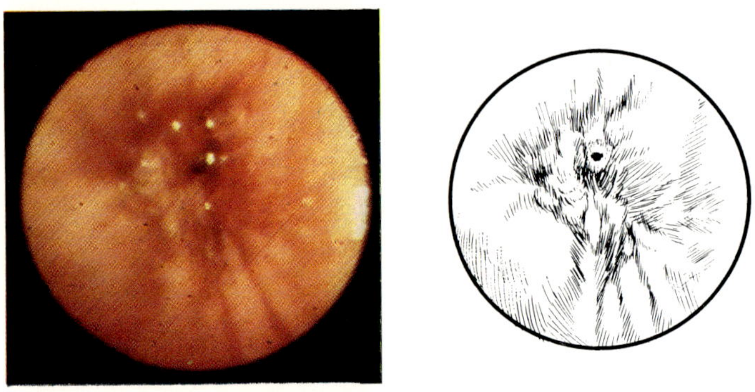

**Fig. 140 Narrowing and infiltration:** The proximal portion of the left upper division bronchus is narrowed by enlarged extrinsic lymph nodes. Distally, the bronchus is narrowed by an exposed tumor. Cartilaginous rings are not visualized. The mucosal surface is irregular and the blood vessels are engorged. These findings are due to carcinomatous infiltration.

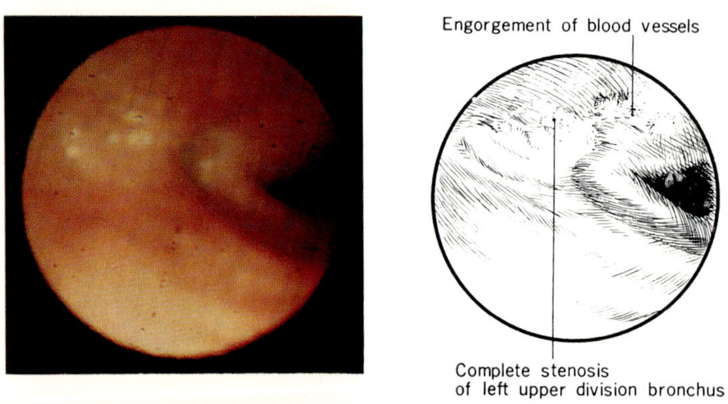


**Fig. 141 Stenosis** (tuberculous): The left upper division bronchus is completely stenosed with reddening and blood vessel engorgement of the surrounding area. Later, the stenosis was confirmed by resection as caused by pulmonary tuberculosis.

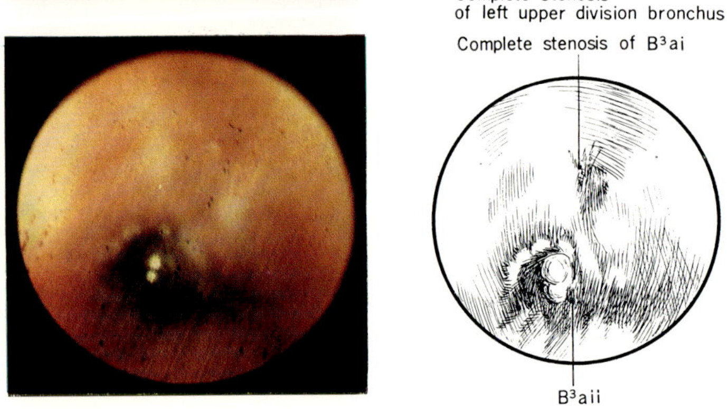


**Fig. 142 Stenosis** (caused by lung cancer): The right $B^{3}$ai is completely stenosed and $B^{3}$aii is partially obstructed by an exposed tumor. Adenocarcinoma frequently causes this type of stenosis.

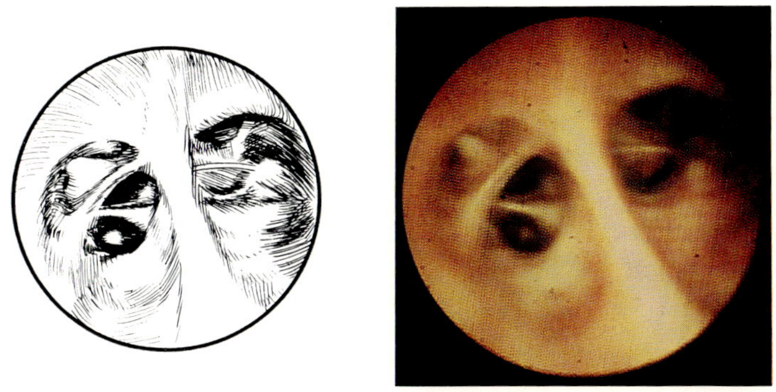

**Fig. 143 Ectasis:** The septa are sharper, enabling one to visualize the distal bronchial divisions easily. This is bronchiectasis.

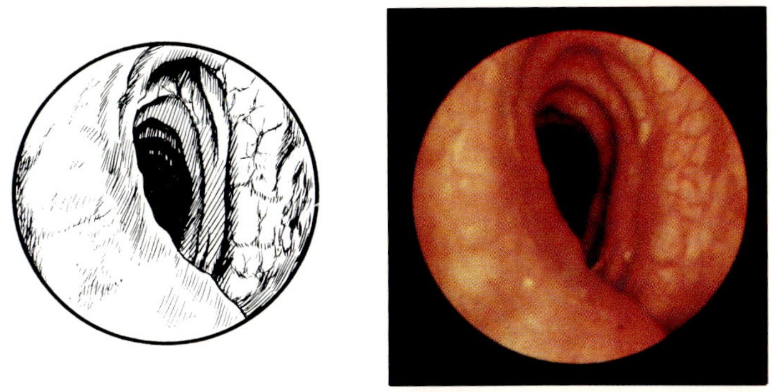

**Fig. 144 Compression of a major bronchus:** The trachea is compressed from the posterior lateral wall and the lumen is distorted to an inverted teardrop form. There is marked engorgement of vessels. This displacement of the trachea is due to a mediastinal tumor.

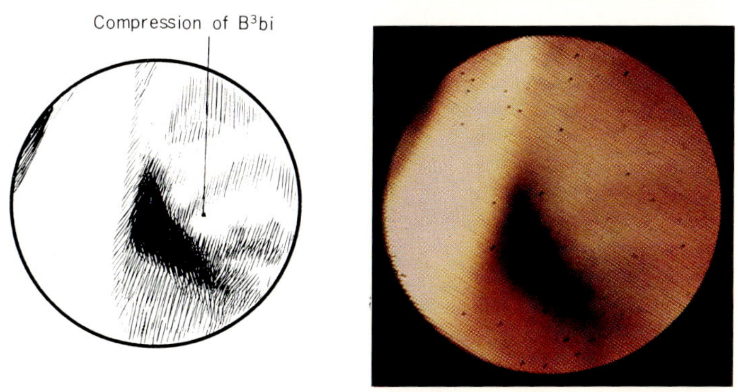


**Fig. 145 Compression of a small bronchus:** The right lateral wall of the right $B^3$bi, though its mucosa is normal, is narrowed by extrinsic pressure. This case was confirmed to be an enlarged pulmonary artery.

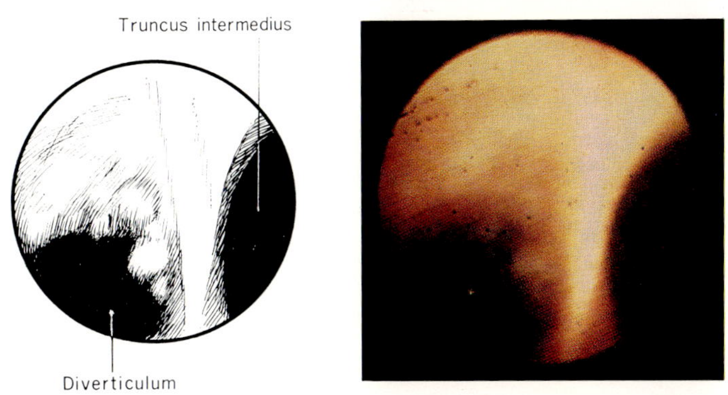


**Fig. 146 Abnormal bifurcation due to a diverticulum:** A diverticulum is located at the left side of the right truncus intermedius. The diverticulum measures about 5 mm in diameter at the orifice and 7 mm in length. This was confirmed by bronchogram.

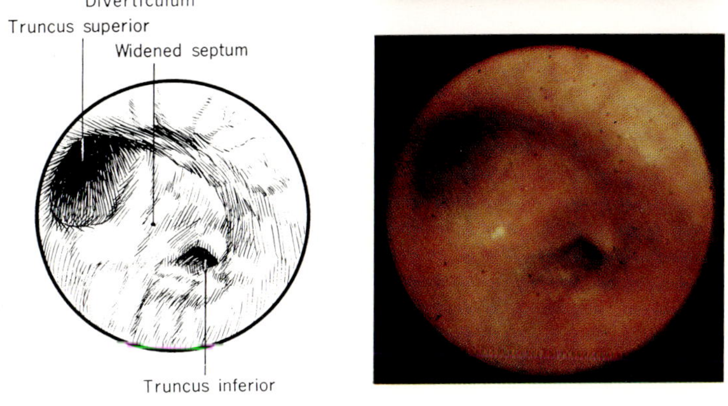


**Fig. 147 Widened septum:** The keel-like widened carina between the truncus superior and inferior of the left upper lobe is so thickened that the two orifices are displaced widely. The truncus inferior is stenosed. A cancerous lymph node was found beneath the bifurcation.

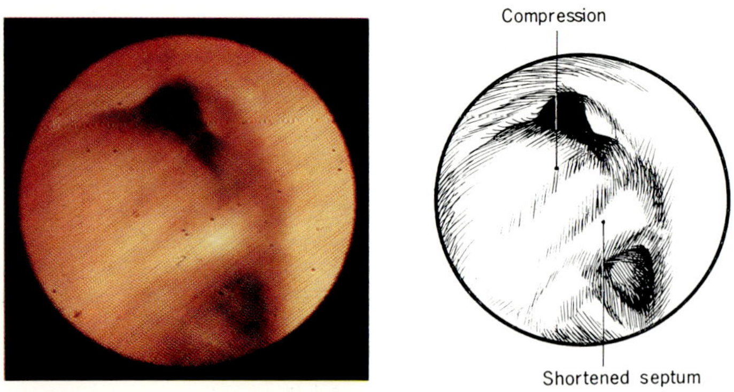


**Fig. 148 Compressed and shortened septum:** The bifurcation, which forms the branching into the left $B^6$ and the truncus basalis, is compressed antero-medially, due to extrinsic pressure from an enlarged gland. Although the bronchial mucosa remains normal, the septum is shortened.

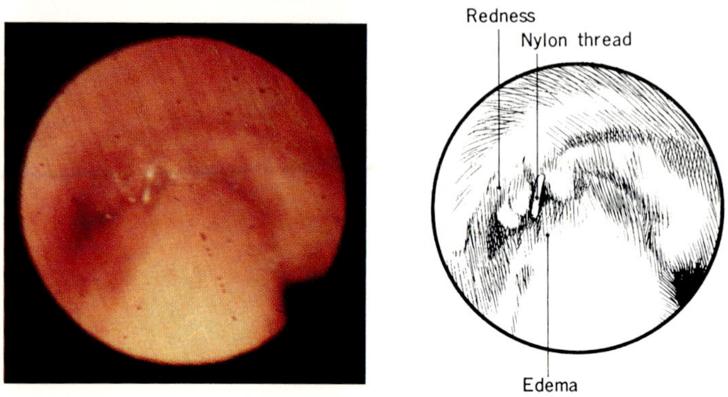


**Fig. 149 Bronchial stump:** The bronchial stump two hours after a left pneumonectomy. Notice the nylon threads. The bronchial stump is reddened and edematous.

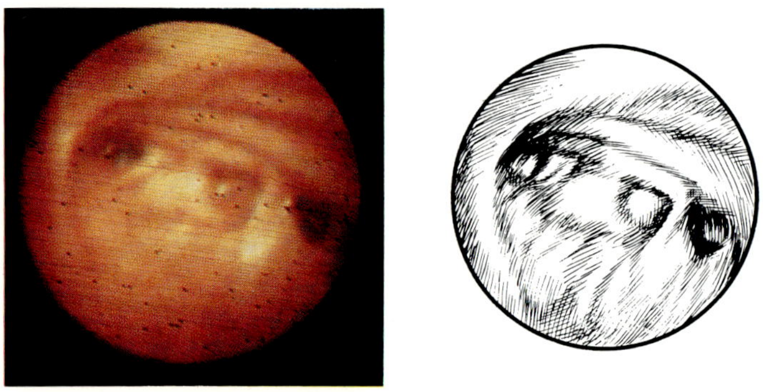

**Fig. 150 Bronchial stump:** A bronchial stump two months after right pneumonectomy, closed by interrupted end sutures. The depressions are not fistulae.

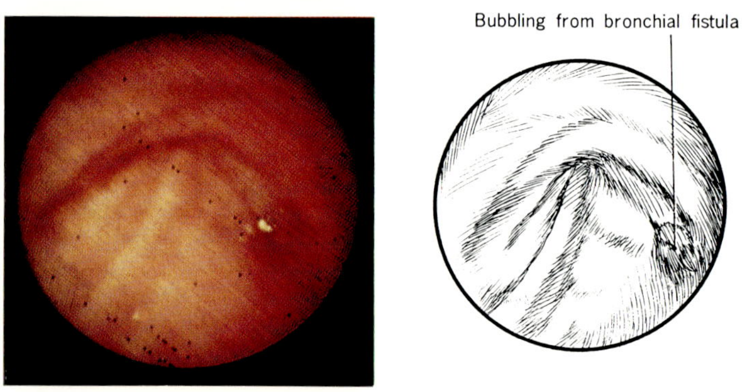


**Fig. 151 Bronchial stump:** A bronchial fistula resulting from a left pneumonectomy. There is redness, swelling and bubbling from the right angle of the wound.

### c. Abnormal substances in the bronchial lumen

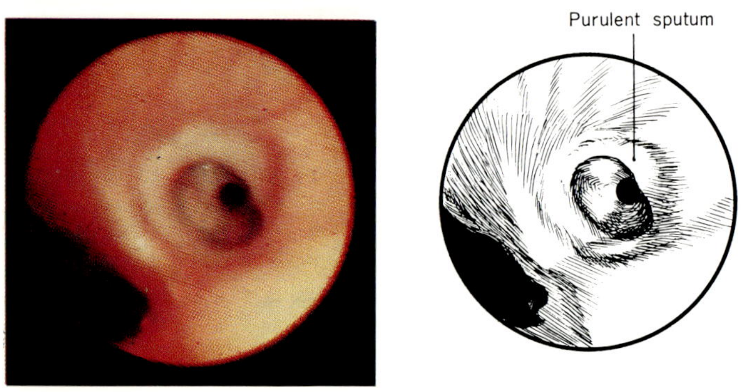


**Fig. 152 Secretions:** Purulent sputum surrounds the orifice to the right $B^8$. Similar picture is noted at the deeper bifurcation.

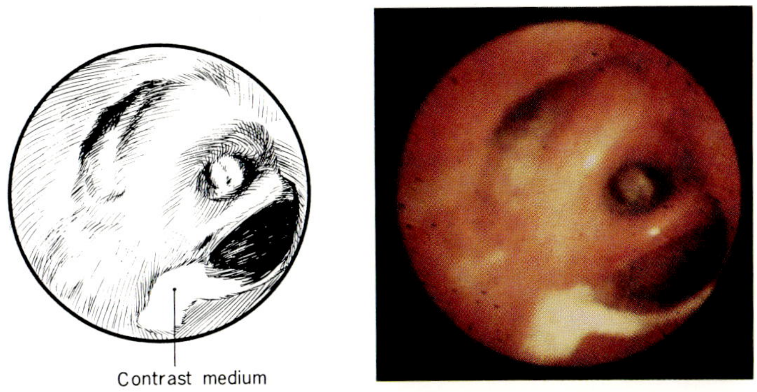


**Fig. 153 Secretions:** The white secretion-like material within the left upper lobe bronchus is residual contrast medium. Secretion on the posterior wall of the upper division bronchus is thin sputum. The entrance to B$^4$ is reddened and swollen. Diagnosis: Pulmonary suppuration.

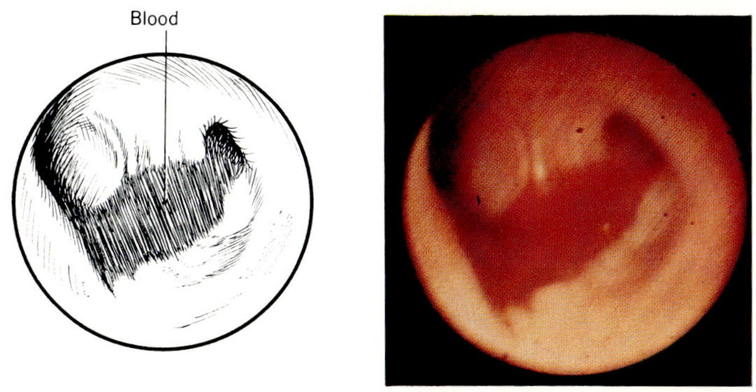


**Fig. 154 Blood:** Lung cancer found in the periphery of the right B$^2$. Blood is seen flowing out of the stenotic upper lobe bronchus into the truncus intermedius.

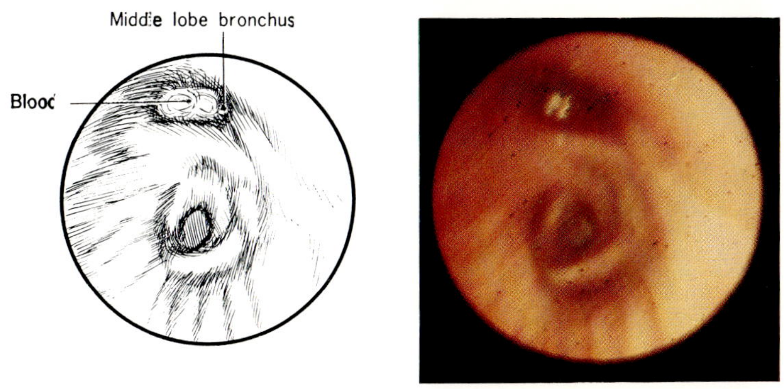


**Fig. 155 Blood:** The middle lobe bronchus is obscured by blood.

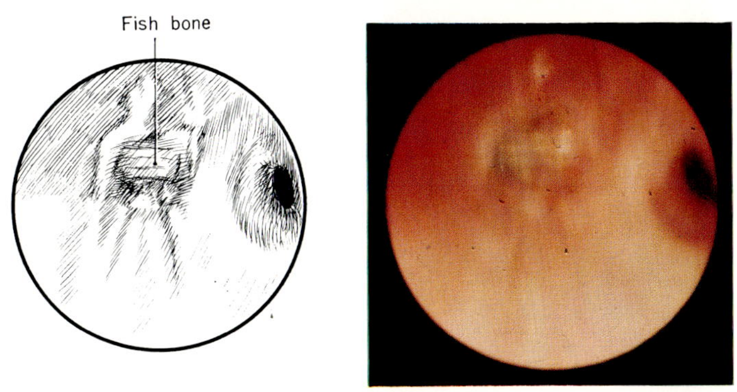


**Fig. 156 Foreign body:** A fish bone impacted into the anterior wall of right B$^8$aii, which is stenosed as the result of inflammation caused by the foreign body.

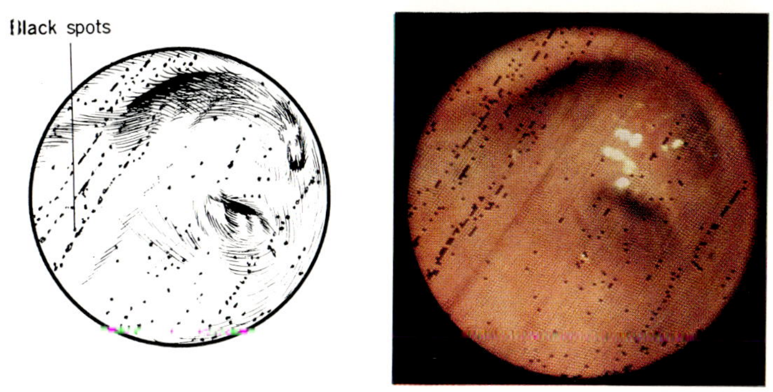


**Fig. 157 Broken glass fibers:** Black spots mean that glass fibers in the body of the bronchoscope are damaged.

# BRONCHOSCOPY REPORT

Patient : __________ Age : _____ Sex : _____

Chart No. : __________ In-patient (Ward No. _____), Out-patient

Premedication : __________ Anesthesia : __________

Intubation : Rigid tube, Flexible tube, Transnasal or Oral

Apparatus : Rigid telescope, Flexible bronchofiberscope (MACHIDA, OLYMPUS)

Pathology { Histologic specimen, Cytologic specimen<br>Instruments : Rigid brush, Flexible brush, Small biopsy forceps, Small currettes, Washing, Others

Bacteriology : Routine, T. B. B., Fungal, Others

Records { Camera : Olympus-Pen F, Olympus SC-16, Kowa camera SQ, Others<br>Cine-film : 8 mm, 16 mm<br>Color T. V. : V. T. R.

| Bronchoscopic findings | | Tumor | Necrosis | Ulcer | Infiltration | | | Obstruction | Stenosis | Compression | Redness | Swelling | | | | Normal |
|---|---|---|---|---|---|---|---|---|---|---|---|---|---|---|---|---|
| | | | | | Engorgement of blood vessels | Irregular mucosa | Unclearness of br. cartilage | | | | | | | | | |
| Affected br. | | | | | | | | | | | | | | | | |
| Related br. | | | | | | | | | | | | | | | | |
| | | | | | | | | | | | | | | | | |
| | | | | | | | | | | | | | | | | |

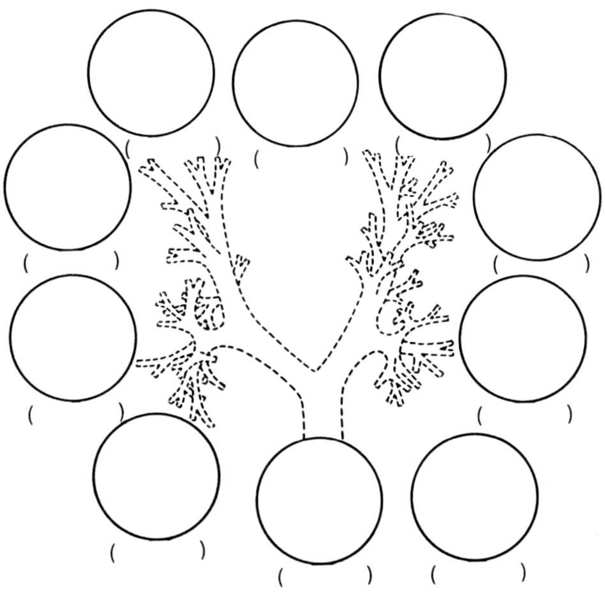

Bronchoscopic diagnosis : __________

Location of the lesions : __________ (Bronchial degree : _____)

Examiner : __________ Sign : __________

**Fig. 158** This is the English version of the form which is used in the National Cancer Center Hospital, Tokyo. The schematization of the bronchofiberscopic findings is absolutely indispensable together with the branching order of the lesions in any of the ten circles. It is also necessary for the cine film and/or the camera film to be conveniently classified for the bronchial findings to be well grasped more accurately.

# VII. Achievements with the Flexible Bronchofiberscope in Lung Cancer

## CASES OF LUNG CANCER

Seven hundred and forty-three cases of lung cancer were examined at the National Cancer Center Hospital during the 4 years from January, 1967 to December, 1970. Of these 743 cases, 676 (91 %) were subjected to bronchoscopic examination. The flexible bronchofiberscope was utilized in most of these cases, except for a few cases in the early part of 1969 with tumors in the major bronchi, when the conventional rigid bronchoscope was used. The 67 cases who were not bronchoscoped were either too ill to tolerate the procedure or refused to undergo the examination.

## CLASSIFICATION OF BRONCHOSCOPIC FINDINGS IN LUNG CANCER

In Chapter VI, a classification of bronchoscopic findings has been listed. In lung cancer, it may be advantageous to adopt another classification of bronchoscopic findings which are directly or indirectly associated with the tumor.

*A. Findings directly associated with lung cancer*

1) Tumor
   a. Tumor mass
   b. Necrosis
2) Infiltration
   a. Engorgement of blood vessels
   b. Irregularity of the bronchial mucosa
   c. Unclearness (indistinct) of the cartilage
3) Obstruction

*B. Findings indirectly associated with lung cancer*

1) Stenosis
2) Narrowing or compression
3) Swelling
4) Redness

*C. No findings or other findings*

Of the above findings, the most disputable is "infiltration" (A-2). In infiltration due to lung cancer, it is important to stress that all three findings are present ; (namely, a : engorgement of blood vessels, b : irregularity of the bronchial mucosa and c : unclearness of the bronchial cartilages). On the other hand, in inflammatory conditions such as pulmonary tuberculosis or bronchitis one may find just one or two of these infiltrative changes.

"Obstruction" (A-3) itself is a primary pathological condition but oftentimes it is difficult to distinguish it from post inflammatory cicatricial stenosis. If obstructive stenosis is coexistent with the three changes mentioned under "infiltration", this is further corroborative evidence in favor of lung cancer.

## BRONCHOSCOPIC FINDINGS AND THEIR LOCATIONS

The locations of the abnormal bronchial findings are plotted diagrammatically (Fig. 159). Of the 676 cases, 558 (82.7 %) had positive direct findings indicative of cancer distributed throughout the bronchial tree from the major bronchi to IV and V order of branching. The bronchoscopic findings were negative in 45 (6.6%)

out of 676 cases of lung cancer. With the conventional rigid bronchoscope, the detection rate was less than one half (30 to 40 %) of that obtained with the flexible instrument.

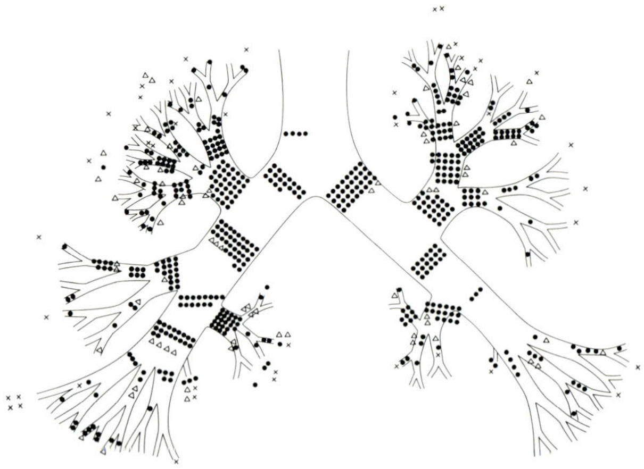

• Direct findings····558 cases (82.7%)
△ Indirect findings···73 cases (10.8%)
× Invisible··················45 cases (6.6%)
Total·······················676 cases

**Fig. 159** Locations of abnormal findings in lung cancer.

# RELATIONSHIP BETWEEN BRONCHOFIBERSCOPIC FINDINGS AND HISTOPATHOLOGICAL CLASSIFICATION

Of these 743 cases, squamous cell carcinoma was found in 305 (41.0%); adenocarcinoma in 264 (35.5%); undifferentiated large cell carcinoma in 118 (16.0%) undifferentiated small cell carcinoma in 52 (7.0%), and others, 4 (0.5%) cases. These figures include those cases that were not bronchoscoped.

| Order of branching | 0–I | II | III | IV | V | VI– |
|---|---|---|---|---|---|---|
| –20 (mm) | ●●● | ●●●●● □□ | □ | | | ×× |
| 21–30 | ●●●●● ●●●●● ※ | ●●●●● △△ | ●●●● □ △ ※ | ● △△ | ● □□□ △ | ××× ※ |
| 31–40 | ●●●●● ●●●●● □ ×× | ●●●●● ●● □□ △△ × | ●●●● × | ●● □□ × | □ △ | △ × ※ |
| 41–60 | ●●●●● ●●●●● ●●●●● ●●●●● ●● □ △△ ※※ | ●●●●● ●●●●● ●●●●● ●●●●● ●●● □□□ △△△ × ※※ | ●●●●● ●●●●● ●●●● □□□□□ □ △ ×× ※ | ● □□ △ ※ | ● × ※※ | ×× ※ |
| 61– | ●●●●● ●●●●● ●● □ △△△ | ●●●●● ●●●●● ●●● □□ △ ×× | ●● □□□ △ | ●●●● □ | | ● × ※ |
| Atelectasis | ●●●●● ●●●●● ●●●●● ●●●●● ●●●●● ●●●●● ●●●●● ● □□□□□ □□ △ ×× | ●●●●● ●● □□□ × | ● × | | | |
| Infiltrative tumor | ●●●●● ●●●● | ●● □ | ● | | | |

● Tumor visualized □ Obstruction △ Stenosis
× No finding ※ Unexamined

**Fig. 160** Locations and sizes in squamous cell carcinoma.

### a. Squamous cell carcinoma (Fig. 160)

Fourteen of the 305 cases were not bronchoscoped. Tumors were visualized in 201 (69 %) out of the 291 cases subjected to bronchoscopy. Obstructions were noted in 43 (15 %); narrowing or compression in 23 (8 %) and negative findings in 24 (8 %).

When these tumors are analyzed to their size and location in the bronchial tree, 164 cases (81.6 %) were visualized in the major, lobar or segmental (II order of branching) bronchi. Tumors of any size may occur at any position in the branching order. In the presence of atelectasis, an exposed tumor is a characteristic finding by bronchoscopy.

### b. Adenocarcinoma (Fig. 161)

Of the 264 cases of adenocarcinoma, 31 were not bronchoscoped. Of the 233 cases bronchoscoped, tumors were found in 72 cases (31.0 %); obstruction in 97 cases (41.6 %); stenosis in 32 cases (13.7 %) and in 32 cases (13.7%) the examinations were entirely negative.

In general, in the major and segmental bronchi, the tumors themselves can be recognized. However, beyond this level, the presenting finding is usually an obstruc-

| Order of branching | 0-I | II | III | IV | V | VI- |
|---|---|---|---|---|---|---|
| -20(mm) | ● | △ | ● □□□□ △ ※ | ● □□□ × ※ | ● □ | □ ××××× ※ |
| 21-30 | ● | ●●●●● □ △ | ● □ △△△ | ●●● □□□□□ □□□□ △ ×× ※※※ | ● □□ △ ×××× ※※※ | △ ××××× ×× |
| 31-40 | ●●●● □□□ | ●●●●● ●●●●● ●● □□□□□ □□ △ ※ | ●●●●● □□□□□ □□□ △△△ × | ●●● □□□□□ □□□□□ □ △ | □□□ △ × ※ | ××××× ※※ |
| 41-60 | ●●● □ ※ | ●●●●● ●●●● □□□□□ □□□□□ □ △△ | □□□□□ □□ △△ ※※ | ● □□□□□ □□□ △△△ ※ | ● □ ×× ※ | ××× ※※※ |
| 61- | | ● □□ △ | ●●● □□□□□ △△ ※ | △ ※※※ | □ △ × | |
| Atelectasis | ●●●●● ●●● □□ ※※※※ | ● □□ | ● | | | |
| Infiltrative tumor | ●●●●● □□ △△ ※ | □ △△△ | | | ※ | |

● Tumor visualized □ Obstruction △ Stenosis
× No finding ※ Unexamined

**Fig. 161** Locations and sizes in adenocarcinoma.

| Order of branching | 0-I | II | III | IV | V | VI- |
|---|---|---|---|---|---|---|
| -20(mm) | | | ●● | | ※ | |
| 21-30 | □ ※ | ●● | ●● | ● | △ ※※ | ×× |
| 31-40 | ●●●●● ●● | ●●● □□ | ●● □□ | ● □□ ※ | □□ △ ※ | ※ |
| 41-60 | ●●●●● ●●● □ ※ | ●●●●● △△ ※※※ | ●●●●● ●● □□ | ● □□ | ● △△ ※ | △ × ※ |
| 61- | ●●●●● ● ※ | ●●● □□ | ●●● □ △△ ※ | □ ※ | | |
| Atelectasis | ●●●●● ●● □□□ △△ ※※ | △△ | | | | |
| Infiltrative tumor | ※ | □ | | | | |

● Tumor visualized □ Obstruction △ Stenosis
× No finding ※ Unexamined

**Fig. 162** Locations and sizes in undifferentiated large cell carcinoma.

tion. On the other hand, usually, the lesion of adenocarcinoma is not often recognizable bronchscopically as a tumor but as an obstruction. The adjacent part of the bronchus is normally obstructed, with vascular engorgement, irregular mucosa and unclearness of the bronchial cartilages. A tumor is sometimes dimly seen in the deeper part of such obstructions.

**c. Undifferentiated large cell carcinoma** (Fig. 162)

Ninteen of the 118 cases of undifferentiated large cell carcinoma were not bronchoscoped. Bronchoscopically, tumor was found in 61 cases (62%); obstruction in 22 cases (22%); stenosis in 13 cases (13%) and negative findings in 3 cases (3%).

A large cell carcinoma may be found in any part of the bronchus. When seen through the flexible bronchofiberscope, its appearance is intermediate between squamous cell carcinoma and adenocarcinoma. Furthermore, it often presents as a polyp which can be recognized bronchoscopically. In some cases, infiltration of the base of the polyp can be demonstrated.

## CYTOLOGICAL ACHIEVEMENTS WITH A FLEXIBLE BRONCHOFIBERSCOPE

Instruments for obtaining cytological specimens have evolved through three stages. During the first period from January to December, 1967, the implement was a "drill", needle with a small head (p. 14; Fig. 24). From January, 1968 to June, 1969, a small brush was utilized. During the last period, a small hinged curette and a small biopsy forceps were developed. The choice between these two latter instruments depends upon the location and type of lesion (p.47). Fig. 163 lists the years when the various instruments were used, and the rates of definitive diagnoses yielded by the respective instruments. It is noted that with the "drill", the positive yield was 73% (54 out of 74 cases). During the second period when the brush was utilized, the positive yield increased to 83.4% (126 out of 151cases). With the small curette and biopsy forceps, the definitive diagnostic rate has been further improved to 90.3% (165 out of 183 cases). According to the newest data during the recent two years between Jan. 1971–Dec. 1972, the definitive diagnostic rate has been improved to 95.7% (242 out of 253 cases).

There are two reasons for this improvement of positive yield. During the first and second periods, cytological specimens were obtained by Tsuboi's transbronchial biopsy method, using the "drill" or brush through Metra's catheter under fluoroscopy. In the third and fourth period, the small implements were passed through the flexible bronchofiberscope and so utilized.

The second reason for the improved positive yield is that, in addition to the above, the flexible bronchofiberscope can be maneuvered with exactness. If a tumor is exposed, biopsy can be performed under direct vision. If not, the small curette can be advanced precisely to the focus under X-ray TV fluoroscopy and a specimen obtained.

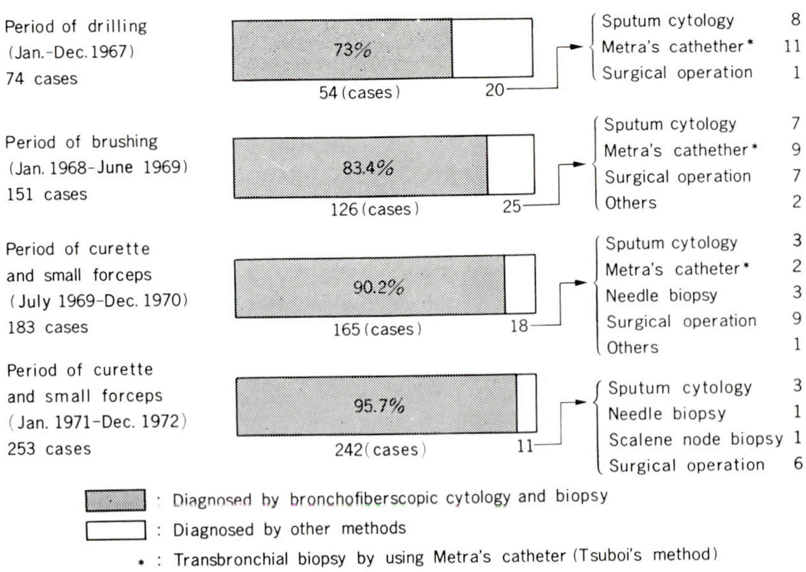


**Fig. 163** Rates of definitive diagnoses of lung cancer (since the development of bronchofiberscope).

# DEFINITION OF EARLY LUNG CANCER

Early lung cancer, surgically excised, implies a complete cure and a normal survival. In defining early lung cancer,one must consider three factors : 1) the presence or absence of metastases, 2) the survival rate and 3) location of the lesion. It is difficult to determine whether or not a tumor can be classified as early lung cancer by presurgical findings, by a study of the surgical specimen, or even inspection of the intrathoracic cavity because of the possible presence of distant metastases.

We have studied the relationship of tumor size with the incidence of lymph node metastasis (Fig. 164). In tumors less than 20 mm in diameter, the incidence of lymph node metastasis was 0.9 % ; whereas in tumors larger than 20 mm in diameter, the incidence of lymph node metastasis rose to more than 35.0 %. This led us to the present definition of early lung cancer : the tumor in the resected specimen being less than 20 mm in diameter, with no evidence of pleural metastasis (P0), no lymph node metastasis (L0) and no distant metastasis (M0).

Let us examine the 5 year survival rates of two groups : 1) those cases of early lung cancer with no determinable metastasis (P0, N0 and M0) and 2) those cases in which there is evidence of metastasis in at least one of the three locations : P, N and M. In the former group, the survival rate is far greater than 2), being 80 %. However, in defining early lung cancer, since complete cure and normal survival are expected, it seems that the present definition must be altered. We propose that in early lung cancer, the tumor must be measured less than 10 mm in the resected specimen. Such cases might truly be representative of early lung cancer.

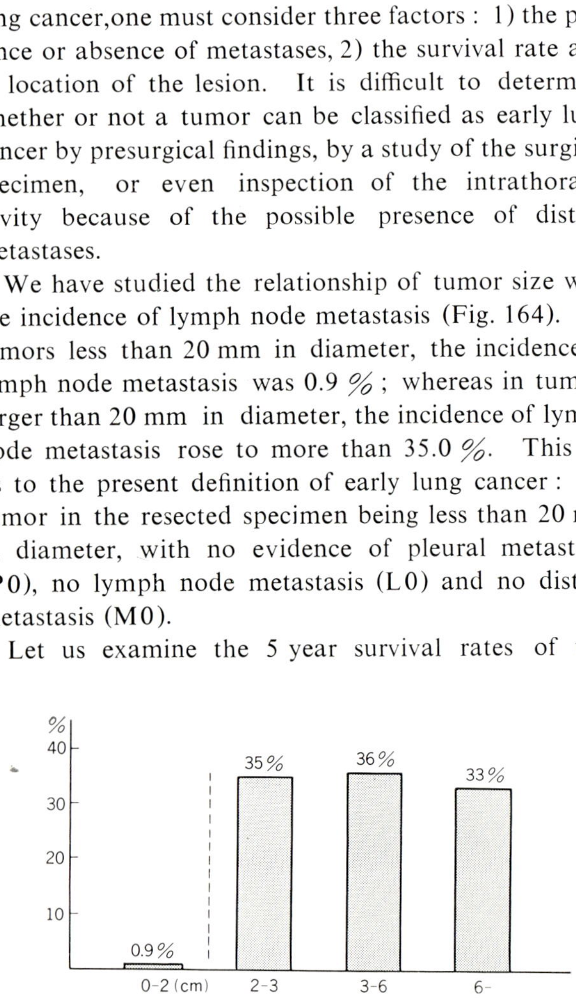


**Fig. 164** Tumor size and lymph node metastasis (E. Tsuboi, 1970).

The traditional definition "less than 20 mm in diameter in the resected specimen" is applicable only if the focus is in the peripheral part of the lung. If the lesion is located near the hilum and the tumor is growing within the wall of a major bronchus, the definition is usually not applicable as the tumor may not be identifiable in a routine chest X-ray. Papanicolaou in 1951 coined the term "occult carcinoma" in patients with a positive sputum cytology and negative chest X-rays. Locating these lesions have up to now been the clinician's dilemma. However, the flexible bronchofiberscope has greatly simplified the problem of seeking out exact location of these lesions.

As the result of our clinical experiences with these various tum. s, we are defining hilar and peripheral early lung cancers separately :

1) An early lung cancer of the hilar type is a case in which histopathologically the tumor remains within the bronchial wall with P0, N0 and M0.
2) The peripheral type of early lung cancer is defined as a case in which the tumor is less than 20 mm in diameter with P0, N0 and M0.

# RESULTS ON EARLY LUNG CANCER

Among 1,013 cases of primary lung cancer from 1962 to 1972, 19 cases were categorized as early lung cancer in accordance with the definition described in the chapter VI.

These 19 cases can be further classified into various categories. By location 8 were hilar type and 11 peripheral. By combined histology and location, the hilar types were all squamous cell carcinoma, while the peripheral types were varied —2 squamous cell carcinoma, 8 adenocarcinoma and 1 large cell carcinoma (Table 3).

**Table 3** Classification of Early Lung Cancer (National Cancer Center).

| | Hilar type (lesion is localized within segmental bronchus) | Peripheral type (lesion is localized more peripherally than subsegmental bronchus) |
|---|---|---|
| July 1962–Dec. 1966 | 2 | 4 |
| Jan. 1967–Dec. 1972 | 6 | 7 |
| Total | 8 | 11 |
| Squamous cell carcinoma | 8 | 2 |
| Adenocarcinoma | — | 8 |
| Large cell carcinoma | — | 1 |
| Total | 8 | 11 |

Since our successful introduction of a flexible bronchofiberscope in 1966 the new endoscope has been utilized clinically. This has greatly improved the diagnostic rate of lung cancer at its early stage. The numbers of detected cases during 4.5 years from the latter half of 1962 to the end of 1966, will be compared with those detected during 6 years from 1967 to the end of 1972. Cases of hilar type, for instance, discovered in the former 4.5 years were 2, while in the latter 6 years, the number increased to 6. This increase is presumed to be attributed to the improved facilities for the diagnosis of early lung cancer of the hilar type.

Consideration will be directed to survivals in the early lung cancer up to the present (Table 4). Patients with the hilar type are all surviving and, of 11 patients with the peripheral type, 10 are still living. Of course, it must be admitted that the estimation is not definitive since these are relatively recent cases.

**Table 4** Prognosis of Early Lung Cancer (diameter less than 20 mm).

| | | Hilar type | Peripheral type |
|---|---|---|---|
| P 0, N 0 | Alive | 8 | 10 (3) |
| | Dead | 0 | 1 (1) |
| | Total | 8 | 11 (4) |
| P (+), N (+) | Alive | 0 | 5 (2) |
| | Dead | 4 | 14 (4) |
| | Total | 4 | 19 (6) |

( ): Survivals of peripheral type over five years.

Cases in which the diameter of the resected tumor is less than 20 mm yet whose P and N are both +, will be compared. The statistics show that all 4 cases of hilar type died but that 5 of the peripheral type are surviving with 14 dead. It will be understood that, even if the diameter of tumor is less than 20 mm, cases which fall in the category of early lung cancer in terms of P and N (both zero) and cases P (+) and N (+) make definite differences in survival rate. As Table 4 shows, 5-year survival rates are listed in brackets only for cases of the peripheral type. In the right column of the upper figures 3 cases of early lung cancer out of 4 are still living. That is, the longer than 5-year survival rate is as high as 75 %. On the other hand, as the right column of the lower figures show, 2 cases out of 6 are still living (both cases being P (+), N (+), diameter less than 20 mm). This shows lower survival rate as compared with the rate of P 0, N 0, peripheral type.

# CHARACTERISTICS OF EARLY LUNG CANCER OF HILAR TYPE

Of the 8 cases of early lung cancer, hilar type, 2 were diagnosed before the flexible bronchofiberscope was developed, and 6 after. This implies that the increase in number of diagnoses may be attributed to the use of the flexible bronchofiberscope. One may argue that carcinomatous manifestations are present in areas where they may be visualized with a rigid bronchoscope. Yet the increase in number, the author believes, should be ascribed to the efficiency and accuracy in discovering carcinoma with the flexible bronchofiberscope.

A few common features are found among these cases.

1) Patients are in general older than 40 and mostly males.
2) They are all smokers, consuming more than 20 cigarettes a day. Some are heavy smokers consuming more than 50 cigarettes a day.
3) All the patients have sputum slightly stained with blood. This was their chief complaint.

**Table 5** Hilar Type of Early Lung Cancer.

| Total | July, 62–Dec., 66 | Jan., 67–Dec. 72 |
|---|---|---|
| 9 | 2 | 7 |

Chest X-ray Finding

| Negative | Atelectasis | Obstractive pneumonia |
|---|---|---|
| 3 | 3 | 3 |

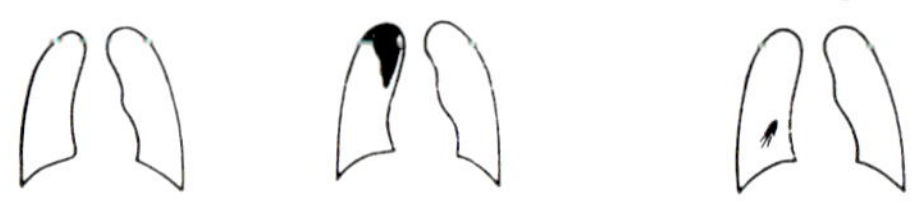

4) Their chest X-ray films reveal a minimum of abnormal shadows. For example: 3 cases show no abnormality, 3 cases show a very slight tumor shadow, and 3 cases a shadow suggestive of pneumonitis obliterans (Table 5).
5) Some definitive abnormality or abnormalities were found by bronchofiberscopy. Bronchofiberscopic cytology and histology were positive for cancer cells in all cases.
6) Pathologic findings obtained from the resected lung have been those of squamous cell carcinoma. Tumors are all localized and limited to the bronchial wall, without infiltration into the lung parenchyma.

The postoperative follow up of these cases of early lung cancer is relatively short, ranging from one to five years. They are all squamous cell carcinoma, and a longer survival period is expected.

## HOW TO FIND EARLY LUNG CANCER

No discussion is necessary that unless discovered at an early stage, lung cancer cannot be treated successfully. The recent improvements in the techniques of diagnosing lung cancer are matter of marvel. The bronchofiberscope in particular, has enabled not only the early discovery of lung cancer of the hilar type, but also the definitive diagnosis of peripheral lesions has been made much easier. The recent mass survey of cancer by means of photofluorography was conducted concurrently with the survey for pulmonary tuberculosis. As a result of this survey, some cases of early *peripheral* types of lung cancer were discovered. However, discovery of early *hilar* tumors is very difficult, as a tumor smaller than 15 mm in diameter in the hilar region is rarely demonstrable in chest roentgenogram. This suggests that two separate procedures must be established for finding (a) early *peripheral* tumors and (b) early *hilar* tumors.

### a. Procedures for finding early peripheral lung cancer (Fig. 165)

Any abnormal peripheral shadow on the chest X-ray appearing in the semi-annual mass survey should be initially studied by tomograms, then by bronchograms. The bronchography must be selective, with the contrast medium entering the peripheral branch bronchi for accurate localization. Following this, bronchofiberscopic curettage of the lesion under fluoroscopic guidance is performed to obtain a specimen for cytologic diagnosis. Persistent efforts to improve one's skill and technique will be rewarded by a diagnostic accuracy rate approaching 80 % even in early peripheral lung cancers. However, if the cytology proves negative though the lesion is still highly suspicious of cancer, one may resort to needle biopsy under fluoroscopic control. Lastly, exploratory thoracotomy may be necessary in some cases for diagnosis and treatment.

### b. Procedures for finding early hilar lung cancer (Fig. 166)

The X-ray film is usually negative in the early cancer of the hilar type. However, one often finds increased linear markings which may fan out from the hilar region where the tumor is located, suggesting a pneumonitis. This, we feel, is a very important clue in finding an early hilar tumor.

Early peripheral tumors rarely give rise to symptoms. Contrariwise, in early hilar tumors, subjective symptoms such as a chronic long-standing cough, expectoration of sputum which is often blood streaked, may occur. If these symptoms occur in a heavy smoker or in one exposed to industrial hazards in the form of bronchial irritants, they should not be neglected. Any of these symptoms or X-ray findings should lead one to suspect a hilar tumor.

Initially, repeated cytological examinations of the sputum are done. We have been interested in the technique of Frost of Johns Hopkins University, who has been utilizing sputum induced with Hanks' solution in an isolated booth for this purpose. Any patient reported to have a sputum cytology of Papanicolaou Class III or higher is subjected to a bronchofiberscopic

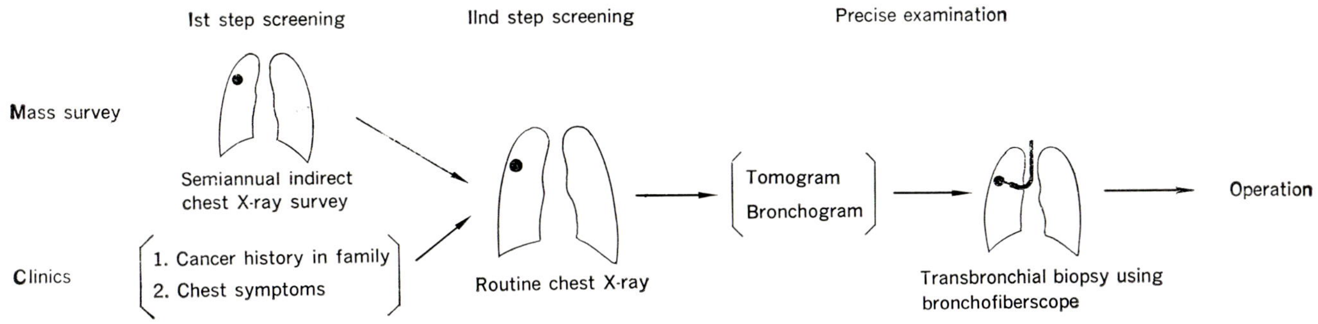


**Fig. 165** Diagnostic procedures of peripheral lung cancer.

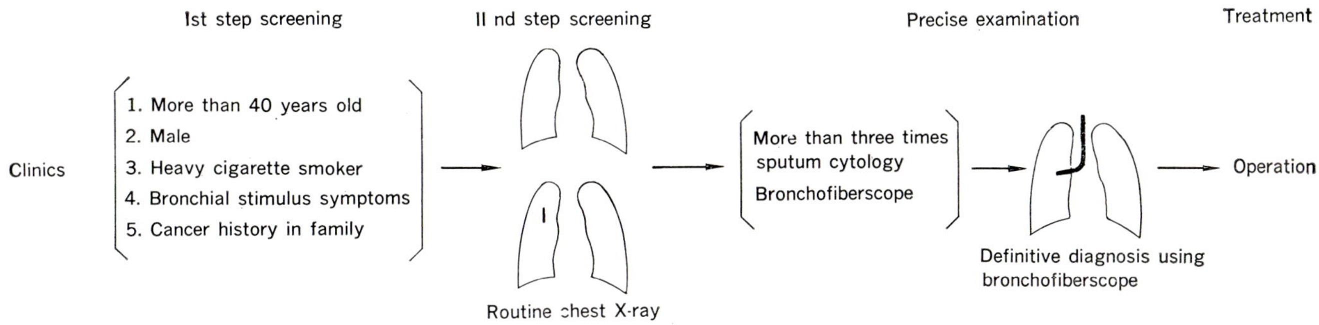


**Fig. 166** Diagnostic procedures of hilar lung cancer.

examination. Furthermore, any male over the age of 40, who has a long standing cough and is a heavy smoker must undergo a bronchofiberscopy in order to find an early hilar lung cancer. This is particularly the case if he has been raising blood streaked sputum.

In conclusion, in order to discover early lung cancer of the hilar type, diagnostic priority is first placed on the patient's subjective symptoms and then his environmental conditions must be taken into consideration.

# VIII. Therapeutic Bronchofiberscopy

## SIGNIFICANCE

Therapeutic roles played by bronchofiberscopy include:

1) Removal of foreign bodies
2) Aspiration and removal of sputa or secretions
3) Bouginage of narrowed or occluded portions of the bronchus
4) Local application of therapeutic agents
5) Emergency relief of airway obstruction

Since foreign bodies in most cases lodge in a major bronchus, the conventional rigid bronchoscope can be used to better advantage than the bronchofiberscope, the larger lumen of the former allowing the use of larger forceps. However, if a foreign body is lodged more peripherally in a segmental or a smaller bronchus, the bronchofiberscope is advisable (as in case 57, Part II).

Therapeutically, the bronchofiberscope is utilized for aspiration and removal of secretions, and also for the local application of medications. In the United States in recent times, the bronchofiberscope is frequently used therapeutically to relieve airway obstruction due to thick secretions, particularly in pulmonary diseases characterized by inadequate ventilation, such as in pulmonary suppuration, bronchiectasis, chronic bronchitis and pulmonary emphysema. Another important and effective use of the bronchofiberscope is in treating and relieving postoperative atelectasis. Thus in the following, the importance of bronchofiberscopy in relieving bronchial obstruction and inadequate ventilation will be emphasized (Fig. 167).

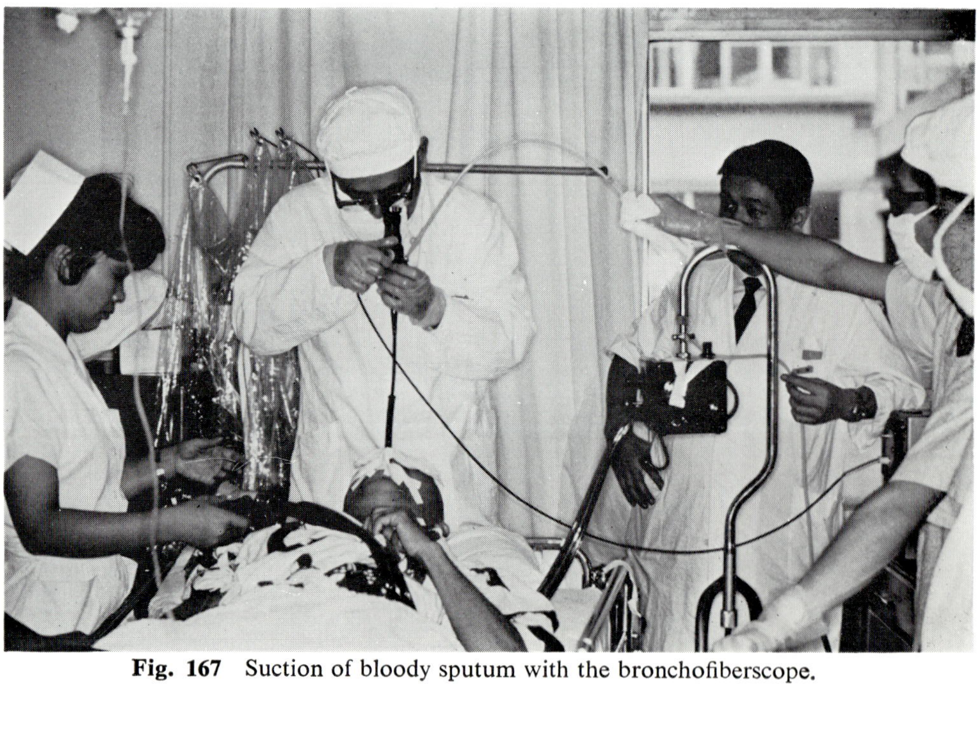

**Fig. 167** Suction of bloody sputum with the bronchofiberscope.

## ADVANTAGES

The advantages of the bronchofiberscope over the rigid bronchoscope are: the ease of introducing the instrument with minimal discomfort to the patient in either the sitting or supine position, and the ease of aspiration and removal or secretions as well as local application of therapeutic agents. It can be introduced through a tracheostomy opening or an intratracheal tube in the seriously ill patient in the surgical recovery room or intensive care unit after the instillation of a small amount of a topical anesthetic. Attachments are available for delivering a constant supply of oxygen during aspiration of secretions to prevent hypoxia.

## IMPORTANT POINTS OF TECHNIQUE IN THERAPEUTIC BRONCHOFIBERSCOPY

The intratracheal tube must be utilized in every case, except when introducing the scope through a tracheostomy cannula or incision. Olympus bronchofiberscope is better suited for the latter purposes than the Machida make, as its body is more flexible. If Machida scope is being utilized through a tracheostomy, it should be introduced through the incision after temporarily removing the cannula (Fig. 168). When the bronchofiberscope is introduced through a cannula, the outer surface of the fiberscope should be annointed with olive oil or some water soluble lubricant such as Xylocaine jelly® prior to its insertion.

When bronchofiberscopy is performed on a case of respiratory failure, the procedure is performed through a closed system with a constant supply of oxygen by means of a respirator. In these cases, a cuffed intratracheal tube must be used (Fig. 169). The proximal end of the intratracheal tube must also be made air tight to prevent the leakage of oxygen.

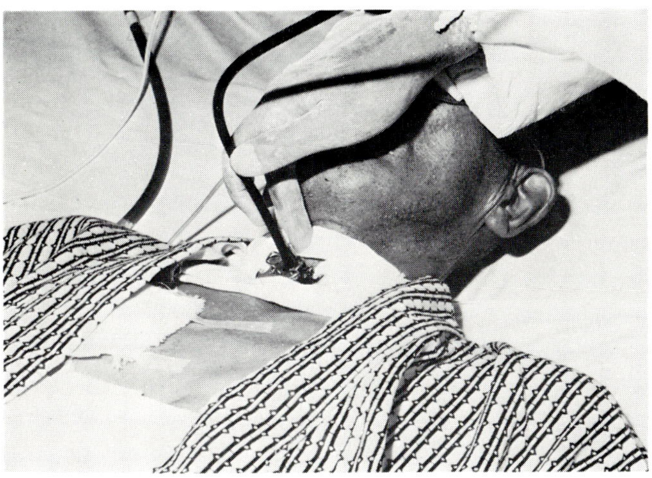

**Fig. 168** Fiberscope being intubated into the cannula at the incised opening after tracheotomy.

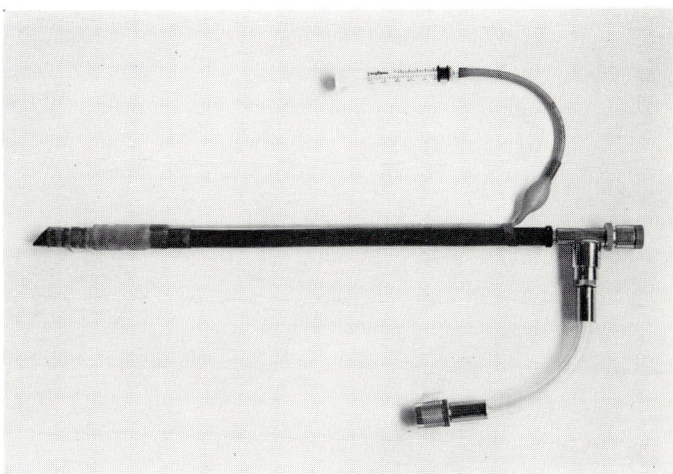

**Fig. 169** Tracheal tube with a cuff and two-way adaptor.

## SUCTIONING

Ordinarily, the 5 mm bronchofiberscope with its 1.4 mm channel is adequate in aspirating sputum or other secretions of moderate to moderately thick viscosity. For very thick secretions, the bronchofiberscopes with larger channels such as Machida 6mm scope (FBS-6) equipped with a 2.2 mm channel or Olympus B model (BF-B) with a 1.9 mm channel are utilized to better advantage. When using the larger scopes for suctioning, one must realize that the cross section area of the airway is reduced, thus respiratory exchange may be embarrassed. It is very important that sufficient oxygen be delivered at all times. Occasionally, one finds it necessary to remove the bronchofiberscope and deliver supplemental oxygen through the tracheal tube.

Suctioning must be performed under direct vision at all times, and one must be careful he does not aspirate all of the intrabronchial air during the procedure. In aspirating, the tip of the scope should just come in contact with the secretions The tip should not be allowed to come in contact with the bronchial mucosa, as this may cause mucosal hemorrhage.

"Synergistic bronchoscopic aspiration" (JACKSON) is occasionally necessitated. In this procedure, the patient is made to cough actively, or made to cough by irritating the bronchus with the aspirating tip in order to expel secretions in the peripheral portions of the bronchial tree.

Markedly suppurative secretions may thicken and harden, causing bronchial obstruction. If repeated aspiration is unsuccessful, one may introduce a proteolytic enzyme such as acetylcysteine onto the obstructing material to liquefy it. If the channel in the 5 mm bronchofiberscope should become clogged with thick secretions, the instrument should be withdrawn and the channel cleansed out and cleared by irrigation with a syringe.

One must pay extra care and caution when aspirating occluded bronchi, as these areas are frequently inflammed and readily subject to hemorrhage. The same care and caution must be exercised in the so-called trans-occlusion suctioning. In this maneuver, the tip of the bronchofiberscope is thrusted through the stenotic or occluded portion of the bronchus for aspirating accumulated secretions. This procedure is done only when tomograms or bronchograms reveal findings indicating that the bronchus in question is obstructed and the peripheral portion of this bronchus is filled with secretions.

## CASES ILLUSTRATING BRONCHOFIBERSCOPIC THERAPY

**Case A (55, male)**

A left pneumonectomy was performed for a primary lung cancer. Two hours postoperatively, atelectasis of the right upper lobe was found on the chest X-ray (Fig. 170) taken in the recovery room. The intratracheal tube was immediately introduced after local anesthesia and the 5 mm bronchofiberscope was utilized for active suction. Bloody secretions were obtained on repeated aspirations. The second chest X-ray film (Fig 171) showed a shadow suggesting the presence of a moderate amount of residual secretions in the peripheral bronchi of the upper lobe. Bronchofiberscopic aspiration was continued, and the third chest X-ray film (Fig 172) taken immediately after this revealed a clear right upper lobe. This postoperative atelectasis was caused by sputum spilling over into the contralateral lung due to inadequate bronchial cleansing during the course of the surgery. If this atelectasis had not been corrected, it is highly probable that the patient might have been lost as the result of pulmonary insufficiency. This case illustrates one of the most important application of therapeutic bronchofiberscopy.

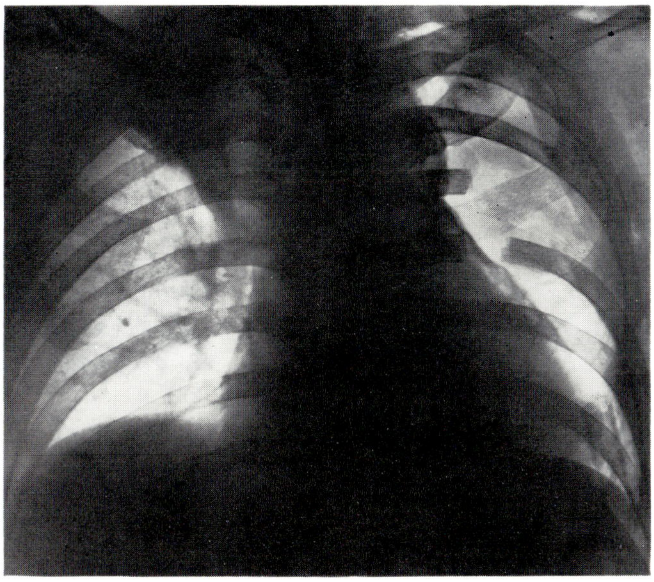

Fig. 170

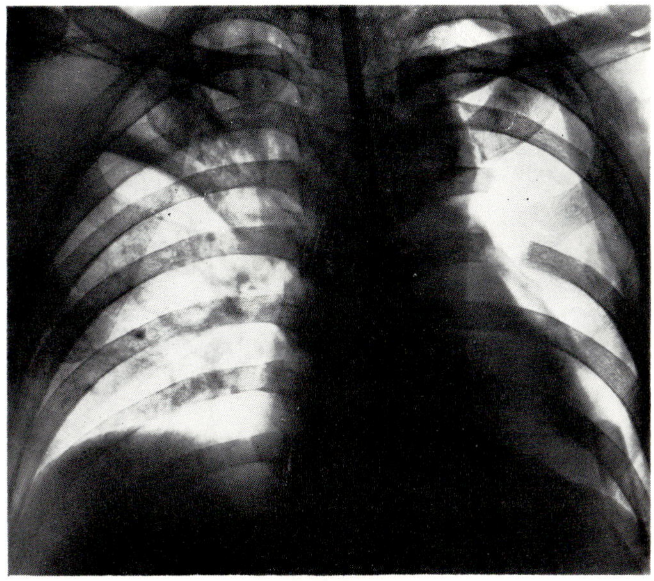

Fig. 171

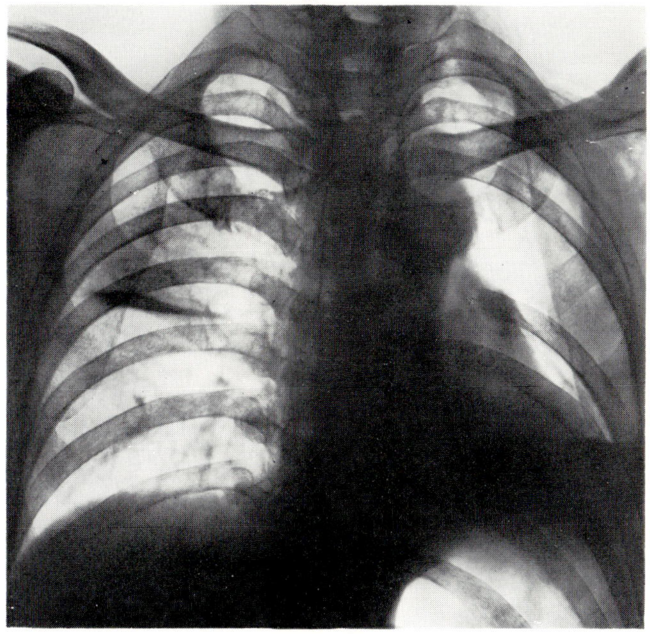

Fig. 172

**Fig. 170** The X-ray film before bronchofiberscopy.
**Fig. 171** The second X-ray film after first bronchofiberscopy.
**Fig. 172** The X-ray film immediately after second bronchofiberscopy.

### Case B (54, male)

This patient underwent complete extirpation of the thoracic esophagus, cervical esophagostomy and jejunostomy for cancer of the middle third of the esophagus.

The preoperative chest X-ray film (Fig. 173) revealed a small nodular infiltration in the right upper lung field due to fibrosing tuberculosis. Pulmonary function findings revealed a slight degree of respiratory failure and a slight reduction in the pulmonary diffusing capacity.

The postoperative chest X-ray (Fig. 174) revealed satisfactory re-expansion of the right lung. The patient was not able to raise any sputum. On the second postoperative day, atelectasis was recognized in the right middle and lower lung field (Fig. 175). Immediate therapeutic bronchofiberscopy was instituted after appropriate local anesthesia using the 6 mm bronchofiberscope. A constant supply of oxygen was delivered through the respirator. The right main bronchus was found to be filled with purulent secretions. This was aspirated, then the entire middle and lower lobes until each segmental bronchus was clearly seen. Immediately after this procedure, a chest X-ray (Fig. 176) revealed an airbronchogram with some clearing of the atelectasis although the peripheral bronchi were still clogged with secretions. The patient, however, was now able to cough and expectorate effectively. Three hours following the bronchofiberscopic aspiration, moderate re-expansion was noted in the middle and lower lobes (Fig. 177). Chemotherapy was given concurrently. By the third day after bronchofiberscopy, with continued effective cough and expectoration, the chest X-ray revealed the lungs to be well expanded and clear (Fig. 178).

Arterial blood gas records were obtained during the pre and post-broncofiberscopic periods. On the first postoperative day, it disclosed a slightly elevated $PCO_2$ and a low pH consistent with respiratory acidosis, suggesting a decreased volume of ventilation. The $PO_2$ was lower than the preoperative level. All of these figures indicate a gradually developing postoperative atelectasis (Fig. 179)

On the second postoperative day just prior to the therapeutic bronchofiberscopy, the $PO_2$ was still low in spite of a markedly decreased $PCO_2$ level denoting arteriovenous shunting or obstruction of oxygenation of the arterial blood. This is assumed to be evidence of the presence of postoperative atelectasis.

Immediately following the therapeutic bronchofiberscopic aspiration, the $PO_2$ and $PCO_2$ were found to be approaching normal, consistent with a gradual improvement of the atelectasis.

On the 5th postoperative day the shadow on the chest X-ray film was improved and at the same time the respiratory profile was restored to normal

This case illustrates the relationship between the

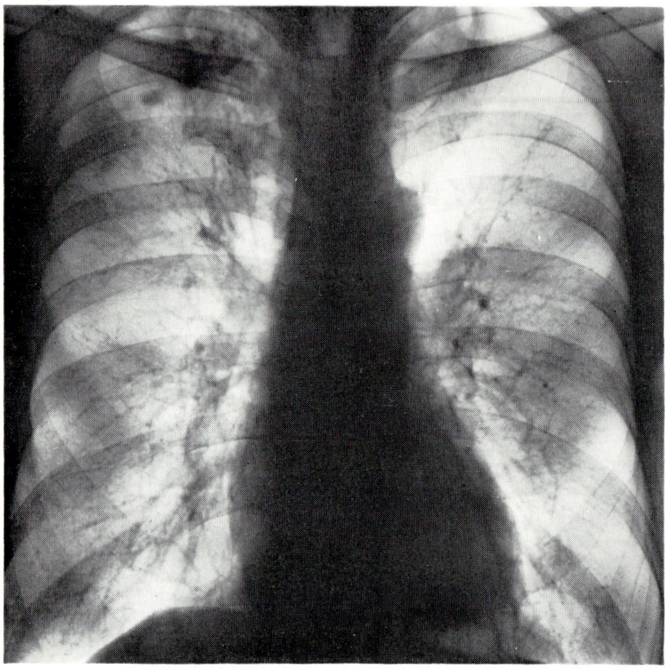

**Fig. 173** The X-ray film before the surgical operation.

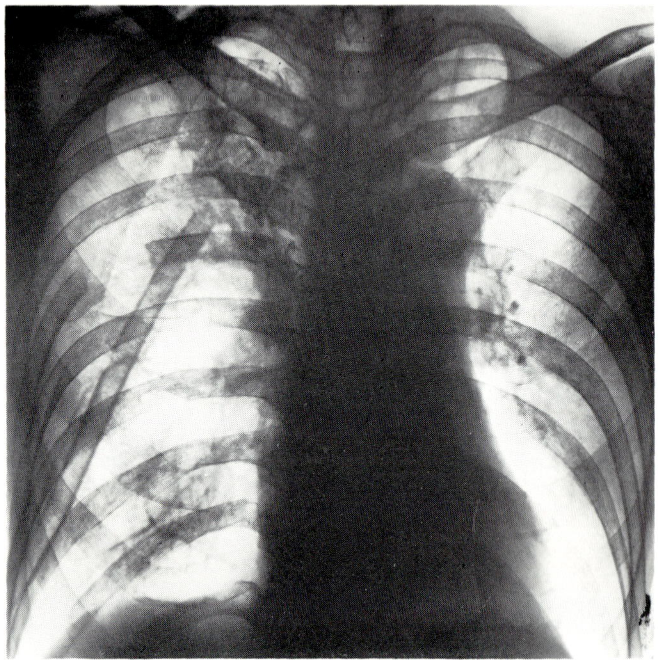

**Fig. 174** The X-ray film immediately after the operation.

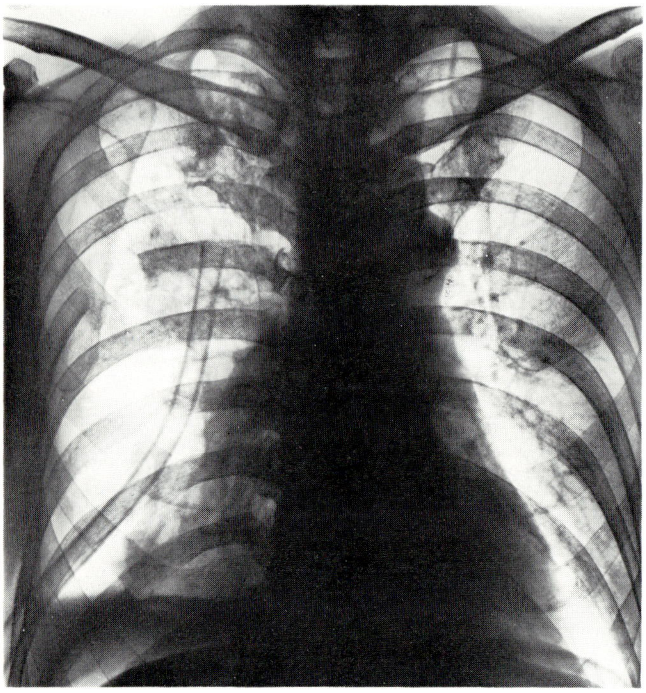

**Fig. 175** The X-ray film one day after the operation.

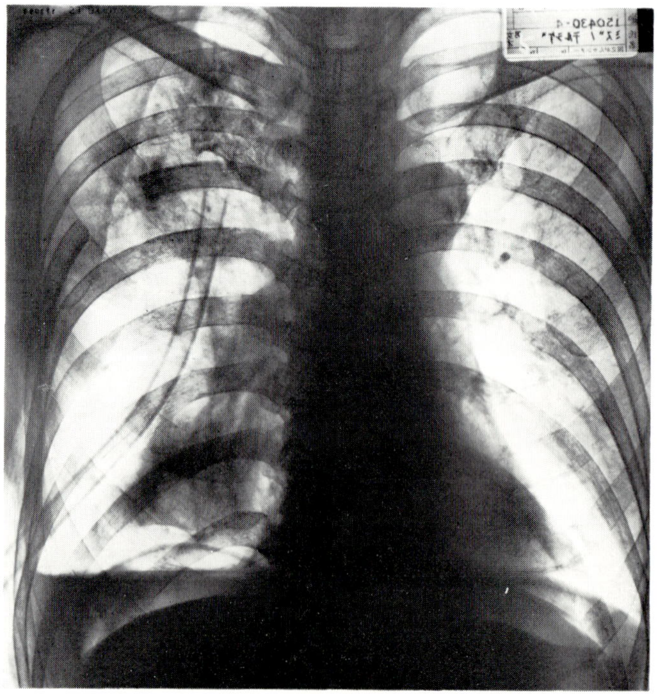

**Fig. 176** The X-ray film immediately after bronchofiberscopy.

arterial blood gas studies (respiratory profile) and the extent of atelectatic involvement of the lung. After the therapeutic bronchofiberscopy, with improvement of the atelectasis, the respiratory profile was found to approach normal values. Also, the procedure assisted the patient in establishing an effective cough with expectoration of sputum.

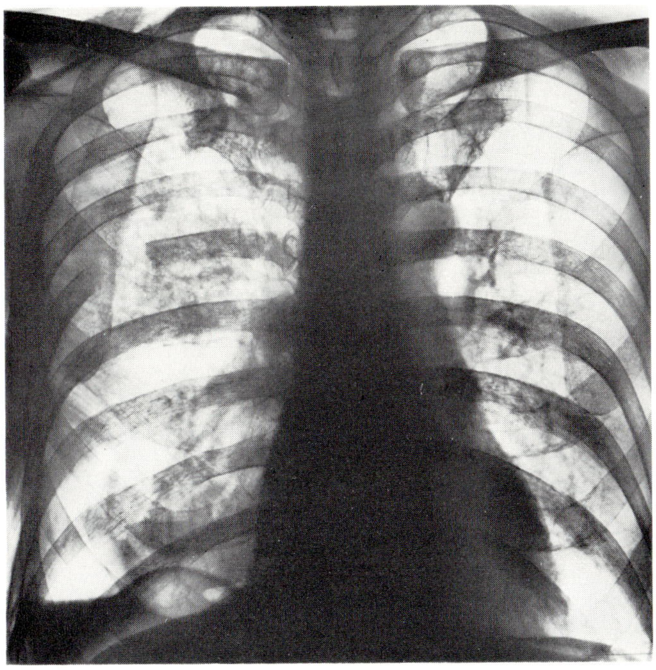

**Fig. 177** The X-ray film three hours after bronchofiberscopy.

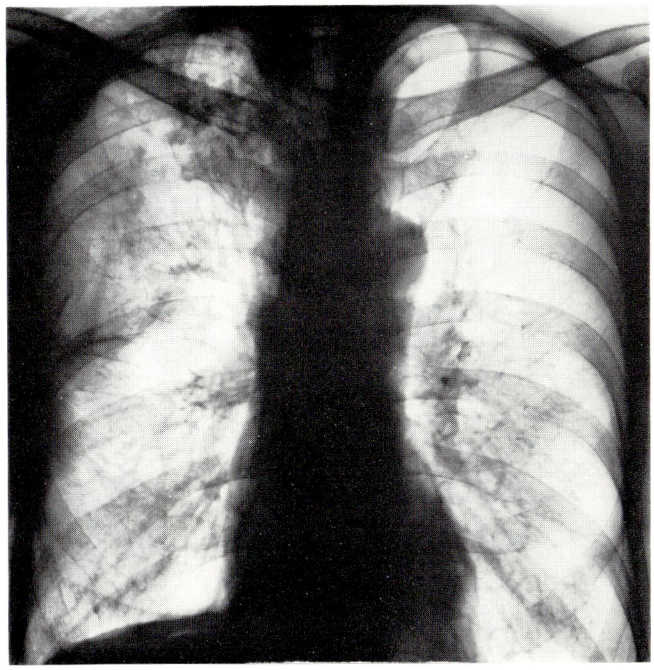

**Fig. 178** The X-ray film three days after bronchofiberscopy.

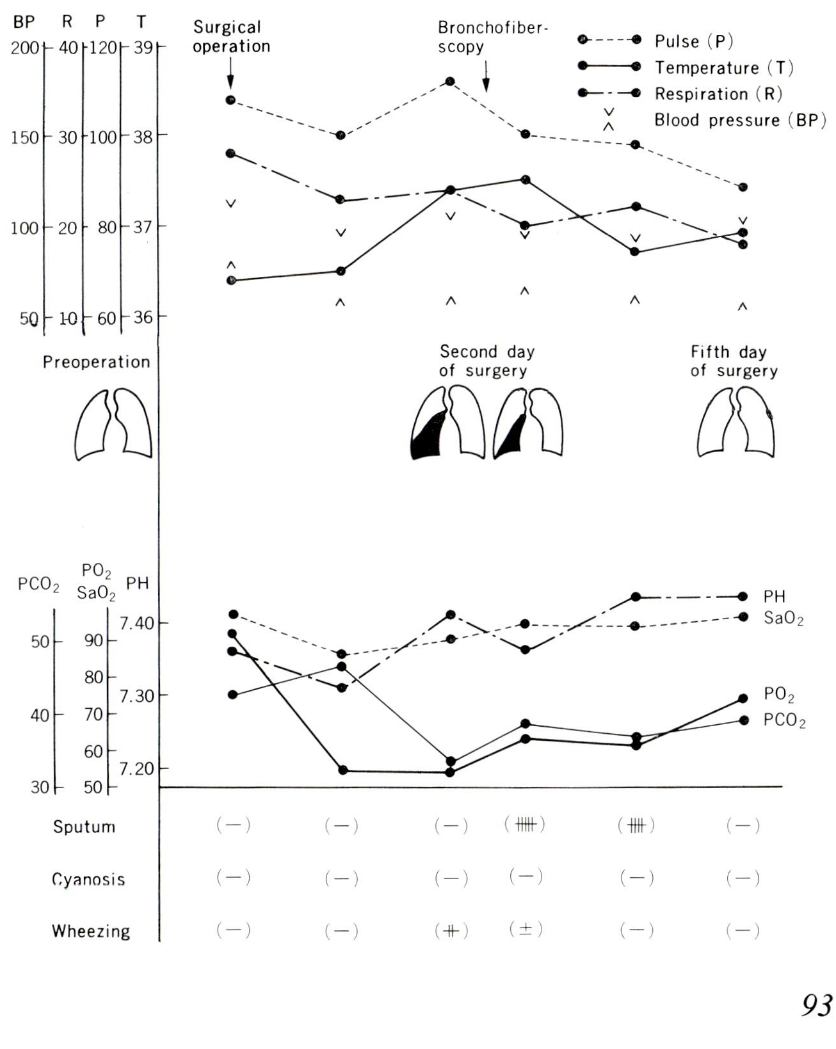


**Fig. 179** Clinical records.

# Part 2
# CASE PRESENTATION

## I. Lung Cancer and Metastatic Lung Tumor

## Case 1 Lung Cancer, Early Stage – Hilar Type (64, male)

**Chief complaints :** Bloody sputum.
**Definitive clinical diagnosis :** Squamous cell carcinoma by bronchofiberscopic biopsy.
**Pathological diagnosis :** Squamous cell carcinoma at the orifice of $B^6$ and carcinoma in situ in the middle lobe bronchus.
**Case history :** The patient, though robust and healthy by nature, had influenza-like symptoms with bloody sputum a year and a half ago, and the symptoms continued for 9 months. Six months ago, the bloody sputum recurred. Bronchoscopic findings suggested the presence of lung cancer, and the patient was referred to our hospital. At the time of admission there was no bloody sputum. The patient had been a smoker for forty years, averaging 50 cigarettes a day.

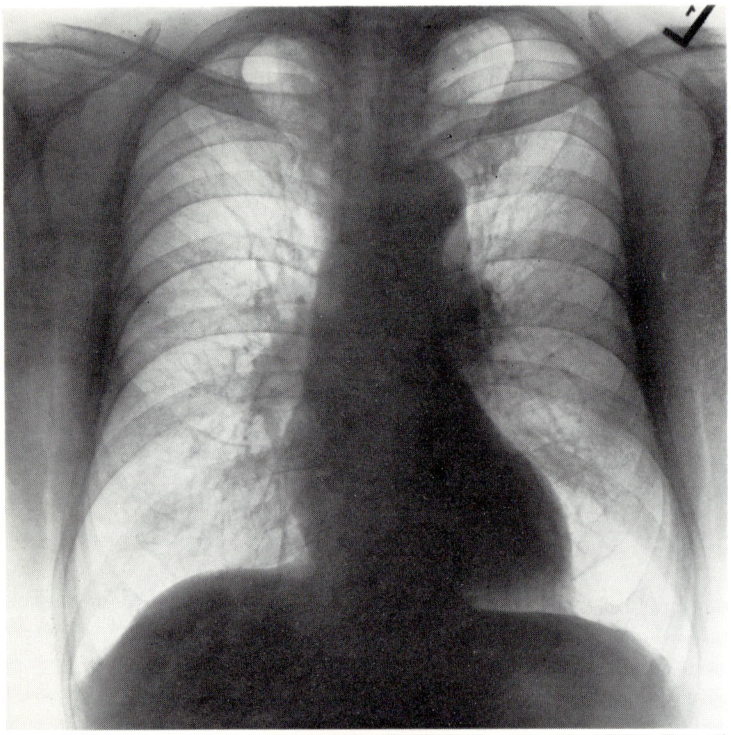

**Fig. 180 Chest X-ray, frontal :** No abnormality found in the pulmonary hilum nor in the periphery.

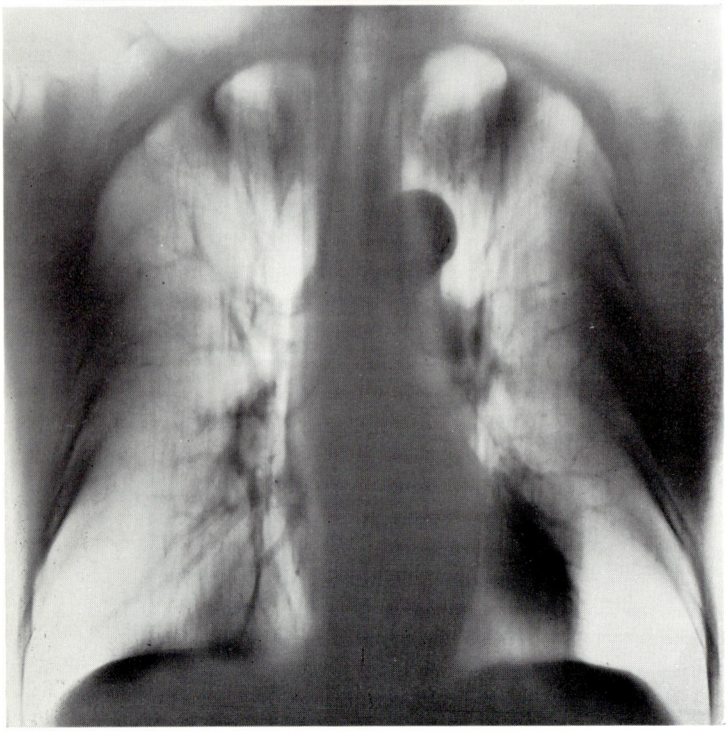

**Fig. 181 Tomogram :** No tumor-suggestive shadow or change detectable in the hilum or elsewhere in the tomogram taken 11 cm from the posterior chest wall.

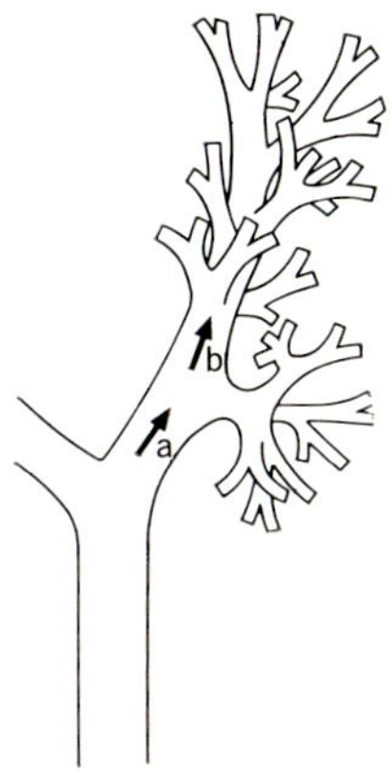


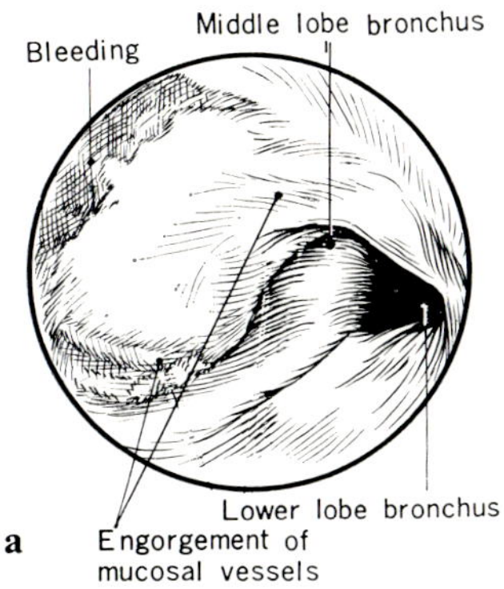


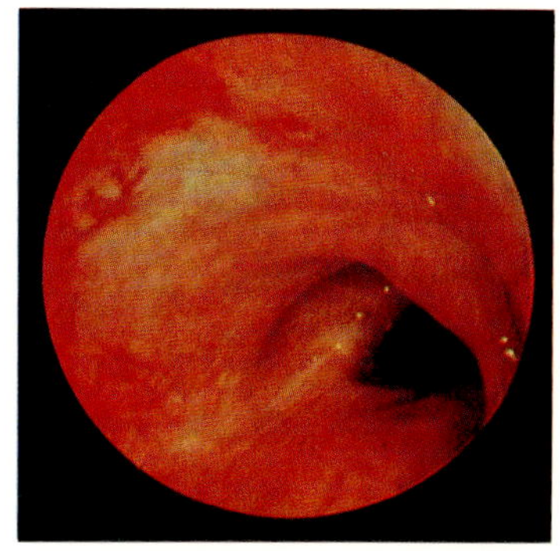

182 a

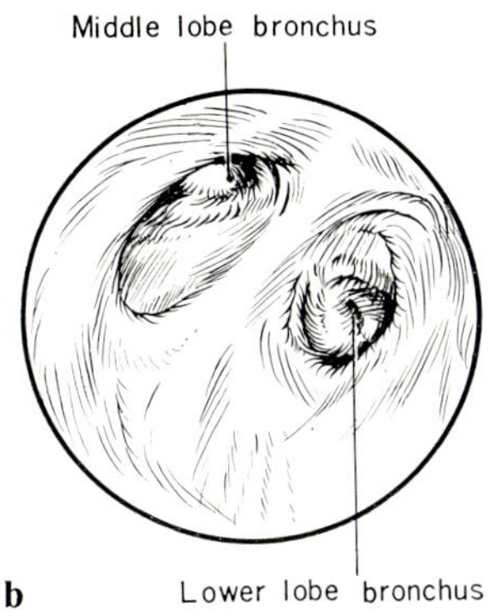


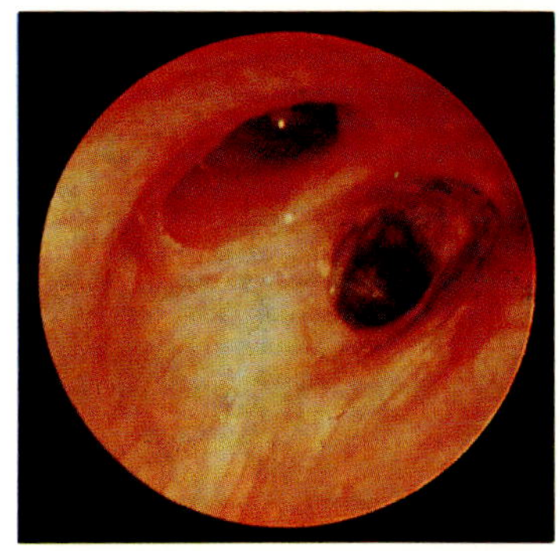

182 b

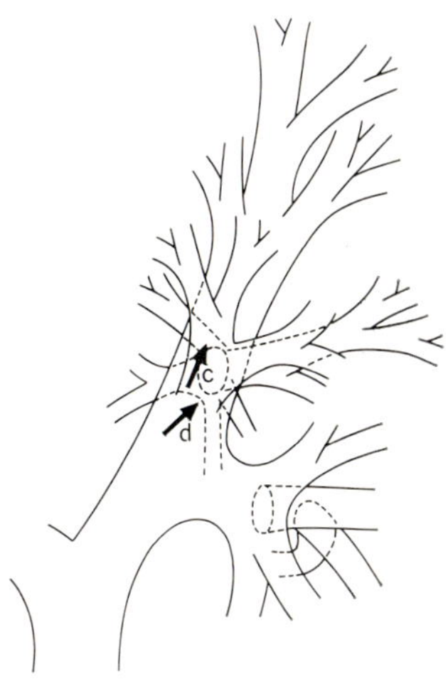


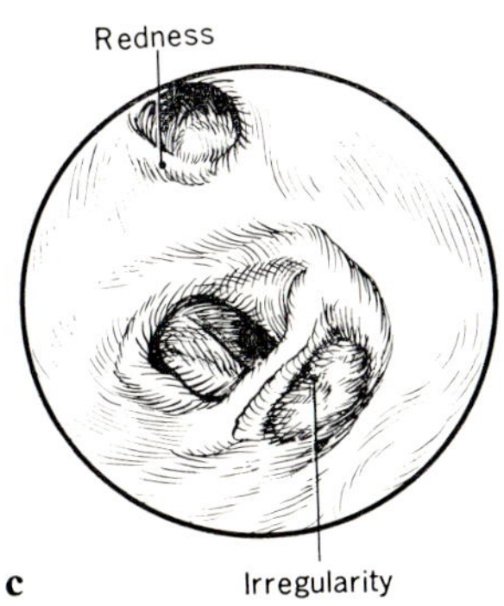


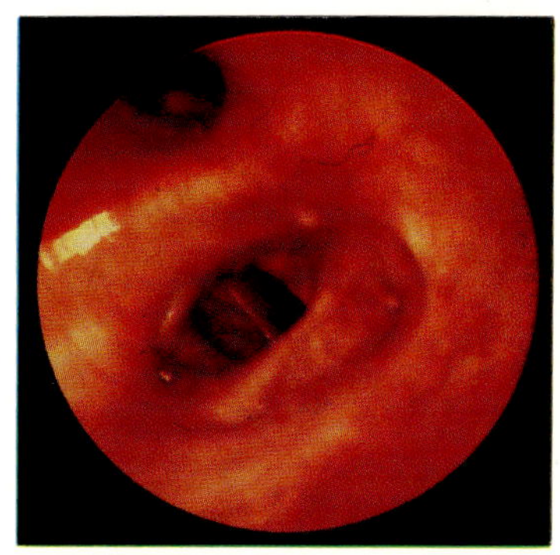

182 c

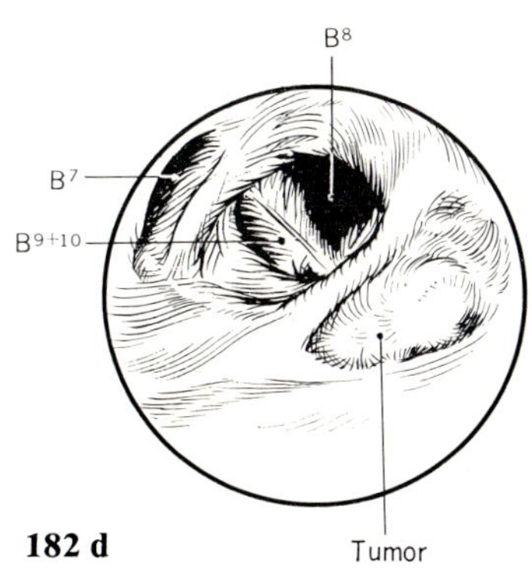


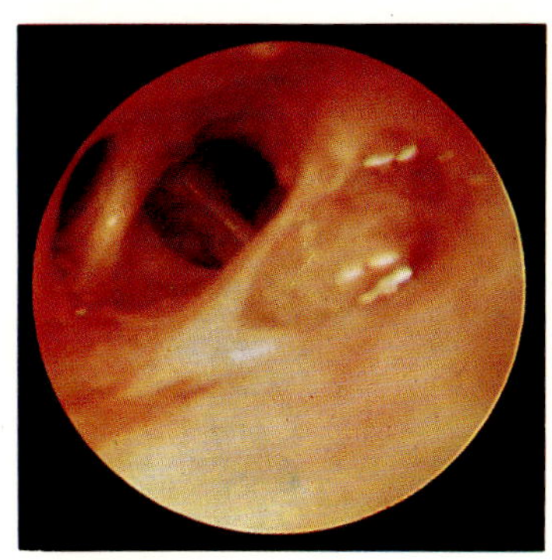

182 d

**Fig. 182 Fiberscopic findings:**

**a.** From the main bronchus to the truncus intermedius there are generalized irregularity of mucosa, indistinct bronchial cartilages and engorgement of blood vessels.

**b.** In the truncus intermedius reddening is intense particularly on the right wall and blood vessels are engorged.

**c.** The orifice of the lower lobe bronchus is irregular in shape. Intense reddening is observed on the posterior wall of the middle lobe bronchus.

**d.** A prominent tumor, slightly swollen, smooth surfaced and whitish-yellow, is located at the orifice of $B^6$. Biopsy specimen was obtained from this area.

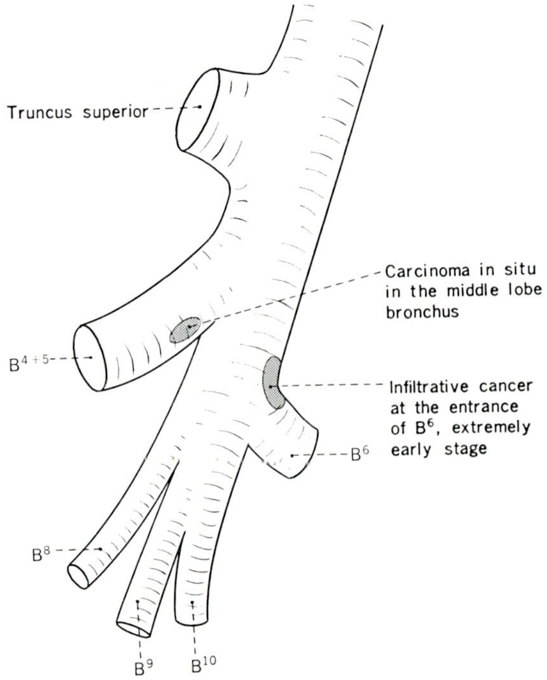


**Fig. 183 Traced schema**

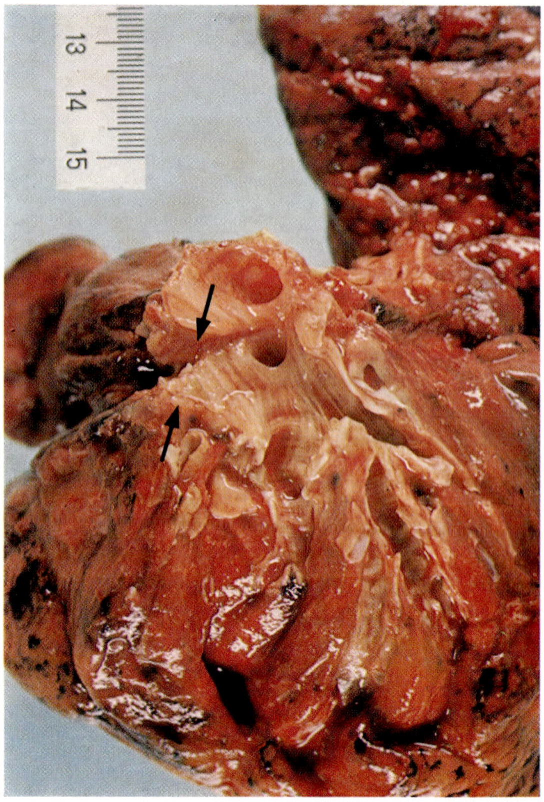


184 a

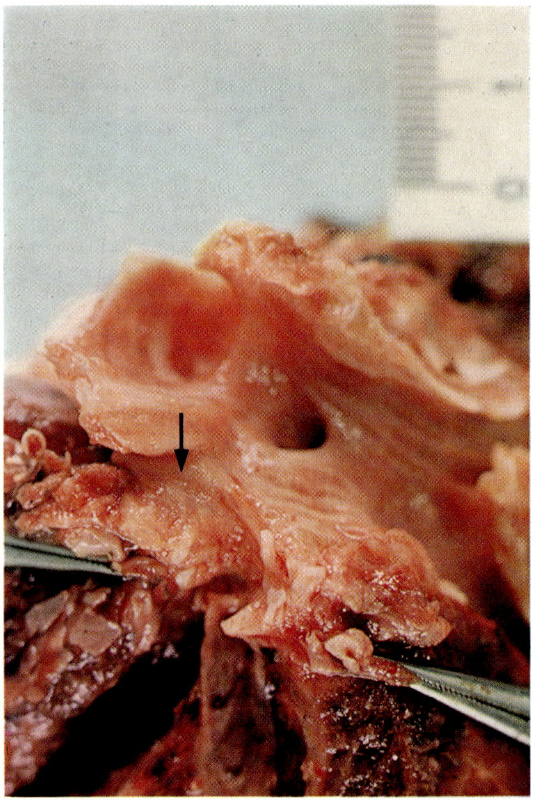

184 b

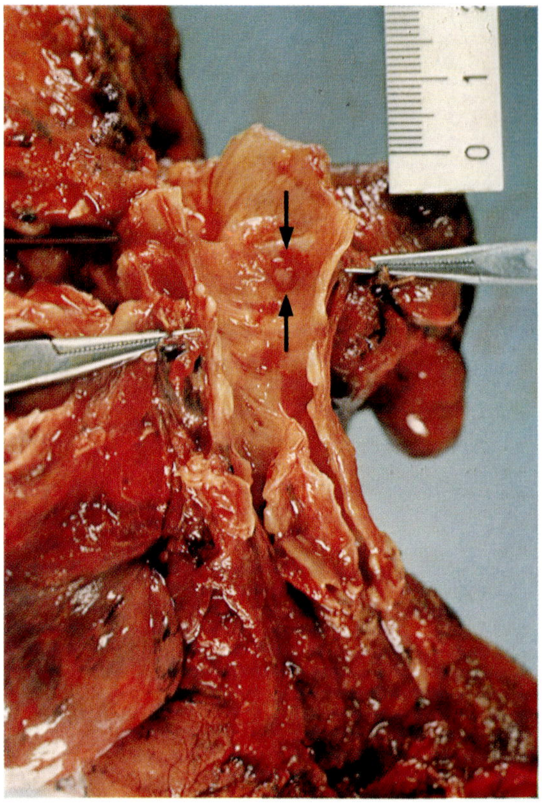


184 c

**Fig. 184 Macroscopic findings:**

**a.** Resected specimen. Right middle-lower lobectomy was performed.

**b.** Contact print of a fresh specimen showing the lower lobe bronchus to $B^6$. The entrance of $B^6$ is slightly narrowed. The mucosa is rough and has lost the epithelial fold for 3–4 mm. No change is found in color.

**c.** Contract print of a fresh specimen in which the middle lobe bronchus was exposed. A reddened lesion, 7×4 mm in size, is located about 10 mm from the entrance of the bronchus and appears to be eroded or ulcerated.

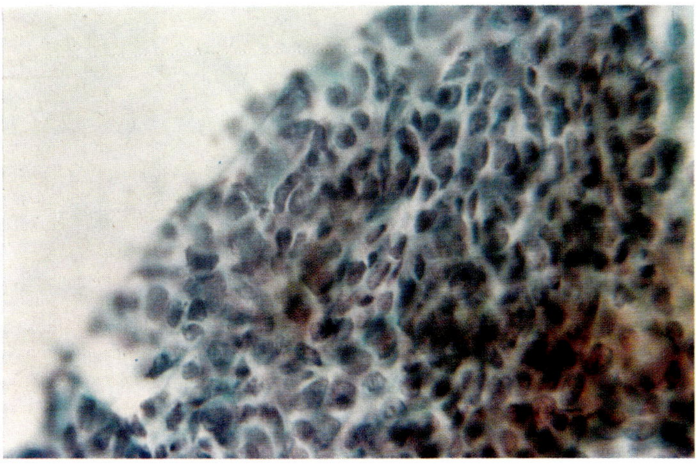

**Fig. 185 Cytodiagnosis** (Papanicolaou stain) : The sputum obtained two days after bronchofiberscopy yielded cells of squamous cell carcinoma. An irregularly cumulated cluster of cells with dense nuclei. Each nucleus is malformed and varies in size. ×350

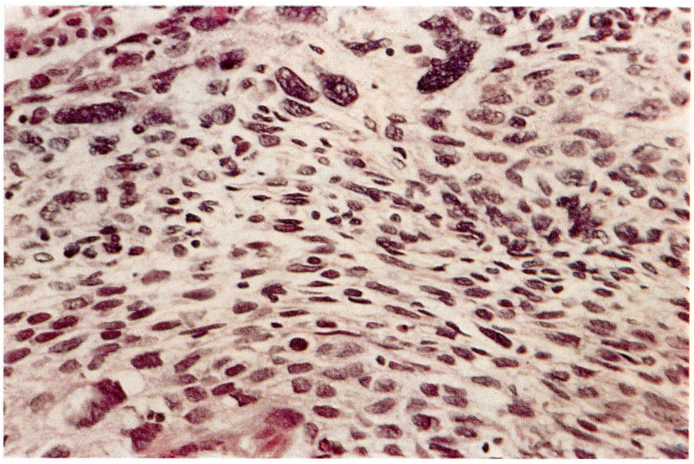

**Fig. 186 Bronchofiberscopic biopsy :** Atypical cells are arranged haphazardly or flowing in a vortex fashion, accompanied by capillary vessels. No keratinization.

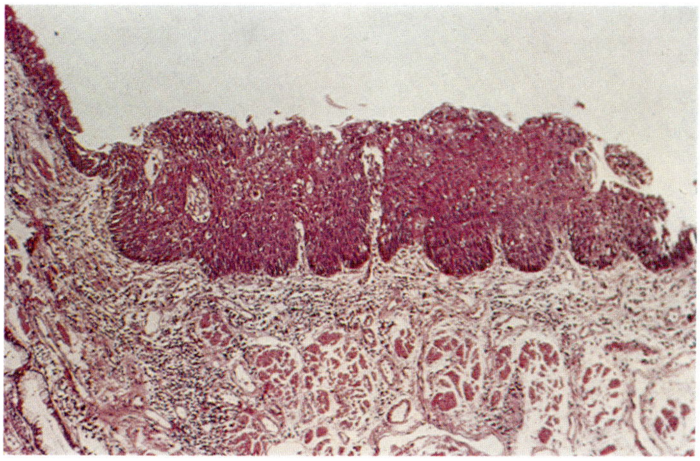

**187 a**

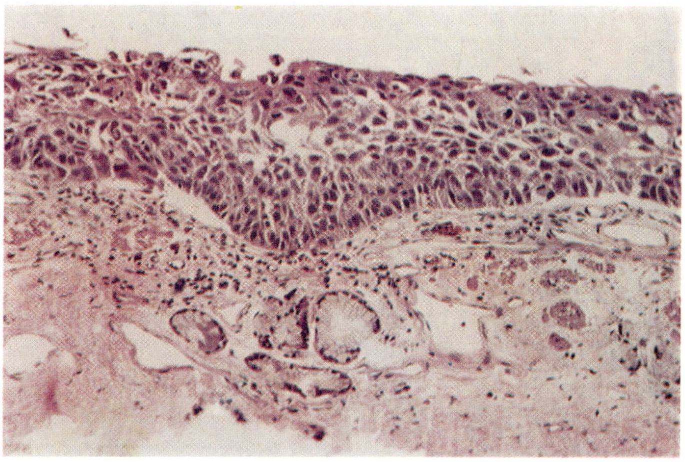

**187 b**

**Fig. 187 Microscopic findings :**

**a.** Histology of the change around the entrance of $B^6$. Atypical cells have proliferated downwards considerably in a regular fashion as if forming a rete ridge of the skin. The change is in a flat form and 4 times as thick as ciliated epithelium. Diagnosis : Early infiltrative cancer.

**b.** Findings in the middle lobe bronchus, somewhat similar to the preceding one, reveal the changes of the duct epithel but no sub-epithelial infiltration. Diagnosis : Squamous cell carcinoma in situ. The two changes had no pathological linkage with each other.

## COMMENT :

This case of a male heavy smoker with the complaint of blood-stained sputum did not reveal any abnormality on the chest X-ray. Bronchofiberscopy was performed three times. The first time, a tumor was suspected but cytology and biopsy specimens were negative. Ten days later, the lesion was not clear ; however, this time the cytology and biopsy specimens were positive for squamous cell carcinoma from the orifice of $B^6$. Bronchofiberscopy was performed the third time (Fig. 182) to confirm the previous findings. In an extremely early lung cancer diagnosis by biopsy is difficult. At the same time it is also hard to identify the location where biopsy diagnosis or cytodiagnosis can be obtained even with the use of a bronchofiberscope. This case reveals the extreme difficulty in correlating the pathology with the bronchofiberscopic findings. A carcinoma in situ in the middle lobe bronchus was not discovered before the surgery.

## Case 2 Lung Cancer, Early Stage – Hilar Type (47, male)

**Chief complaint :** Bloody sputum.
**Definitive clinical diagnosis :** Squamous cell carcinoma by bronchoscopic biopsy.
**Pathological diagnosis :** Keratotic squamous cell carcinoma.
**Case history :** The patient produced bloody sputum in November, 1965, was roentgenographed and treated for tuberculosis. Repeated bloody sputum in July, 1966, and the patient was referred to our hospital. He smoked 20–30 cigarettes a day for the past 20 years.

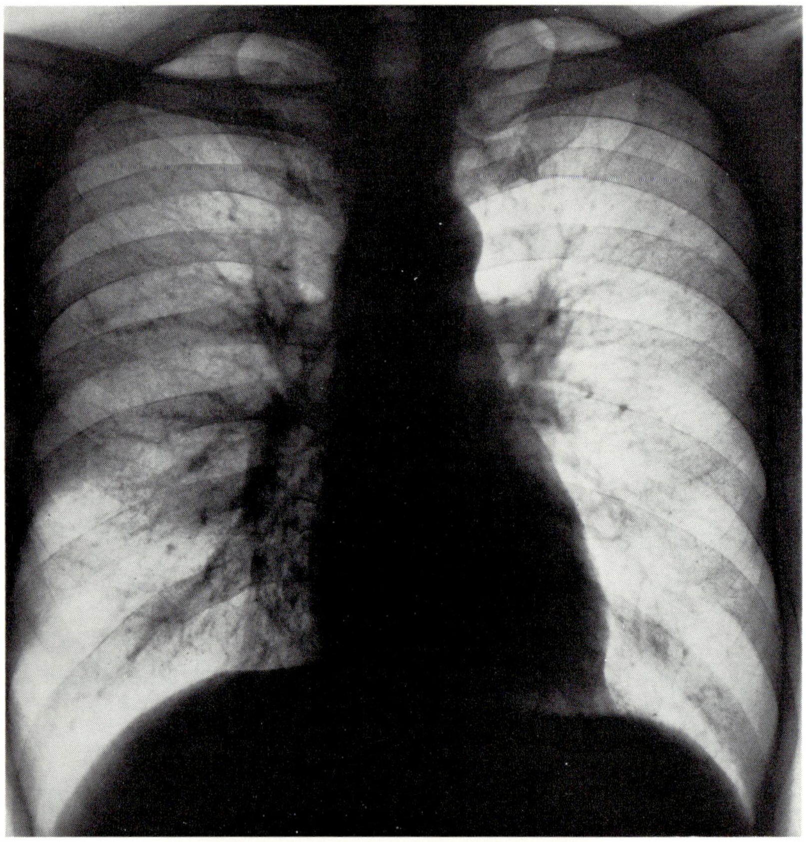

**Fig. 188 Chest X-ray, frontal :** No abnormality in the hilum nor lung fields bilaterally.

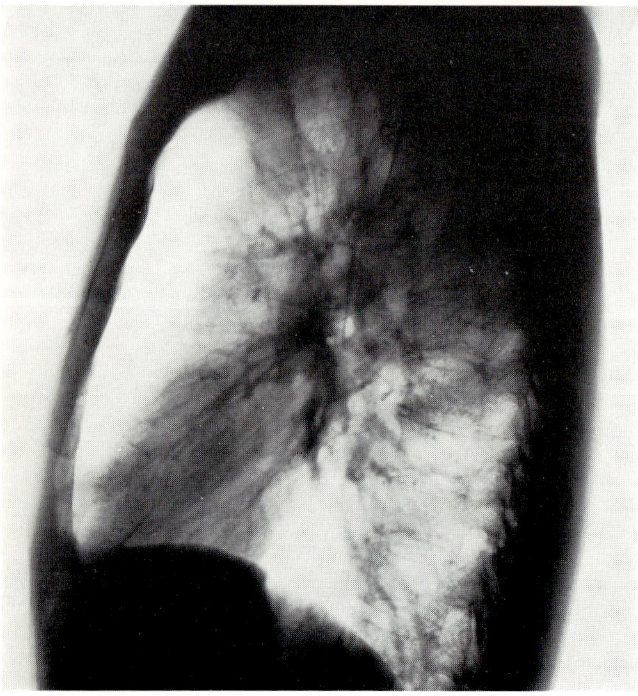

**Fig. 189 Chest X-ray, lateral :** No specific findings noted.

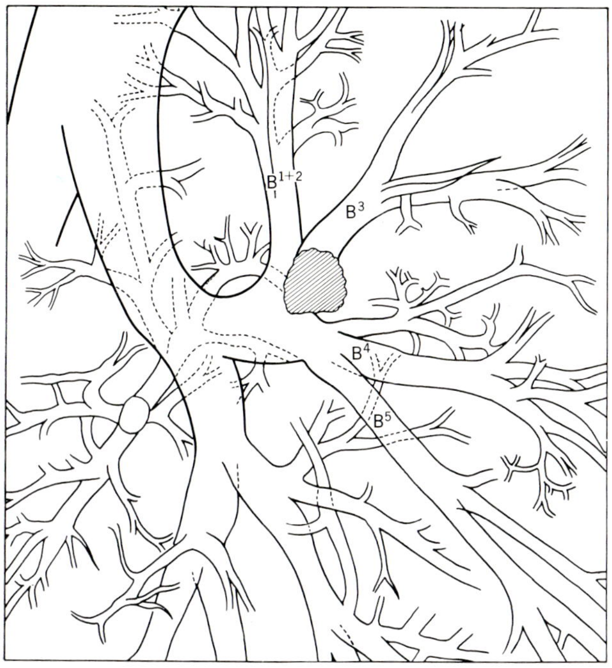


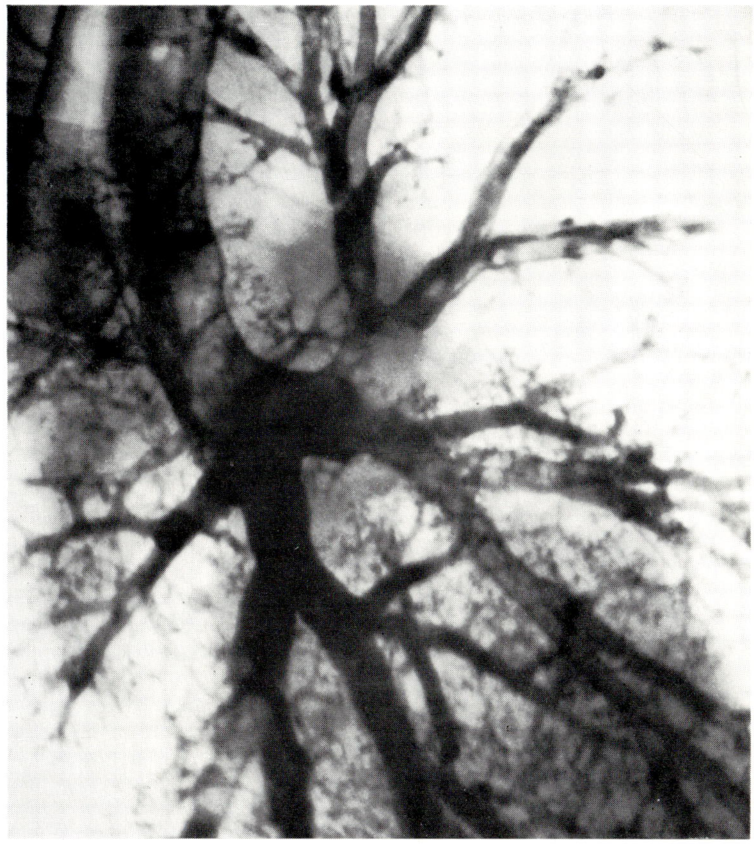

**Fig. 190 Left bronchogram, oblique :** Indented shadow defect, as if gnawed by a rat, is present in the left upper division bronchus with narrowing.

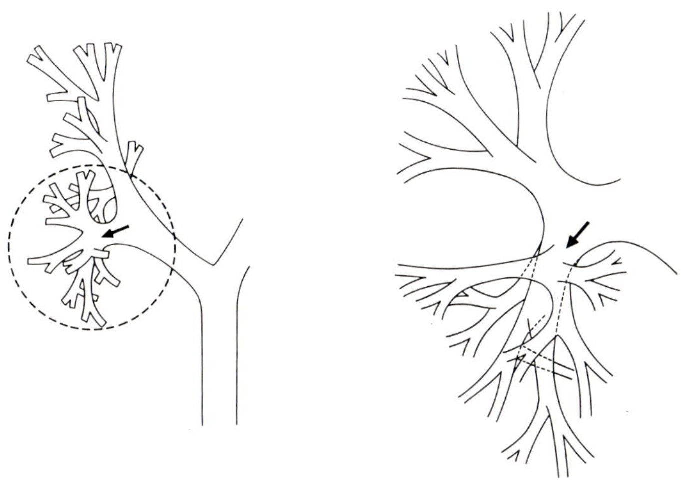

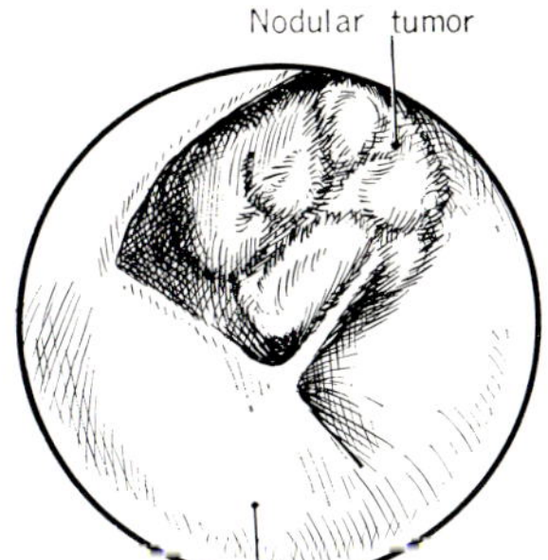


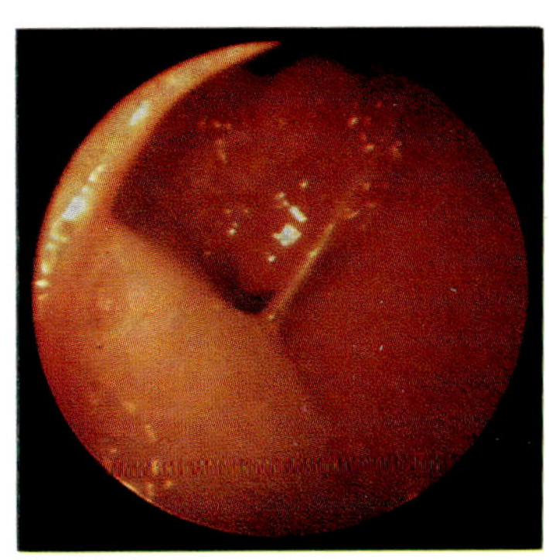

**Fig. 191 Bronchoscopic findings :** A tumor with an uneven surface is seen in the left upper bronchus with no visible necrosis (at the time of this examination, a rigid bronchoscope was used, and the picture was taken through the lateral viewing telescope).

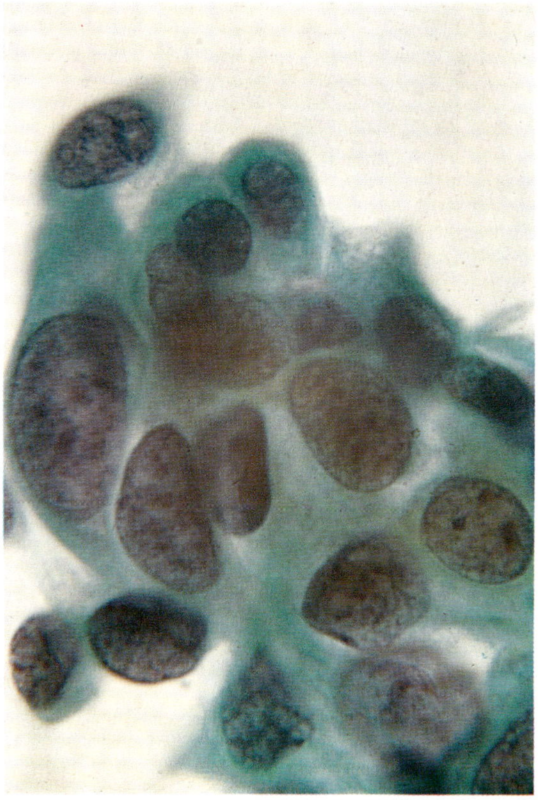

**Fig. 192 Cytodiagnosis :** Bronchoscopic cytological specimen. The cytoplasm is orange in color, the nuclear membrane is irregularly thickened with roundness partially lost. The distribution of chromatin is not uniform, and nucleoli are indistinct. The cells are of squamous cell carcinoma.

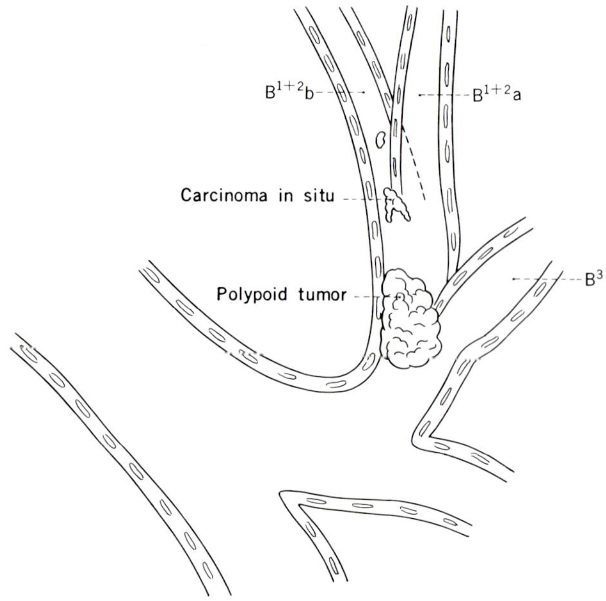


**Fig. 193 Traced schema**

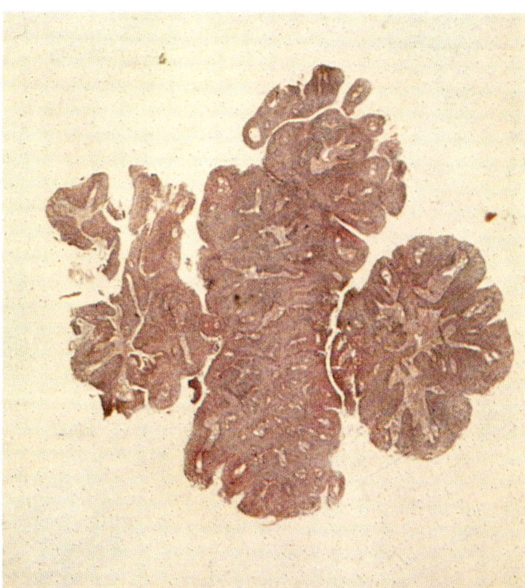

**194 a**

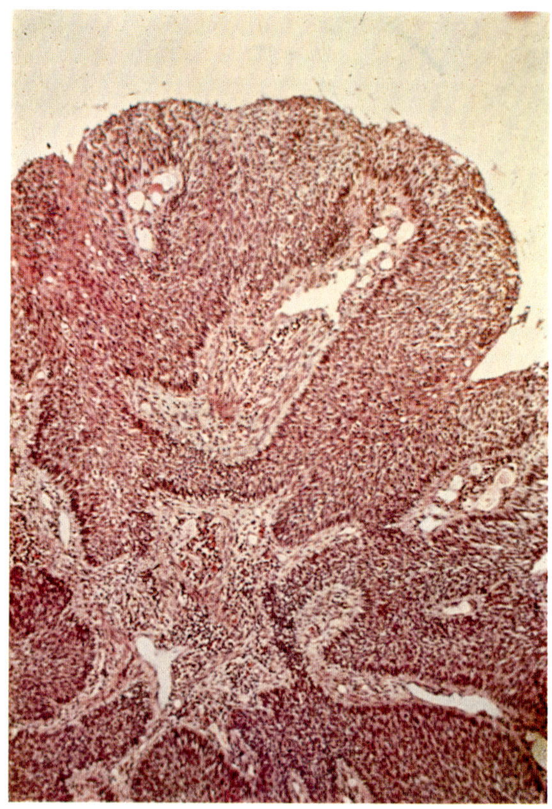

**194 b**

**Fig. 194 Microscopic findings :**

**a.** Specimen of the entire cut surface of the papillary polypoid tumor.

**b.** Enlarged part of Fig. 194 a. The tumor resembles a basal cell carcinoma in pattern. Keratotic trend is also recognized. Diagnosis : Keratotic squamous cell carcinoma.

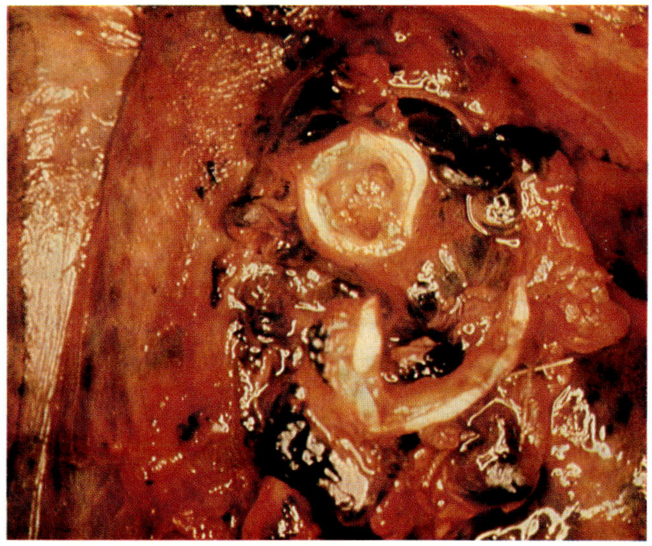

**Fig. 195 Macroscopic findings:**
**a.** Fresh resected specimen. The transverse section of the left upper division bronchus at the middle of the plate. A fragile polypoid tumor, 6 mm, is seen in the lumen.

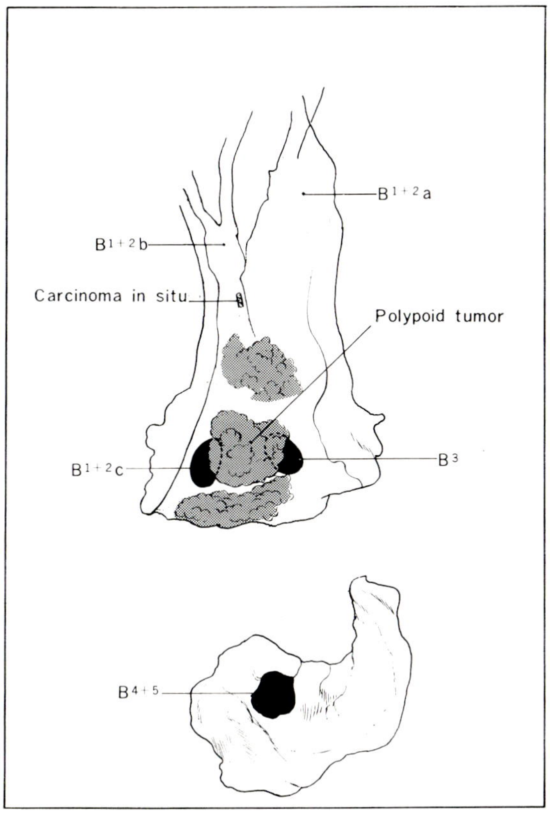


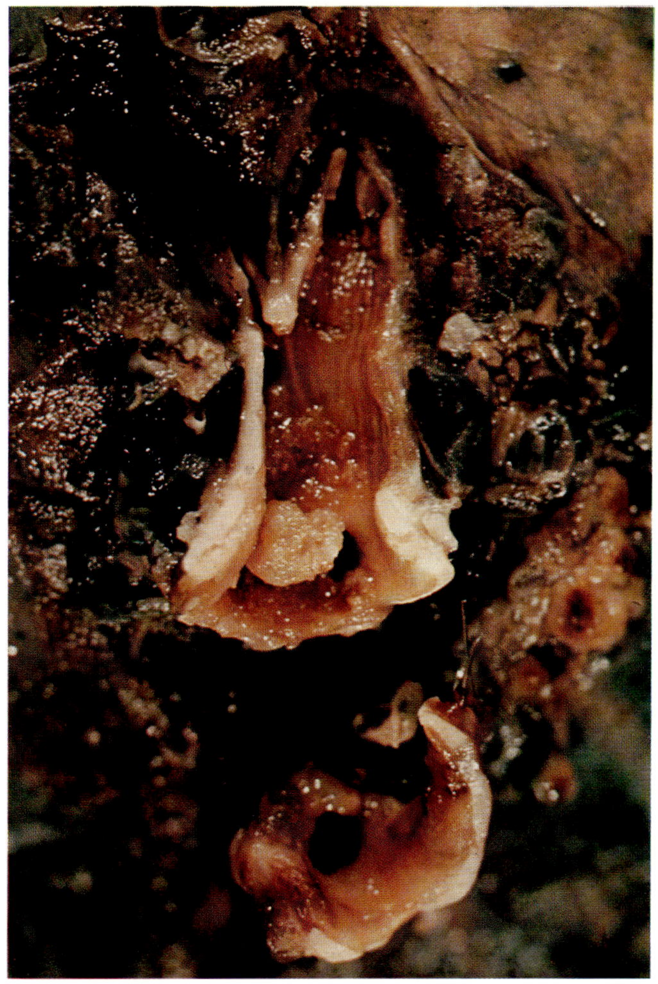

**b.** Upon opening $B^{1+2}$, a polypoid tumor is near the entrance of $B^{1+2}c$ and $B^{3}$. The tumor infiltrates from the upper division bronchus to $B^{1+2}a+b$. The infiltrated area is $15 \times 10$ mm. The mucosa here is granular and moderately protuberant.

**COMMENT:**

Bloody sputum was the chief complaint but no finding was detectable by routine chest X-ray. A shadow defect was present on the bronchogram, following which the tumor was seen by bronchoscopy and definitively diagnosed by biopsy. When the patient was admitted to our hospital, flexible bronchofiberscopy was not yet available. In view of the fact that the above findings were obtained by rigid bronchoscopy, a flexible bronchofiberscope would have supplied us with better endoscopic pictures and a tumor in this location would have been easily found.

## Case 3 Lung Cancer, Early Stage – Hilar Type (55, male)

**Chief complaint :** Coughing with sputum.
**Definitive clinical diagnosis :** Anaplastic carcinoma by bronchofiberscopic curettage.
**Pathological diagnosis :** Keratotic squamous cell carcinoma.
**Case history :** Since October, 1969, the patient had heavy cough and sputum. In January, 1970, he had a high fever, 39°C, and bloody sputum for the first time. He then came to our hospital for examination. He has a history of smoking more than 50 cigarettes a day for the past 30 years.

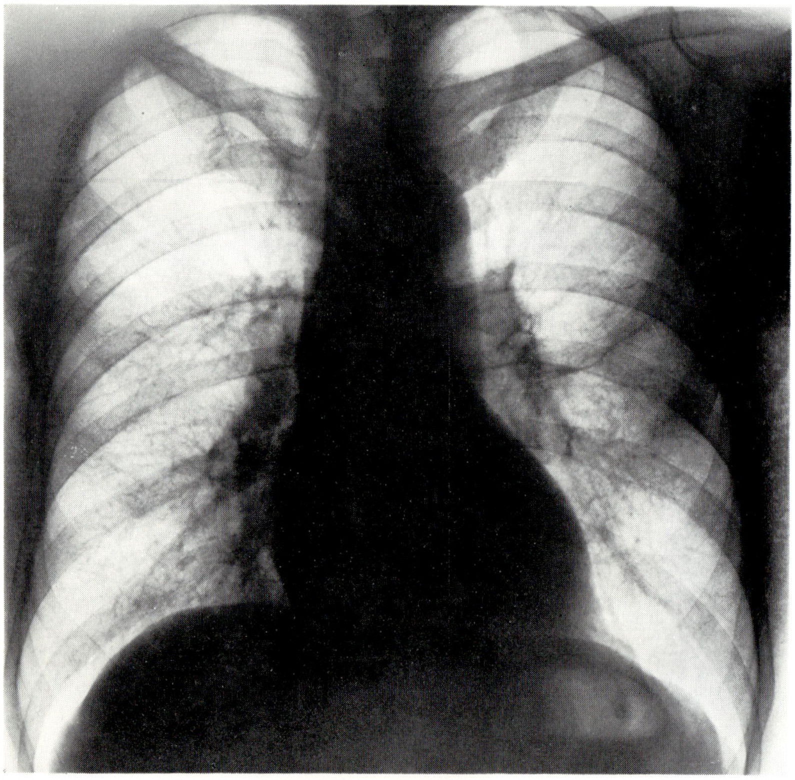

**Fig. 196 Chest X-ray, frontal :** Practically no abnormality is detectable.

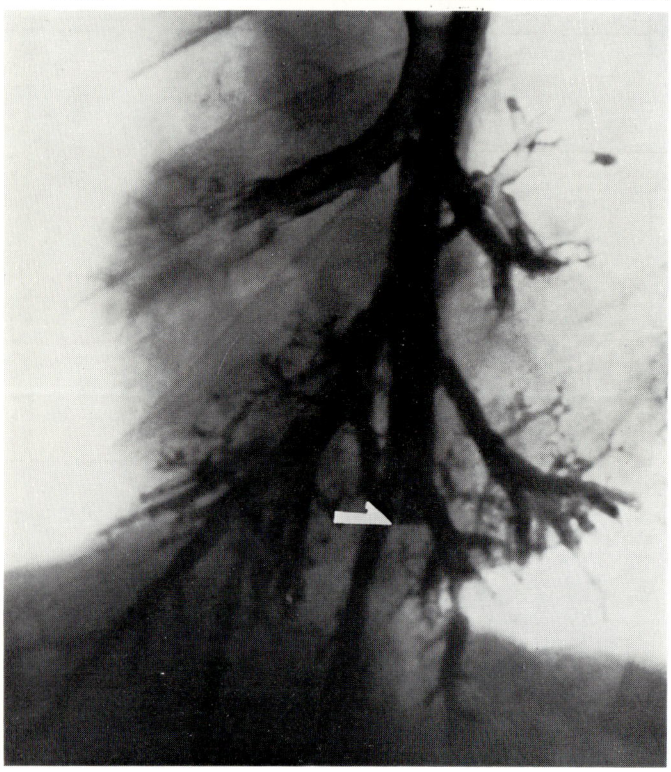

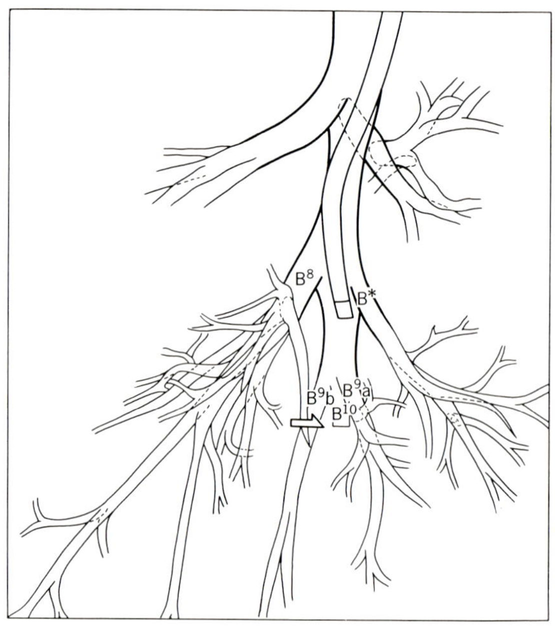


**Fig. 197 Right bronchogram, oblique :** Obstruction is noted at $B^{10}$ (arrow).

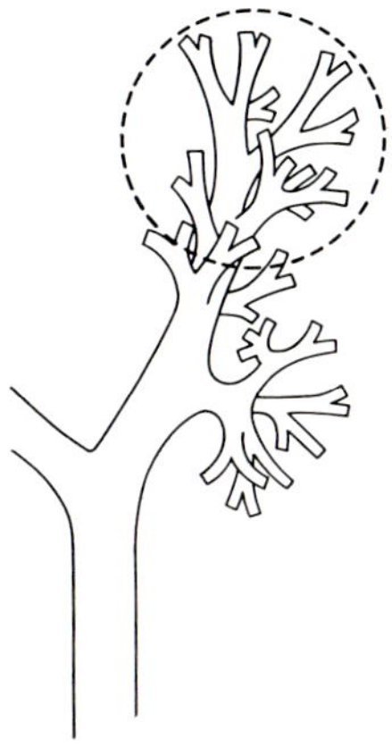

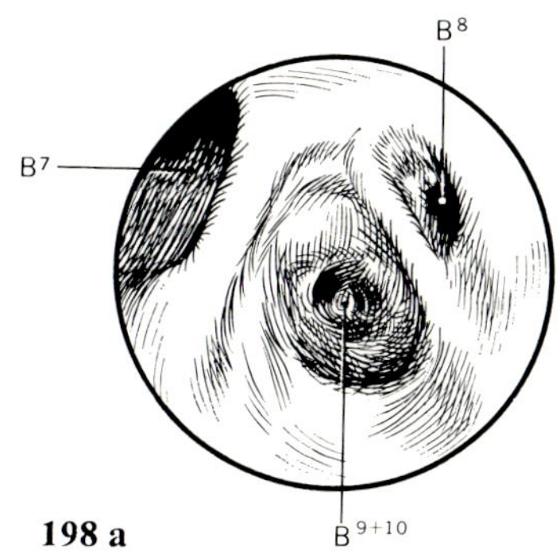


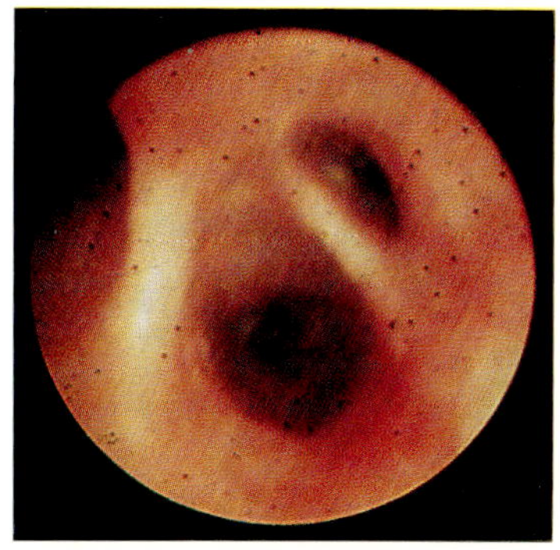

198 a

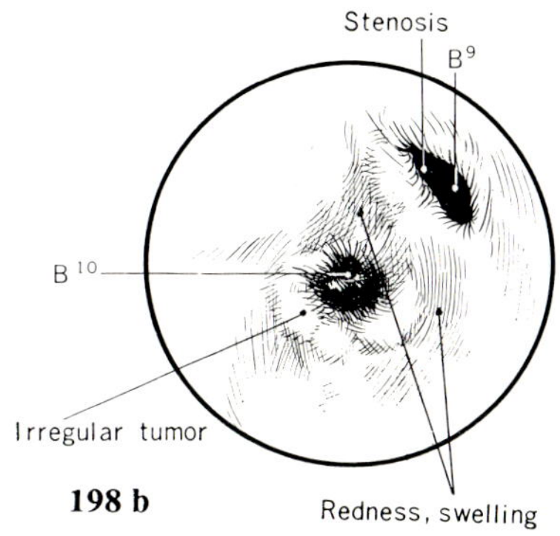


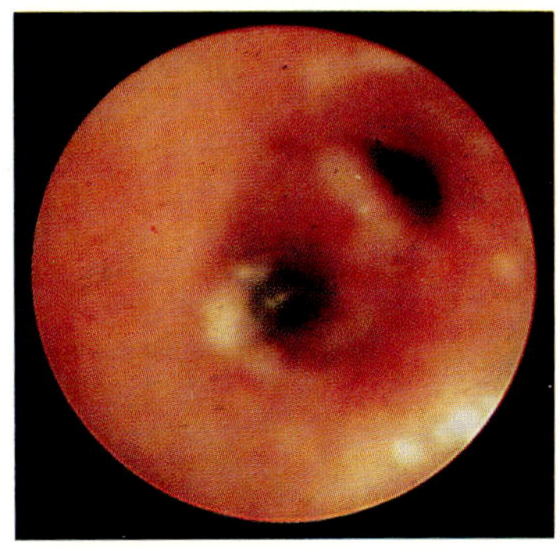

198 b

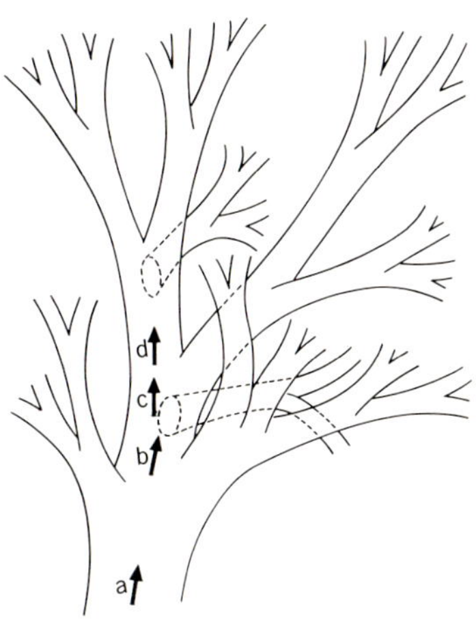


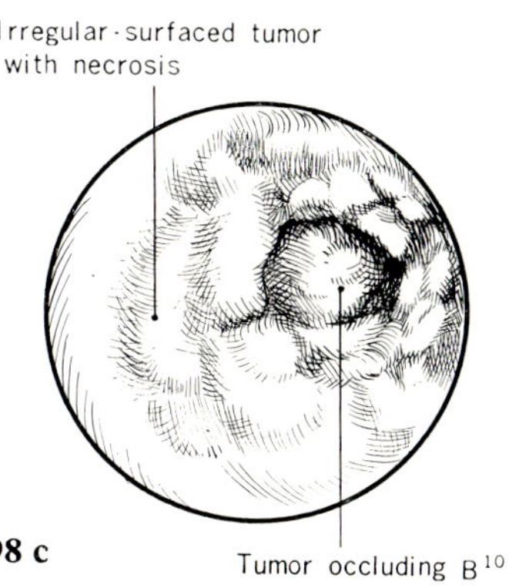


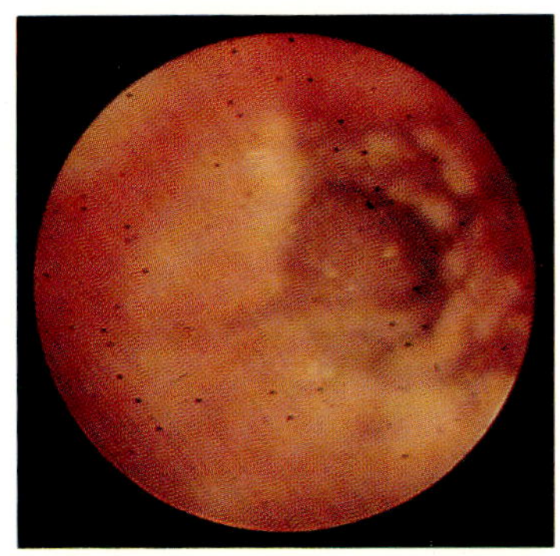

198 c

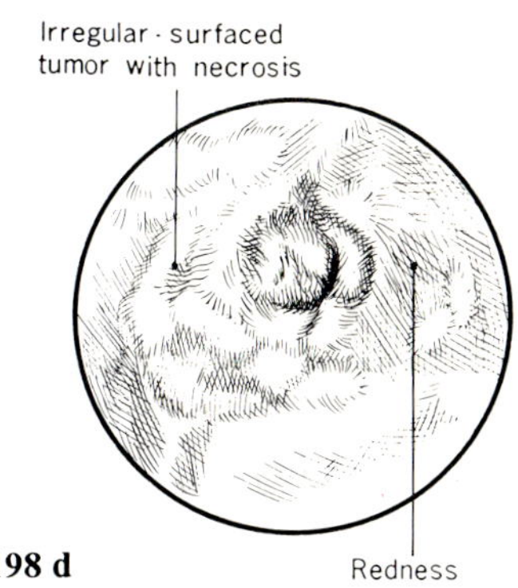


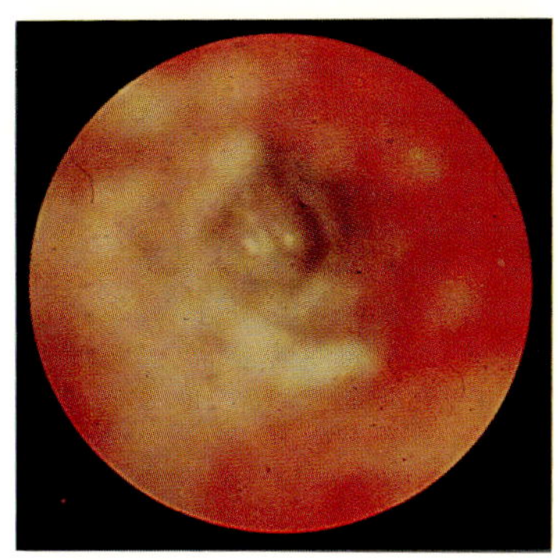

198 d

**Fig. 198 Fiberscopic findings :**

**a.** The mucosa at the orifice of $B^{9+10}$ is slightly reddened.

**b.** Stenosis is present and the mucosa is reddened at the orifice of $B^9$. The $B^{10}$ orifice is reddened and swollen, and the left lateral wall is irregular.

**c.** In the $B^{10}$ lumen a tumor with uneven surface is visualized on the left wall and the deeper lumen is stenosed by another tumor with an uneven surface. Small tumors are scattered on the right wall,

**d.** Still deeper, the lumen is almost completely surrounded with tumors, but those on the left wall are more intense.

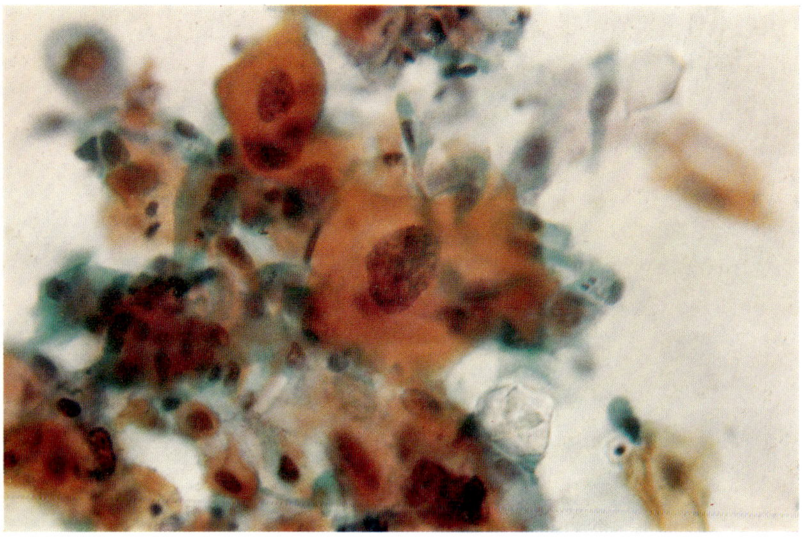

**Fig. 199 Cytodiagnosis:** Bronchofiberscopic curettage. The cytoplasm is brilliant orange. The nuclear chromatin shows irregular condensation and is hyperchromatic, while cytological examination on the sputum was negative on five occasions.

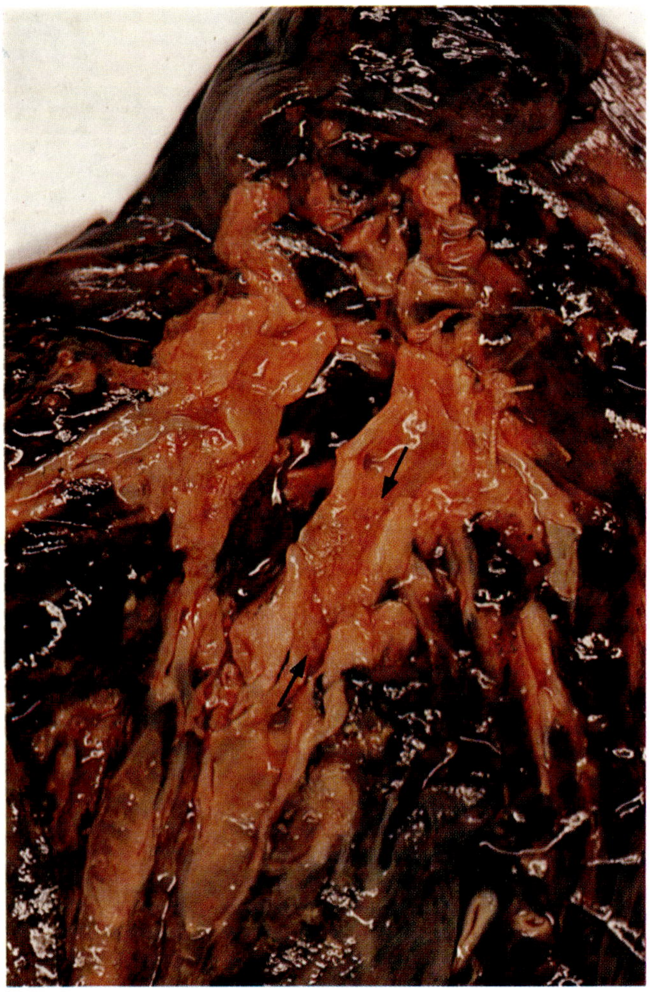

200 a

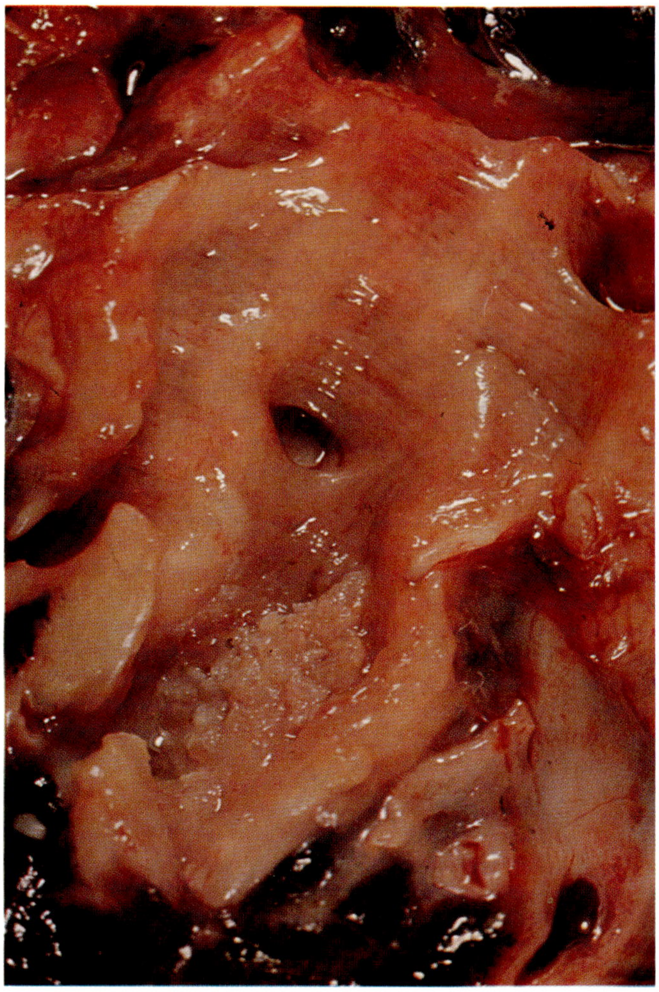

200 b

**Fig. 200 Macroscopic findings:**

**a.** $B^{10}$, laid open, is obstructed by a small lesion (arrow) which is within the bronchial wall. The peripheral bronchi are ectatic and full of purulent secretions.

**b.** Contact print of the central part of the lesion. The irregular surfaced cancer has infiltrated the inner wall of $B^{10}$.

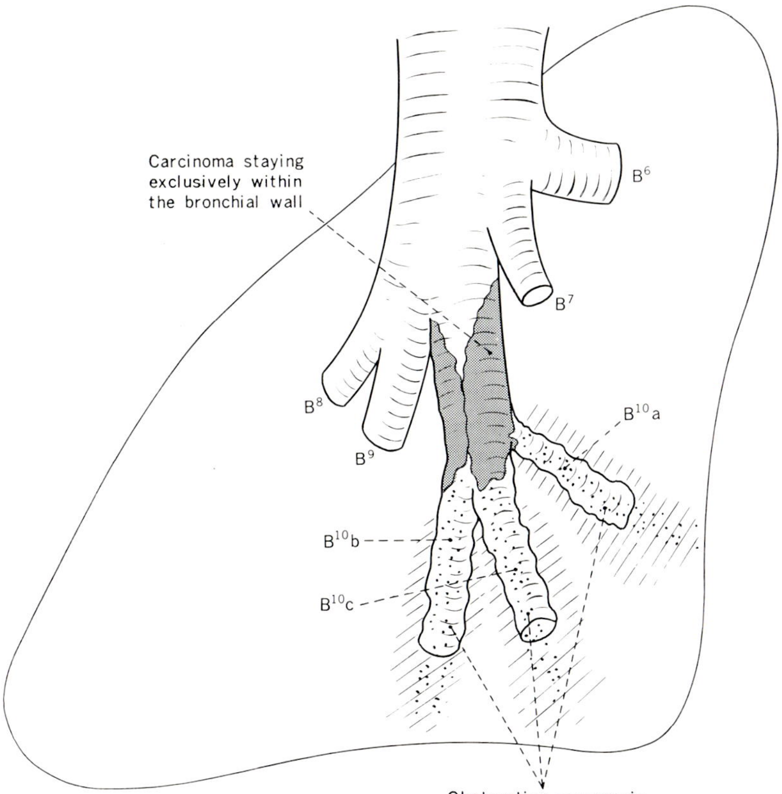


**Fig. 201 Traced schema :** Cancerous lesion, 20 mm in extent, is within the $B^{10}$ bronchial wall. The lumen is nearly obstructed and the peripheral branches (**$B^{10}$a, $B^{10}$b** and **$B^{10}$c**) are involved in obstructive pneumonia.

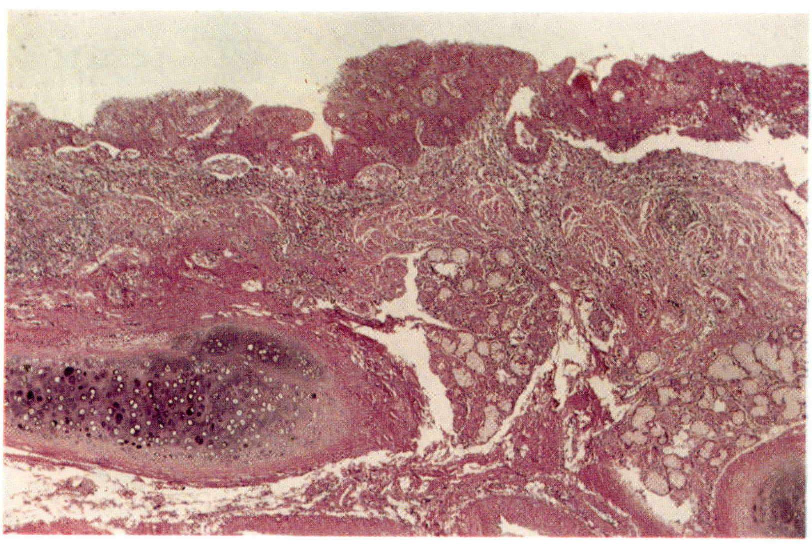

**202 a**

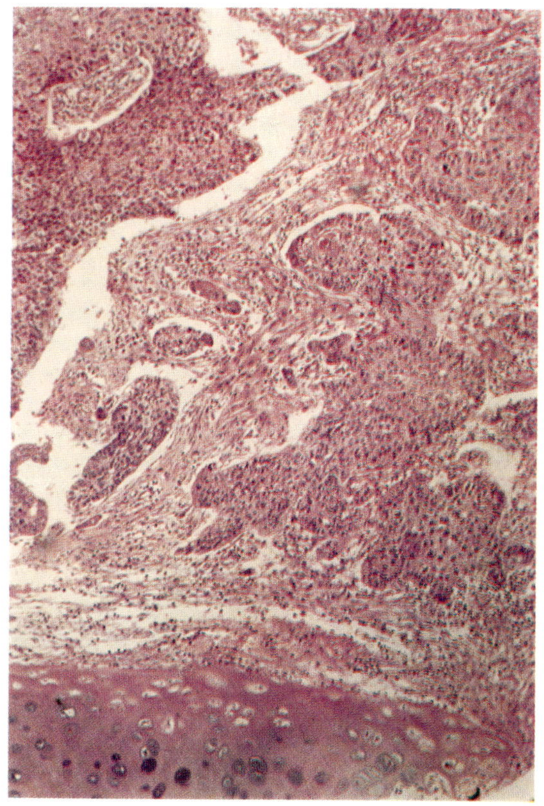

**202 b**

**Fig. 202 Microscopic findings :**

**a.** A micrograph of the peripheral lesion. Squamous cell carcinoma, 1–2 mm in thickness, has superficially infiltrated into $B^{10}$, replacing its epithelium.

**b.** The central part of the tumor has infiltrated the submucosa and further in part into the bronchial cartilage, but remains within the bronchial wall.

## COMMENT :

This is a typical case of early lung cancer of the hilar type, in which definite irregularity of mucosa and the presence of tumors were visualized with a bronchofiberscope. This was suspected because of subjective symptoms of bloody sputum and obstruction of $B^{10}$ by bronchogram. This case best illustrates axiom : Bronchoscopy should immediately applicable in case of the heavy smoker with bloody sputum.

## Case 4 Lung Cancer, Early Stage – Hilar Type (60, male)

**Chief complaint :** Bloody sputum.
**Definitive clinical diagnosis :** Squamous cell carcinoma by bronchofiberscopic biopsy.
**Pathological diagnosis :** Keratotic squamous cell carcinoma.
**Case history :** In May, 1970, the patient had symptoms of flu and in June had blood-stained sputum. A practitioner diagnosed bronchopneumonia with chest X-ray examination. Repeated bloody sputum in July brought the patient to our hospital.

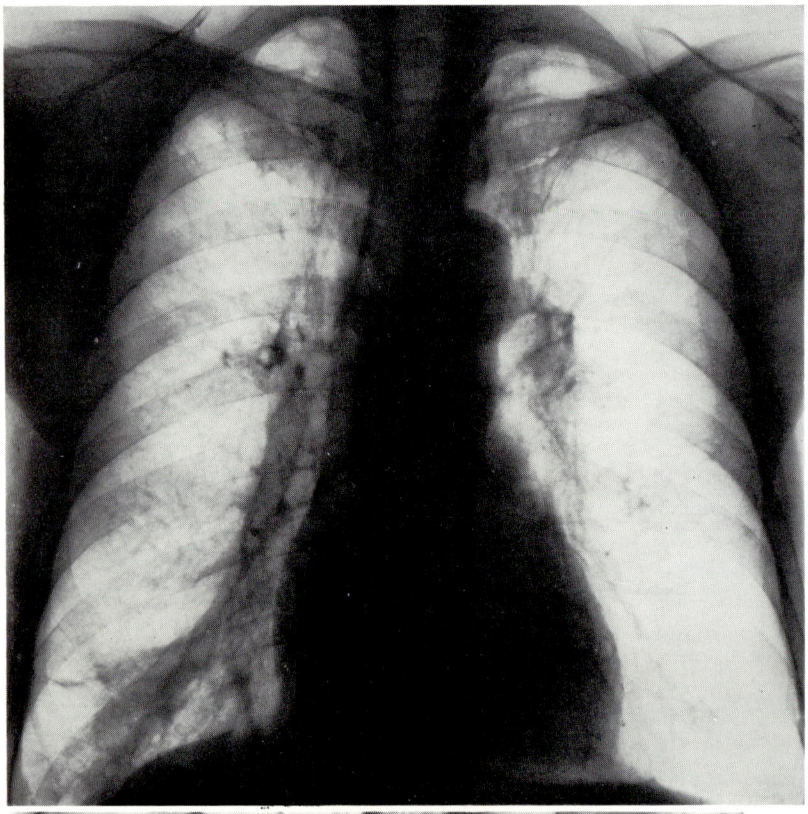

**Fig. 203 Chest X-ray, frontal :** In the right lower lobe lies a broad cord-like shadow. The lumina of $B^8$, $B^9$ and $B^{10}$ appear distended, and the pulmonary parenchyma around these bronchi are fibrotic.

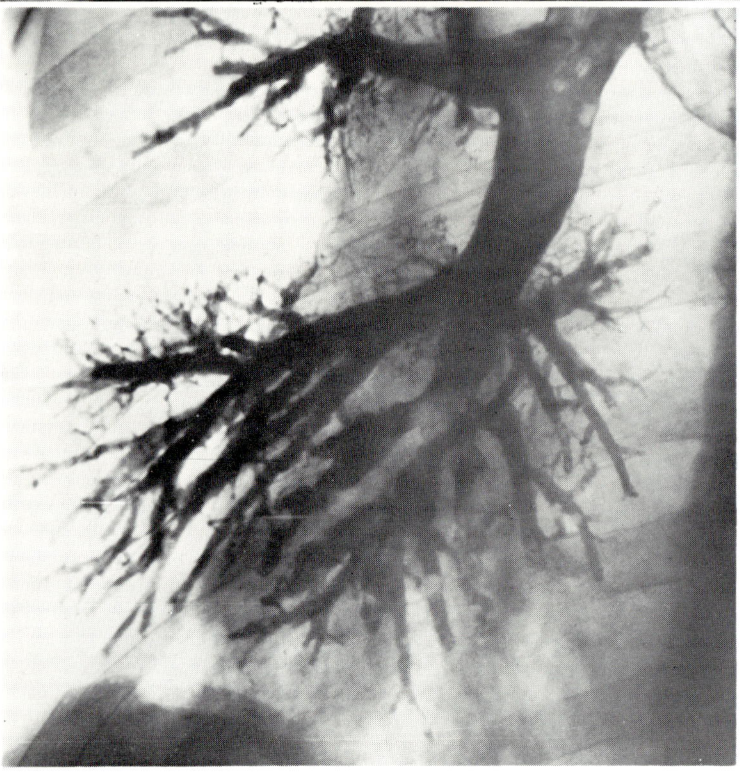

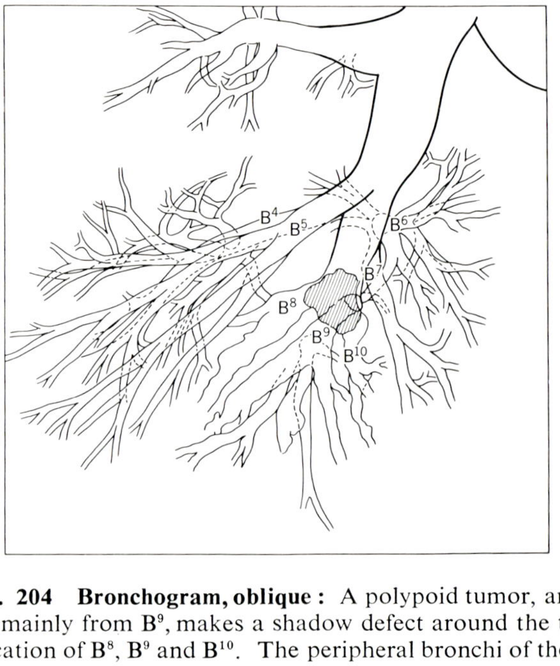


**Fig. 204 Bronchogram, oblique :** A polypoid tumor, arising mainly from $B^9$, makes a shadow defect around the trifurcation of $B^8$, $B^9$ and $B^{10}$. The peripheral bronchi of these three are ectatic, forming several sacs.

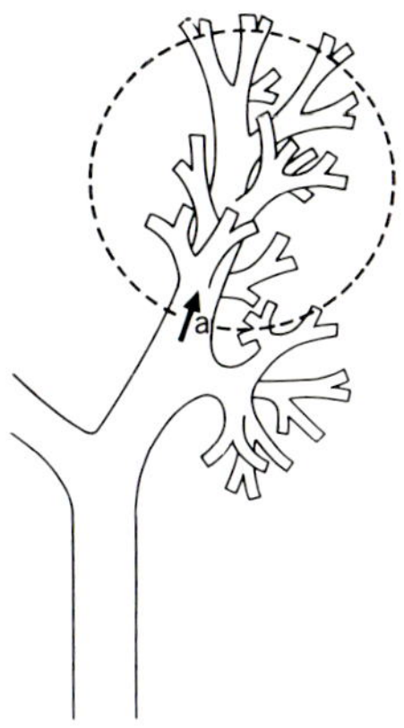


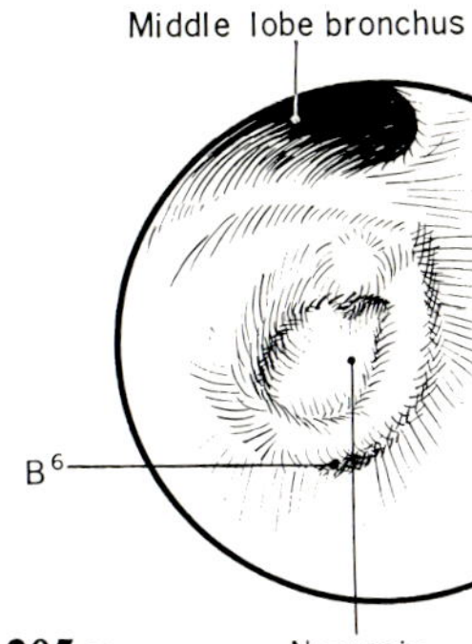


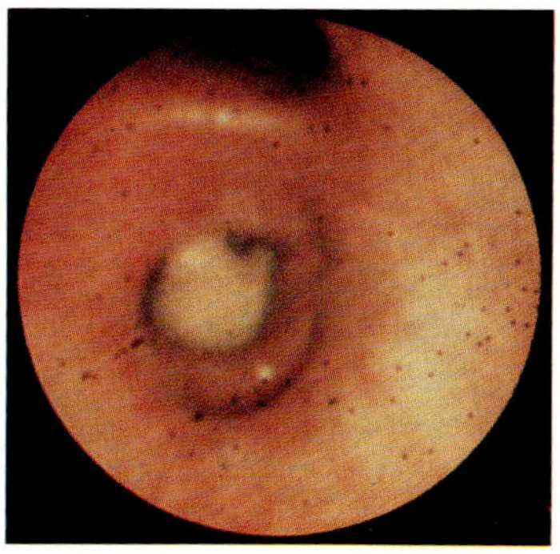

205 a

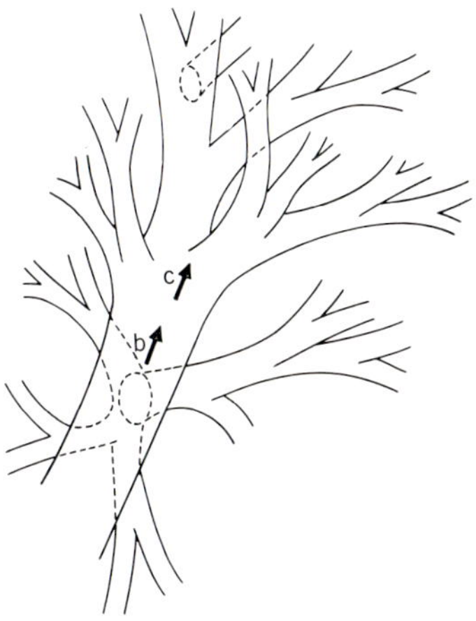


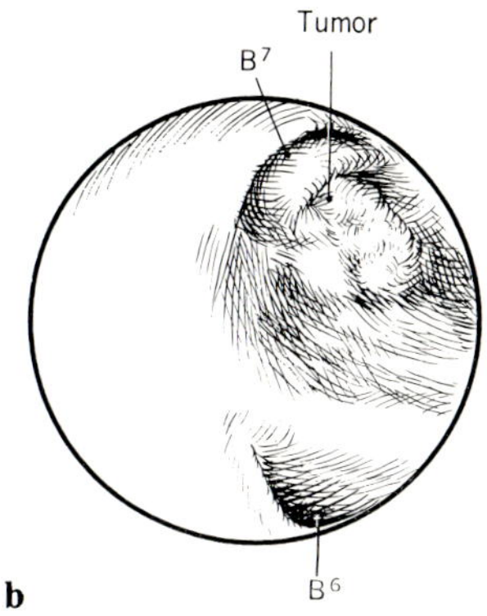


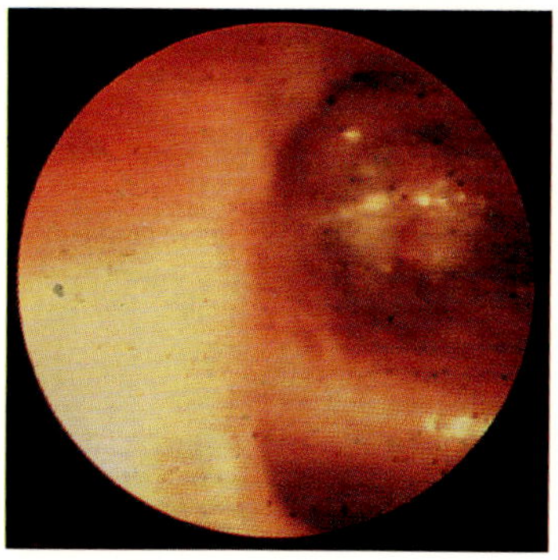

205 b

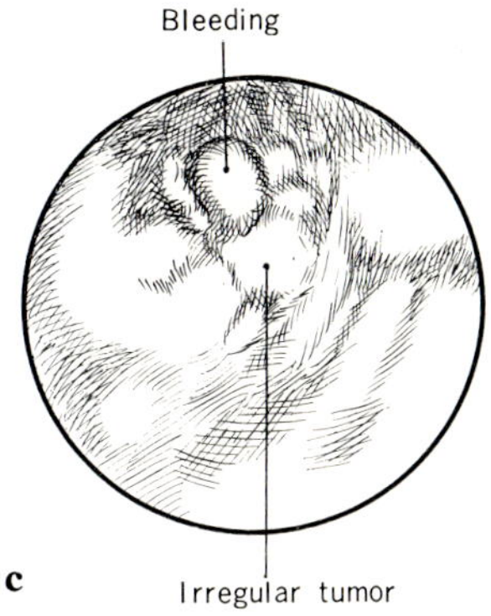


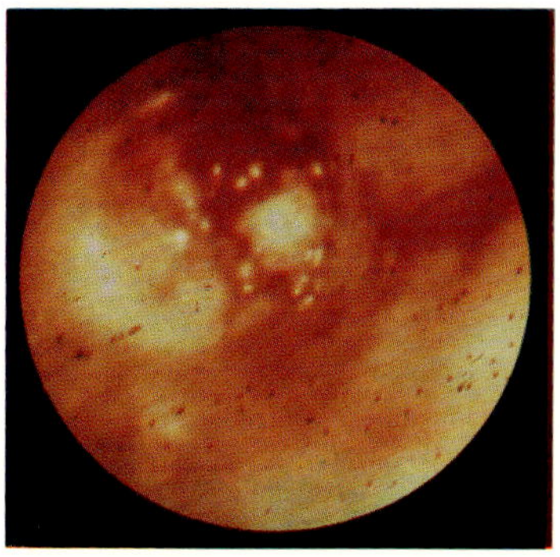

205 c

**Fig. 205 Fiberscopic findings:**

**a.** The basal bronchus is obstructed by necrotic substance. The bronchi around it remain normal.

**b.** An exploration after the removal of the necrosis revealed the lumina of $B^8$, $B^9$ and $B^{10}$ to be almost obstructed by an irregular-surfaced tumor. On the right posterior wall in particular slight infiltrative changes are noted, and on the left posterior wall purulent secretions are present.

**c.** An irregular tumor located at the posterior wall of $B^{8+9+10}$ with some bleeding from the tumor.

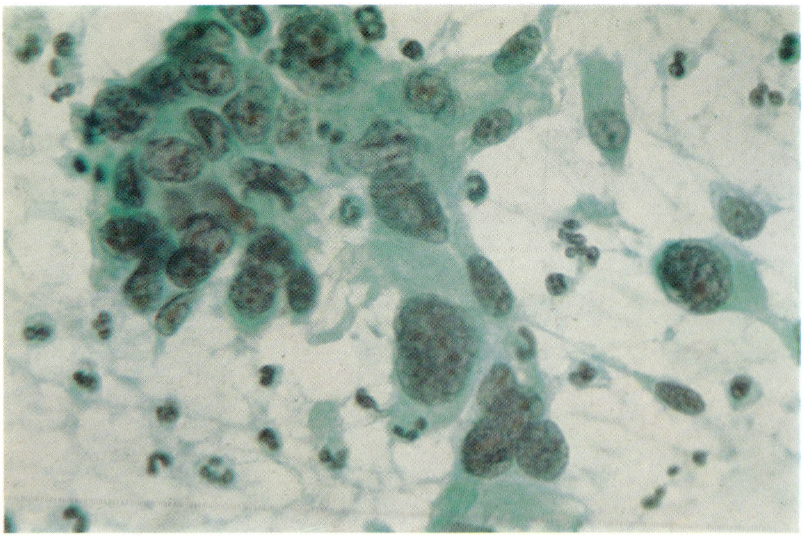

**Fig. 206 Cytodiagnosis :** Bronchofiberscopic curettage. The nuclei are prominently varied in size and malformed. Chromatin is coarse. The nucleoli are red-stained, malformed and scattered in a large number of cells. On the other hand, cytology of sputum, repeated 6 times, was negative.

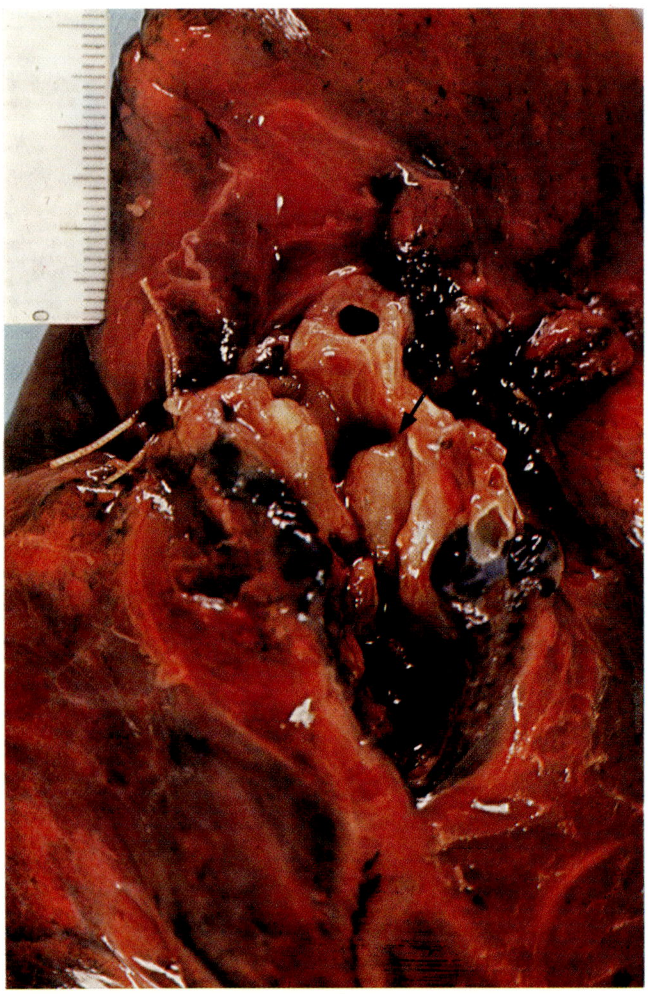

**Fig. 207 Macroscopic findings :** Fresh specimen. A small tumor (arrow) is exposed in the lumen of the right lower lobe bronchus which was partly opened.

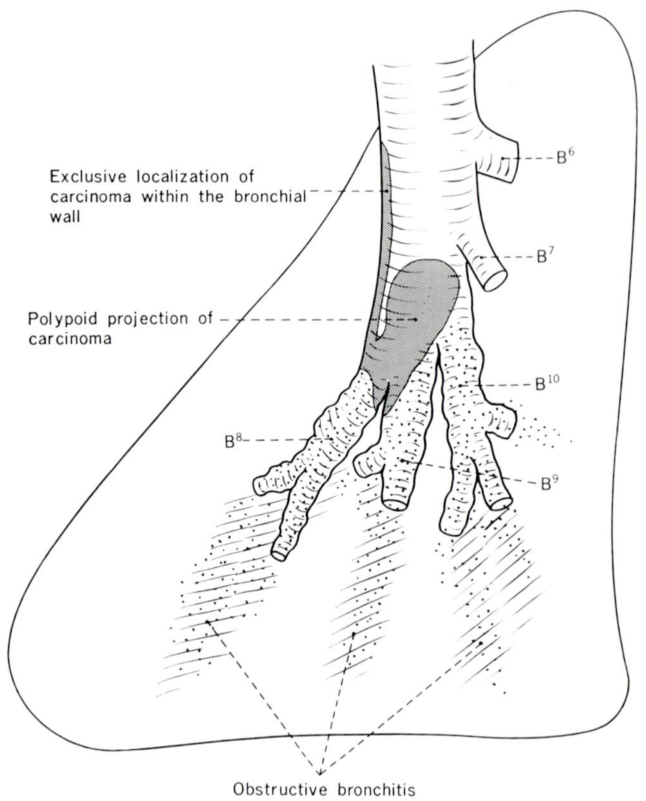


**Fig. 208 Traced schema :** A polypoid tumor protruding from the bifurcation into $B^8$ and $B^9$ nearly obstructs the bronchial lumen. The peripheral areas of $B^8$, $B^9$ and $B^{10}$ are involved in obstructive pneumonia. In some areas, an infiltration has invaded the bronchi proximally along the lumen.

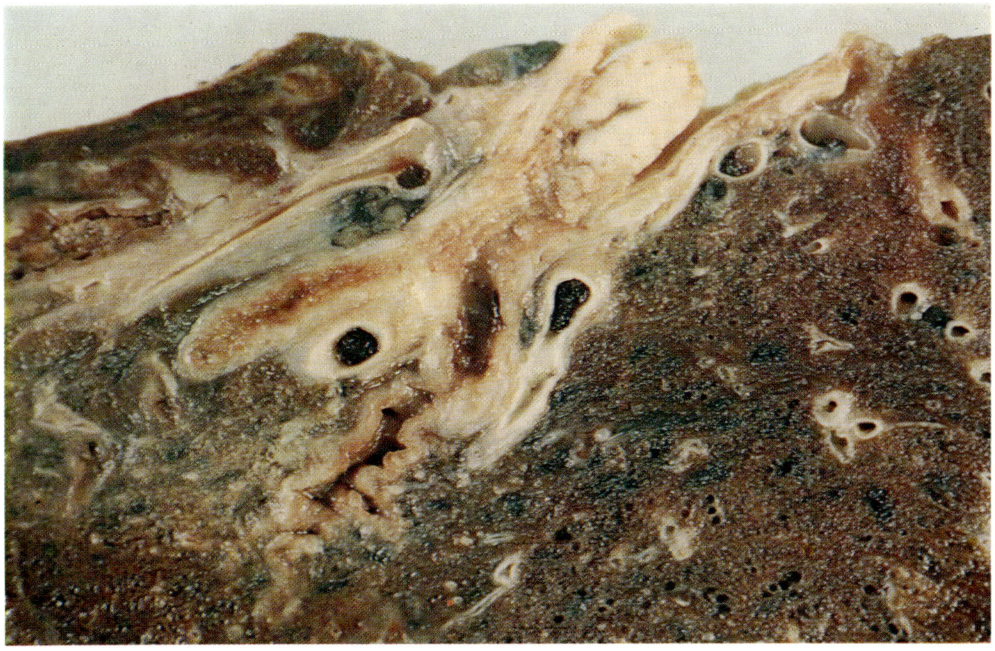

**Fig. 209 Macroscopic findings :** Fixed specimen. The protuberant polypoid tumor, 8×18 mm, barely sticks to the bronchial wall. The peripheral part of the tumor covering $B^8$a and $B^8$b presents an inflammatory lesion suggesting obstructive bronchitis with thickened walls and ectatic lumina, and the lesion extends into the pulmonary parenchyma.

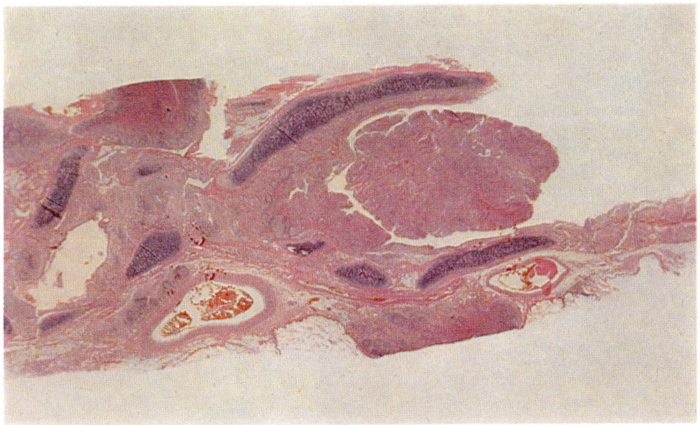

**210 a**

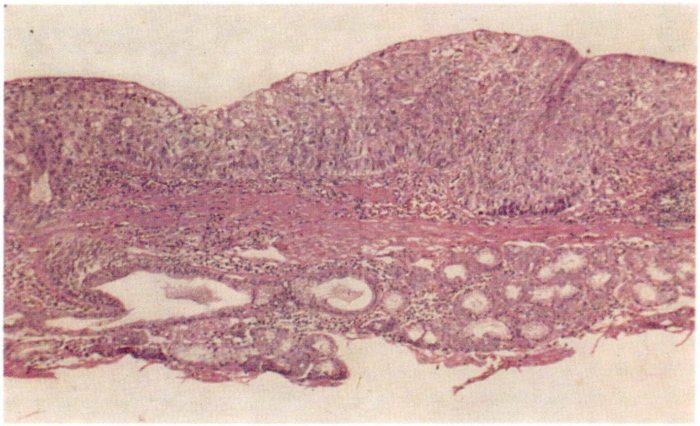

**210 b**

**Fig. 210 Microscopic findings :**
- **a.** Squamous cell carcinoma, less keratinized, has barely infiltrated into the bronchial wall, only reaching the muscular tunic of the mucosa.
- **b.** The tumor has infiltrated partly, replacing the epithelium of the lower lobe bronchus for a distance of approximately 20mm.

## COMMENT :

The chest X-ray film revealed a cord-like shadow but no tumor shadow was obtained. This cord-like shadow was due to inflammation further peripherally from the orifices of $B^8$, $B^9$ and $B^{10}$, caused by bronchial stenosis due to a small carcinoma. Obstcucted pneumonia or bronchiectasis is readily caused by a tumor growing in a major bronchus in this manner. On such an occasion, it is very important to carry out bronchofiberscopic examination, even if a shadow defect is found in the bronchogram. This is one of the examples of early lung cancer located within the bronchial wall. The patient was a heavy smoker with the chief complaint of bloody sputum.

## Case 5 Lung Cancer, Early Stage – Peripheral Type (58, male)

**Chief complaint :** Abnormal shadow was found in a mass survey.

**Definitive clinical diagnosis :** Adenocarcinoma by cytologic examination of sputum, same diagnosis by bronchofiberscopic curettage.

**Pathological diagnosis :** Adenocarcinoma of mucous gland origin.

**Case history :** The patient had been X-rayed by the mass survey annually but no abnomality had been found. One month ago, he was examined by a certain practitioner who X-rayed his chest and referred him to our hospital for further examination. He had no cough nor sputum. His smoking habit was 20–30 cigarettes a day, inhaled deeply, for the past 10 years.

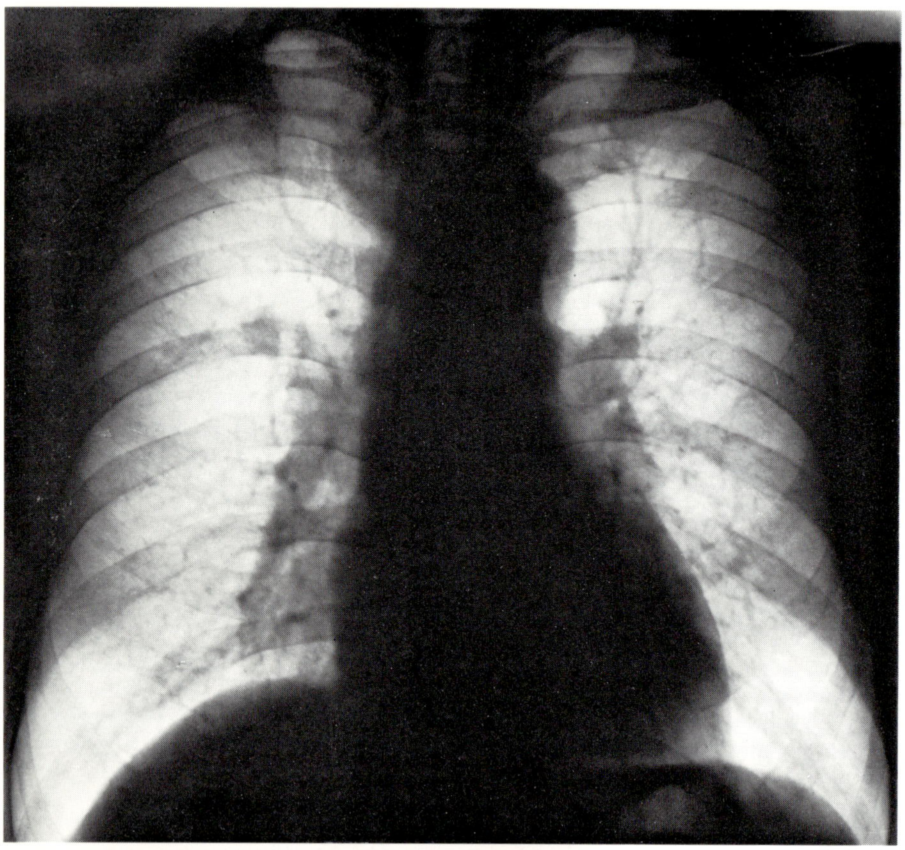

**Fig. 211 Chest X-ray, frontal :** A tumor shadow, 13×13 mm, with relatively distinct periphery, is localized in the middle field.

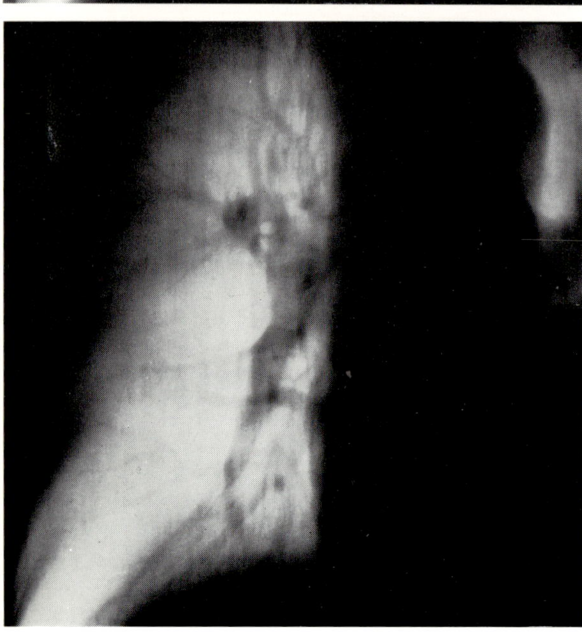

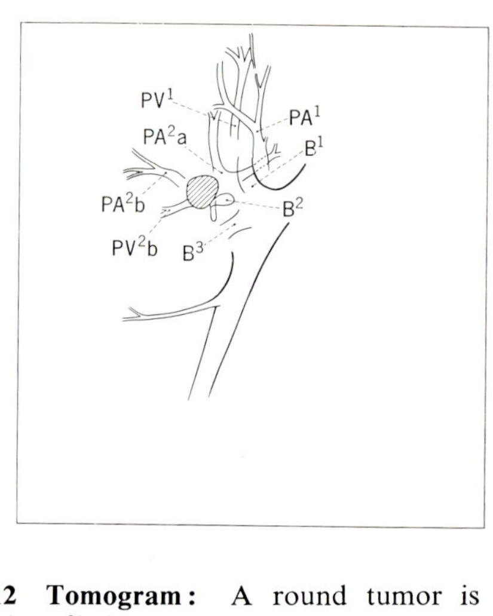


**Fig. 212 Tomogram :** A round tumor is present along the $B^2b$ bronchus and the pulmonary arteries, $A^2a$ and $A^2b$, pass around the tumor.

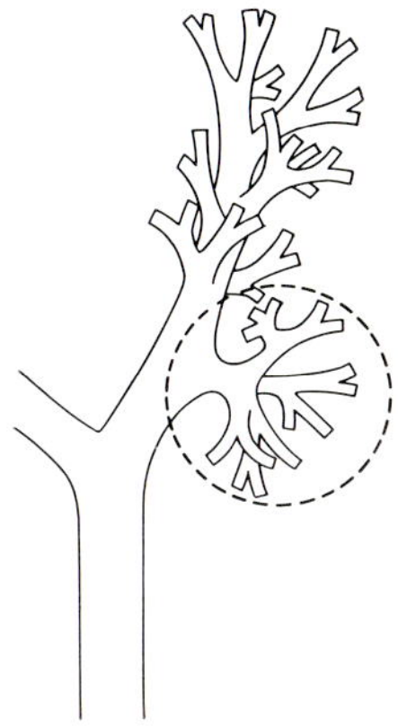

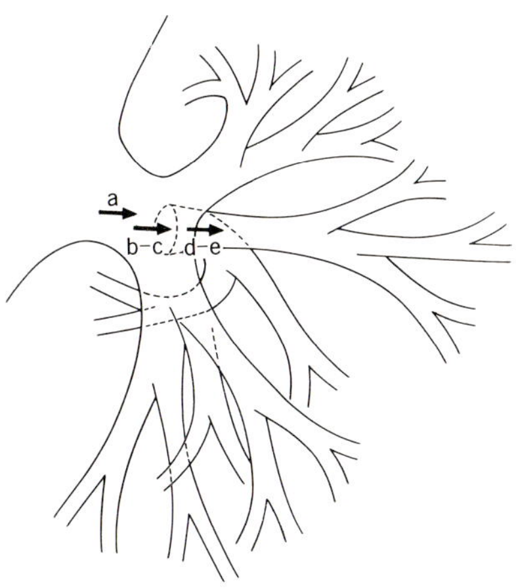


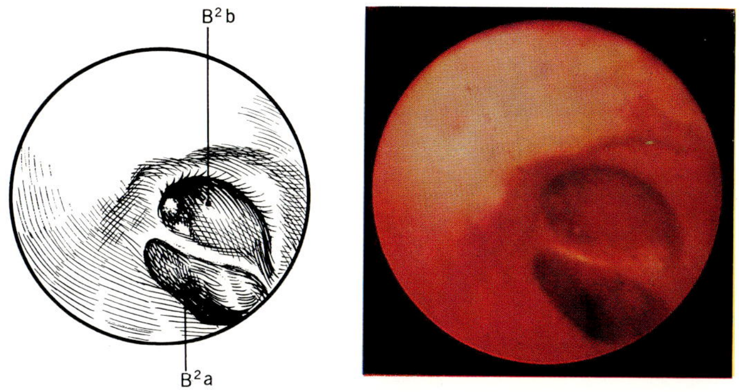


**213 a**

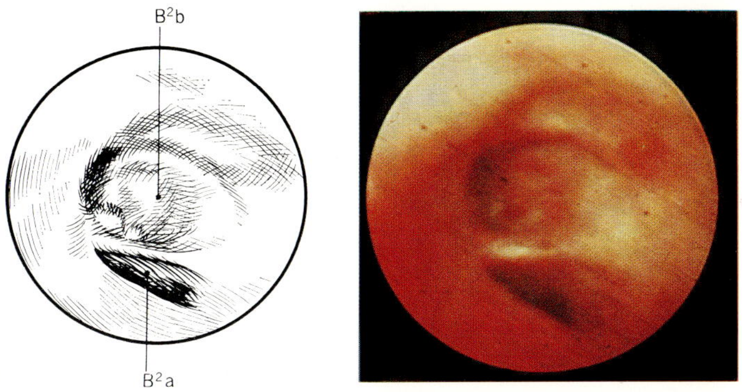


**213 b**

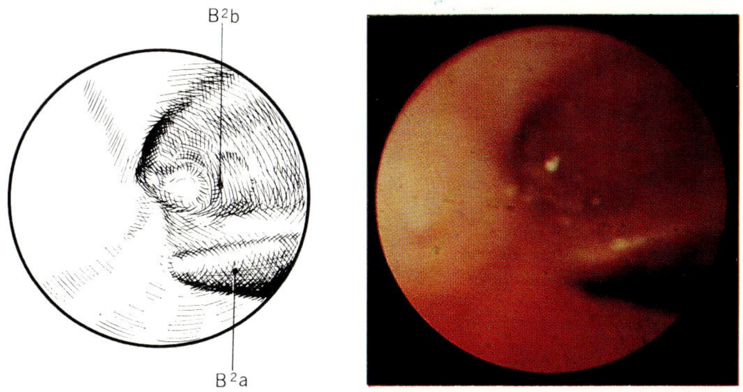


**213 c**

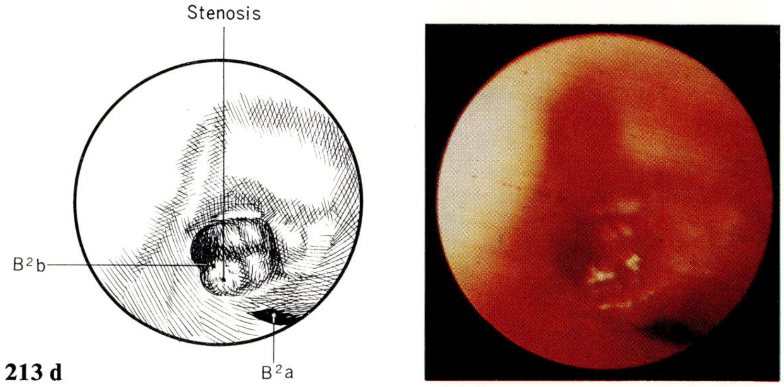


**213 d**

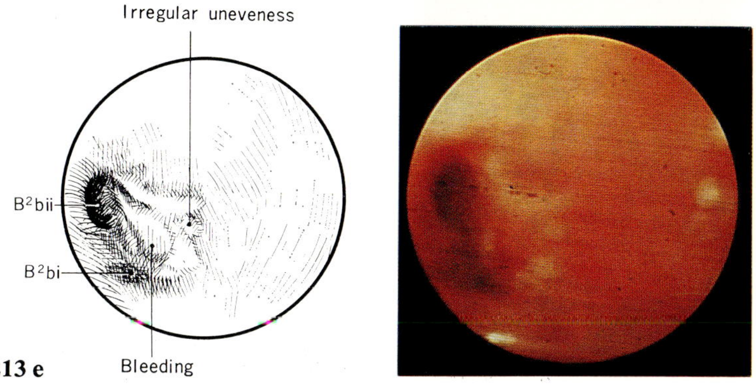


**213 e**

**Fig. 213 Fiberscopic findings :**

**a.** $B^2$ branches off into $B^2a$ and $B^2b$, but the bifurcation is normal.
**b.** Fiberscope advanced deeper into $B^2$.
**c.** $B^2b$ is gradually narrowed.
**d.** $B^2b$ is stenosed at its deeper part and bleeding.
**e.** $B^2b$ bifurcates to i and ii. The mucosa of the right wall at the bifurcation is irregular and the cartilage rings are obscured, and bleeding, $B^2bi$ is completely stenosed.

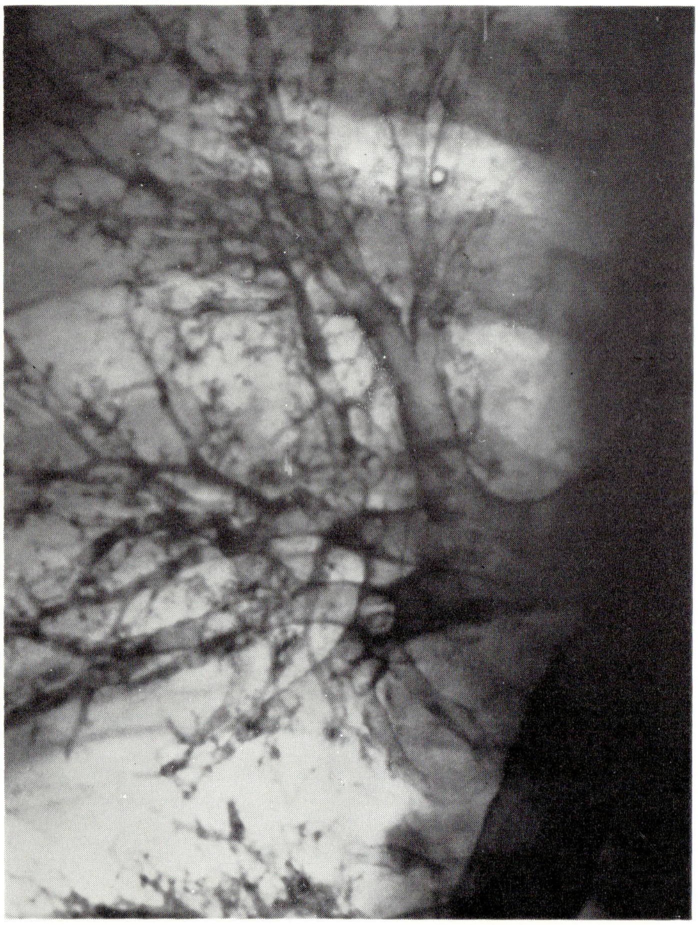

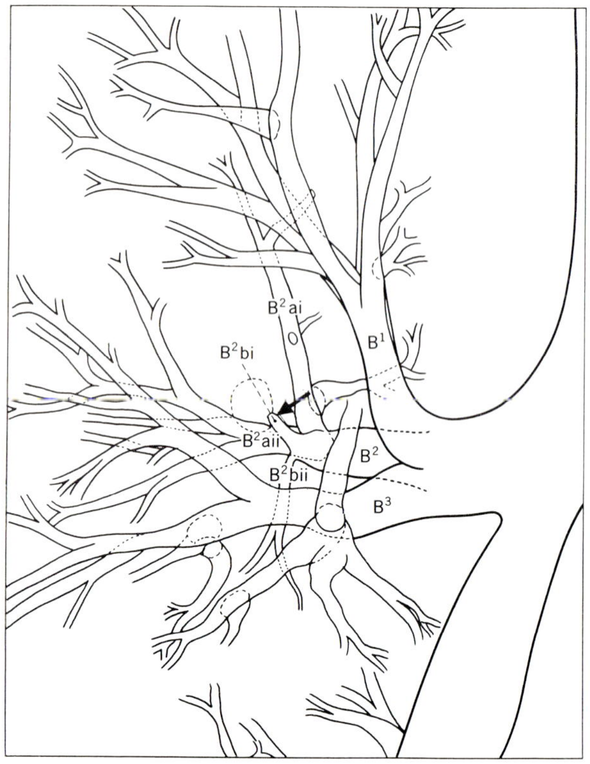


**Fig. 214 Bronchogram, frontal:** $B^2$bi is irregularly obstructed (arrow), $B^2$bii is narrowed, and $B^2$a is almost normal.

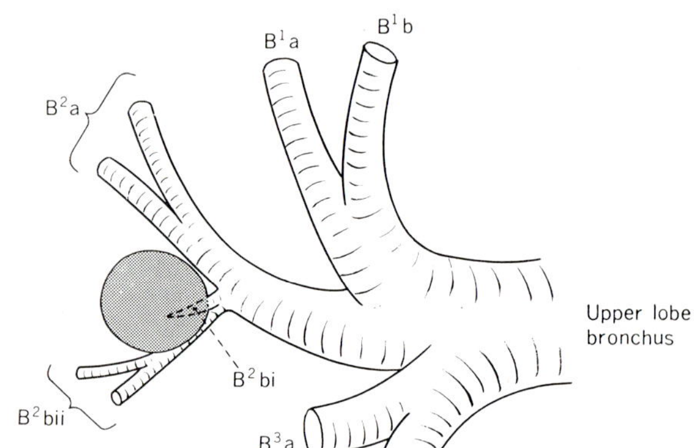


**Fig. 215 Traced schema:** The tumor of 13×11 mm obstructing $B^2$bi and stenosing $B^2$bii.

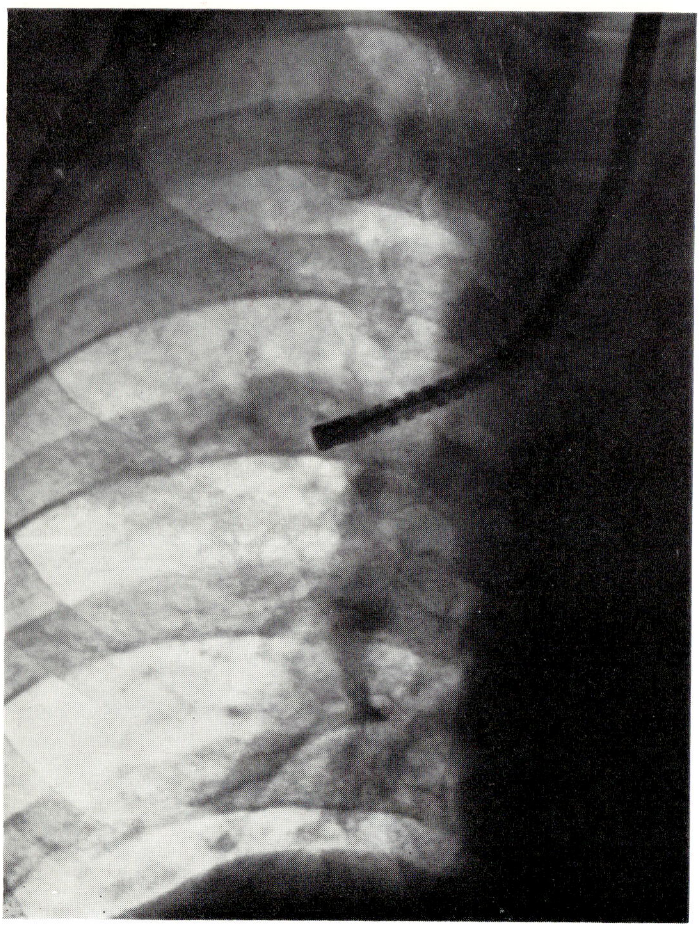

**Fig. 216 Bronchofiberscopy:** A flexible bronchofiberscope, Machida make, 4 mm in diameter, is inserted into $B^2$.

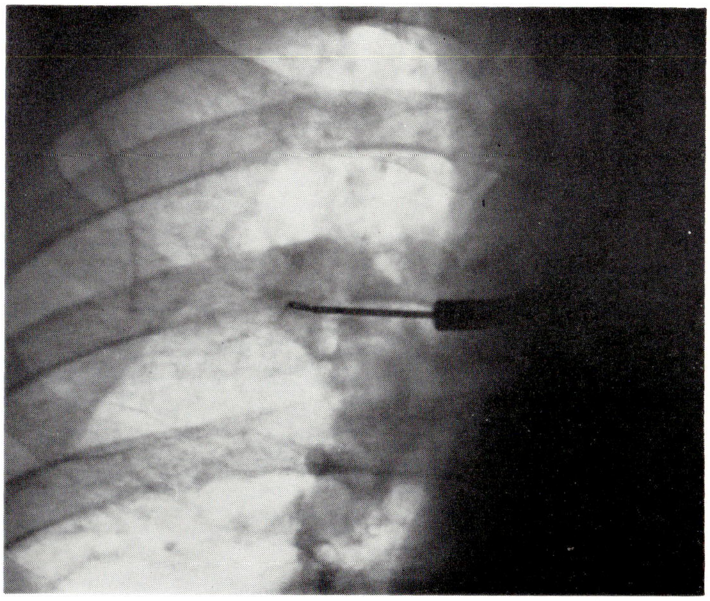

**Fig. 217 Curettage:** A small curette, passed through the 5mm Machida bronchofiberscope channel, enters the tumor.

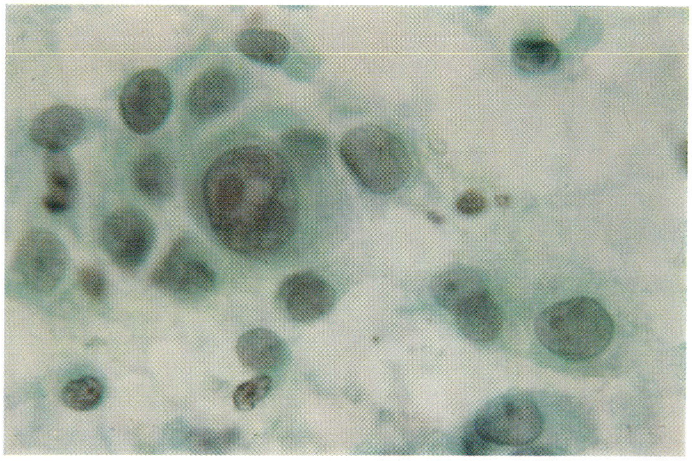

**Fig. 218 Cytodiagnosis:** Adenocarcinoma cells obtained by bronchofiberscopic curettage. Cells are relatively scarce in atypia, but considerably enlarged nucleoli are characteristic. Large cells are present among others.

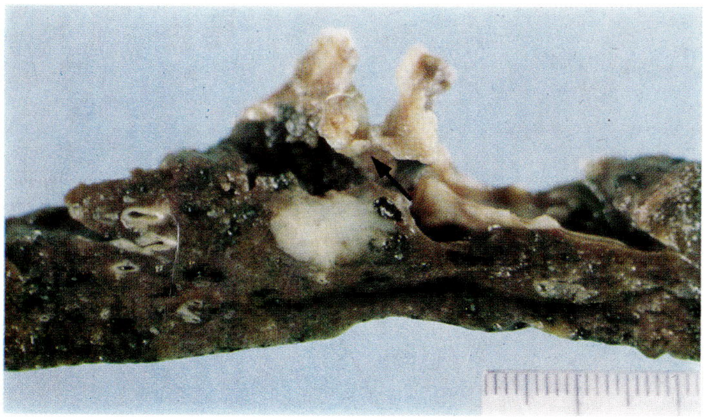

219 a

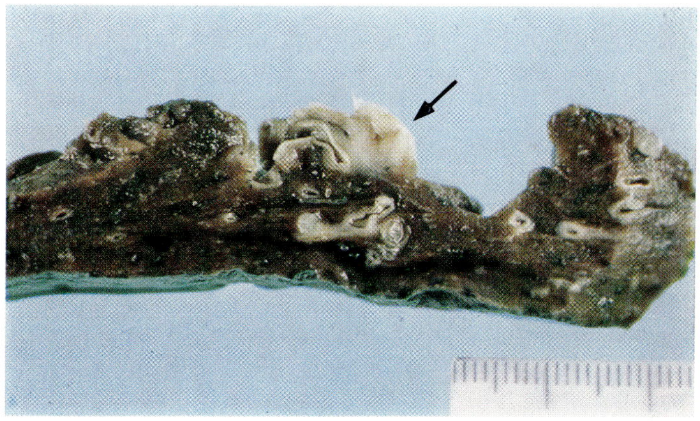

219 b

**Fig. 219 Macroscopic findings:**

**a.** A transverse section of the involved bronchus ($B^2$bi) including the proximal side. The circular tumor, 13×11 mm, with well delineated boundaries is seen. The inside is medullary, homogeneous and ivory-like.

**b.** The involved bronchus is completely destroyed by the tumor (arrow).

**Fig. 220 Microscopic findings:** $B^2$bi surrounded by the cancer has infiltrated completely into the bronchial cartilage, destroying the bronchus and obstructing the lumen irregularly.

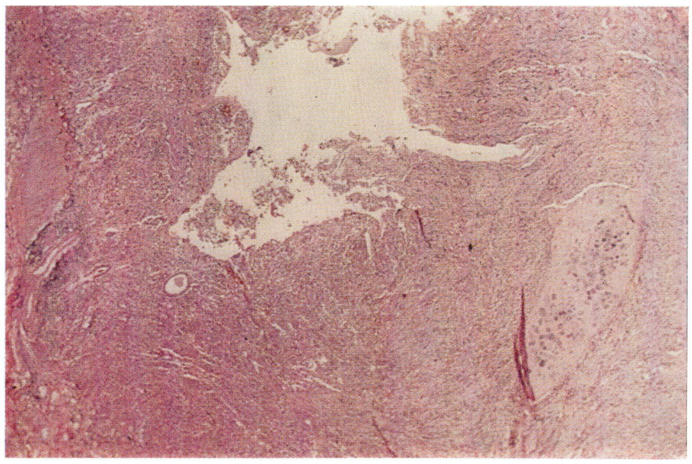

220

## COMMENT:

Even in early stages of peripheral lung cancer, the tumor can be visualized by a flexible bronchofiberscope especially if its location is determined by previous bronchography. Furthermore, definitive cytological diagnosis can be made by curettage of the lesion with a small curette passed through the channel of the bronchofiberscope.

## Case 6 Lung Cancer, Early Stage – Peripheral Type (56, male)

**Chief complaint :** Chest pain.
**Definitive clinical diagnosis :** Adenocarcinoma by bronchofiberscopic curettage.
**Pathological diagnosis :** Papillary adenocarcinoma.
**Case history :** About 30 years ago the patient underwent surgery for tuberculosis on the right lung. About 2 months ago, he was examined for sustained pain in the right chest. An abnormal shadow was found but no definitive diagnosis was made and so visited our hospital. He smoked a little more than 20 cigarettes a day since age 20.

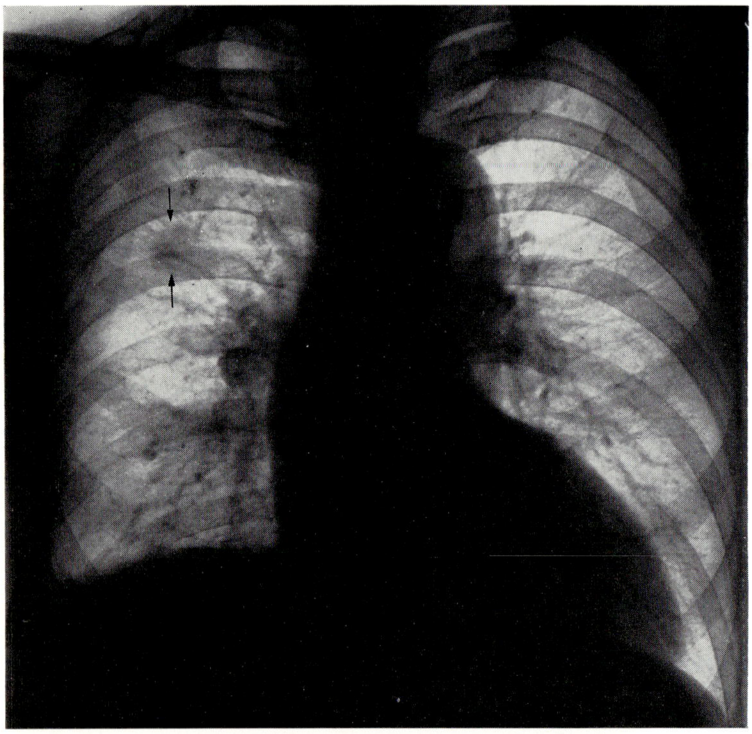

**Fig. 221 Chest X-ray, frontal :** An extremely pale shadow with radiating protrusions on the periphery is observed in the right mid-lung. The presence of pleural indentation is suspected. A lymph node, darkened and calcified, is noted near the hilum.

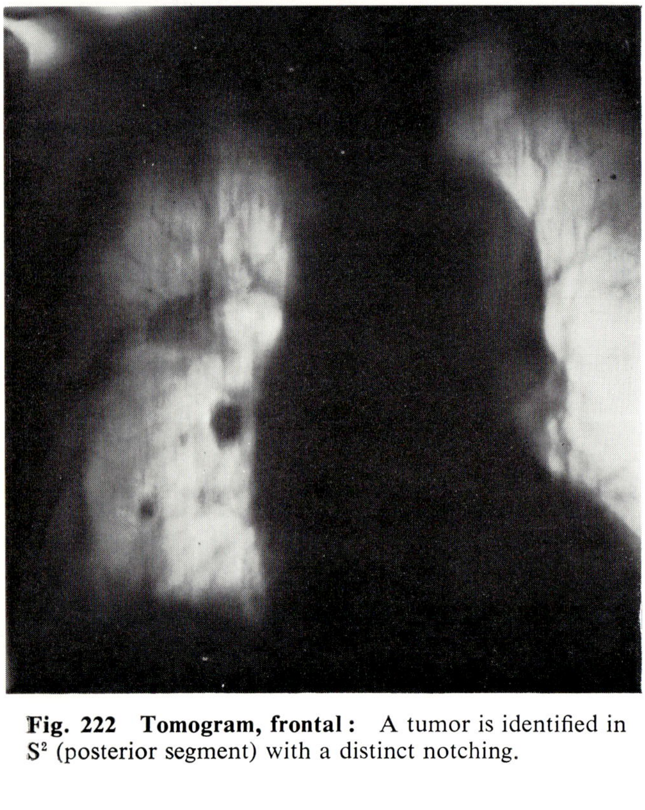

**Fig. 222 Tomogram, frontal :** A tumor is identified in $S^2$ (posterior segment) with a distinct notching.

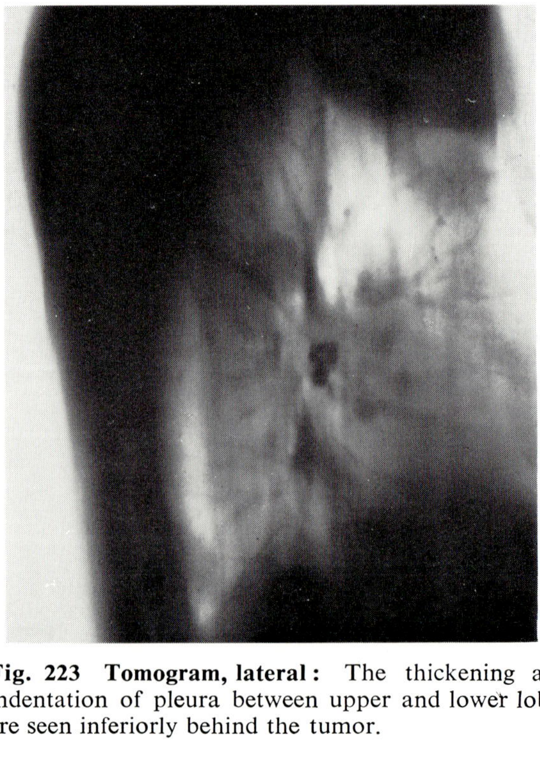

**Fig. 223 Tomogram, lateral :** The thickening and indentation of pleura between upper and lower lobes are seen inferiorly behind the tumor.

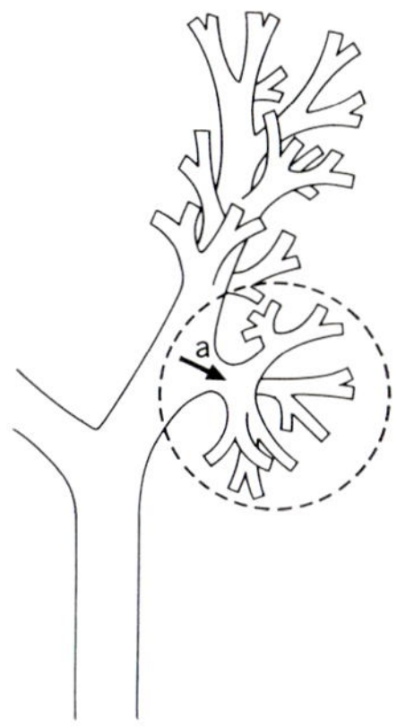


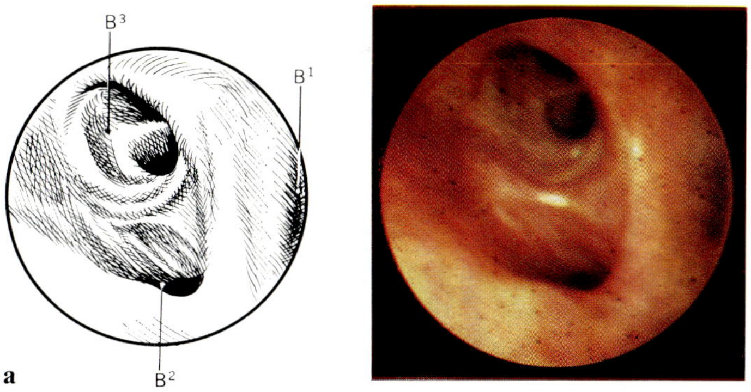


224 a

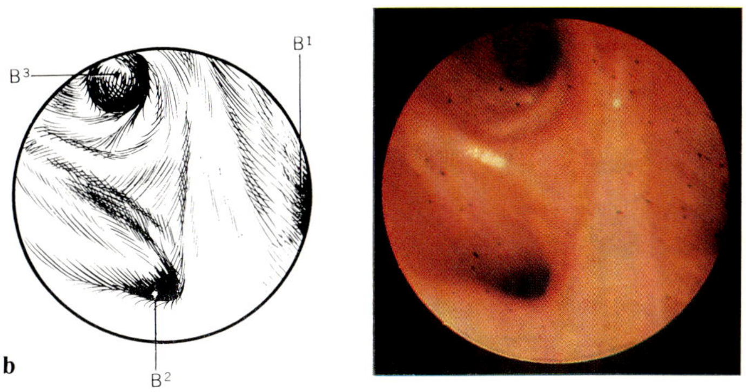


224 b

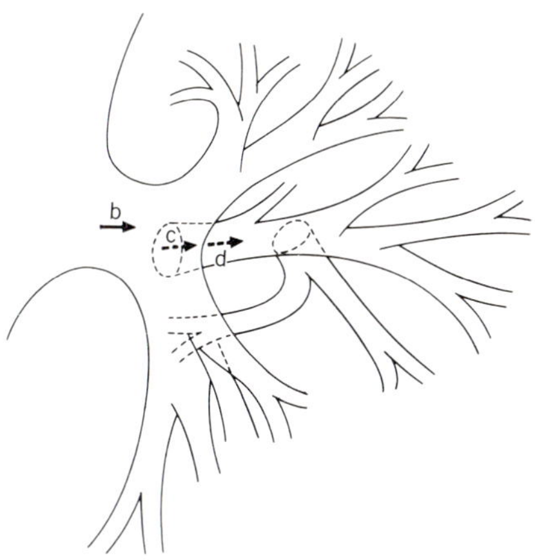


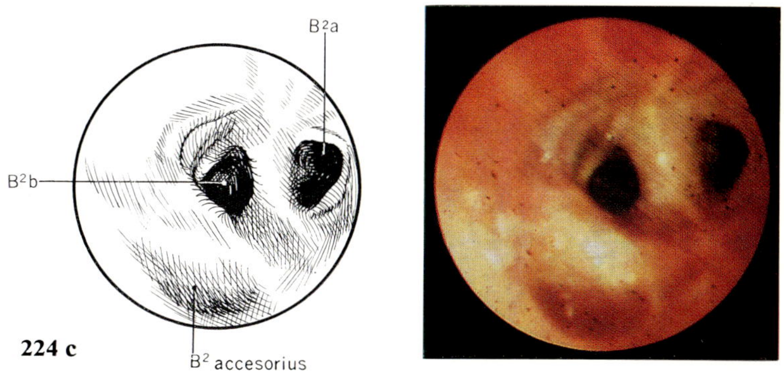


224 c

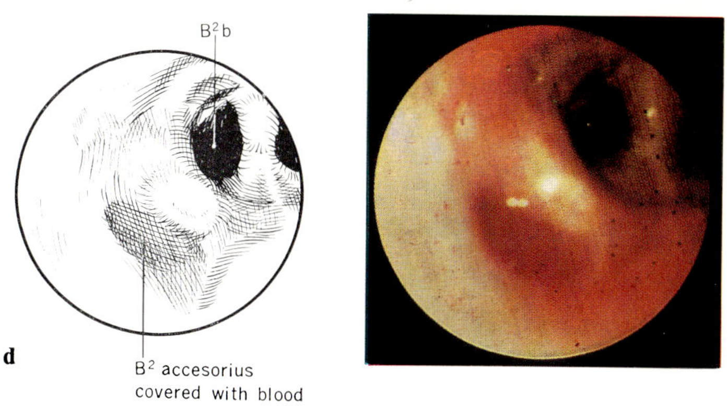


224 d

**Fig. 224 Fiberscopic findings:**

**a.** The upper lobe bronchus branches into $B^1$ and $B^{2+3}$.

**b.** The bronchial mucosa at the orifices of these bronchi is normal.

**c.** $B^2$ bifurcates into $B^2a+b$ and $B^2$ accesorius branch. The bifurcation is a little thickened nearer to $B^2$ accesorius branch.

**d.** $B^2$ accesorius branch is entirely filled with blood. The tumor was located slightly distal to this.

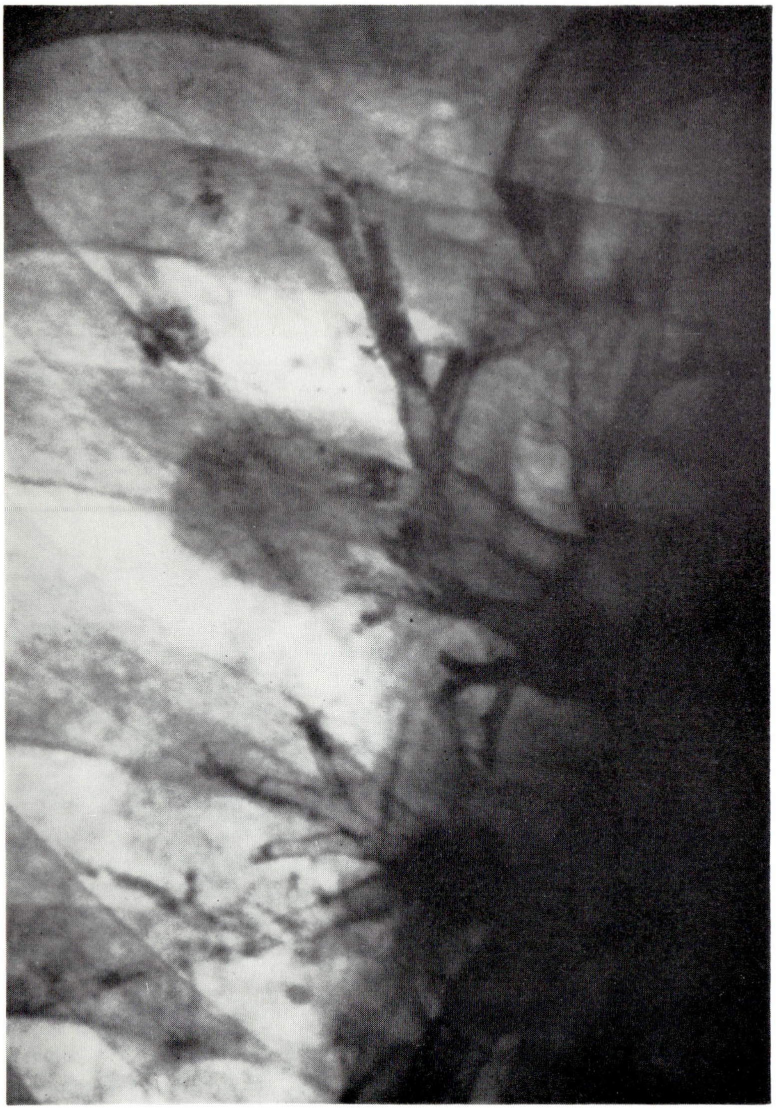

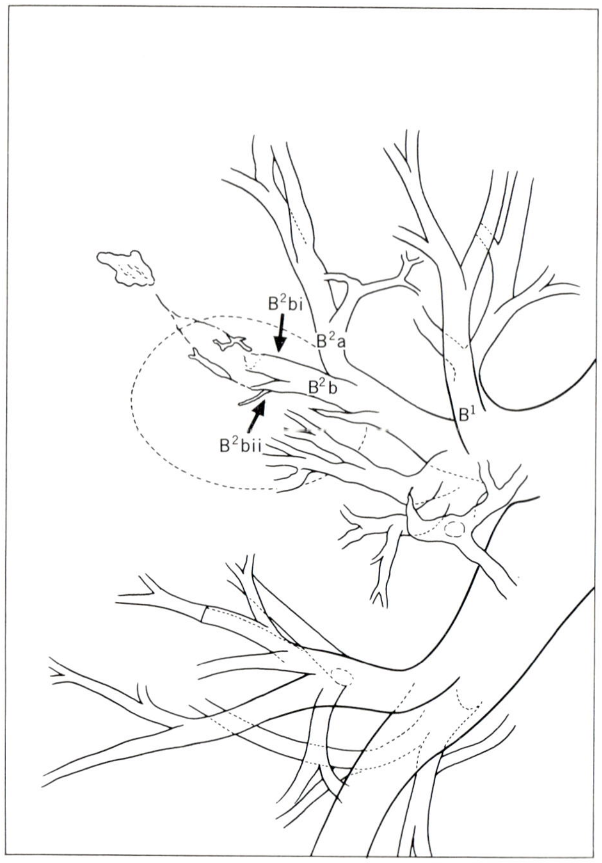


**Fig. 225 Bronchogram, inversely oblique :** The $B^2bii$ is pointed in shape and stenosed (arrow). $B^2bi$ is also sharp and stenosed (arrow). These stenosed bronchi are passing through the tumor. Peripheral bronchiole is seen in the small branch bronchus of $B^2bi$. From these findings the lung cancer can be diagnosed.

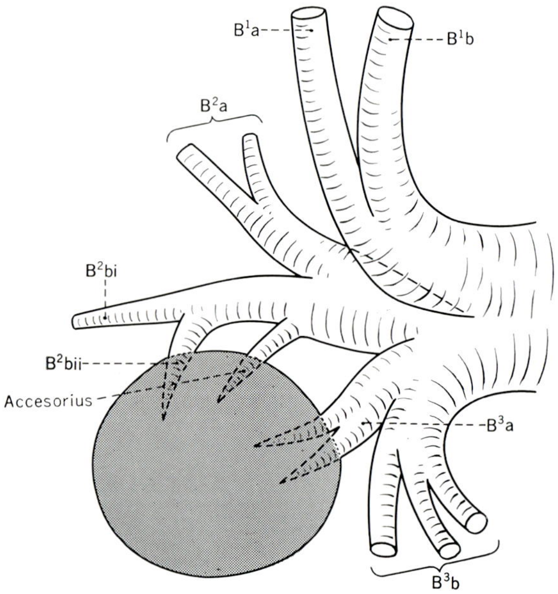


**Fig. 226 Traced schema :** The 20×20mm carcinoma involves 4 bronchi ; $B^2$ accessorius, $B^2bii$, $B^3ai$ and $B^3aii$.

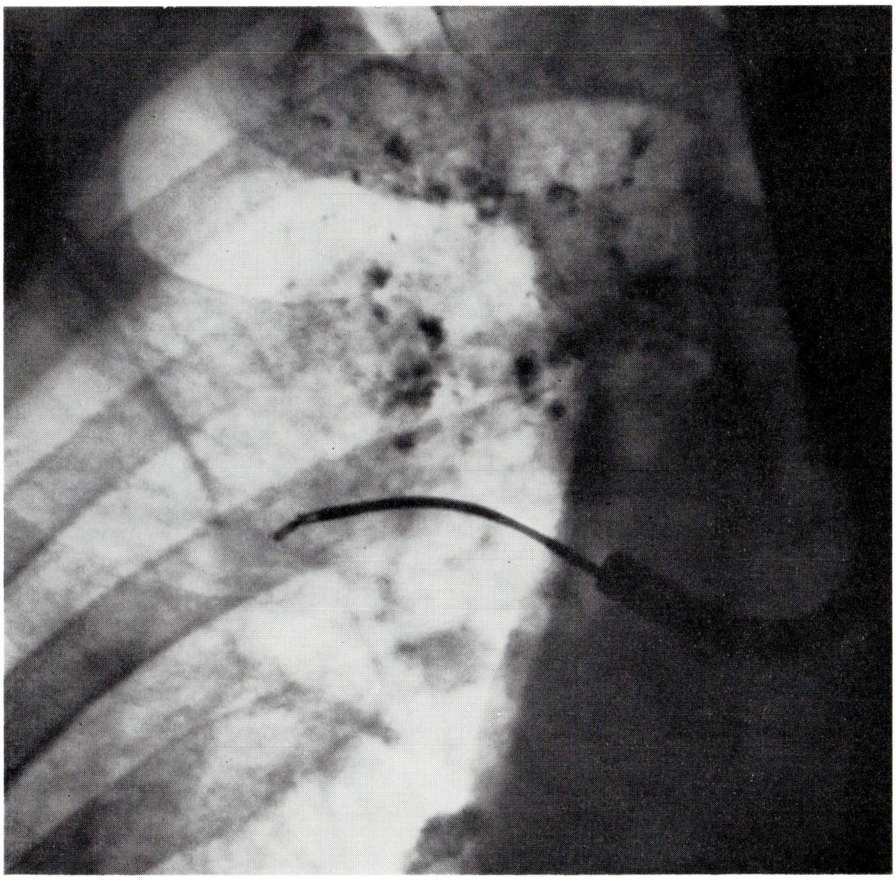

Fig. 227 **Curettage:** The curette is within the tumor.

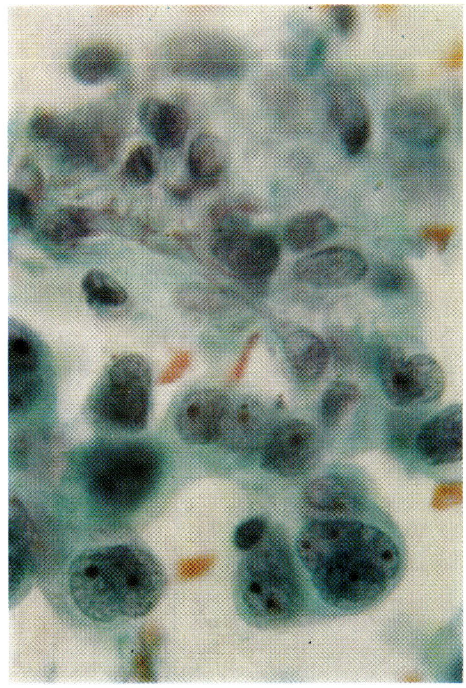

**Fig. 228 Bronchofiberscopic cytological specimen:** Cells are arranged in a papillary formation. Nuclei in individual cells are maldistributed. Round nucleoli are distinctly recognizable.

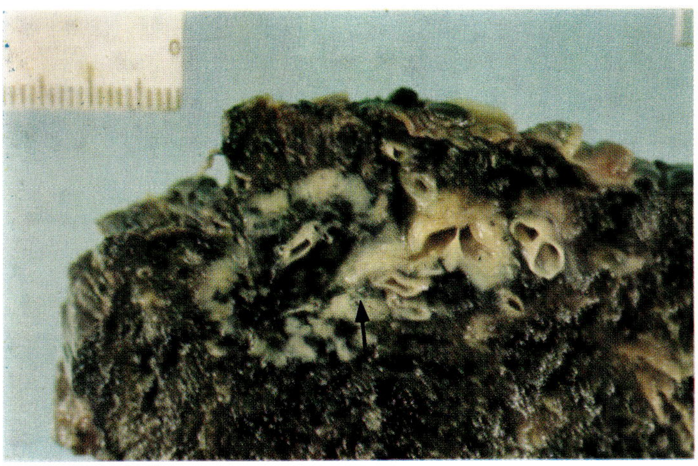

229

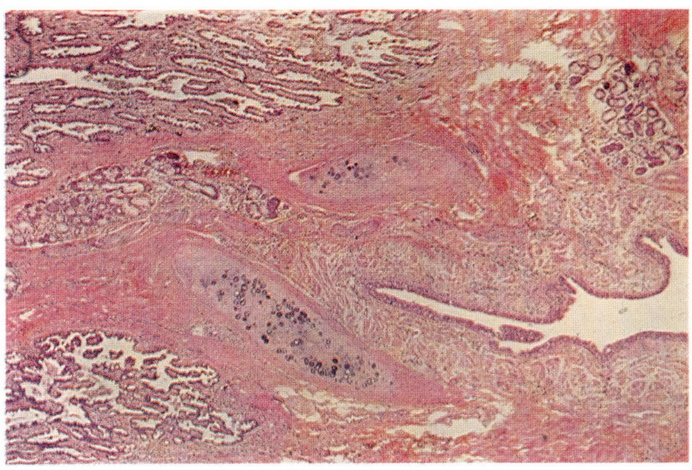

230

**Fig. 229 Macroscopic findings:** The cancer, 20×20mm, has marked anthracosis and fibrosis in the central part. The periphery of the tumor is partly distinct and partly indistinct. One of involved bronchi, $B^2$bii (arrow), remains within the cancer and stenosed pointedly.

**Fig. 230 Microscopic findings:** The affected bronchus is surrounded by cancer and the lumen is narrowed by extrinsic pressure. ×20

**COMMENT:**

This is a peripheral type of a relativery small adenocarcinoma. The bronchial foci indicated by the bronchogram coincide well with findings obtained from the pathological specimen. The endoscopic findings of $B^2$ accessorius branch are those of the lesion nearest the hilum. Note the intact mucosa (Fig. 230) overlying the tumor. This is a feature found frequently in peripheral type of adenocarcinoma.

## Case 7 Squamous Cell Carcinoma (62, male)

**Chief complaint :** Bloody sputum.
**Definitive clinical diagnosis :** Squamous cell carcinoma by sputum cytology.
**Definitive clinical diagnosis on localization :** By bronchofiberscopy.
**Pathological diagnosis :** Squamous cell carcinoma.
**Case history :** The patient was extremely fond of smoking, averagely 50 cigarettes a day for 40 years. He expectorated bloody sputum a month ago, and was examined at a certain large hospital and told that sputum was cytologically positive. The chest X-ray and bronchoscopy failed to show any abnormality. He was transferred to our hospital for further examination with the bronchofiberscope.

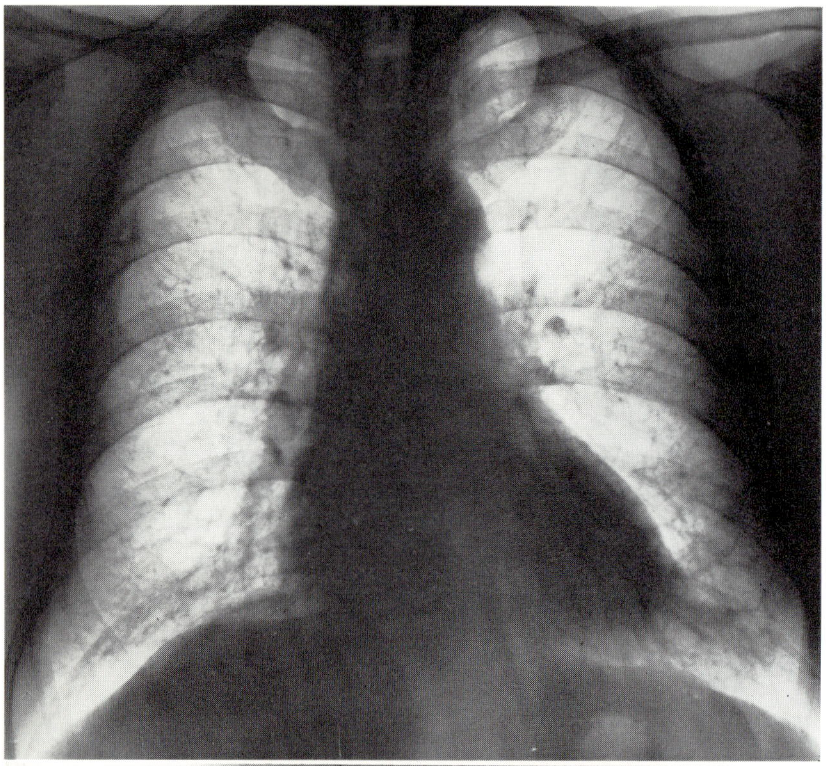

**Fig. 231 Chest X-ray, frontal :** No abnormality noted.

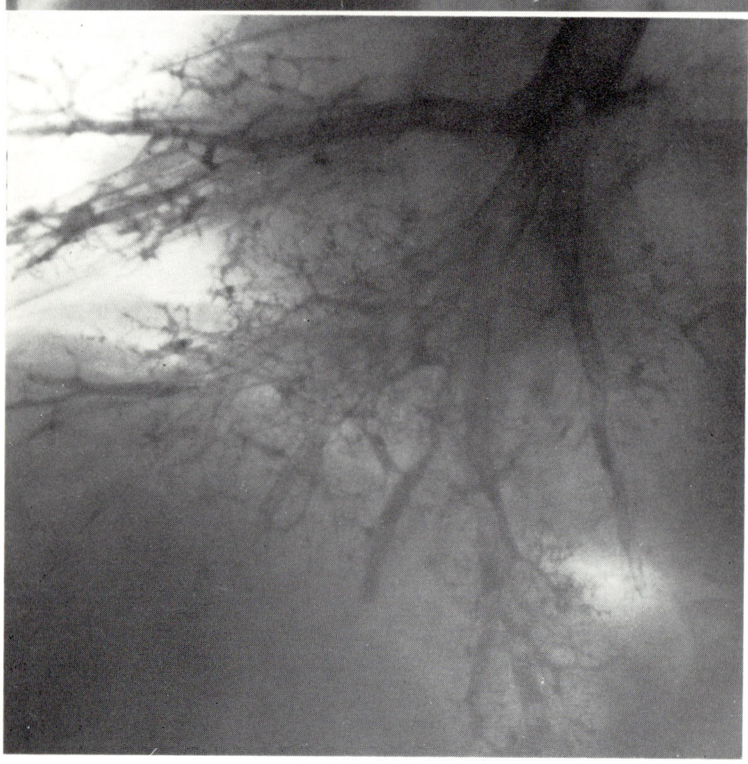

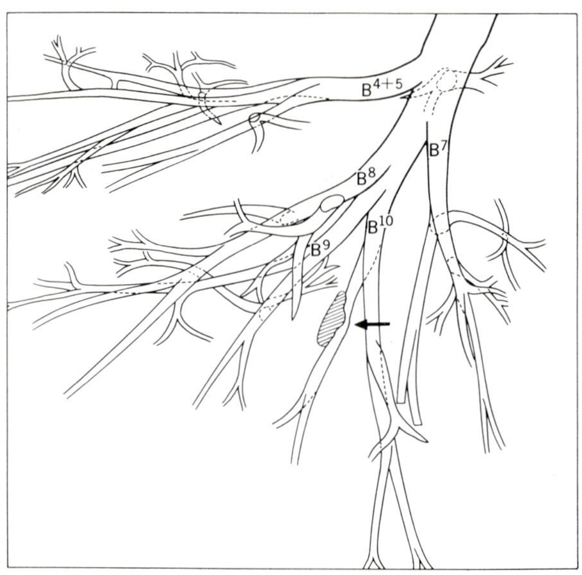


**Fig. 232 Bronchogram :** Stenosis of the right (arrow) $B^{10}c$ accompanied by irregularity of the bronchial wall. No other abnormality.

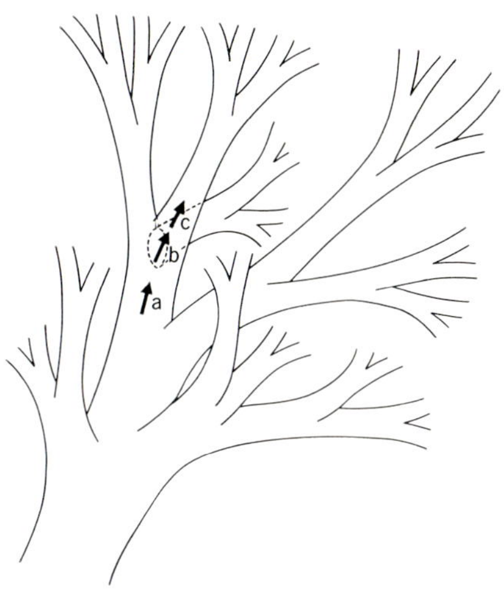


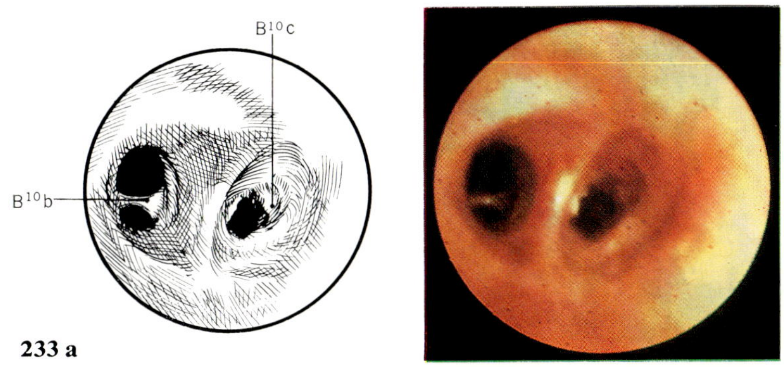


233 a

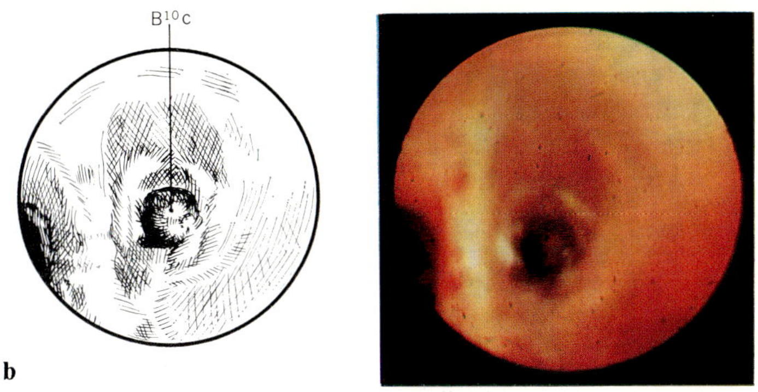


233 b

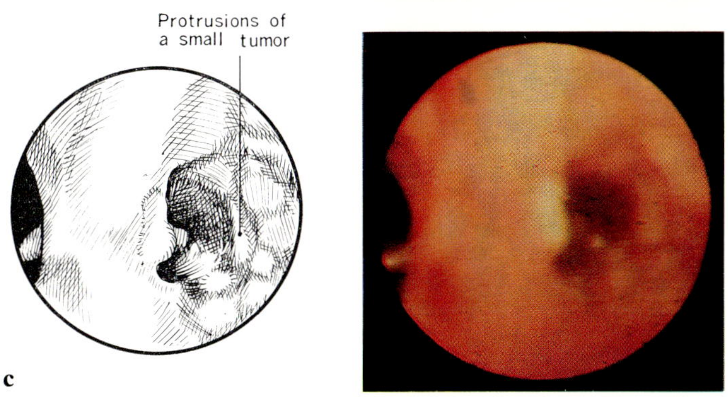


233 c

**Fig. 233 Fiberscopic findings :**

**a.** Since rigid bronchoscopy was negative, the bronchofiberscope was introduced into all subsegmental bronchi bilaterally. This revealed swelling and moderate stenosis in the right $B^{10}$ and slight stenosis in the left $B^{5}b$.

**b.** Following the initial bronchoscopy, the second fiberscopy concentrated on these two lesions. The bifurcation into the right $B^{10}b$ and $B^{10}c$ showed moderate swelling and the deeper part of $B^{10}c$ revealed irregularity of the mucosa. $B^{5}b$ was normal.

**c.** As the bronchofiberscope was advanced farther, $B^{10}$ becomes markedly irregular and rather small tumor-like changes were scattered. It showed the unclearness of bronchial cartilages and markedly reddened. The lesion was diagnosed carcinoma.

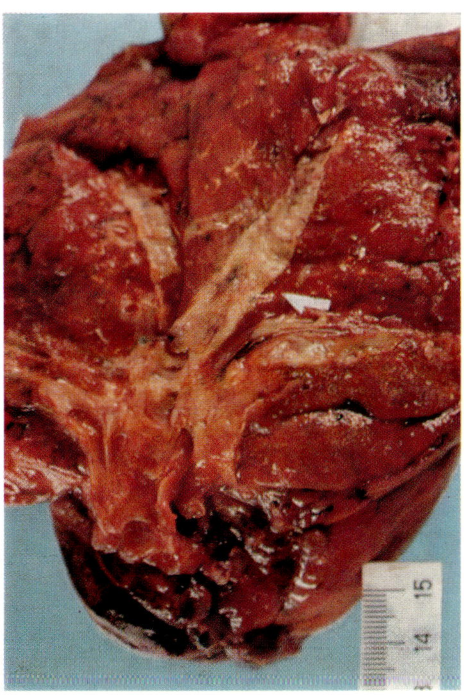

234 a

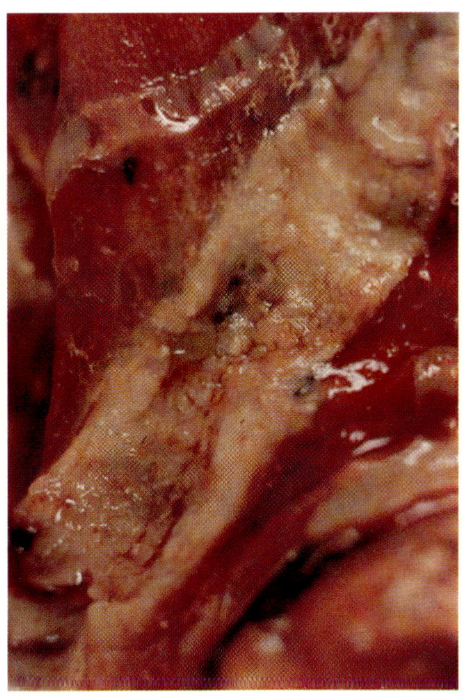

234 b

**Fig. 234 Macroscopic findings :**

**a.** Entire lesion. Fresh specimen showing the changes from the lower lobe bronchus to $B^{10}b$ and $B^{10}c$. Cancer, 20 mm in extent (arrow), was located within the bronchial wall of $B^{10}b$.

**b.** $B^{10}c$ was markedly stenosed by the carcinoma.

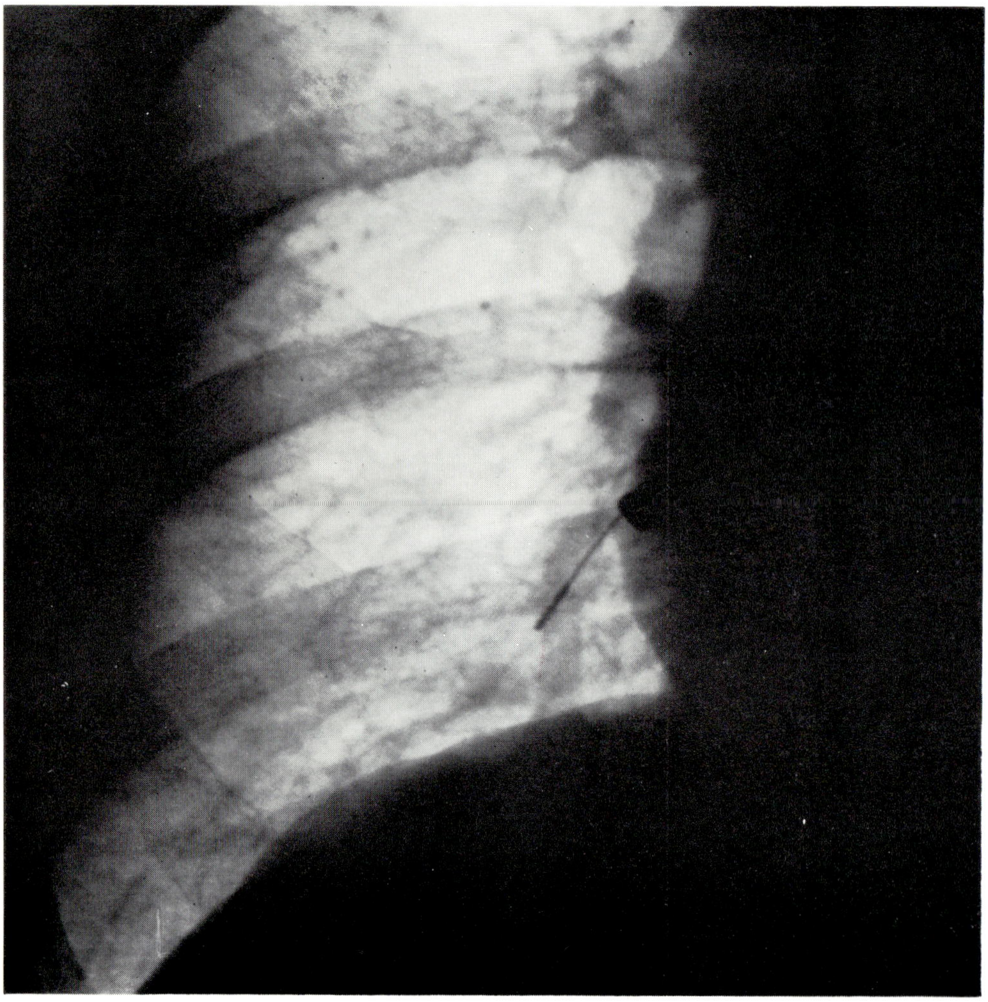

**Fig. 235 Brushing:** A brush intubated into the bronchofiberscope is against the macroscopically confirmed tumor.

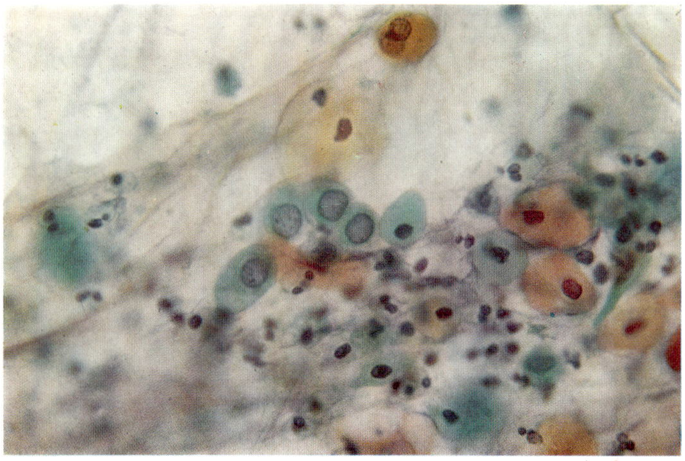

236 a

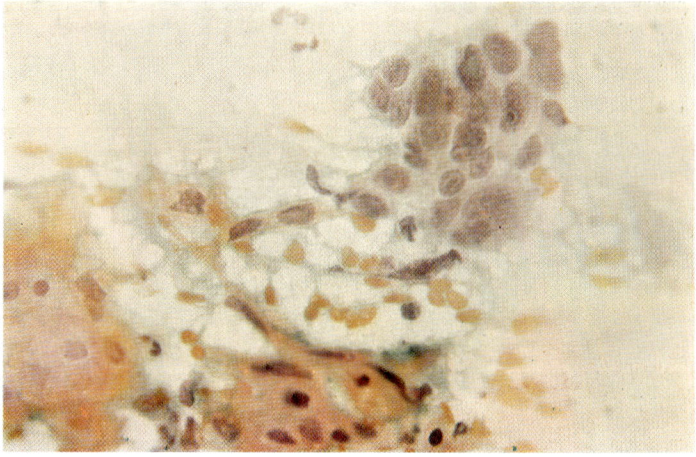

236 b

**Fig. 236 Cytodiagnosis:**

**a.** Sputum cytology. Cells at the central part of this photomicrograph contain the green cytoplasm, have a large N/C ratio and are prominently thickened in the cellular membrane. Some cells indicate pyknosis. At the upper part a cornified cell is seen.

**b.** Cytology from bronchofiberscopic brushing. At the upper part of this photomicrograph is a new cell cluster. In it new cells are conspicuous both in irregularity in size of the nuclei and in malformation. At the lower part are seen cornified cells of fiber cell type.

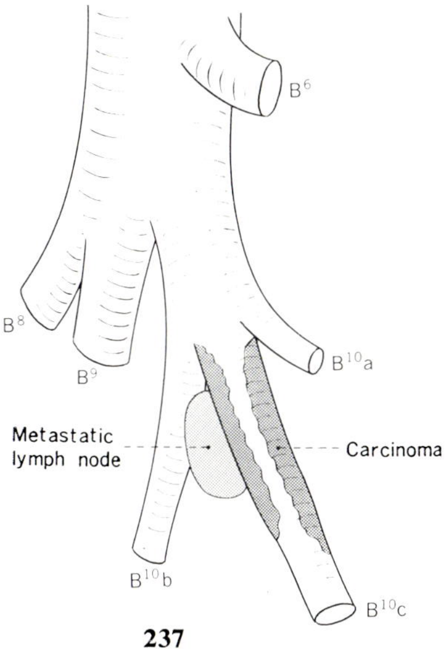


237

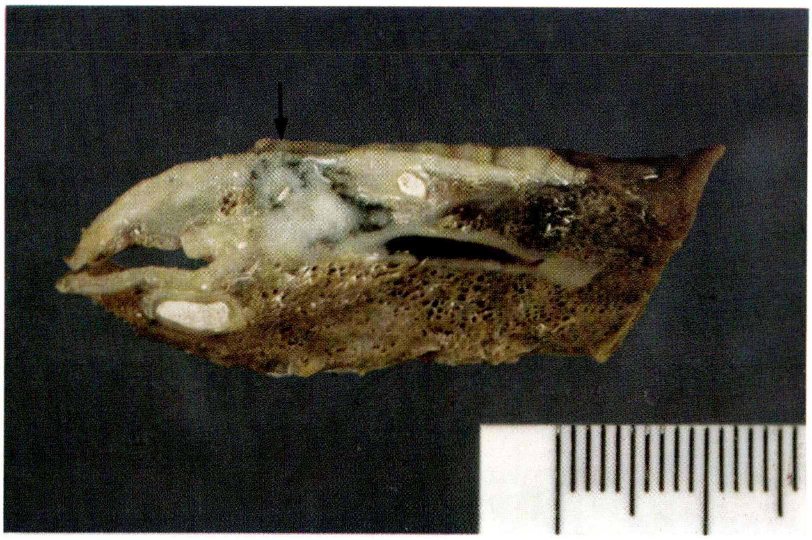

238

**Fig. 237 Traced schema :** The cancer lesion has grown along the inner wall of $B^{10}c$ in an infiltrative fashion and has considerably narrowed the lumen. The lesion is mostly confined within the bronchial wall, but part of it infiltrated the adjacent lymph node directly and metastasized to other lymph nodes at the tracheal bifurcation.

**Fig. 238 Macroscopic findings :** Direct infiltration into the lymph node which is located just below $B^{10}c$.

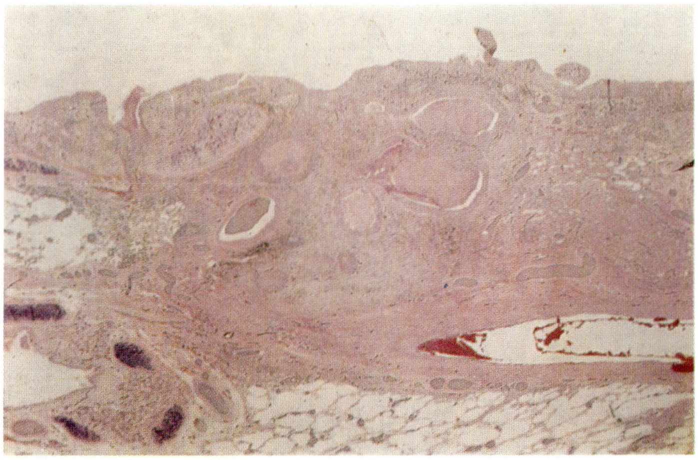

239 a

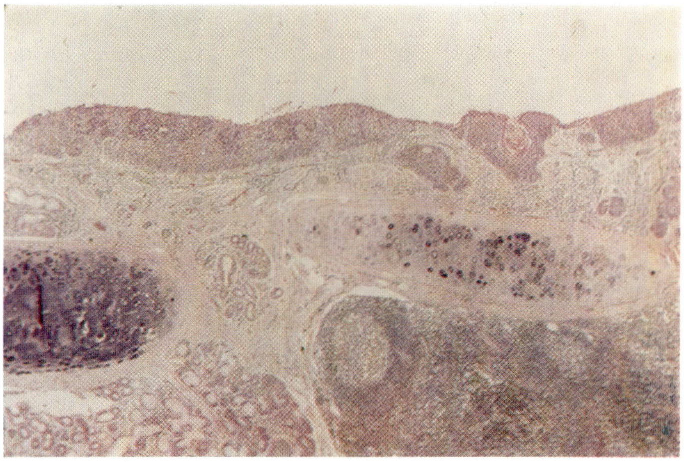

239 b

**Fig. 239 Microscopic findings :**

**a.** Replacement of the epithelium of $B^{10}c$ by keratinized squamous cell carcinoma. The lesion is thus spreading superficial to the bronchial cratilages.

**b.** Direct infiltration of the superficial lesion into the lymph node located immediately below $B^{10}c$.

## COMMENT :

This is a typical case of occult lung cancer in two respects. One is that the patient was a heavy smoker for a long period of time, and the other is that cytological examination of sputum was positive while chest X-ray was negative. It is in such occult cases of lung cancer that bronchofiberscopy plays the most effective role in locating the exact site of the tumor. Although the cancer was found, the lesion had already penetrated the bronchial wall and infiltrated the adjacent lymph node and an enlarged hilar node. The patient died two years after surgical operation. The infiltration into the lymph node and the swelling of the pulmonary hilar lymph node were not found by chest X-ray film nor by bronchoscopy prior to the operation.

## Case 8 Squamous Cell Carcinoma – Radiation Therapy Administered (51, male)

**Chief complaint :** Cough and fever.
**Definitive clinical diagnosis :** Not made preoperatively.
**Pathological diagnosis :** Resected specimen did not reveal any cancer. It is strongly suspected that cancer cells were destroyed by irradiation.
**Case history :** The patient smoked more than 20 cigarettes a day for the past 30 years. Three months ago he developed a cough and fever of 39°C. He visited a university hospital. The chest X-ray revealed a vague flame-like shadow in the left upper lobe (Fig. 240 a). Under rigid bronchoscopy a tumor was not located, nor was a definitive diagnosis made. A month later the chest X-ray revealed an atelectasis of the left lung field (Fig. 240 b), which was highly suggestive of a lung cancer. The lesion was irradiated with $^{60}Co$, total tumor dose 4,000 R. Yet the patient was not reassured with the therapy and visited our hospital (Fig. 240 c) to get a definitive diagnosis. Bronchogram and bronchofiberscopy were performed (Fig. 241). In bronchofiberscopy a tumor was visualized but cytology with a small curette was negative. Lobectomy was performed. Careful examination of the specimen failed to prove the presence of carcinoma. In spite of the latter findings, it is strongly felt that this is a case of carcinoma healed by radiation therapy.

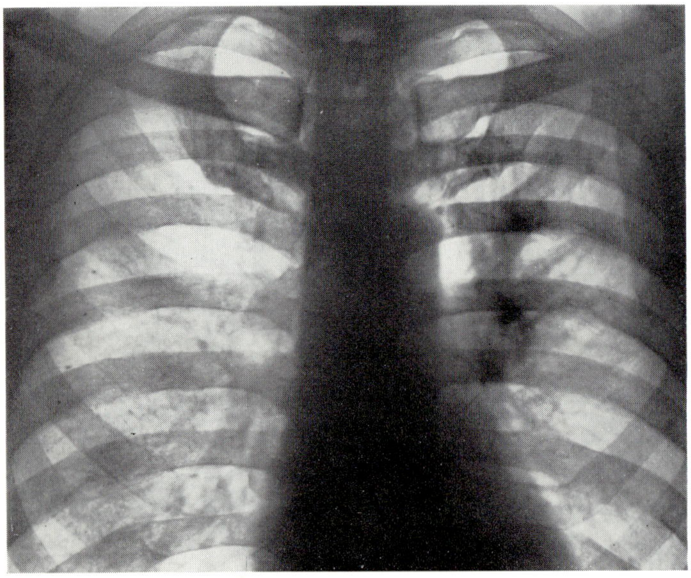

240 a

**Fig. 240 Chest X-ray :**

**a.** *Three months before :* A slight increase in width and density of the left hilum and a flame-like shadow above it are noted. Bronchofiberscopy is indicated when such findings are present on the chest X-ray film.

**b.** *Two months before :* Atelectasis is present in the left upper lobe. The left hemidiaphragm is elevated. Radiation therapy was instituted following this film.

**c.** *At the time of visit to our hospital :* Vascular shadows at the left hilum, although appearing slightly thickened, can safely be judged as normal. Bronchofiberscopy was performed at this time.

**Fig. 241 Bronchogram, oblique, almost lateral view :** The bronchogram was performed in our hospital. The upper division bronchus presents an irregular outline(arrow), particularly in its upper portion. The entrance of $B^{1+2}$ is slightly stenotic. $B^{1+2}c$ is obstructed at the third order of branching. The portion of bronchus from the beginning of $B^3$ to $B^3b$ is irregular. These findings are due to irradiation and should not be confused with manifestations of carcinoma.

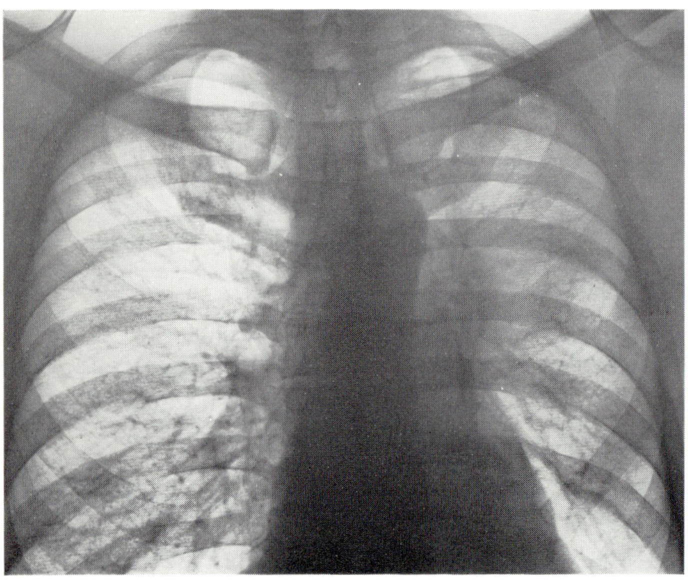

240 b

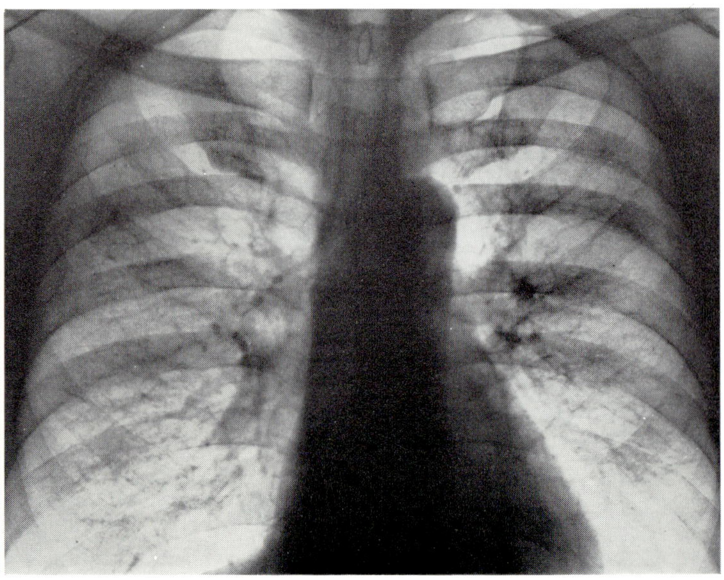

240 c

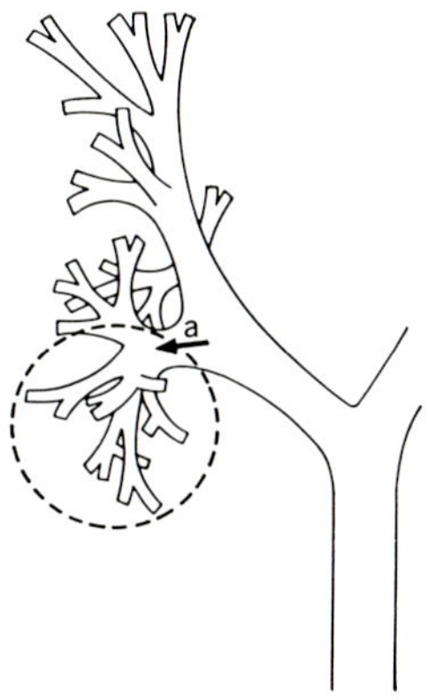


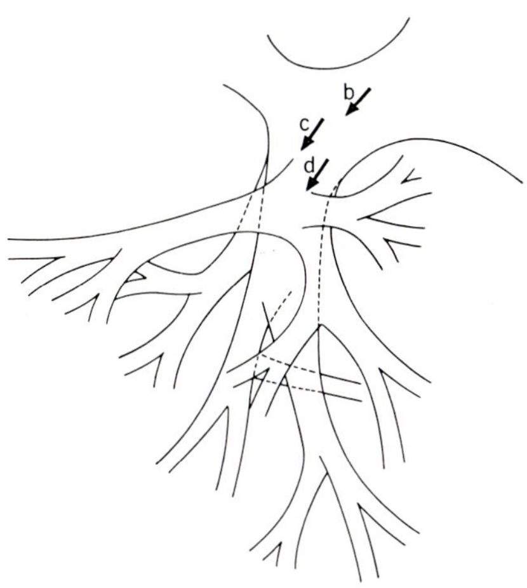


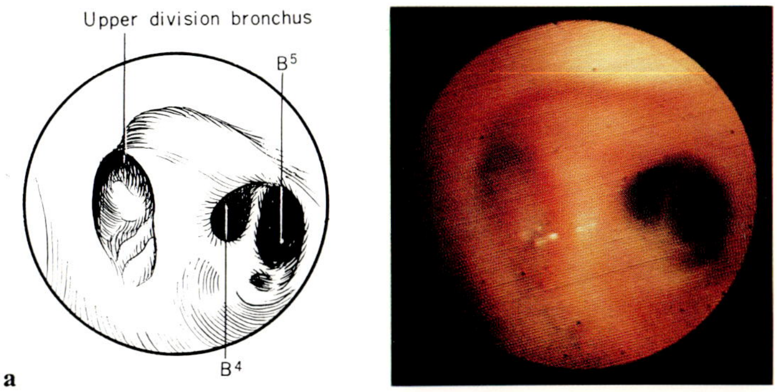


242 a

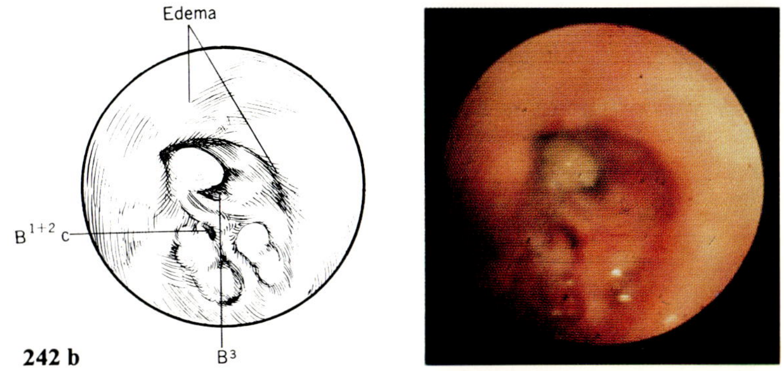


242 b

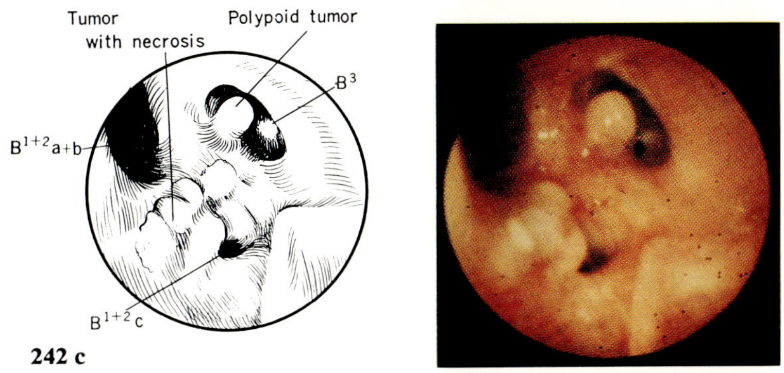


242 c

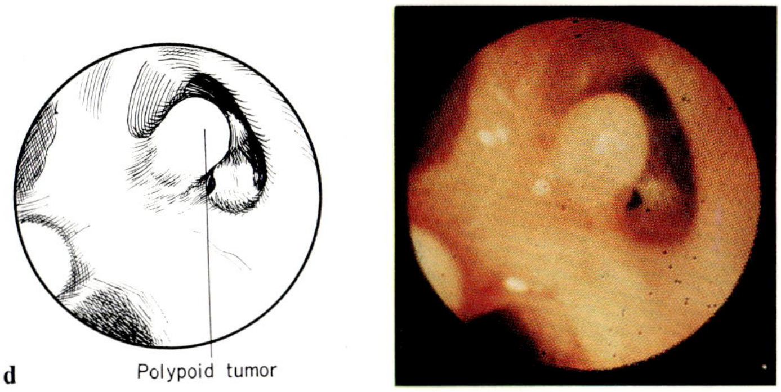


224 d

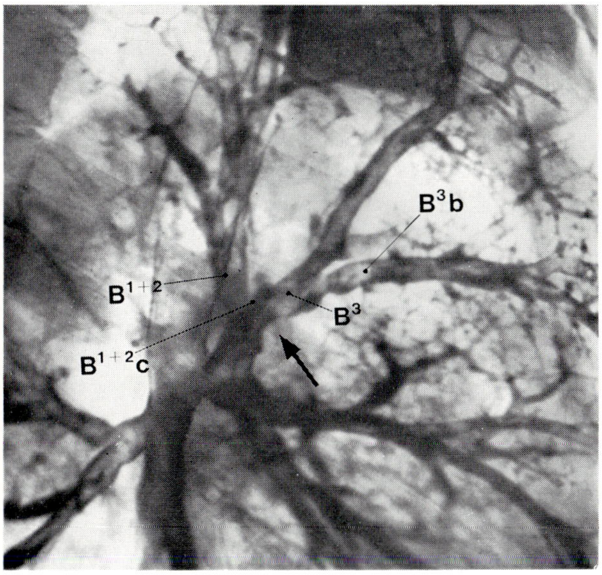


241

**Fig. 242 Fiberscopic findings, after radiation therapy :**

**a.** The upper division and lingular bronchi seen within the left upper lobe bronchus. The orifice of the upper division bronchus is narrowed.

**b.** In the upper division bronchus there is irregularity and edema on the bronchial wall. Note the orifice into $B^{1+2}a+b$ and $B^3$.

**c.** The branching of the upper division bronchus forms a trifurcation into $B^{1+2}a+b$, $B^{1+2}c$ and $B^3$.
Each septum is thickened and inflamed. There is a protuberant tumor with whitish necrosis involving the septum of $B^{1+2}a+b$, $B^{1+2}c$ with partial obstruction of $B^{1+2}c$. There also is a polypoid tumor within the orifice of $B^3$.

**d.** This is the polypoid tumor within the orifice of $B^3$.
Biopsy by means of a small bronchofiberscopic forceps proved negative histologically and cytologically.

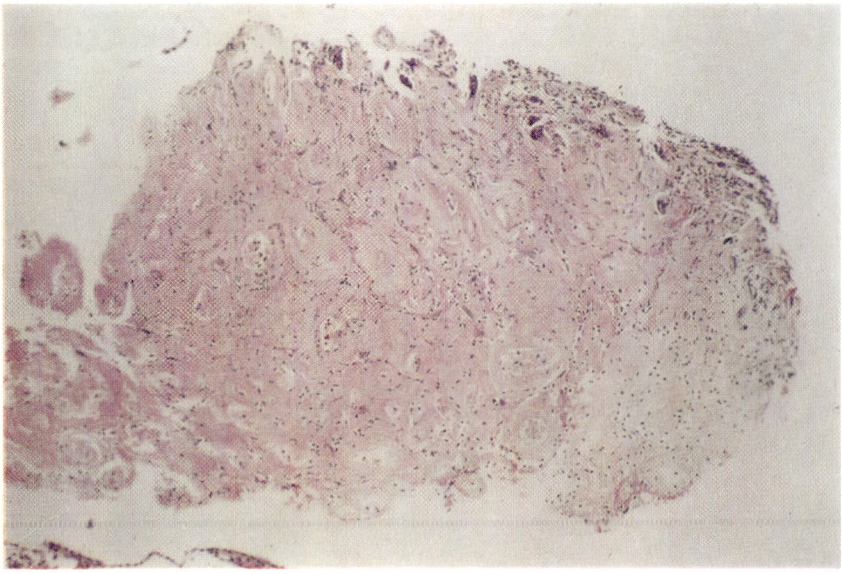

**Fig. 243 Biopsy findings:** Biopsy specimen bronchofiberscopically obtained from the orifice of $B^{1+2}c$. The bronchial epithelium is desquamated. The histological specimen is composed of granulation tissue with hyalinization. No carcinoma is recognized.

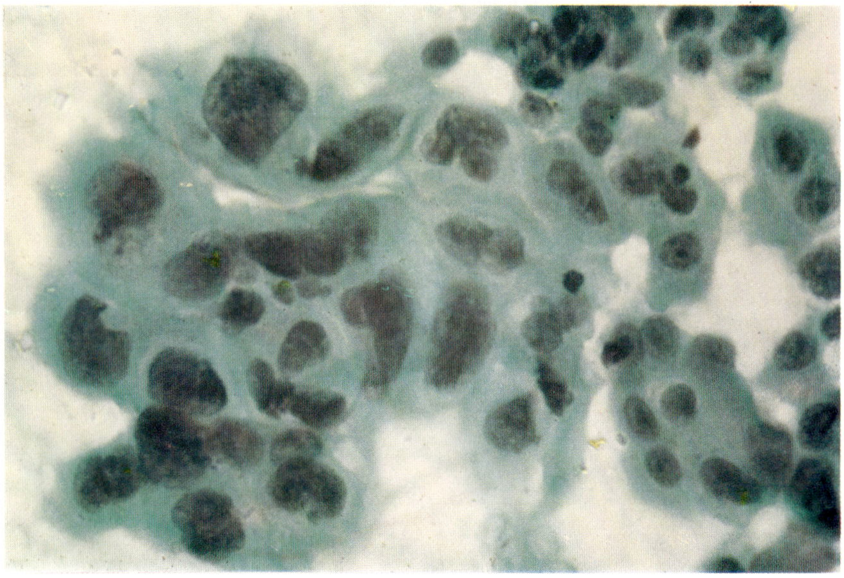

**Fig. 244 Cytodiagnosis:** Cytological diagnoses based on the specimen obtained bronchofiberscopically are negative for cancer cells.

**a.** The post irradiation cytological specimen obtained by bronchofiberscopic curettage reveals the bronchial epithelial cells are enlarged approximately 2 times of the normal cell. The cytoplasm contains a few vacuoles. Although the nuclei are enlarged, the nuclear substance appears essentially normal.

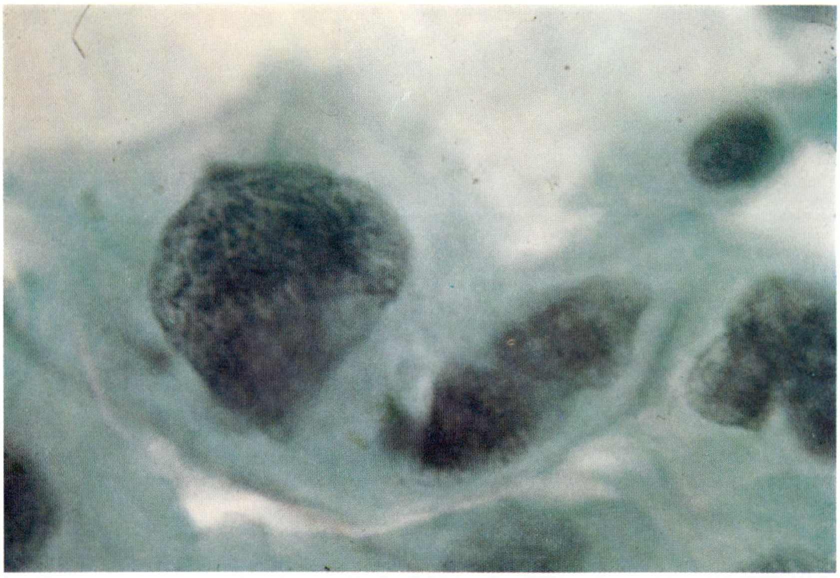

**b.** Enlargement of (a). The cytoplasm is clear. The edge of the cytoplasm is rectangular. No cilia are seen. The nucleus is enlarged and the nuclear substance is reticular. The central cells show lytic degeneration. These pictures are not compatible with a carcinoma.

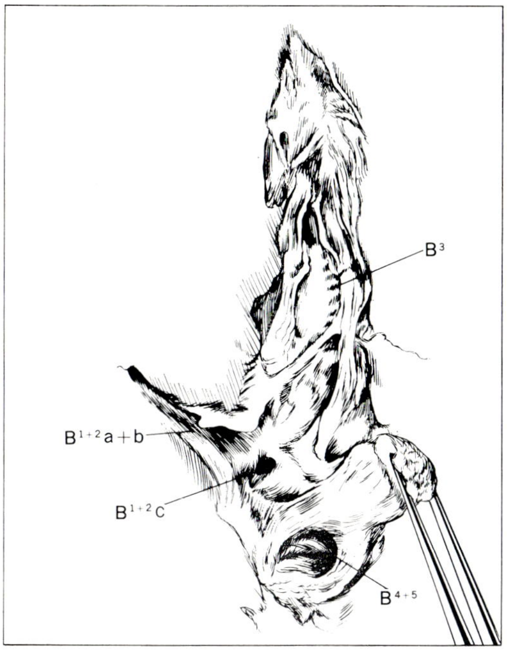


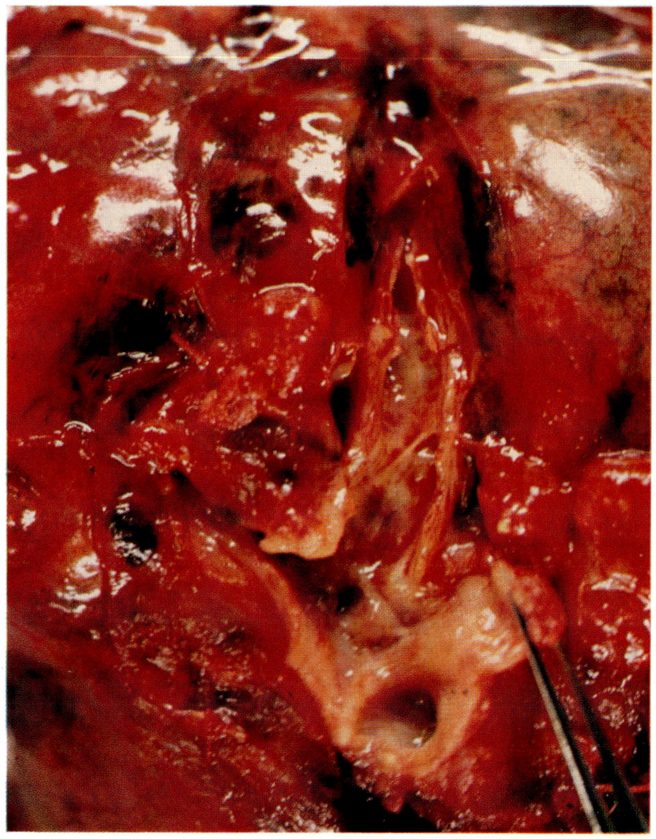

**Fig. 245 Macroscopic findings :** Resected specimen of the affected bronchi. Swelling present at the bifurcation of $B^{1+2}a+b$ and $B^{1+2}c$. The slight stenosis at $B^{1+2}c$ is due to this change. The mucosa from this protuberant area in $B^3$ is coarse.

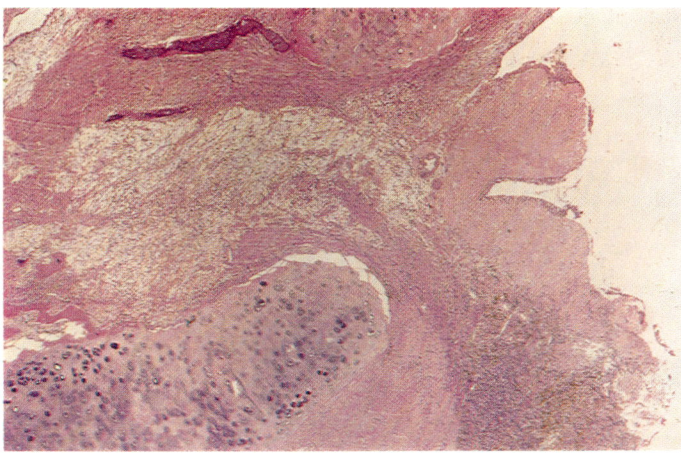

**246 a**

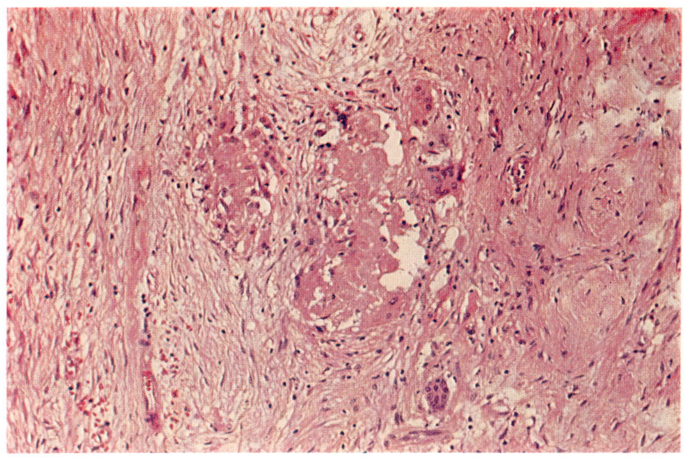

**246 b**

**Fig. 246 Microscopic findings :**

**a.** A section through the tumor involving the septum of $B^{1+2}a+b$ and $B^{1+2}c$ : A polypoid protrusion is present accompanying hyalinized interstices. No bronchial glands are recognized in the thickened mucosa. Froth-like histiocytes are noted adjacent to the cartilages, with areas of ossification.

**b.** Specimen showing granular tissue, with eosin-stained homogeneous substance and giant cells. Histologically, tumor cells were not in any of the specimens, although these microscopic findings indicate that a tumor once existed at this site and was apparently cured by irradiation.

## COMMENT :

This patient had a chief complaint of cough, for which he underwent chest roentgenography and rigid bronchoscopy. Although these examinations were negative, a tentative diagnosis of early cancer was apparently made and he received radiation therapy. Such a case as this is very rare where the pathological findings of the resected specimen can be recognized in the bronchofiberscopic findings after irradiation therapy.

## Case 9 Squamous Cell Carcinoma (56, male)

**Chief complaint :** Cough.
**Definitive clinical diagnosis :** Keratotic squamous cell carcinoma by sputum cytology.
**Pathological diagnosis :** Squamous cell carcinoma.
**Case history :** The patient had been a heavy smoker for more than 30 years. Half a year before, he suffered from influenza, with cough and sputum for several months. About 2 months ago the coughing recurred, accompanied by blood streaked sputum. The chest X-ray was negative but sputum cytology revealed squamous cell carcinoma. Tomograms indicated stenosis of the right major bronchus at the hilum. Bronchofiberscopy revealed a tumor diagnosed as squamous cell carcinoma on biopsy. A right pneumonectomy was performed.

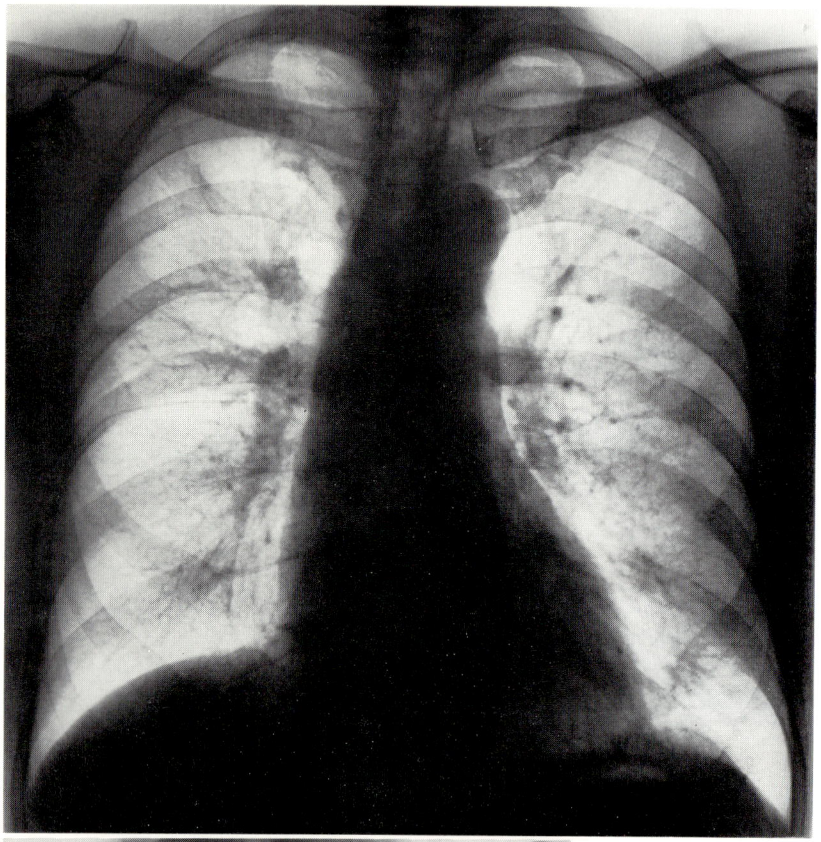

**Fig. 247 Chest X-ray, frontal :** No abnormality noted.

**Fig. 248 Tomogram :** 10 cm level, patient supine. Tomogram demonstrates an air-bronchogram with marked stenosis of the right main bronchus, truncus superior down to the truncus intermedius.

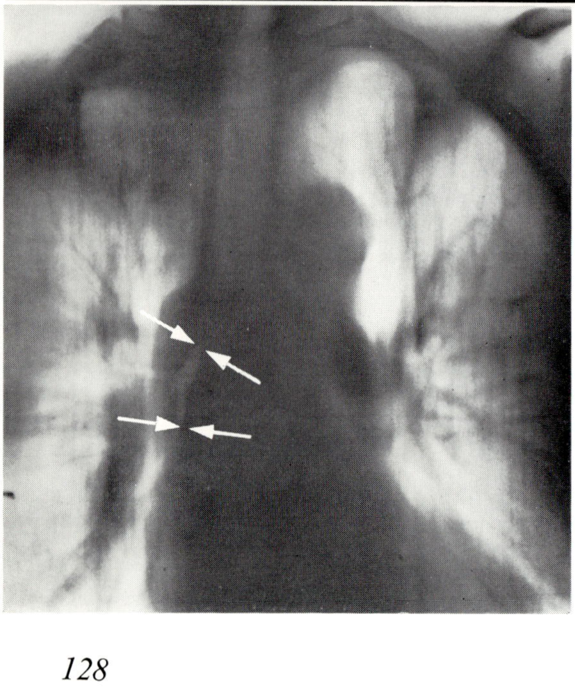

248

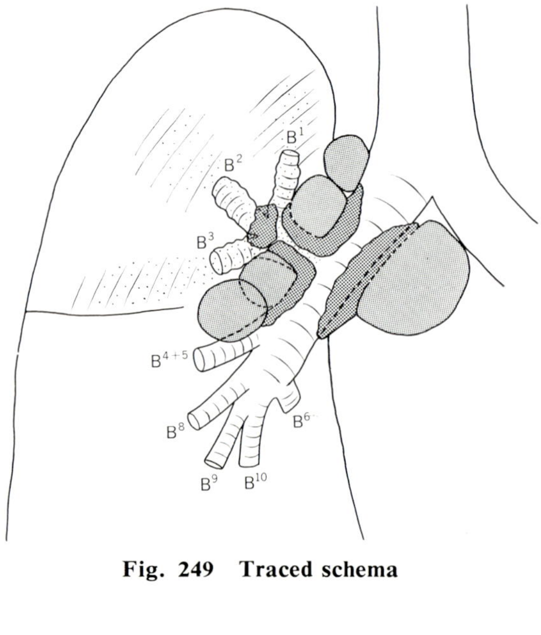


**Fig. 249 Traced schema**

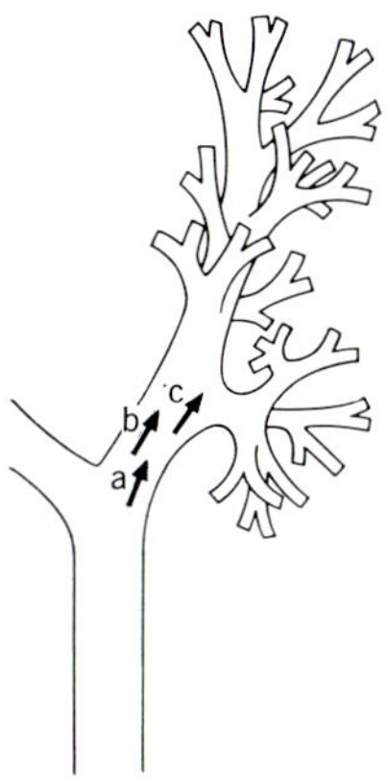


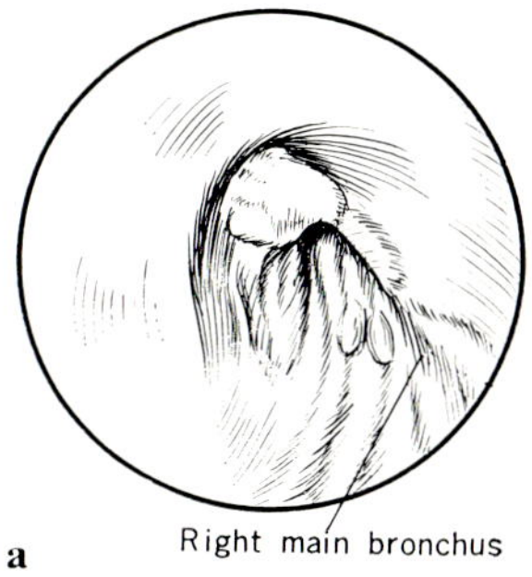


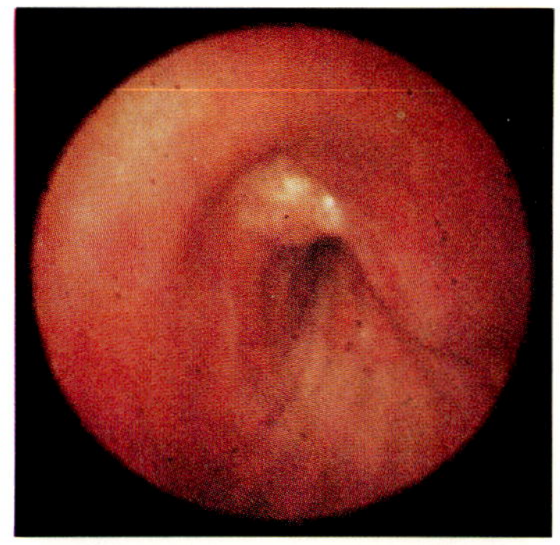

250 a

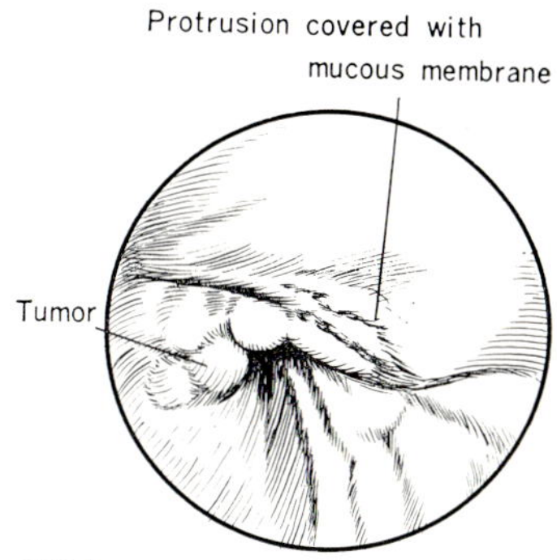


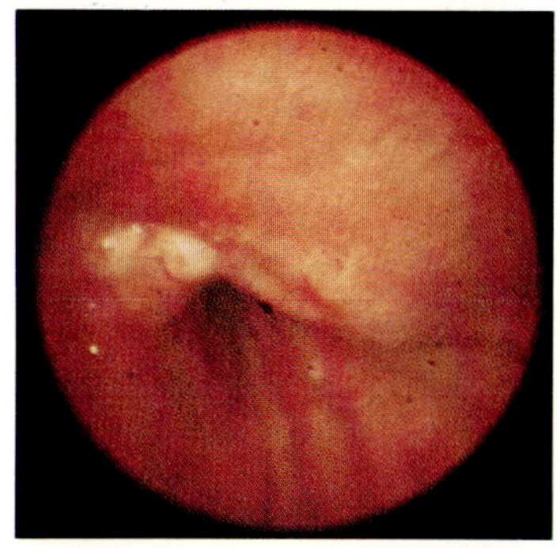

250 b

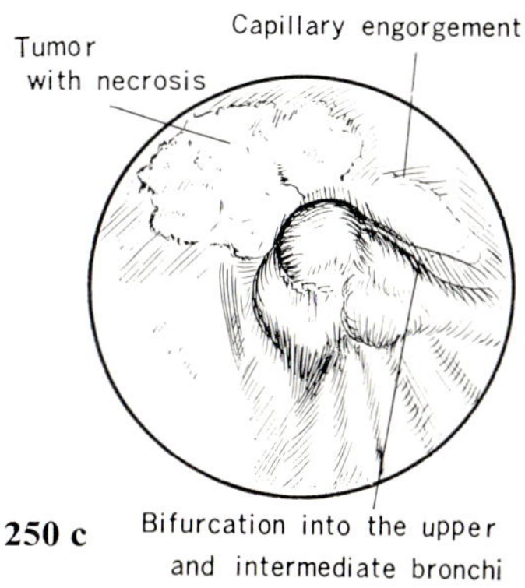


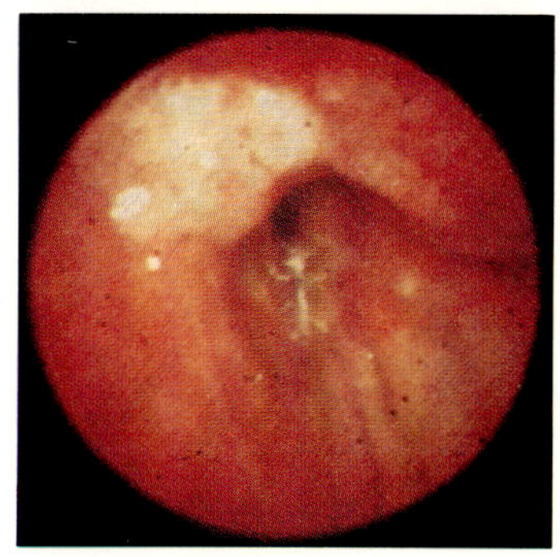

250 c

**Fig. 250 Fiberscopic findings :**

**a.** A tumor is protruding from the anterior wall of the main bronchus and accompanied by necrosis. A protrusion covered with mucous membrane is recognized on the right lateral and posterior walls. This swelling is probably due to compression by an enlarged lymph node.

**b.** The bronchus adjacent to (a). The presence of capillary engorgement of the mucosa overlying the swelling on the right lateral wall of the bronchus is suggestive of carcinomatous infiltration at a deeper level.

**c.** In the deeper recess the bifurcation into the upper and intermediate bronchi is just barely visualized. The septum is thickened and edematous. The bronchofiberscope was denied its further advance from this point.

**Fig. 251 Macroscopic findings :**

**a.** Fresh resected specimen. : A portion of the carcinoma exposed in the lumen.

**b.** The upper and intermediate bronchi are extremely stenosed by the carcinoma and moderately inflamed. The tumor has infiltrated into the interlobar and carinal lymph nodes.

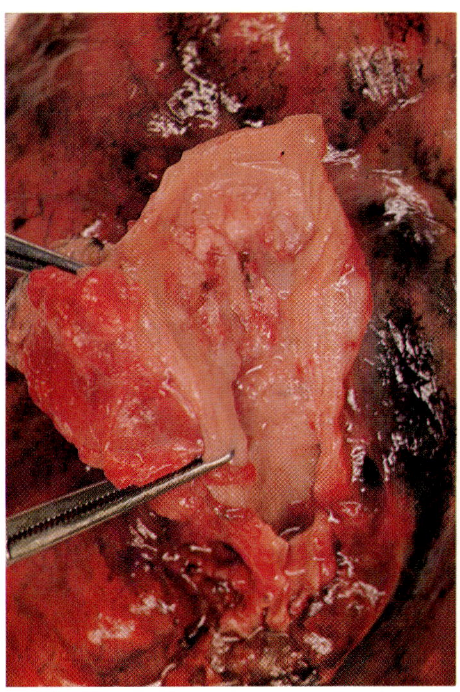

251 a

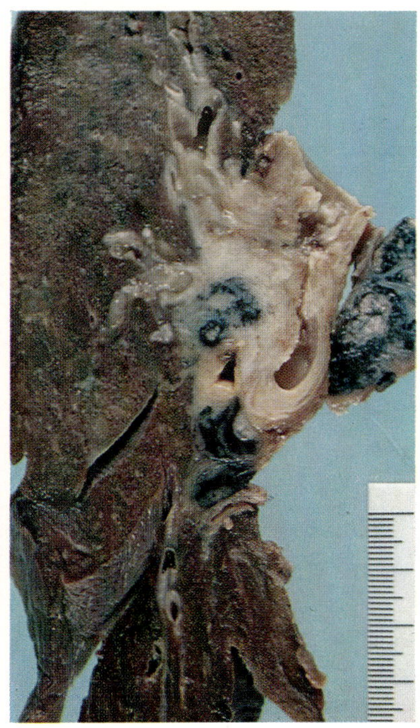

251 b

## COMMENT :

This is a case of squamous cell carcinoma, with no abnormality in the routine chest X-ray but with positive sputum cytology and positive findings on bronchofiberscopy.

## Case 10 Squamous Cell Carcinoma (63, male)

**Chief complaint ;** Bloody sputum.
**Definitive clinical diagnosis ;** Keratotic squamous cell carcioma.
**Pathological diagnosis ;** Keratotic squamous cell carcinoma by sputum cytology.
**Case history ;** The patient had a heavy cough with sputum, and had been treated for bronchitis for two years. Five months before coming to our hospital he had bloody sputum and was treated without any improvement.

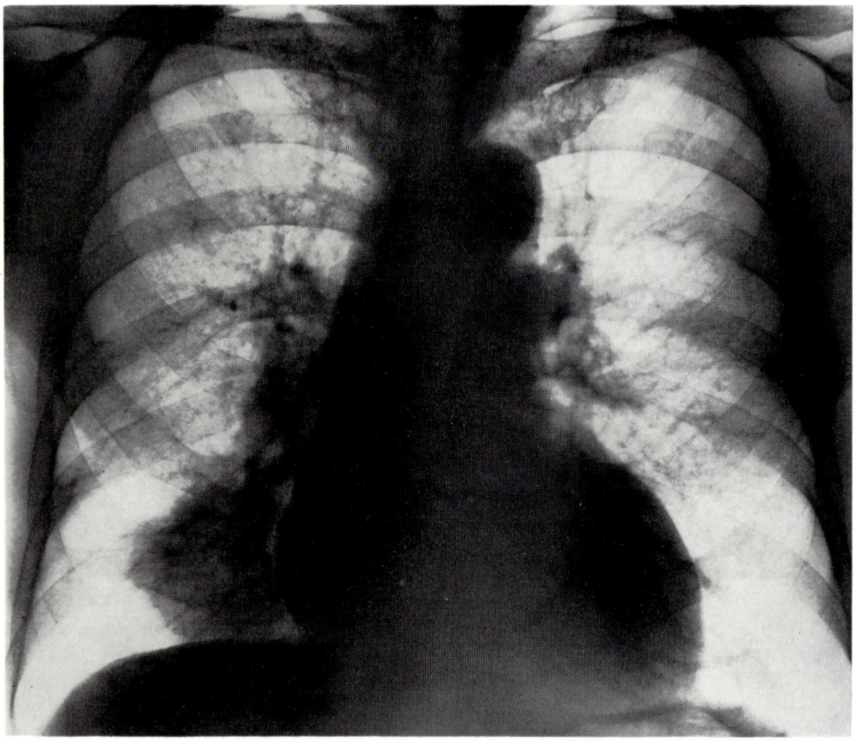

**Fig. 252 Chest X-ray, frontal :** An irregularly shaped tumor, 50×50 mm, with a distinct rim is seen in the right lower lobe. The hilar lymph node is enlarged.

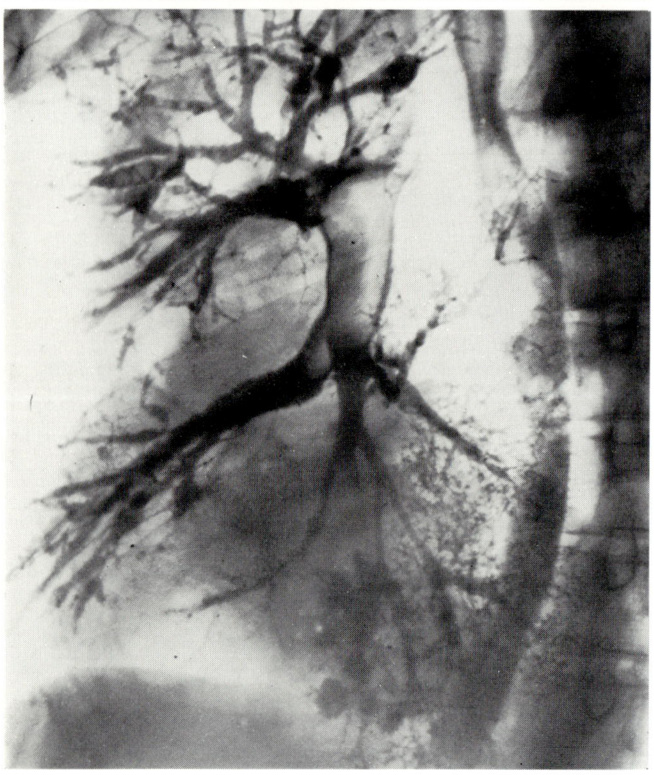

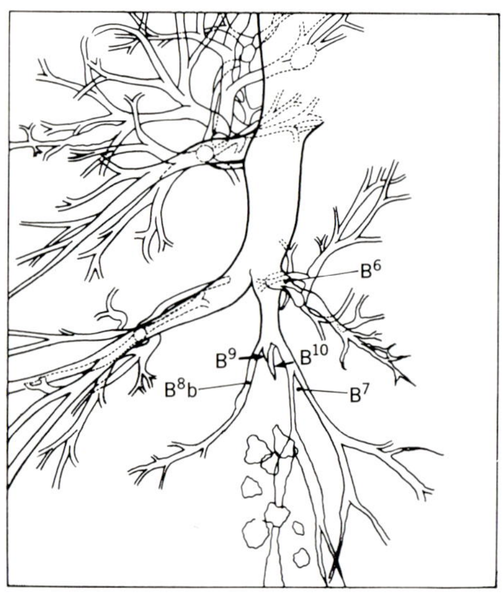


**Fig. 253 Bronchogram, oblique :** The basal bronchus is narrowed, and $B^{9+10}$ is stenosed and obstructed. $B^8$ is in general narrowed ; $B^8$a is stenosed, and $B^8$b is narrowed and compressed by tumor. The tumor arises form $B^{9+10}$. Infiltration has involved $B^8$ and truncus basalis.

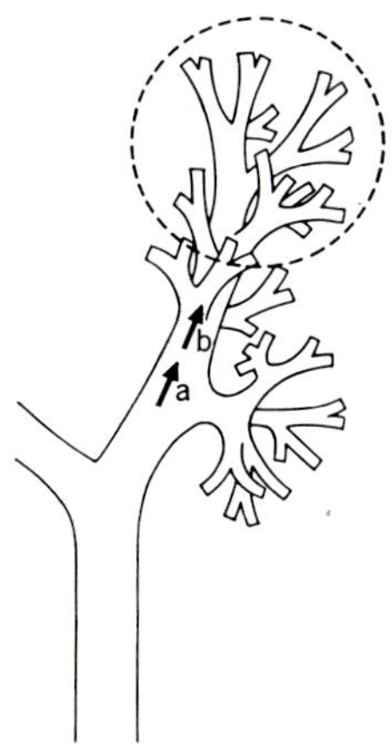


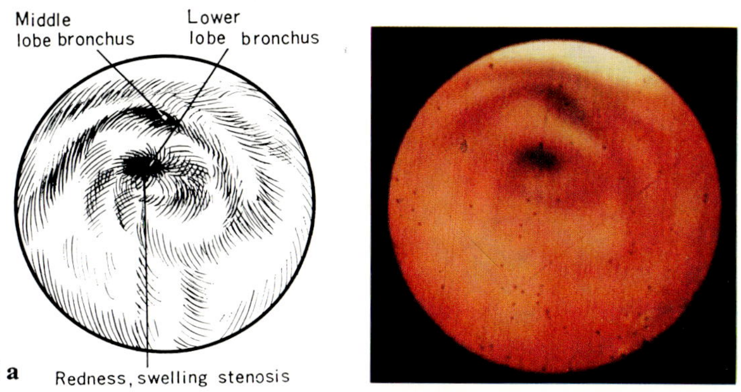


254 a

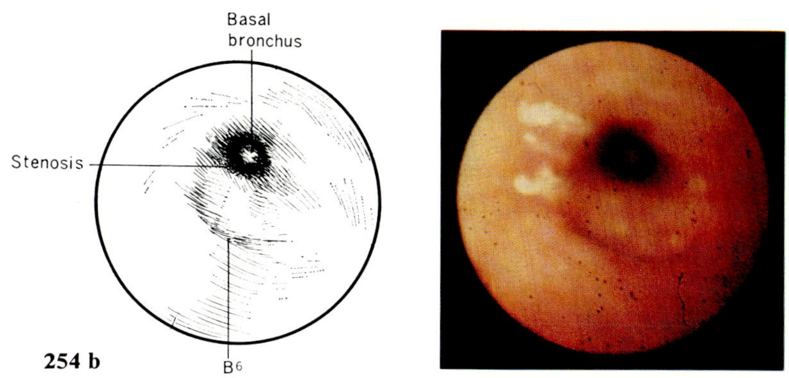


254 b

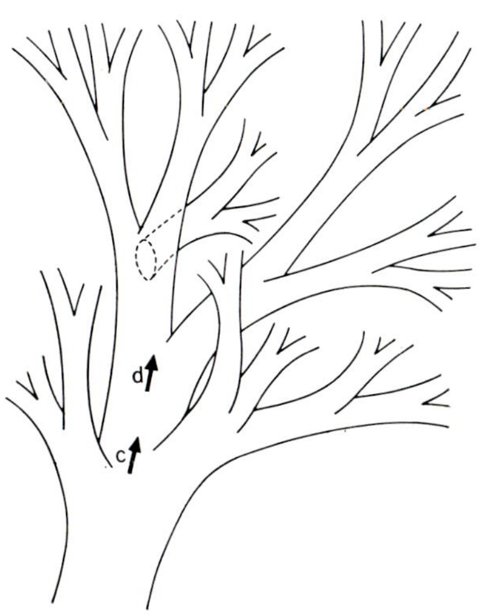


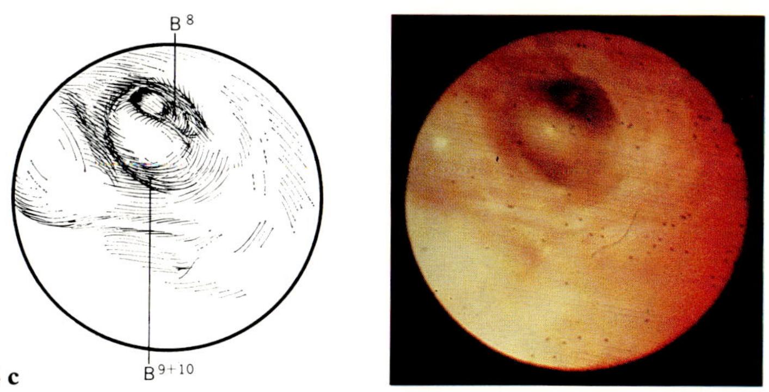


254 c

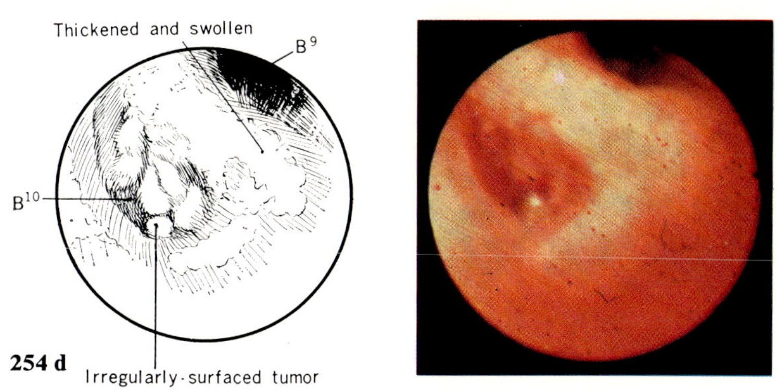


254 d

**Fig 254 Fiberscopic findings :**

**a.** Lower lobe bronchus is stenosed, accompanied by reddening and swelling. The bifurcations of the middle and lower lobe bronchi are thick with swelling.

**b.** The basal bronchus is moderately irregular and the bronchial cartilages are indistinct. Swelling is observed at the bifurcation.

**c.** Marked irregularity of the basal bronchus is visualized. $B^8$ is also stenosed, and $B^{9+10}$ is completely stenosed by tumor.

**d.** When the bronchoscope is further advanced the bifurcation of $B^{9+10}$ is partly visualized. These changes are considered to be the result of carcinomatous infiltration. They coincide perfectly with bronchogram findings.

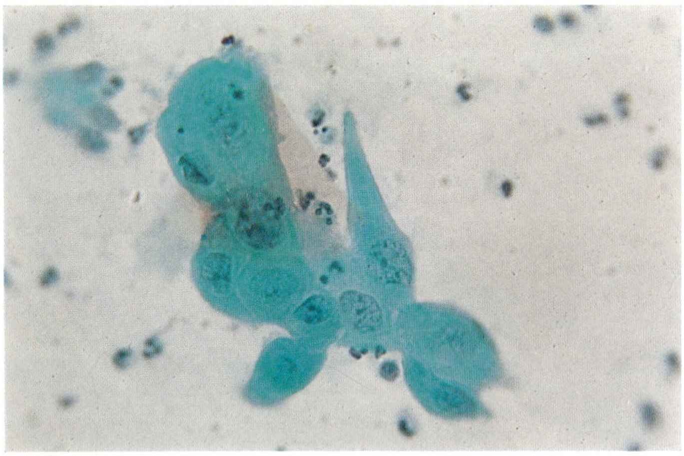

255 a

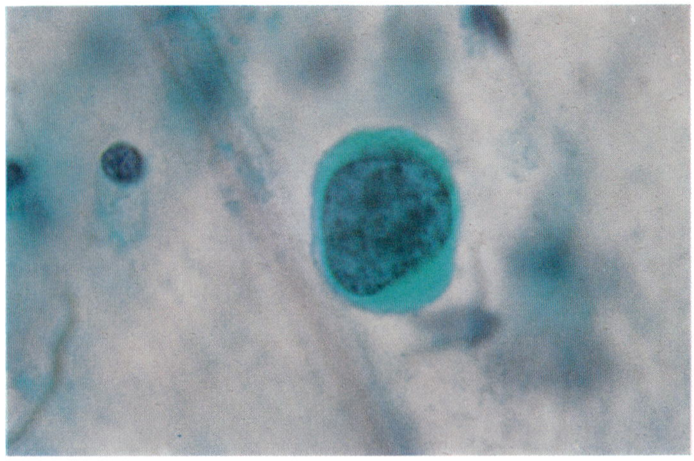

255 b

**Fig. 255 Cytodiagnosis:**

**a.** Bronchofiberscopic curettage. Definitive diagnosis was already established based on sputum, but for the exact differentiation of cell type, cytological diagnosis was made by means of curettage. Multimorphous cells are irregularly connected with each other. Hyperchromatism is not so remarkable, but chromatin is moderately coarse and unevenly distributed.

**b.** Sputum cytology. Large cells show a large N/C ratio, irregular thickening of the cellular membrane, condensation of chromatin, and its uneven distribution. Nucleoli are indistinct.

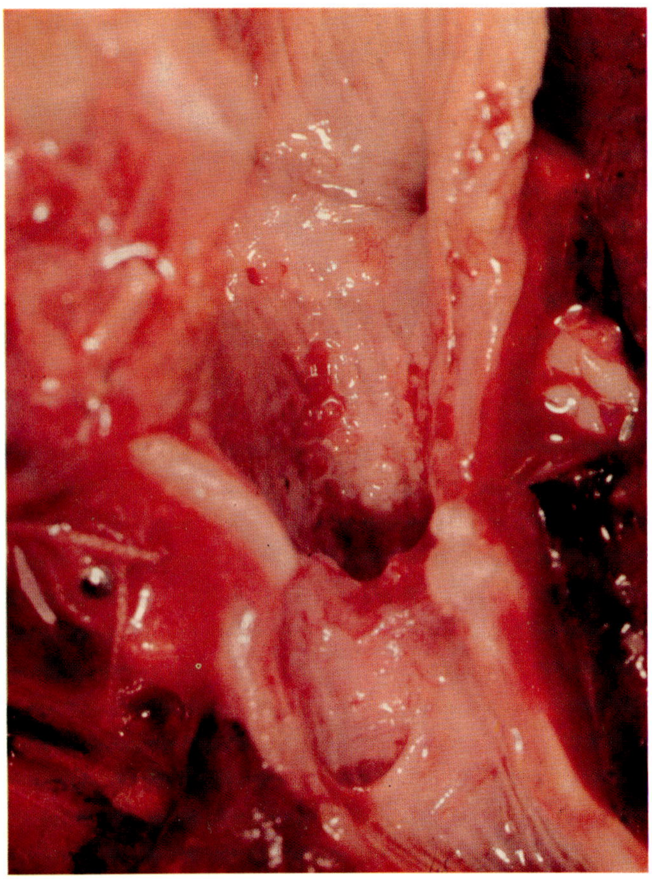

**Fig. 256 Macroscopic findings:**
Close-up view, fresh specimen, showing the lower lobe bronchus to $B^{8}$. The irregularity of the mucosa is prominent from the entrance of $B^{10}$ (at the center) to the lower lobe bronchus. Notice the intraepithelial invasion. The tumor is located more peripherally.

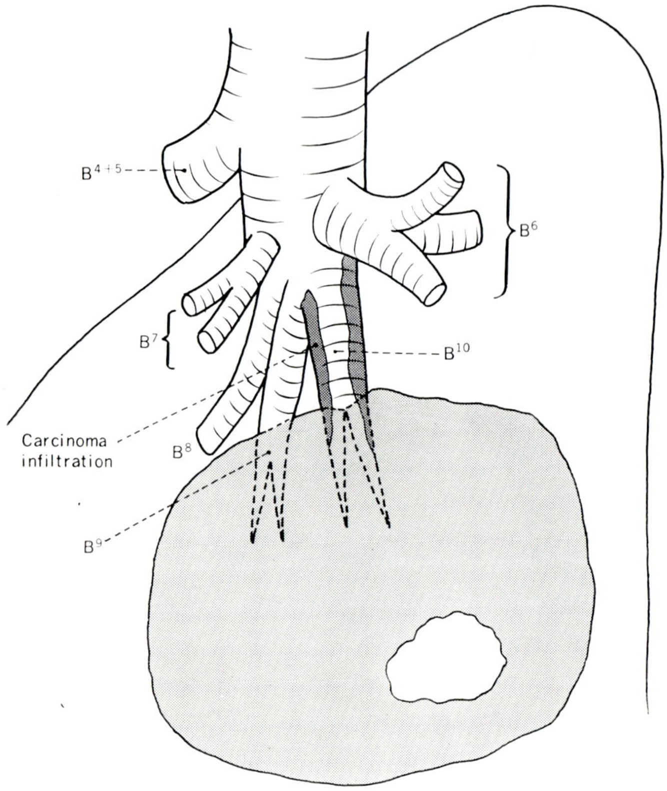


**Fig. 257 Traced schema:** Carcinoma infiltration observed from the entrance of $B^{10}$ to the truncus basalis.

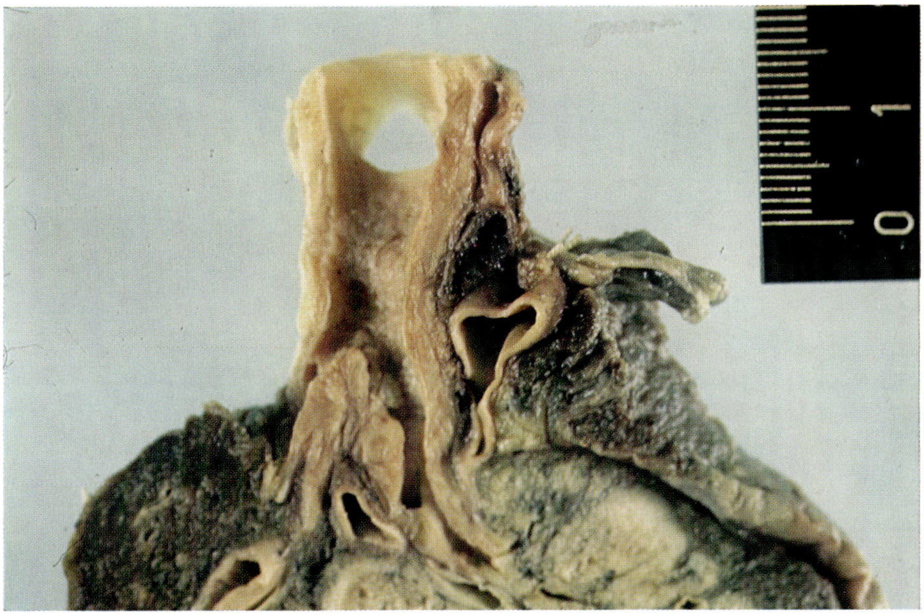

**Fig. 258 Macroscopic findings :** The tumor, 60×40 mm, presents a distinct rim ; the cross section reveals scattered necrotic areas, and relatively rough inner structures. Invaded bronchus ($B^{10}$) with thickened wall passes through the lesion and is stenosed.

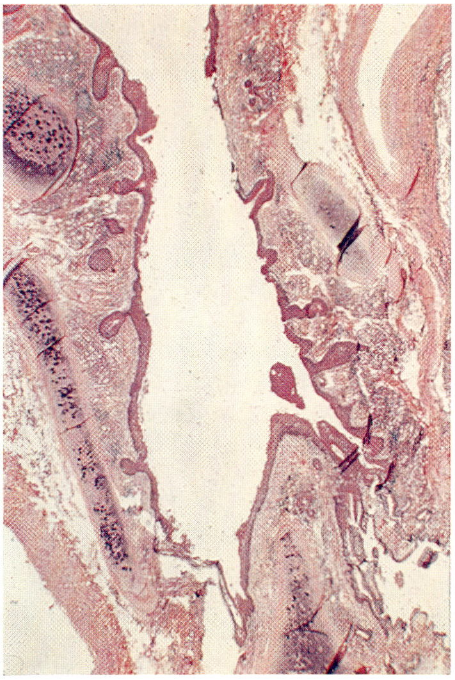

**259 a**

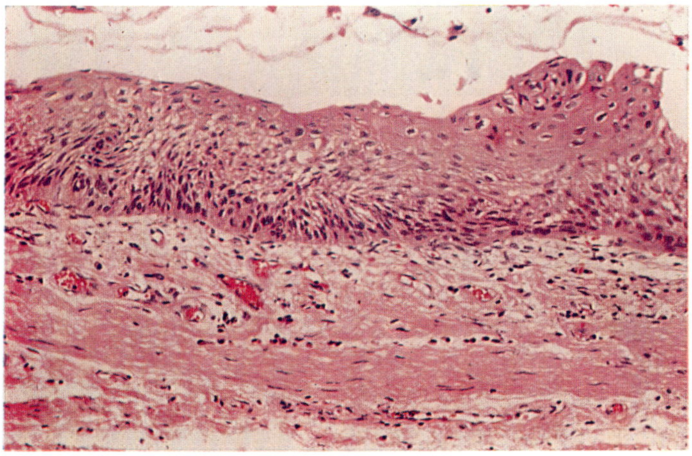

**259 b**

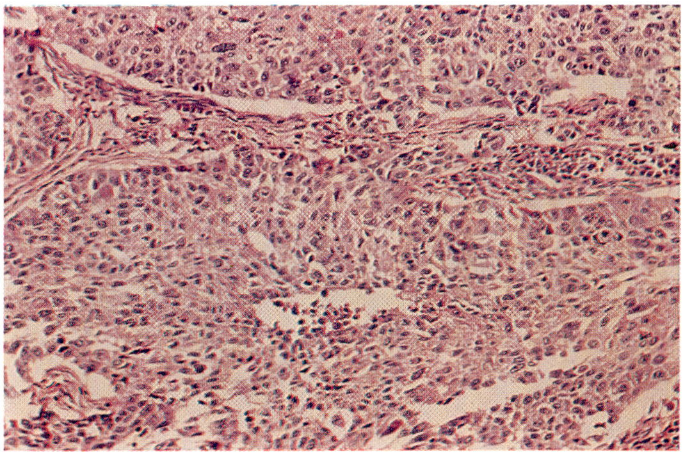

**259 c**

**Fig. 259 Microscopic findings :**

**a.** Histological picture of the intraepithelial invasion. The tumor has superficially and proximally infiltrated the lower lobe bronchus from the affected bronchus, measuring 35 mm in length.

**b.** Enlargement of (a). Keratinized squamous cell carcinoma infiltrates $B^{10}$ and the lower lobe bronchus, replacing the bronchial epithelium.

**c.** The tumor site is composed of slightly keratinized squamous cell carcinoma.

## COMMENT :

As the tumor of squamous cell carcinoma grows, it may infiltrate the hilar bronchus along the mucosa or submucosa. This case is an example of squamous cell carcinoma. Note that the bronchographic and bronchofiberscopic findings coincide well with the pathological findings in the resected specimen.

## Case 11 Squamous Cell Carcinoma (61, female)

**Chief complaint :** Bloody sputum.

**Definitive clinical diagnosis :** Squamous cell carcinoma by bronchofiberscopic curettage.

**Pathological diagnosis :** Moderately differentiated squamous cell carcinoma.

**Case history :** The patient had a severe cough of 4 months duration and consulted a practitioner whose diagnosis was so-called atypical mycobacteriosis. For the past 2 months, she had blood-stained sputum so she came to our hospital.

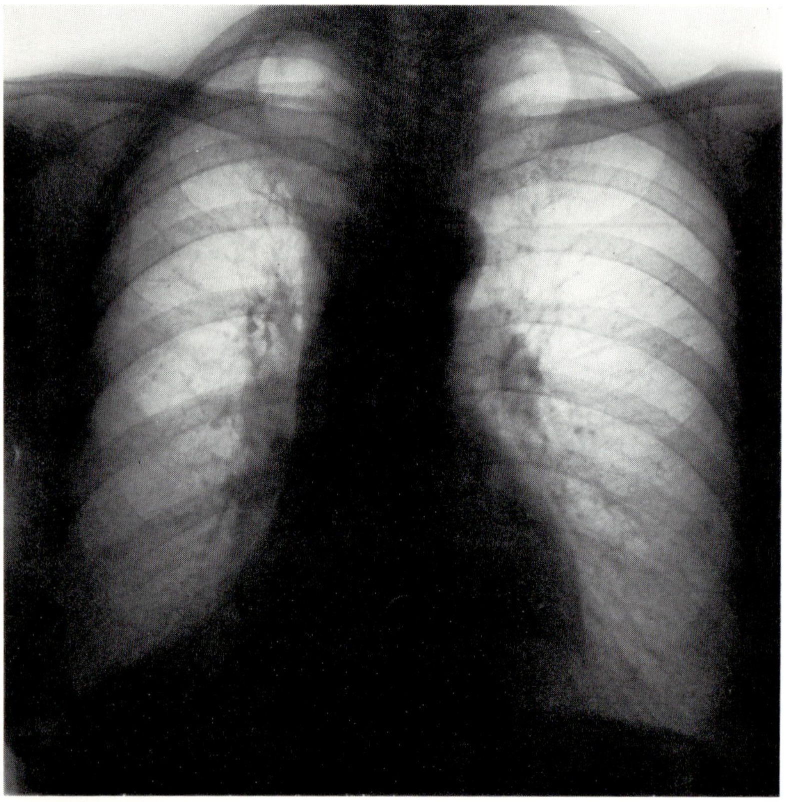

**Fig. 260 Chest X-ray, frontal :** An atelectatic shadow is noted in the medial part of the right lower lung field. This is considered to be due to an atelectasis of the middle and lower lobes, but tumor shadow is not

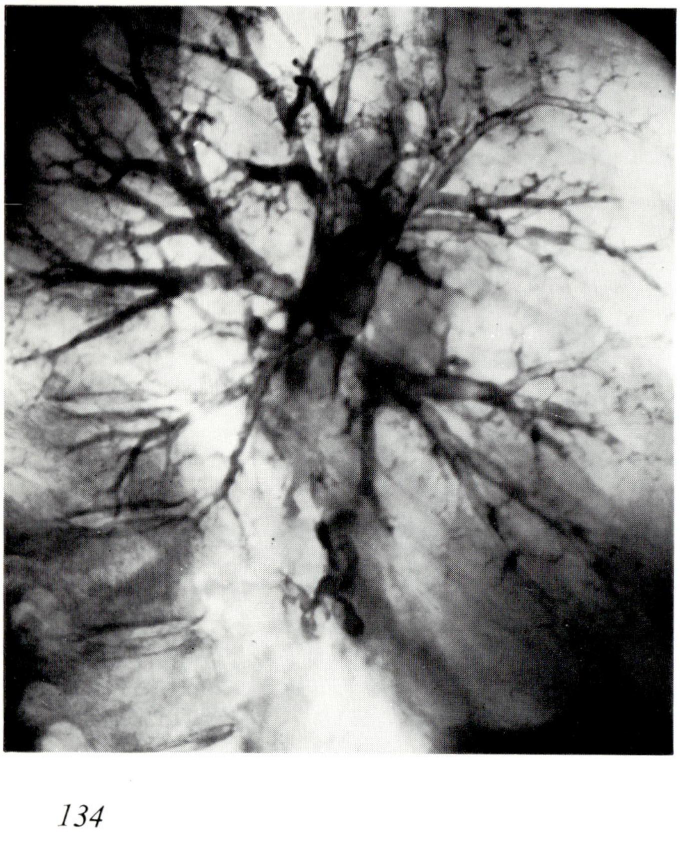

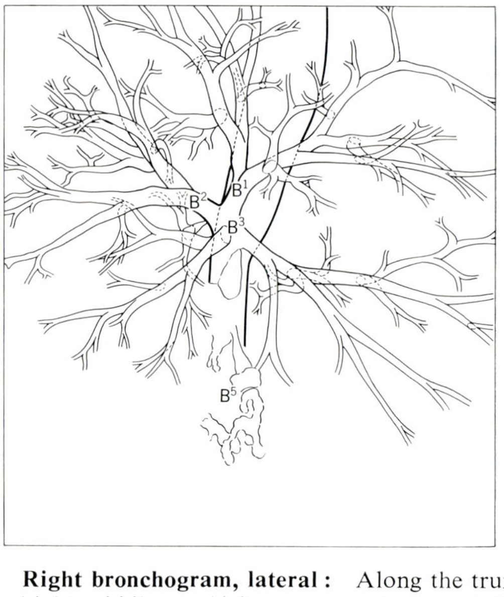


**Fig. 261 Right bronchogram, lateral :** Along the truncus intermedius (right middle trunk) is present a shadow defect considered to be due to tumor. The contrast medium has flowed into the middle lobe bronchus but no further. An ectasis is visible in $B^5$.

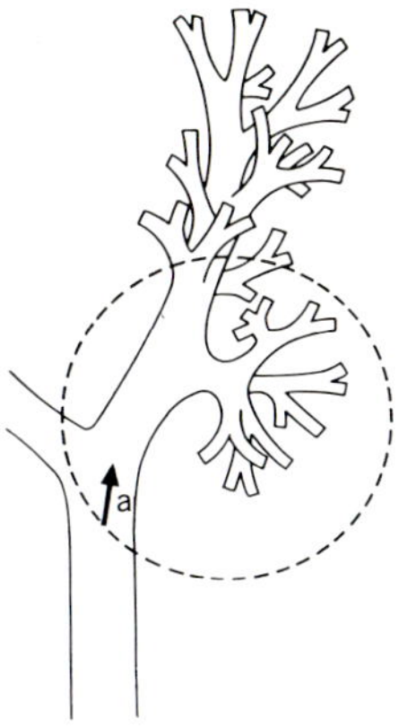


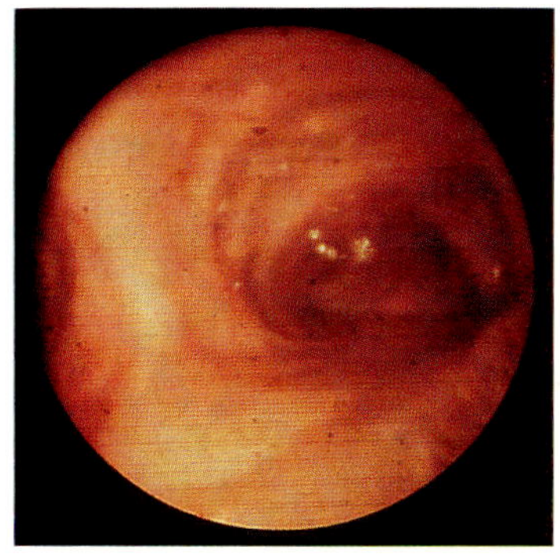

262 a

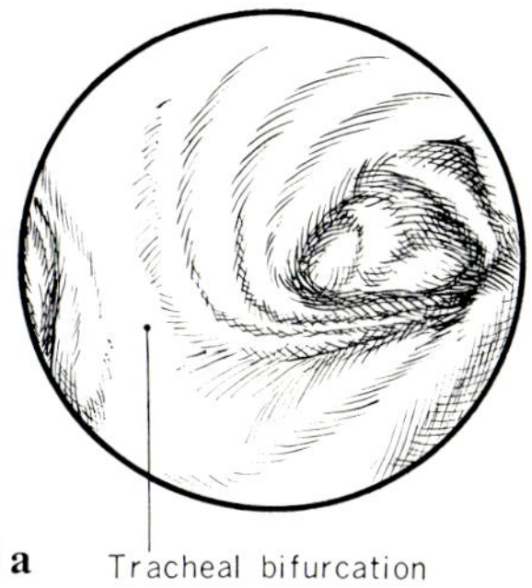


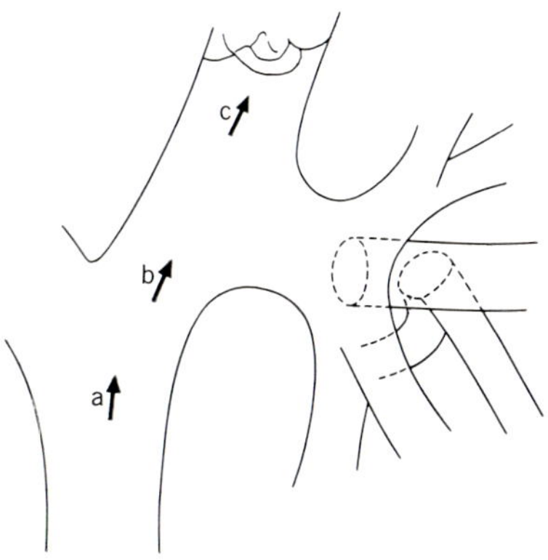


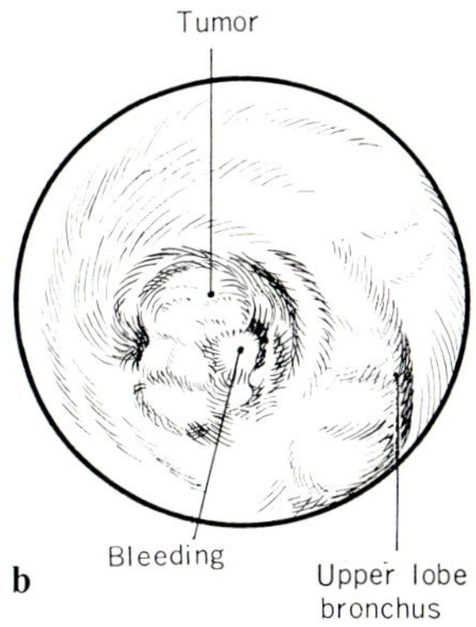


262 b

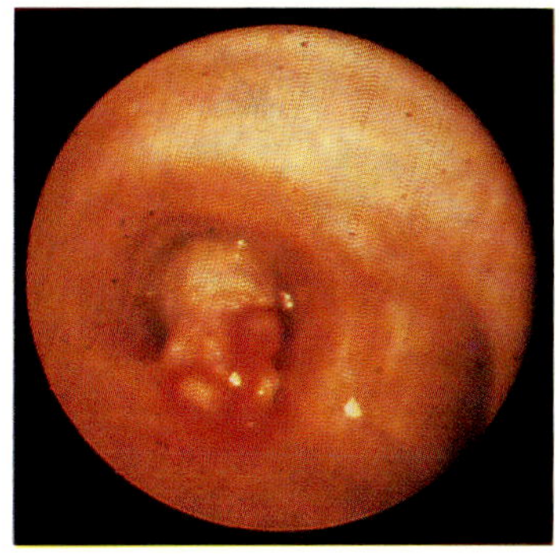

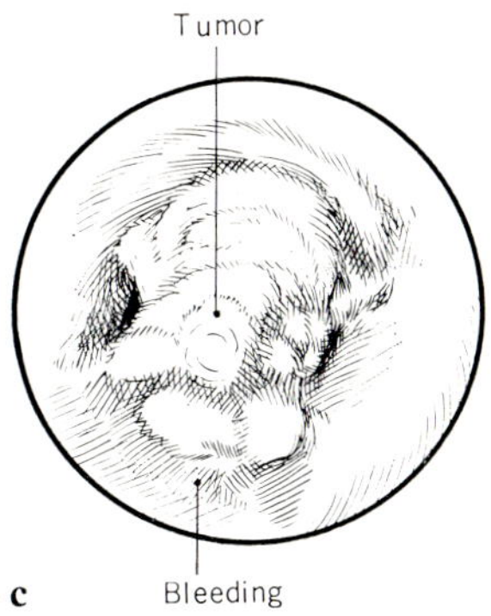


262 c

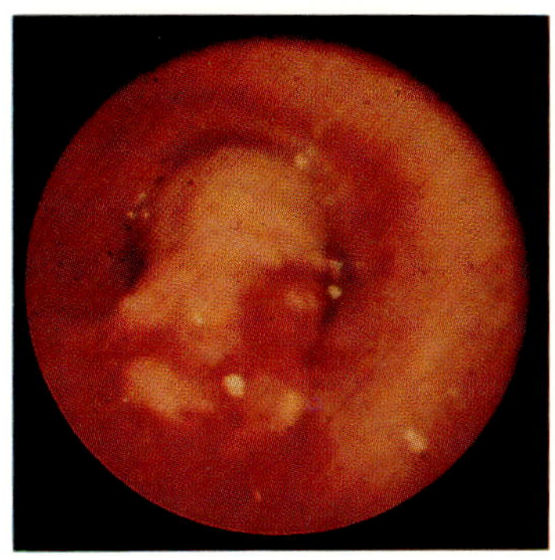

**Fig. 262 Fiberscopic findings :**

**a.** The tracheal bifurcation is normal, and the mucosa of the right main bronchus is also normal.

**b.** The bifurcation into the right upper lobe bronchus and the middle trunk presents a normal but thickened mucosal surface. The orifice of the middle lobe is almost completely occluded by a yellowish-white irregular tumor.

**c.** Tumor infiltration is visualized on the posterior and lateral walls when the scope is advanced farther.

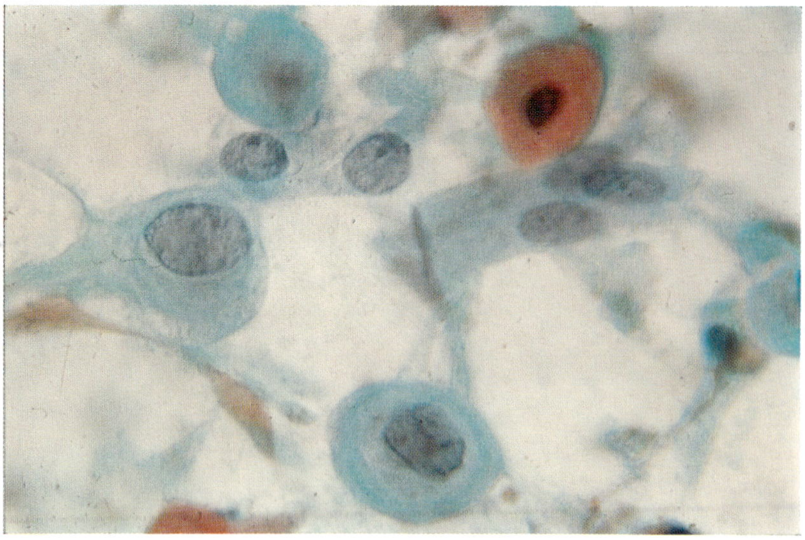

**Fig. 263 Cytodiagnosis:** Cytological diagnoses on three sputum specimens were negative.

**a.** Bronchoscopic curettage specimen. The somewhat circular green cytoplasm contains a stratified structure and a malformed, rugged nuclear membrane with a clear hof surrounding it. An orange cornified cell is present.

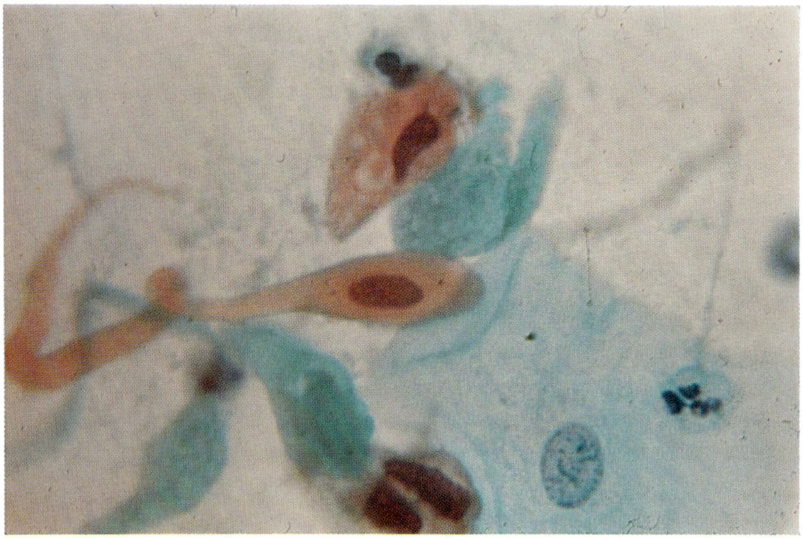

**b.** A so-called tadpole cell, extremely large and brilliant orange in color.

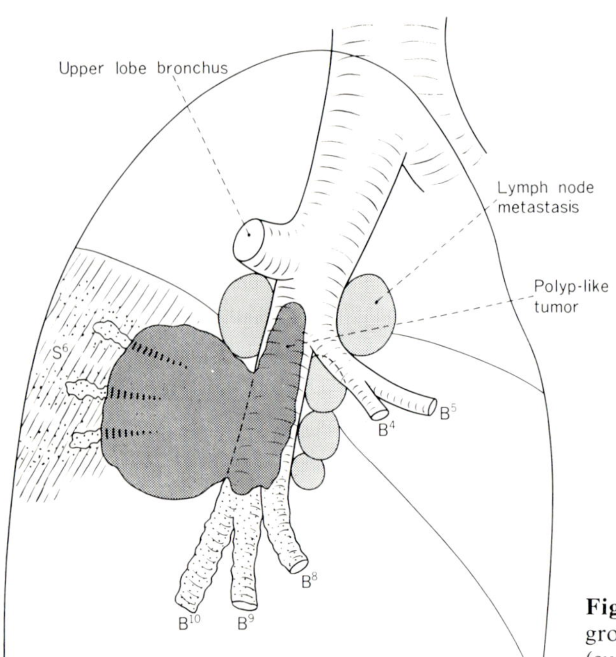


**Fig. 264 Traced schema:** Most of the tumor, which appears to have grown around the entrance of $B^6$, forms a cancer lesion 45×45 mm in $S^6$ (superior segment of lower lobe), jutting out into the lumen in a polypoid fashion. The peripheral bronchi, $B^8$, $B^9$ and $B^{10}$, which are stenosed, present obliterative bronchitis. A pulmonary lymph node is enlarged by metastasis.

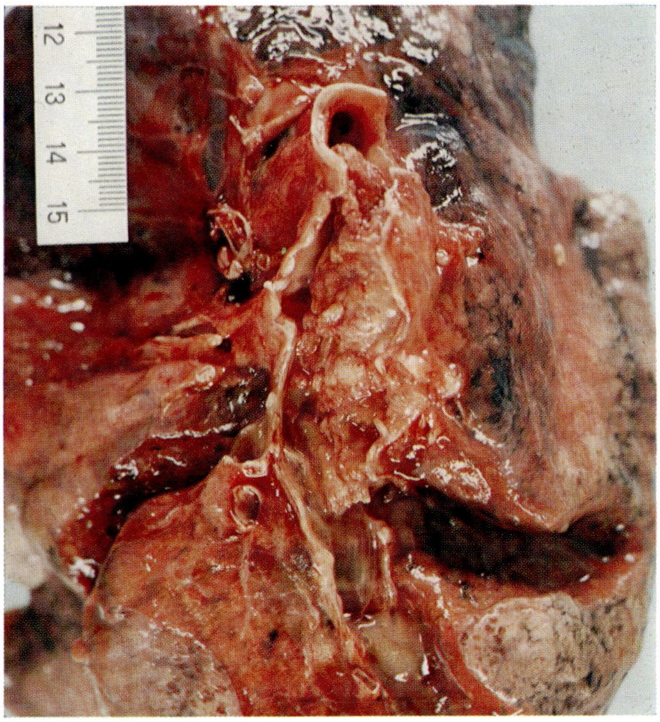


265 a

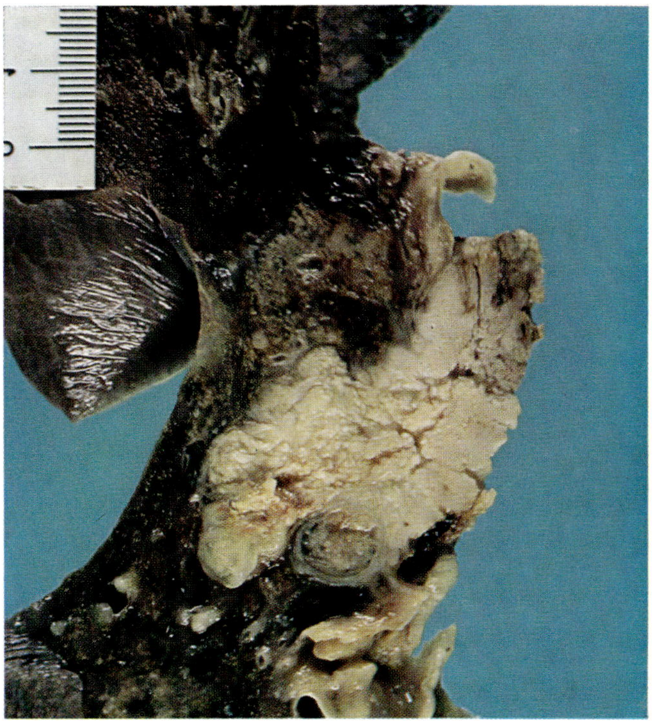

265 b

**Fig. 265 Macroscopic findings :**

**a.** Fresh resected specimen (right lung), exposing the right main bronchus, truncus intermedius and truncus inferior. The proximal side of tumor growth developing along the lumen reaches the bifurcation of the upper and middle lobe bronchi. The lower lobe bronchus is full of purulent secretion.

**b.** Fixed specimen. The part protruding into the lumen and the part infiltrating the lung parenchyma at the superior segment of lower lobe ($S^6$) are visible at the same time. The cut surface of the tumor is full of necrotic tissue and the inner structure is roughened.

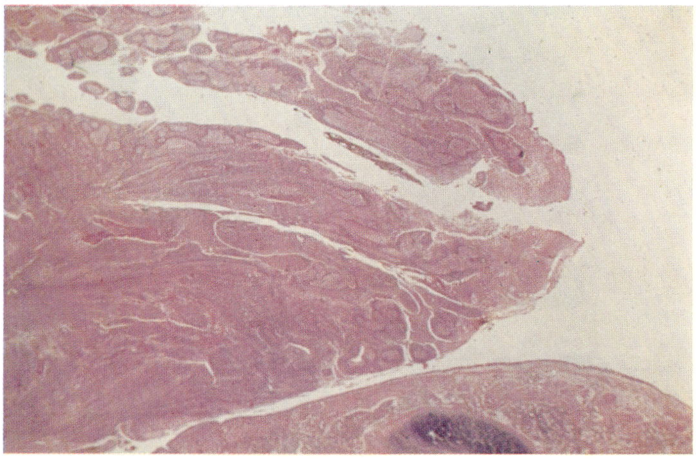

266 a

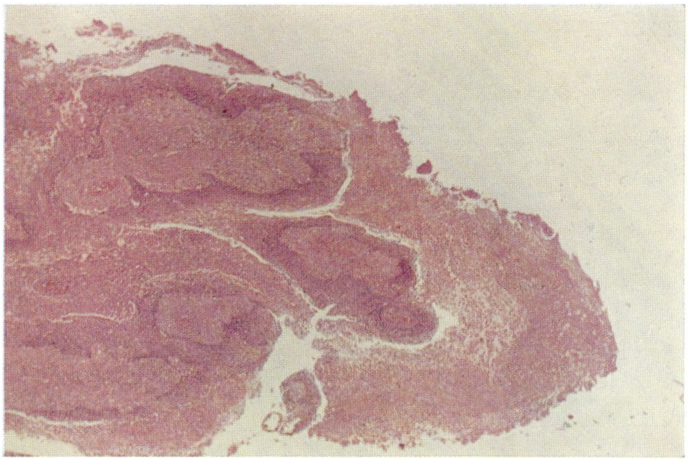

266 b

**Fig. 266 Microscopic findings :**

**a.** Histological picture of the tip of a polypoid projection. Notice squamous cell carcinoma with less keratinized cells.

**b.** Keratotic squamous cell carcinoma is located in the bronchial lumen.

**COMMENT :**

Atelectasis in an adult should always make one suspect the presence of a lung cancer. In this case, a rigid bronchoscope may have been adequate ; however, better pictures can be obtained with the flexible bronchofiberscope.

## Case 12 Squamous Cell Carcinoma (55, male)

**Chief complaint :** Chronic cough.
**Definitive clinical diagnosis :** Keratotic squamous cell carcinoma by sputum cytology.
**Pathological diagnosis :** Moderately differentiated squamous cell carcinoma.
**Case history :** The patient had a chronic severe cough for six months, so had his chest X-rayed, following which he was referred to our hospital.

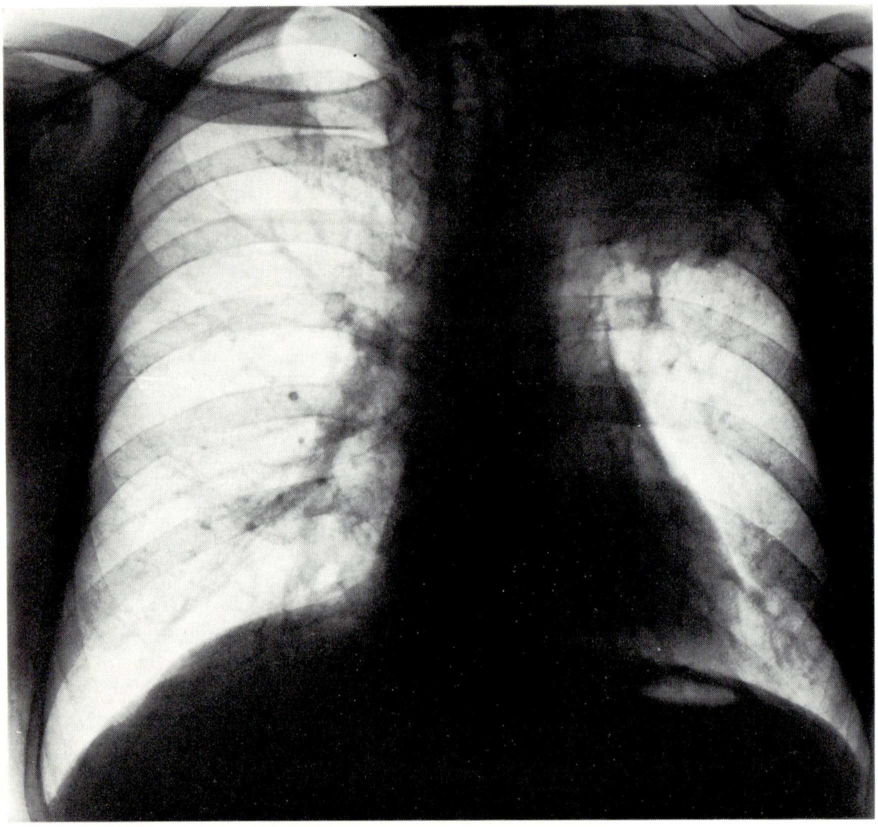

**Fig. 267 Chest X-ray, frontal :** A tumor shadow, 50×50 mm, is seen in the left upper lobe. It is characterized by a distinct outline and probably contains a cavity.

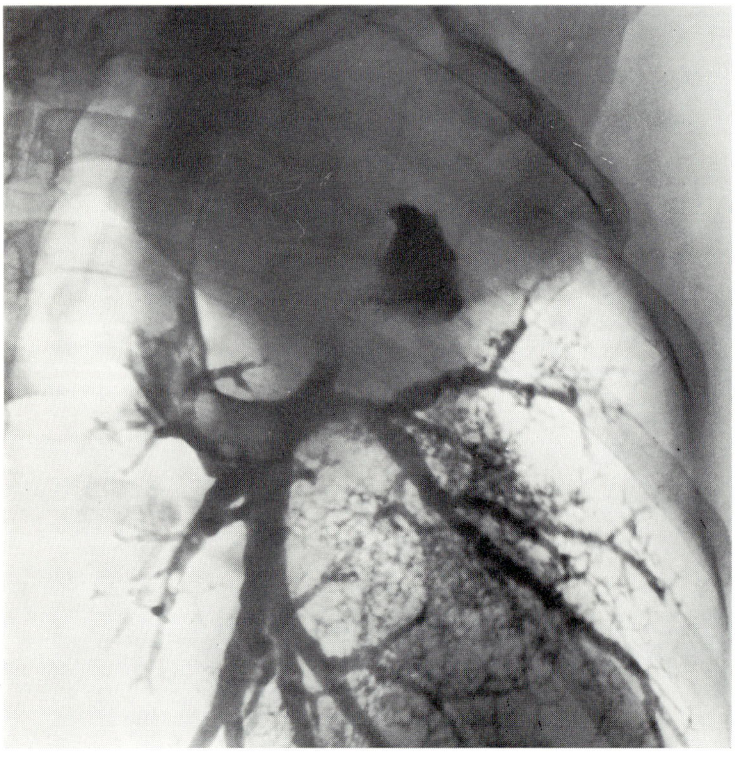

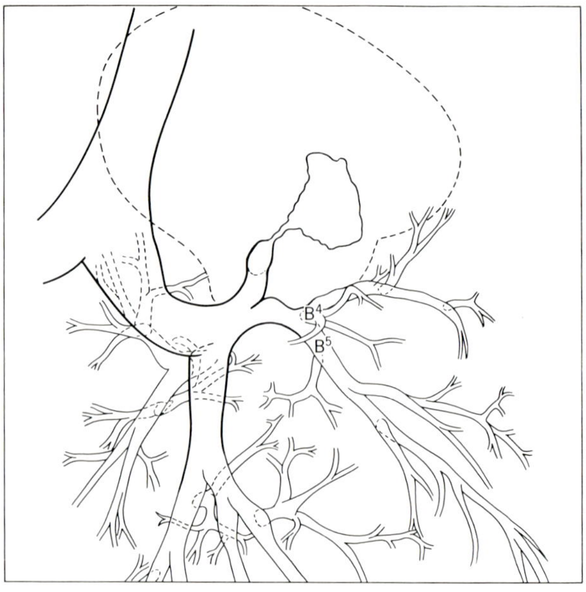


**Fig. 268 Bronchogram, oblique :** Stenosis is located over the upper division bronchus, and a cavity shadow is present in the anterior segment ($S^3$).

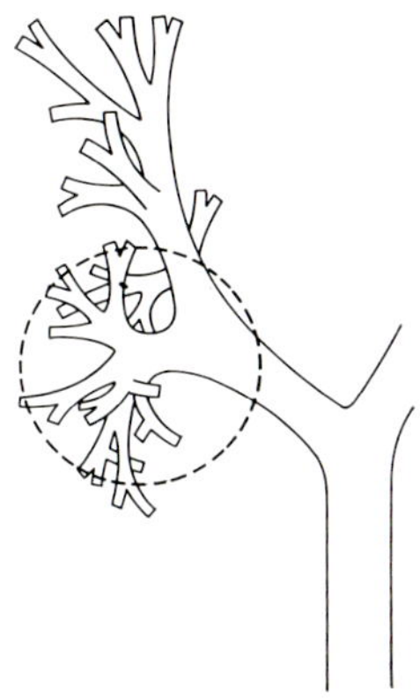

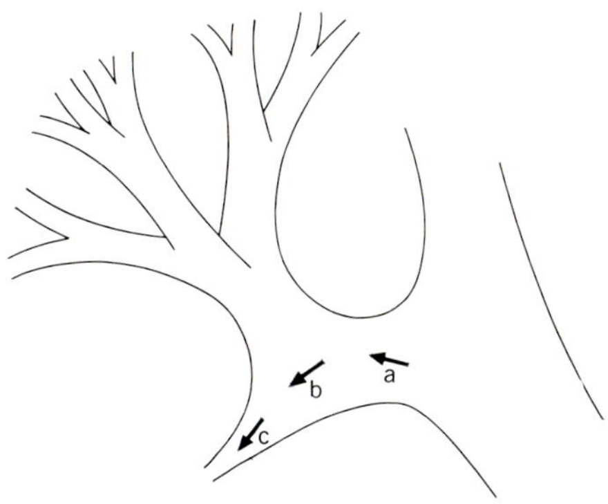


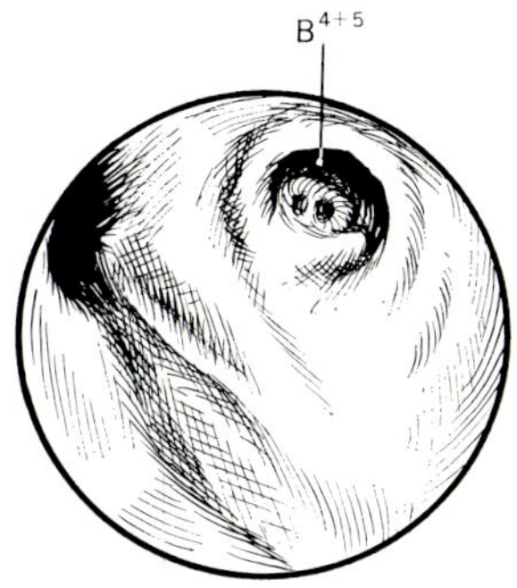


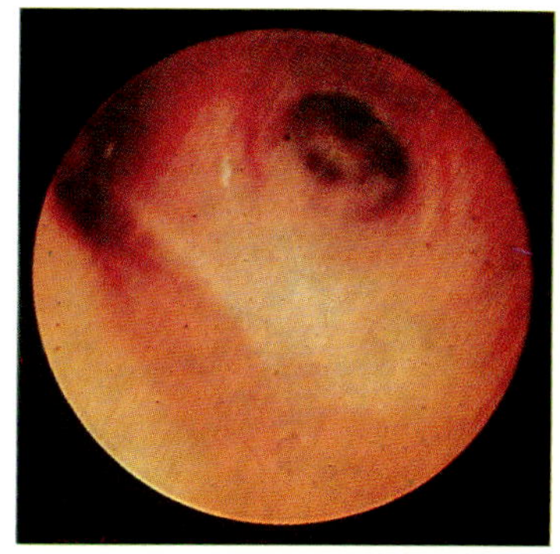

**269 a**

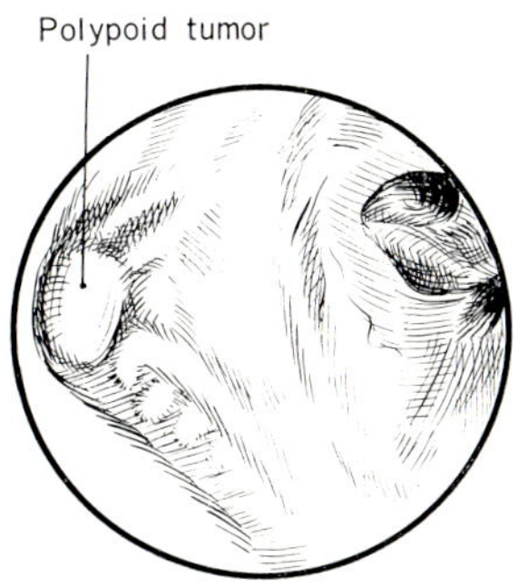


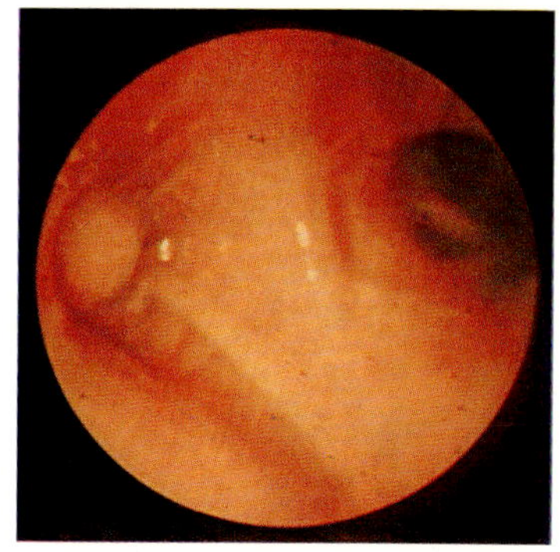

**269 b**

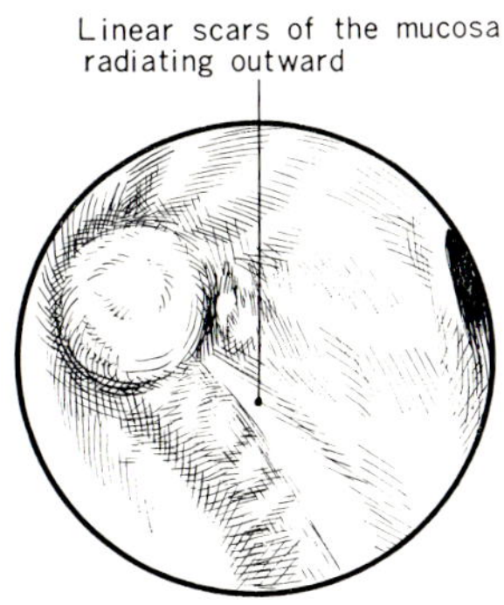


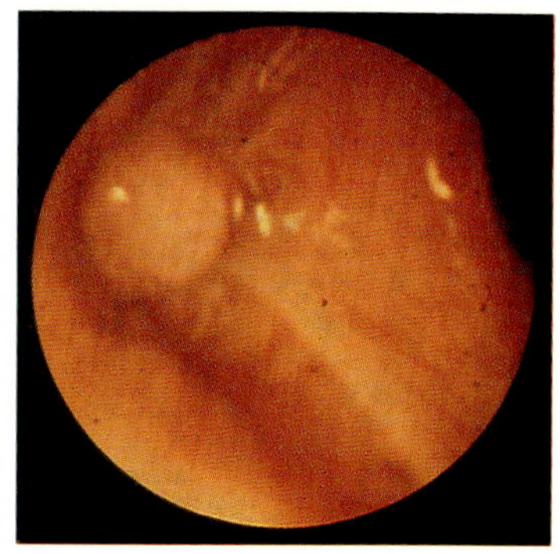

**269 c**

**Fig. 269 Fiberscopic findings :**

**a.** The bifurcation of the upper division bronchus and the lingular bronchus is normal. The upper division bronchus is gradually narrowed.

**b.** At the deeper part of the stenosed upper division bronchus, a smooth-surfaced polypoid tumor is exposed.

**c.** The bronchial mucosa around the basal part of the polyp-like tumor is scar-like with convergence.

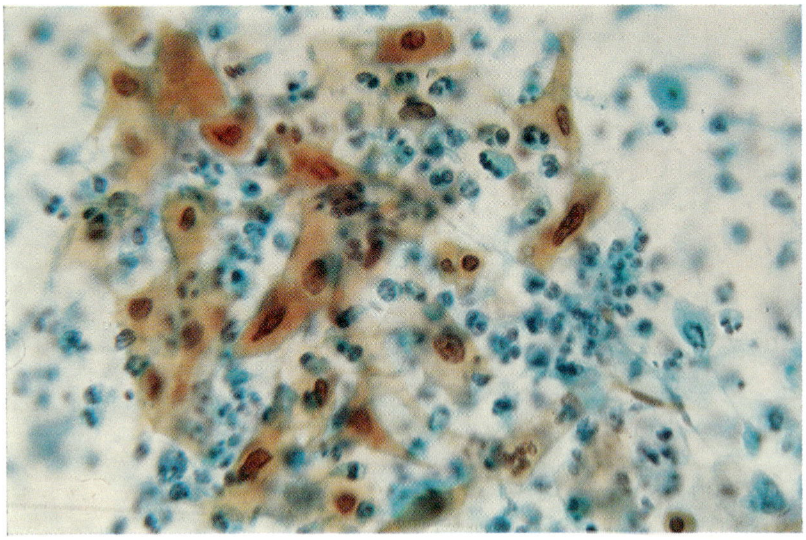

**Fig. 270 Cytodiagnosis:**
**a.** Bronchofiberscopic curettage. The cytoplasm is individually polymorphous and stained orange. The nuclei are varied in size and form. The nuclear membranes are thickened and chromatin is uniformly condensed.

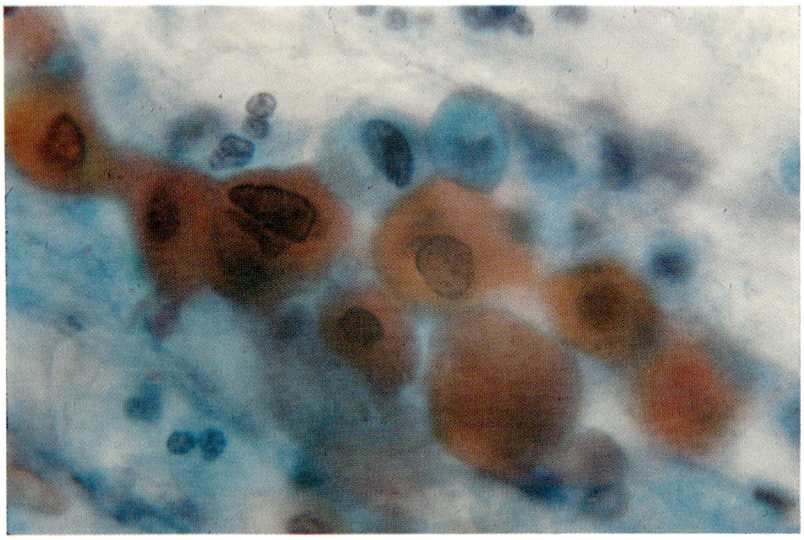

**b.** Sputum cytology. Of three cytologic examinations squamous carcinoma cells were obtained in two. Cells with orange-stained cyotoplasm are intermixed with those with green-stained cytoplasm. A ghost cell also is present.

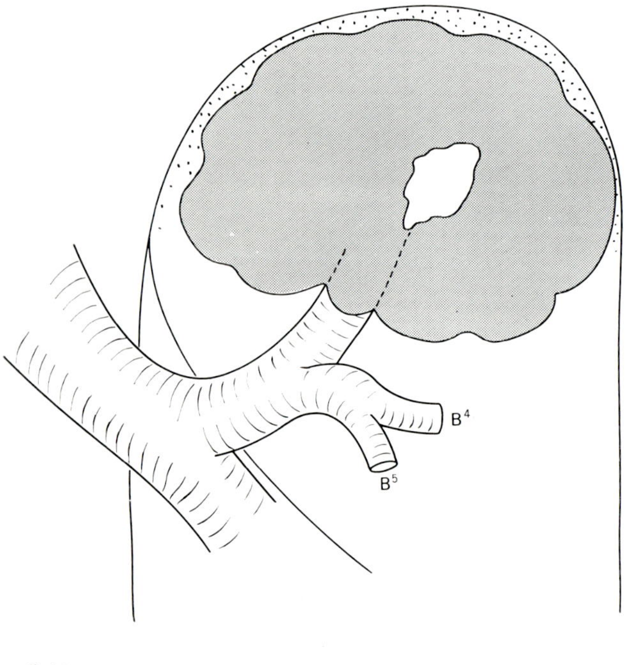


**Fig. 271 Traced schema**

272 a 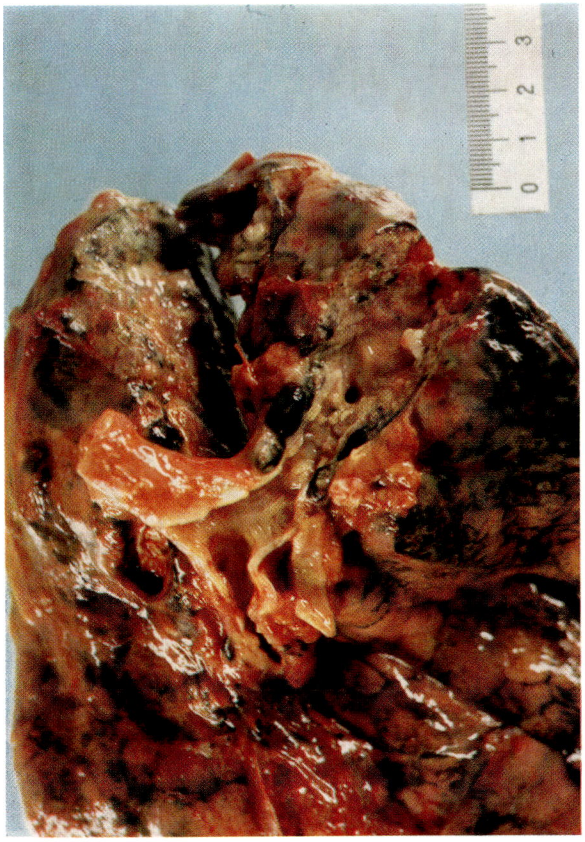

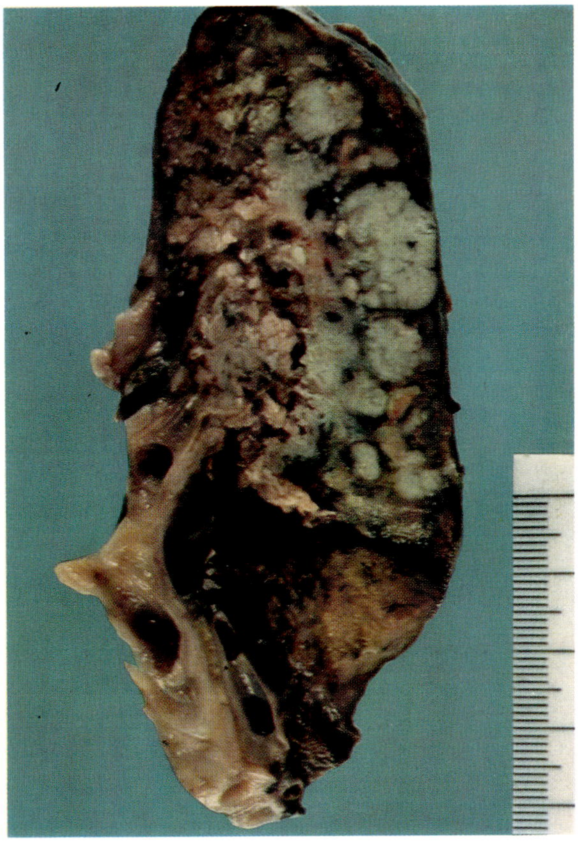 272 b

**Fig. 272 Macroscopic findings :**

**a.** Fresh specimen trimmed, showing the left main bronchus to the upper lobe bronchus. The upper division bronchus points to the center of the tumor containing liquefaction-necrosed substance, gradually destroyed. The tumor is exposed in the lumen.

**b.** Fixed specimen. A relatively large carcinoma, 60×45 mm, is located along the upper division bronchus.

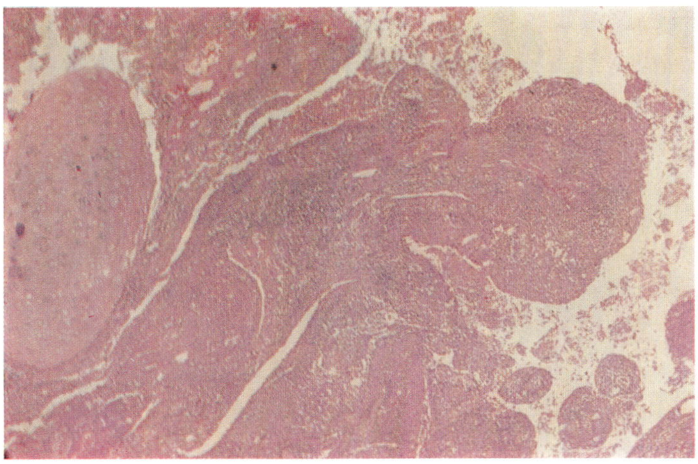

273 a

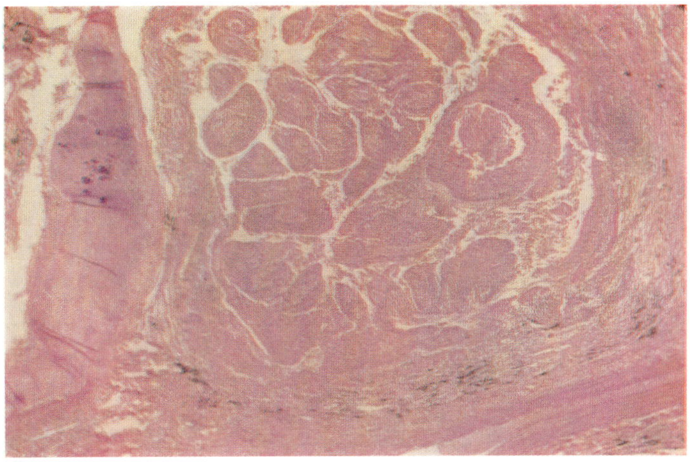

273 b

**Fig. 273 Microscopic findings :**

**a.** Histological picture of the less keratinized squamous cell carcinoma growing and jutting into the lumen in a polypoid manner.

**b.** Squamous cell carcinoma in this case was noted to have protruded into a relatively peripheral bronchial lumen.

**COMMENT :**

A cavity is present on the bronchogram, but this finding alone cannot differentiate between lung cancer and pulmonary tuberculosis. Many cases of this category can be definitively diagnosed by sputum cytology. With a bronchoscope, a tumor may be clearly visualized. The specimen of the resected lung and the bronchoscopic photo revealed the same findings.

## Case 13 Squamous Cell Carcinoma (54, male)

**Chief complaint :** Fever.
**Case history :** The patient had a fever of 39°C three months ago. Chest X-ray revealed atelectasis of the right upper lobe. Thereupon broad spectrum chemotherapy was instituted and temporarily, the atelectasis disappeared. However with the cessation of chemotherapy, the atelectasis recurred so the patient was referred to our hospital. Bronchoscopy disclosed the presence of cancer and a biopsy specimen revealed a squamous cell carcinoma. Radiation therapy was administered.

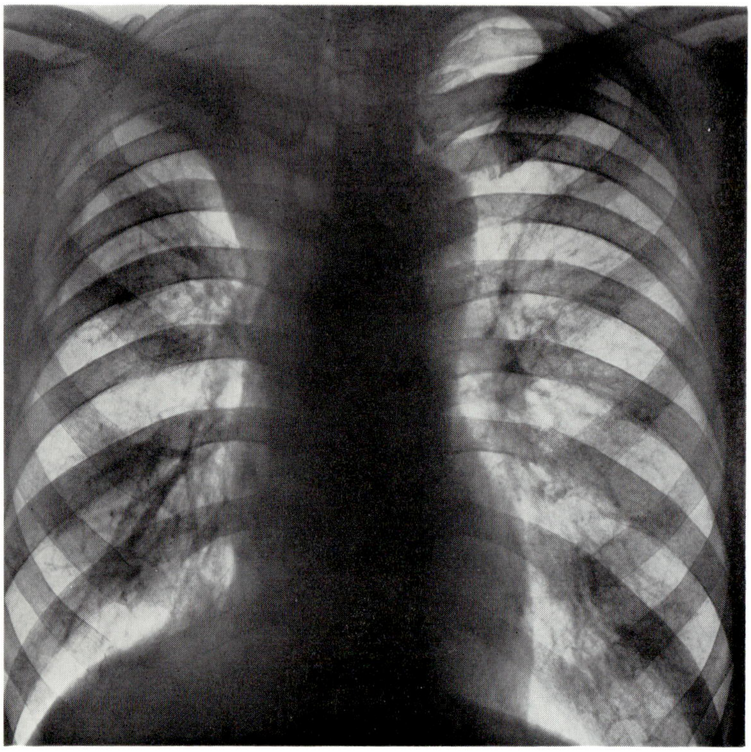

**Fig. 274 Chest X-ray, frontal :** The right upper lobe presents a complete atelectasis. The trachea is slightly retracted to the right. The right diaphragm is elevated.

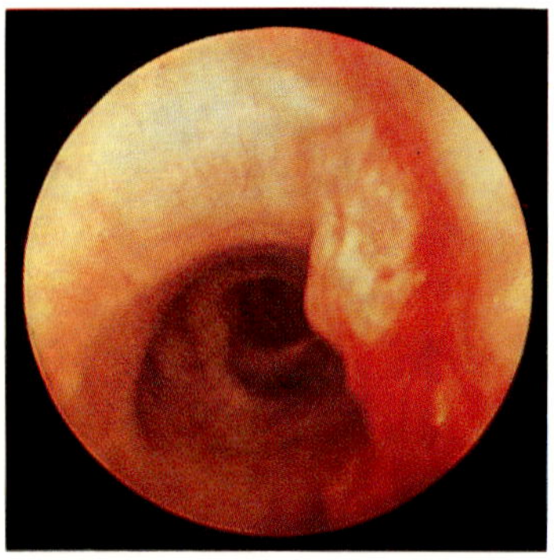

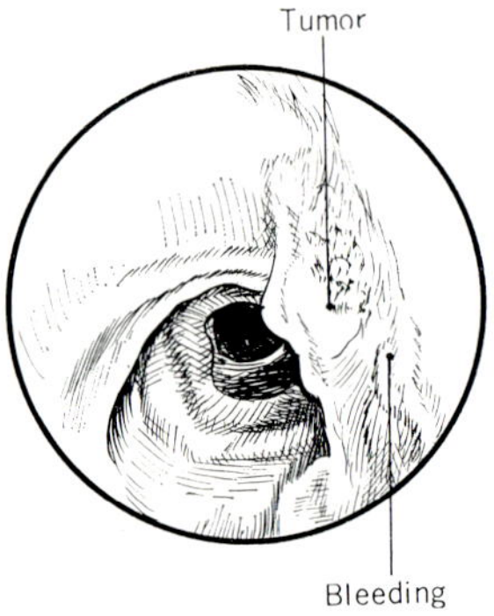


275 a

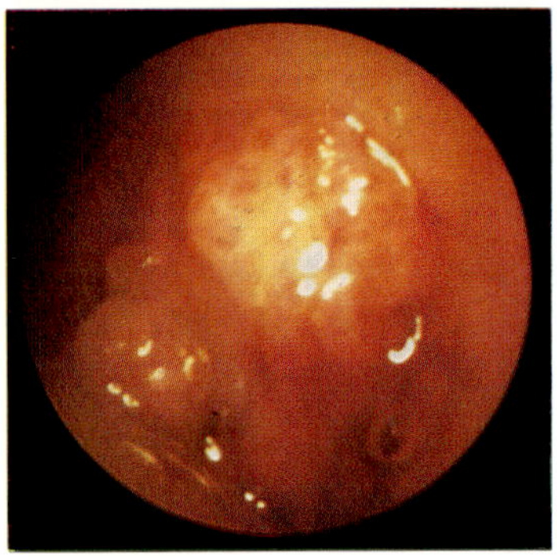

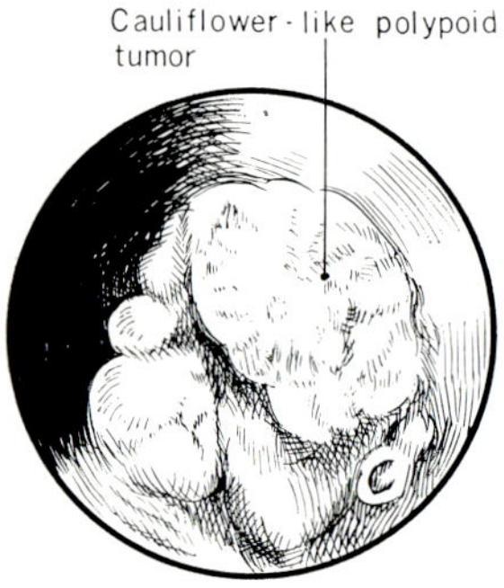


275 b

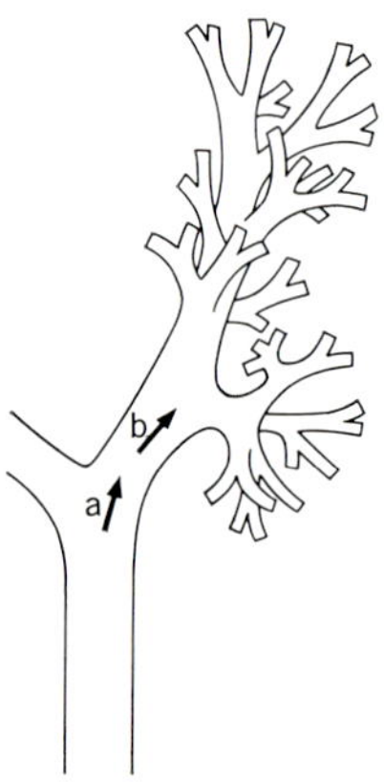


**Fig. 275 Bronchoscopic findings :**
**a.** Rigid bronchoscopy disclosed a tumor arising from the right upper lobe bronchus. The tumor is bleeding.
**b.** A lateral-viewing telescope reveals a polypoid cauliflower-like protrusion of the tumor from the right upper lobe bronchus. There is bleeding from the surface. Biopsy specimen was diagnosed as squamous cell carcinoma.

# Case 14 Squamous Cell Carcinoma (68, male)

**Chief complaint :** Cough and sputum.

**Case history :** Onset 3 months ago with chest pain, cough and sputum, which has become progressively worse. He is a heavy smoker. Chest X-ray shows a 50×50 mm tumor shadow in the right lower lobe. Bronchoscopy revealed a tumor and biopsy led to the diagnosis of squamous cell carcinoma. Both radiation therapy and chemotherapy for cancer were instituted.

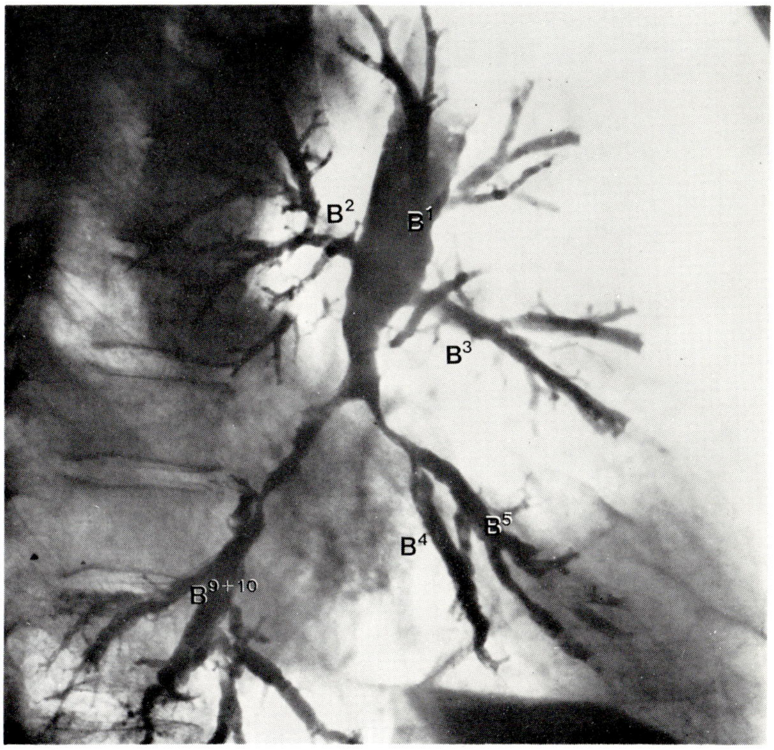


**Fig. 276 Bronchogram, lateral :** The truncus intermedius is compressed and narrowed on both the anterior and the posterior aspects. Irregular stenosis is present ranging from the inferior truncus to the basal truncus. Smooth compression stenosis is demonstrated from the orifice of the middle lobe bronchus to the orifices of $B^4$ and $B^5$.

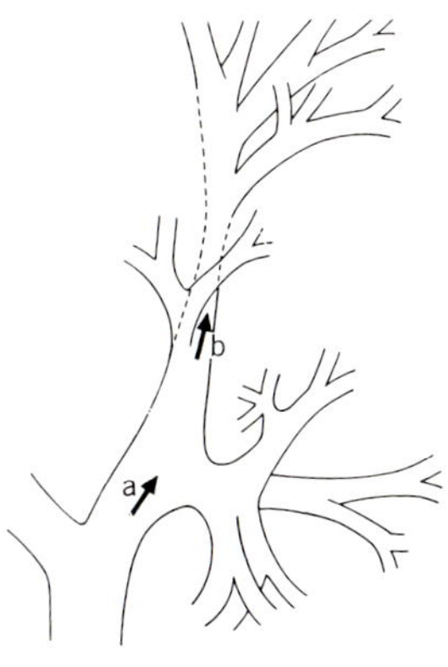


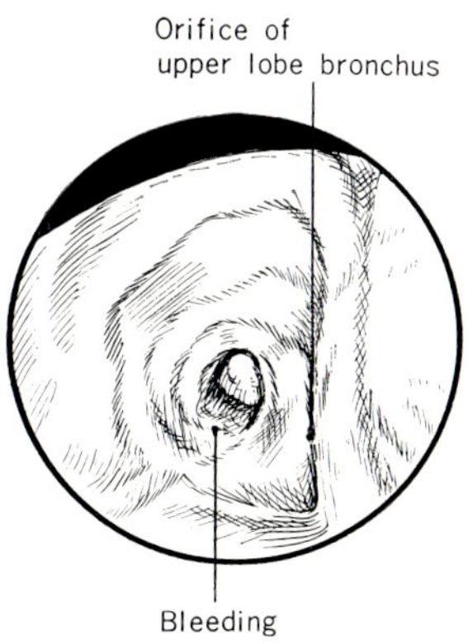


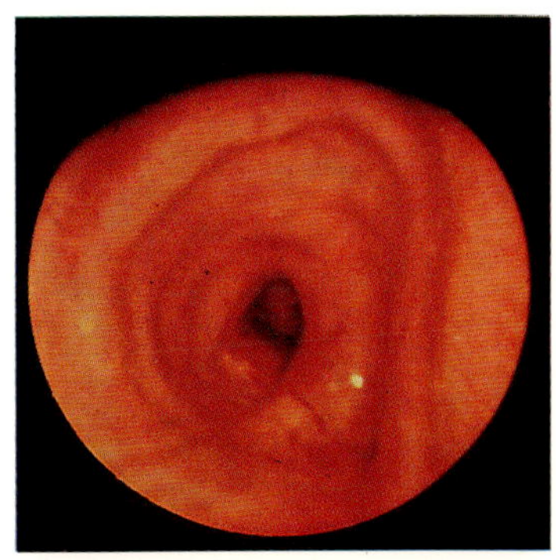

277 a

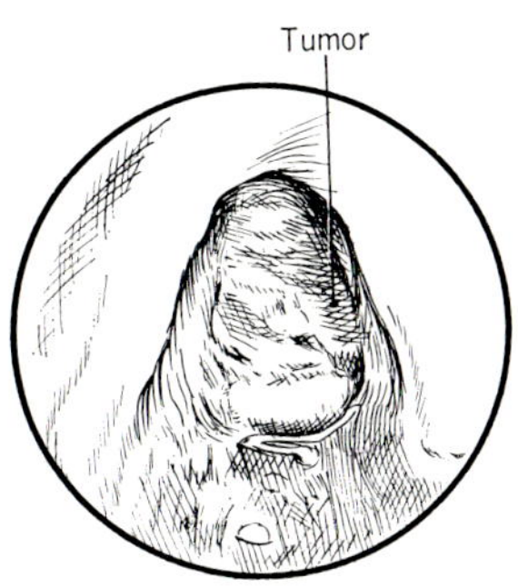


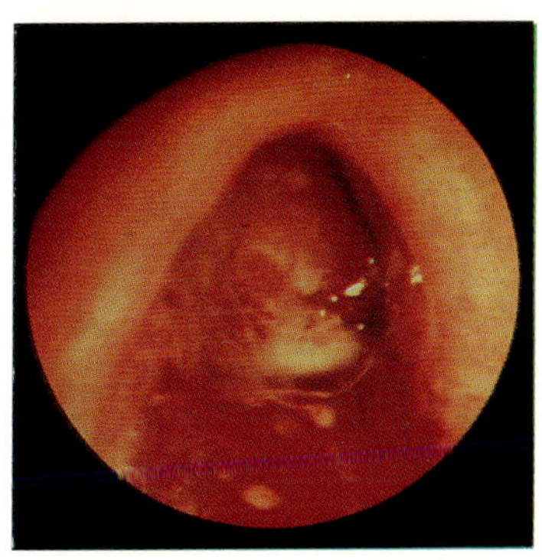

277 b

**Fig. 277 Bronchoscopic findings :**

**a.** A rigid forward viewing telescopic finding reveals concentric stenosis of the truncus intermedius, part of which is stained with blood. The bifurcation of the upper lobe bronchus and the truncus intermedius is thickened.

**b.** Similarly the telescopic picture discloses stenosis of the truncus inferior by a tumor which arises in the lower lobe bronchus. The truncus inferior is obstructed and bleeding. The tumor surface is granular. The middle lobe orifice cannot be identified because of bleeding. With the biopsy specimen, the tumor was diagnosed as squamous cell carcinoma.

## Case 15 Squamous Cell Carcinoma (71, female)

**Chief complaint :** Slight hemoptysis.

**Case history :** Onset 6 months ago with light streaked sputum. Recently as the amount of blood increased, she became alarmed and came to our hospital. The patient, an old female, has been smoking 10 to 20 cigarettes daily, inhaling deeply, for the past 55 years. Bronchofiberscopy disclosed stenosis at $B^3$ and the cytological diagnosis was adenocarcinoma. Left upper lobectomy was performed after two weeks. The pathological diagnosis based on the resected specimen was a poorly differentiated squamous cell carcinoma.

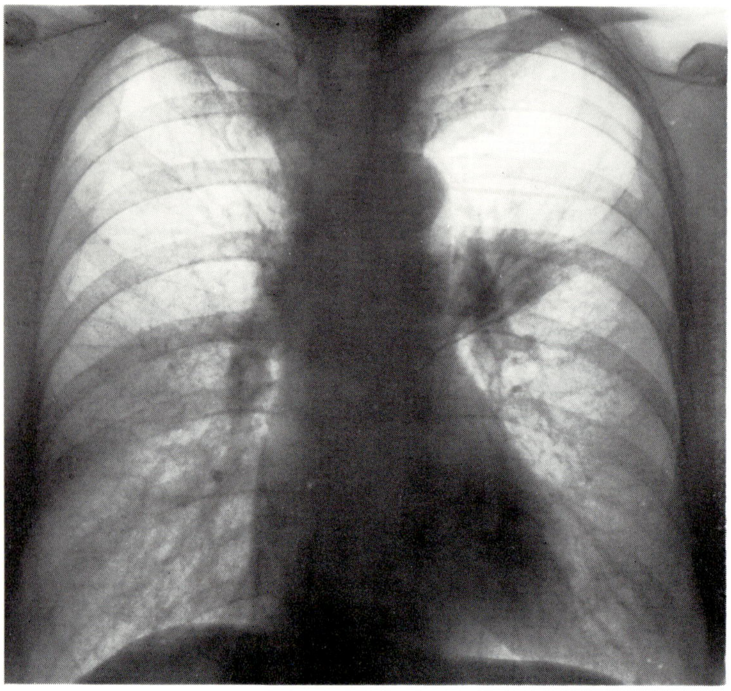

**Fig. 278 Chest X-ray, frontal :** A shadow 30×30 mm with indistinct boundaries is located in the left $S^3$ (anterior segment of upper lobe); a part of the surrounding lung is atelectatic.

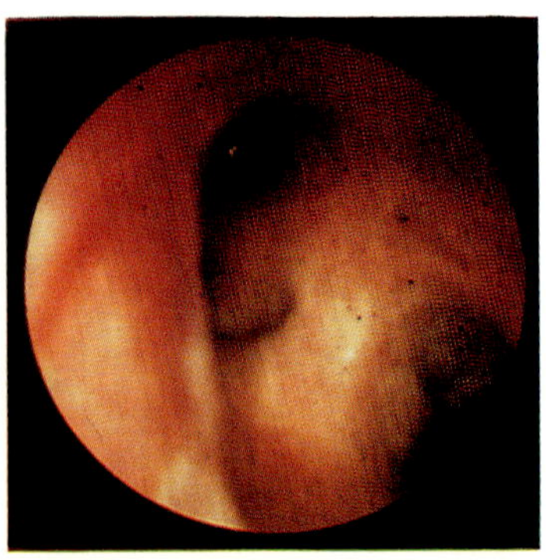

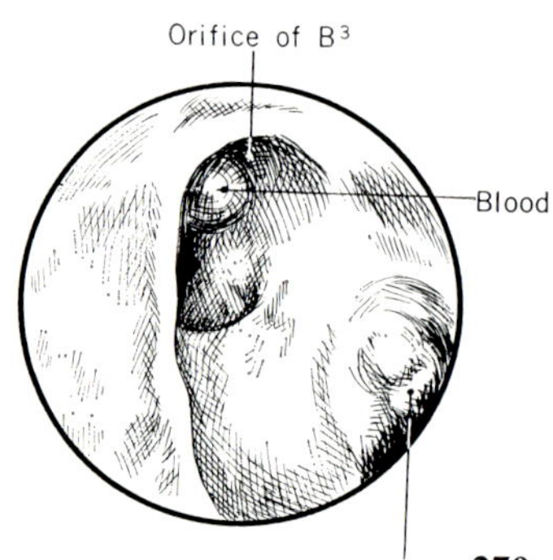


279 a

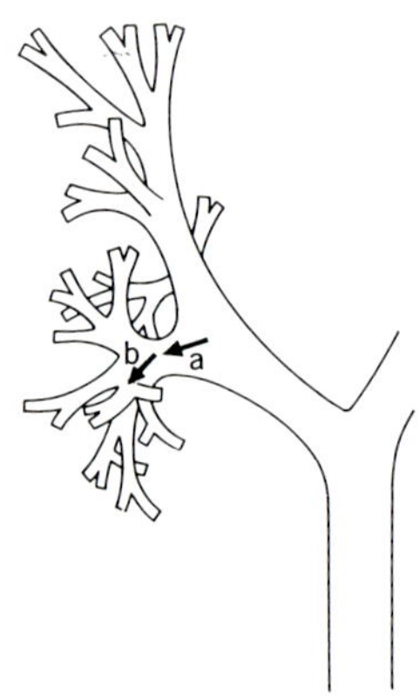


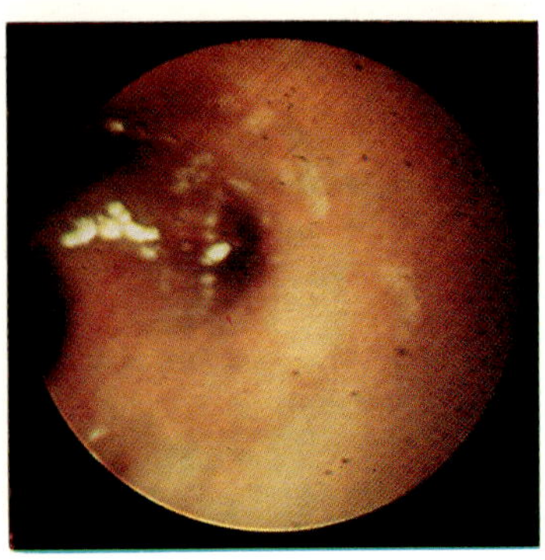

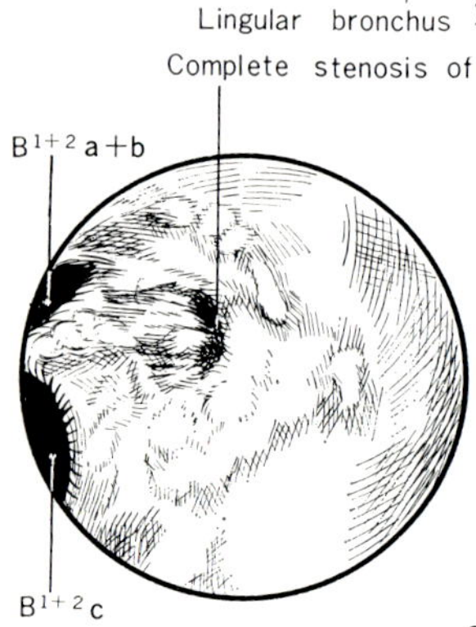


279 b

**Fig. 279 Fiberscopic findings :**

**a.** The upper division bronchus of the left upper lobe is narrowed. The bifurcation of the upper division bronchus and the lingular bronchus is thickened. Superiorly, the orifice of $B^3$ is visible. It contains bloody sputum.

**b.** With the bloody sputum removed, $B^3$ is seen to be completely stenosed. The mucosa is thickened and slightly irregular. The cartilages are obscured. This suggests the presence of carcinomatous infiltration. With bronchofiberscopic curettage, it was diagnosed carcinoma, which was confirmed pathologically in the resected specimen.

# Case 16 Squamous Cell Carcinoma (68, male)

**Chief complaint :** Aphonia.

**Case history :** About 4 months ago the patient suddenly lost his voice so visited a practitioner, who referred him to our hospital. The chest X-ray revealed a tumor shadow in the left upper lobe. With bronchofiberscopy, the case as was diagnosed squamous cell carcinoma.

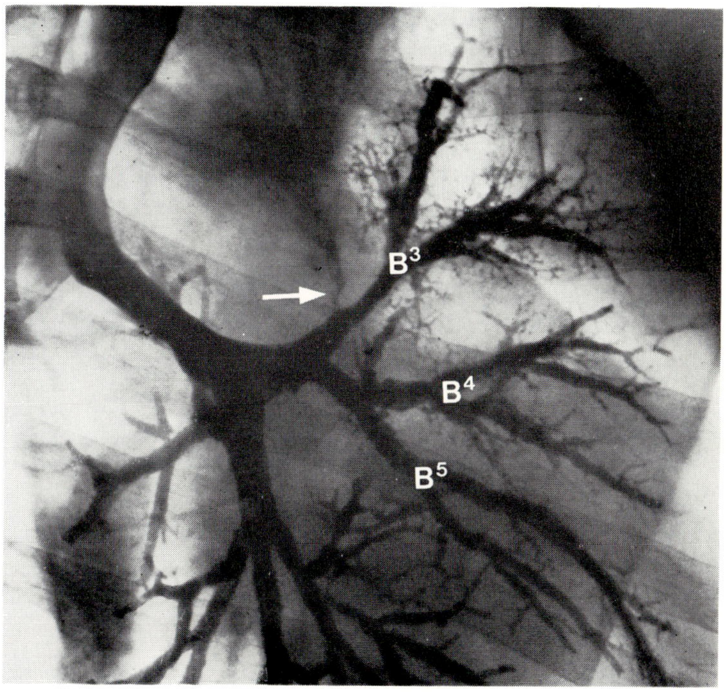


**Fig. 280 Bronchogram, oblique :** The left main bronchus is stenosed. The left main bronchus and the upper division bronchus are curved like a bow. The entrance of $B^{1+2}$ (arrow) is obstructed. Fibrotic strands are seen radiating outward in the periphery of the apicoposteri or segment $S^{1+2}$, suggesting the presence of a tumor obstructing $B^{1+2}$.

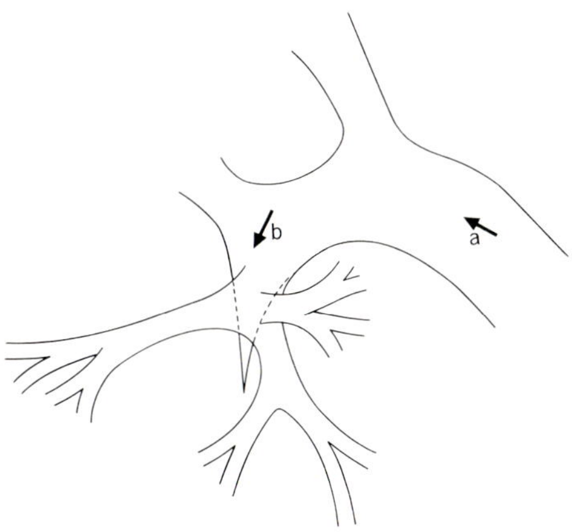


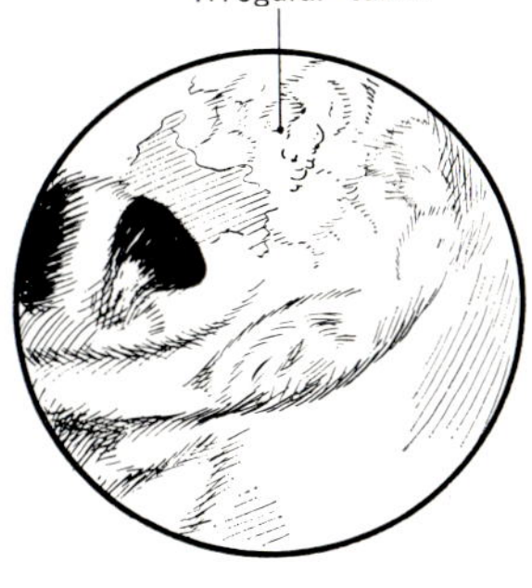


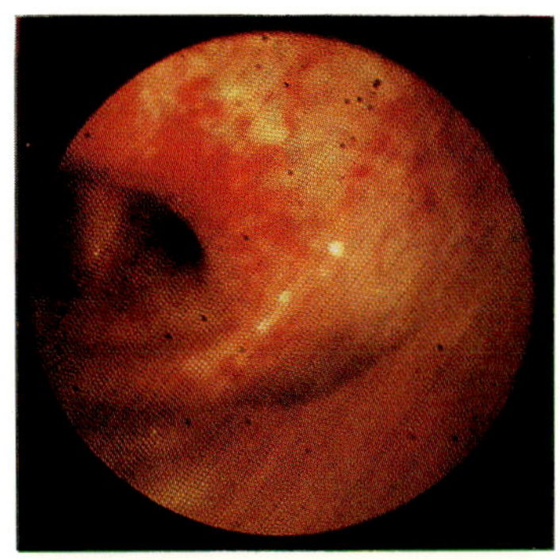

281 a

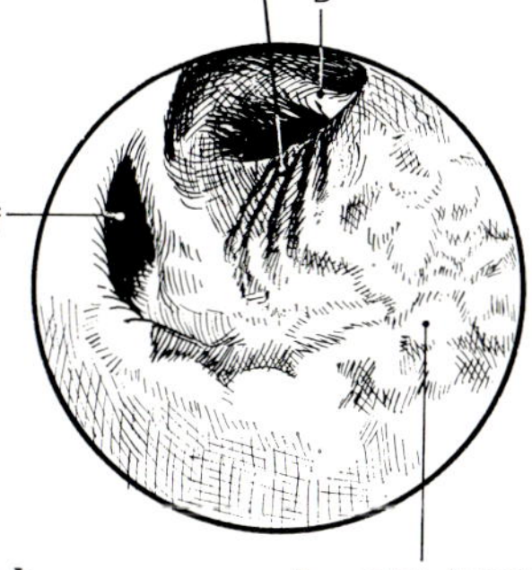


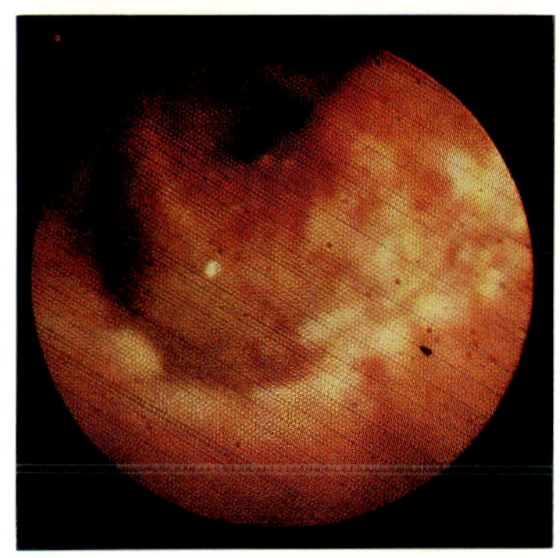

281 b

**Fig. 281 Fiberscopic findings :**

**a.** The anterior wall of the lower part of the left main bronchus is irregular and the cartilage rings are not clearly visualized. This is suggestive of a carcinomatous infiltration in this portion. The upper lobe septum is extremely thickened.

**b.** From the orifice of the upper division bronchus to the bifurcation of $B^{1+2}$ and $B^3$, especially on the posterior wall, irregularity of the mucosa and engorgement of blood vessels are noted. These findings are considered to be the result of cancer infiltration. Marked stenosis is present at the orifice of $B^{1+2}$. Curettage of this region revealed squamous cell carcinoma.

# Case 17 Squamous Cell Carcinoma (63, male)

**Case history :** An abnormal shadow was found in a local mass survey two years ago, but it was left alone. Later the shadow increased in size, so the patient visited our hospital. Definitive diagnosis was made by bronchofiberscopy. Unfortunately, the tumor was inoperable because of extension into, and of compression of the left main pulmonary artery, found by pulmonary angiography. The therapy was irradiation.

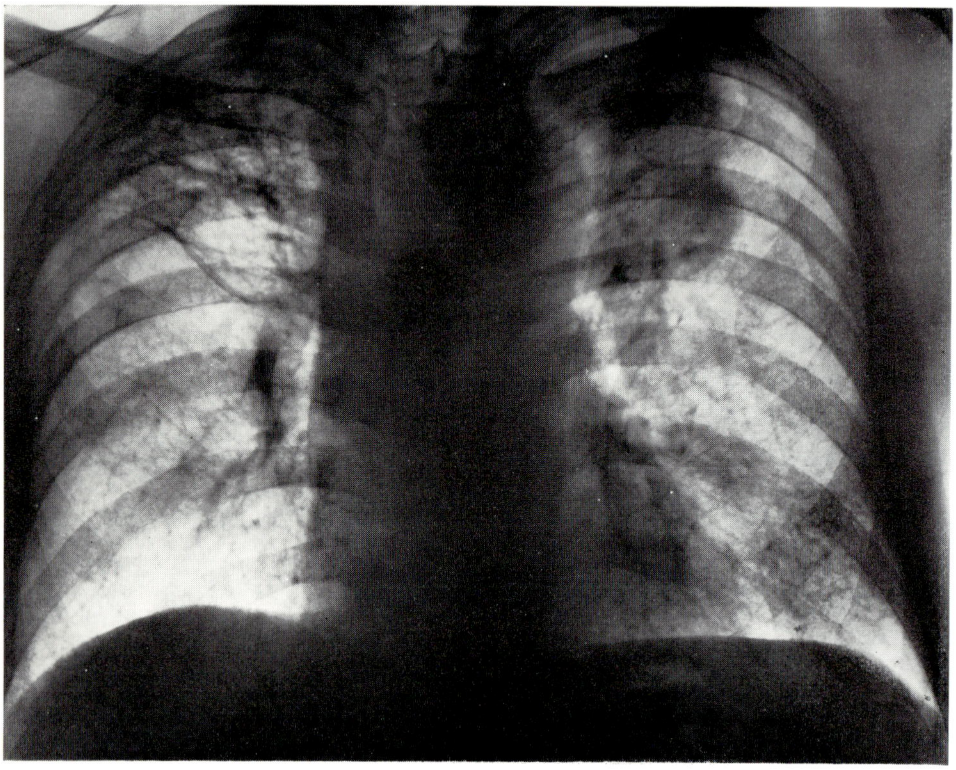

**Fig. 282 Chest X-ray, frontal:** A tumor is located in the left upper lung field. Extensive fibrosis is present in the right upper lung field. The trachea deviates to the right, apparently due to fibrosis.

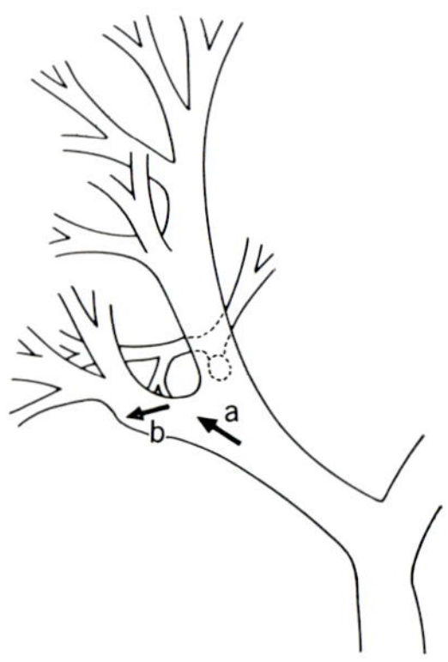


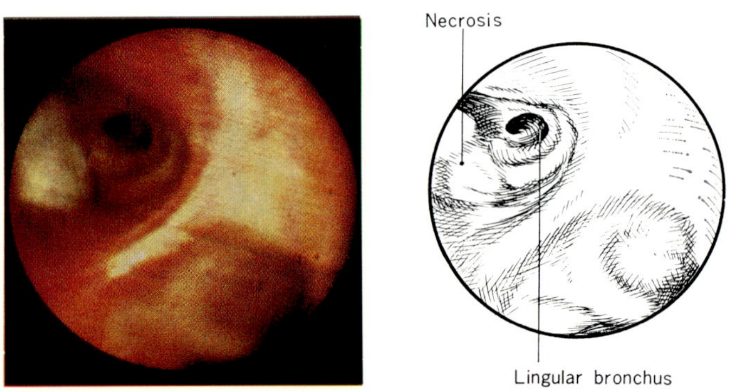


**283 a**

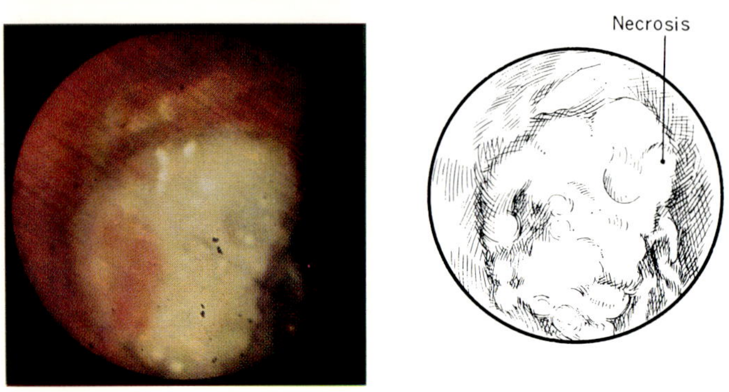


**283 b**

**Fig. 283 Fiberscopic findings :**

**a.** White necrotic substance obstructs the upper division bronchus. The lingular bronchus is normal.

**b.** A tumor with a necrotic surface stenoses the upper division bronchus. No normal structures are visualized in the mucosa orifice of this bronchus. Biopsy specimen with a tiny forceps through the bronchofiberscope, the case was diagnosed as a keratotic squamous cell carcinoma. In a case of necrotic tumor such as this, it is advisable to biopsy the root portion of the tumor projecting from the bronchus instead of the necrotic area. As mentioned previously, examination of necrotic tissue rarely leads to definite pathological diagnosis.

# Case 18 Squamous Cell Carcinoma (38, male)

**Case history :** An abnormal shadow was found by a local mass survey, so the patient visited our hospital. A tumor shadow in the lower part of the right lung is seen on the chest X-ray. Bronchography and bronchofiberscopy were performed. Cytology at bronchofiberscopy diagnosed the case as keratotic squamous cell carcinoma. Radiation therapy was given.

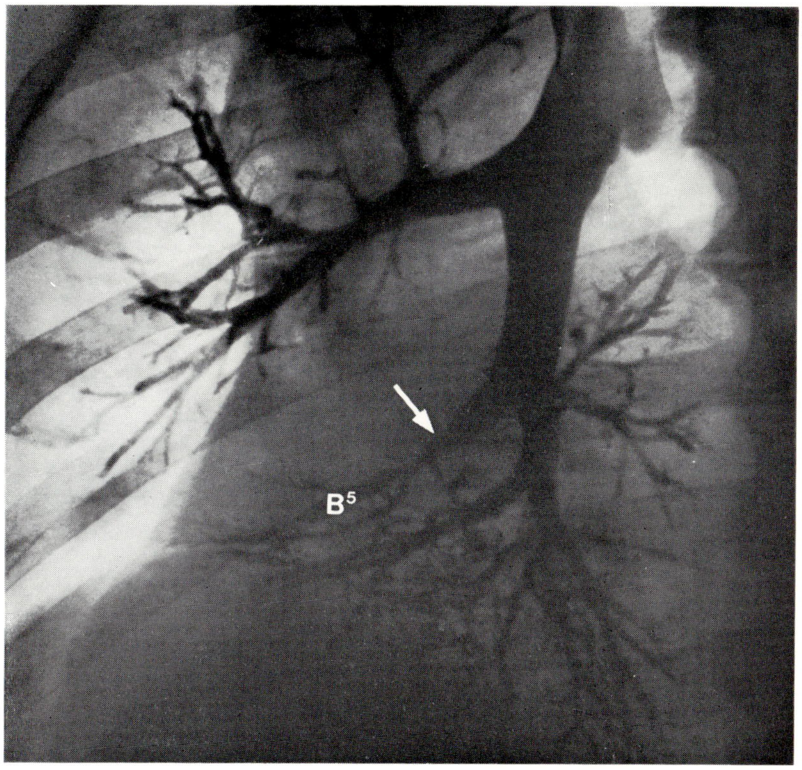


**Fig. 284 Bronchogram, oblique :** $B^4$ is completely obstructed at its orifice (arrow). The entrance of $B^5$ is prominently stenosed.

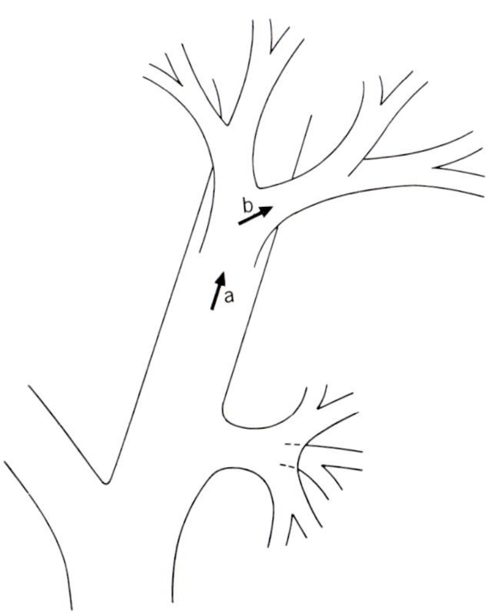


**Fig. 285 Fiberscopic findings :**

**a.** The bifurcation of the lower and the middle lobe bronchi is normal. The orifice of the middle lobe bronchus is fairly normal.

**b.** A tumor with an irregular surface is exposed on the right wall in the middle lobe bronchus, which is stenosed because of it. The site of the tumor is located at the orifice of $B^4$.

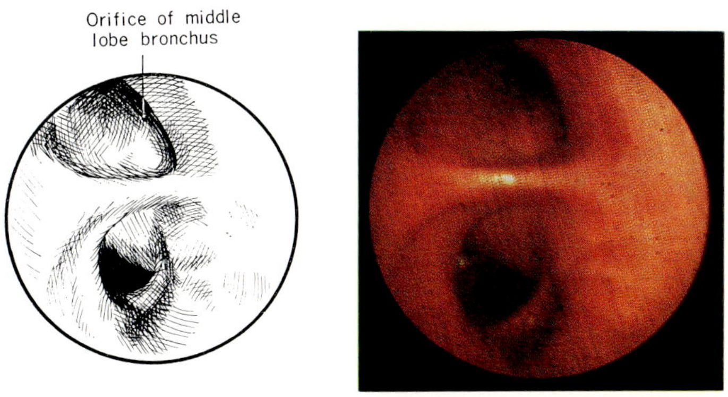


**285 a**

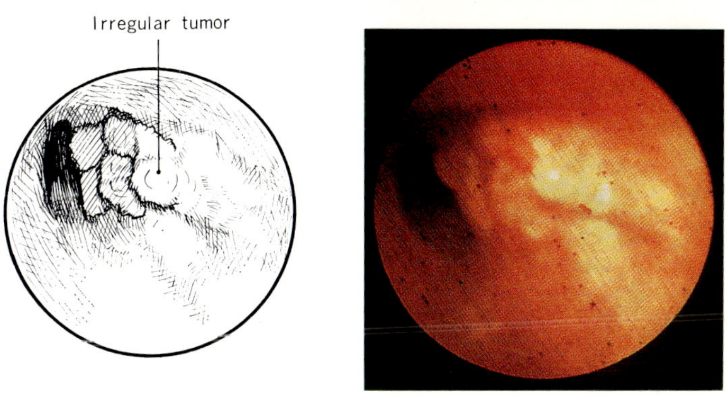


**285 b**

## Case 19 Large Cell Carcinoma (68, male)

**Chief complaint :** Abnormal shadow.
**Definitive clinical diagnosis :** Adenocarcinoma by bronchofiberscopic curettage.
**Pathological diagnosis :** Large cell carcinoma from the resected lung.
**Case history :** An abnormal shadow was found on the chest X-ray at a health check two months ago. Cytological examination of sputum revealed cells suspicious of carcinoma. Patient had no cough. The patient had smoked 30 cigarettes a day for the past 40 years.

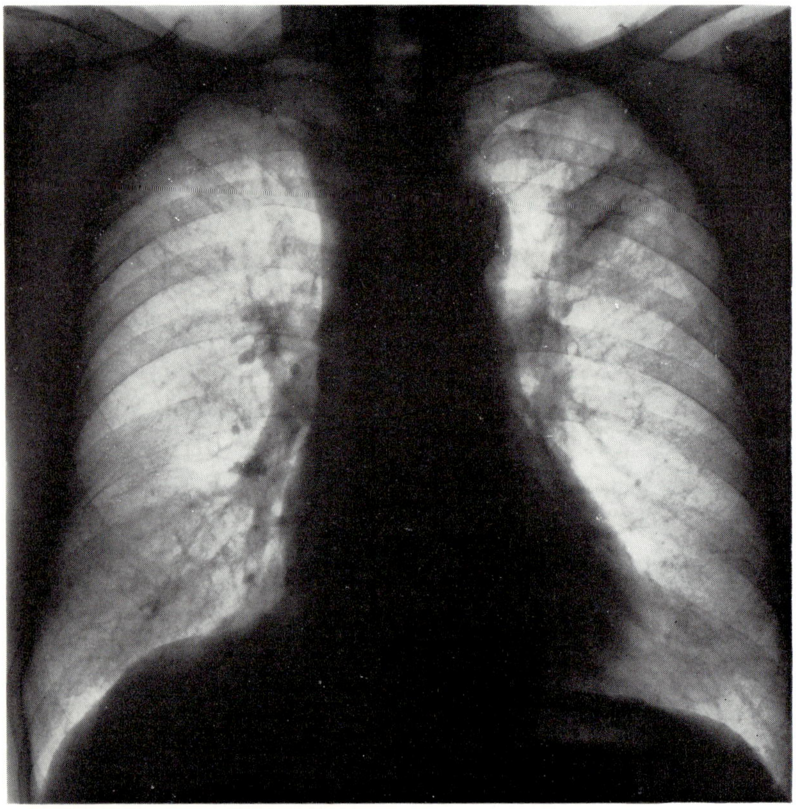

**Fig. 286 Chest X-ray, frontal:** An irregular-shaped shadow extending toward the hilum is seen in the left upper lobe. It is practically homogeneous but contains cord-like linear shadows.

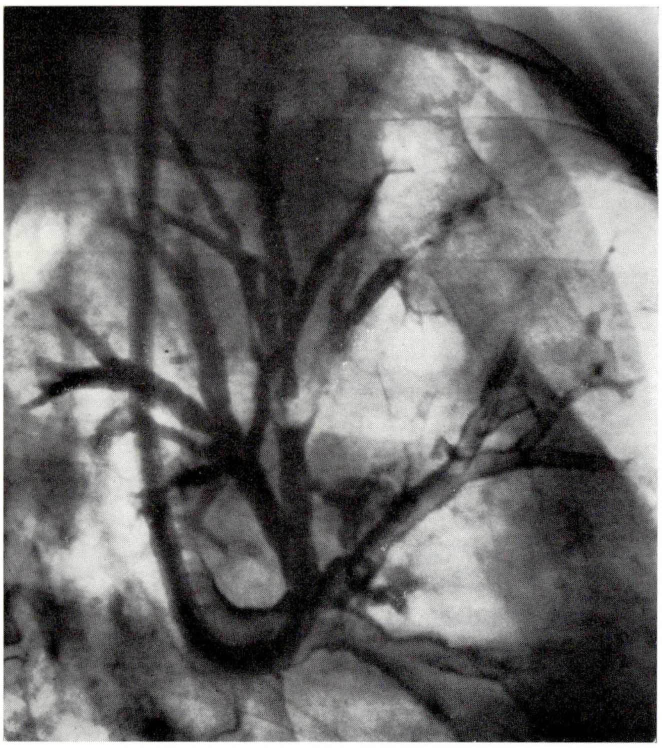

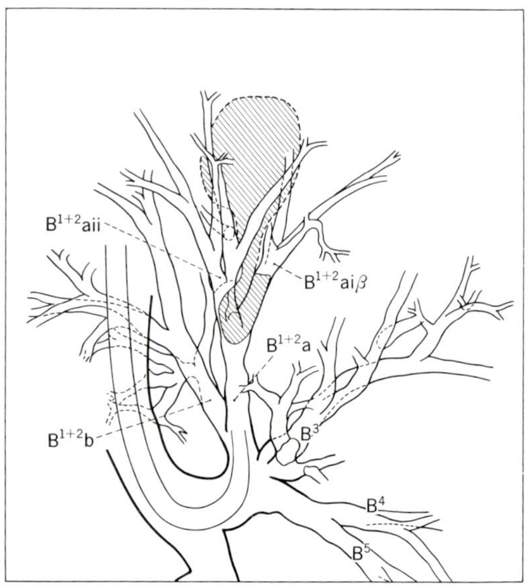


**Fig. 287 Bronchogram, oblique :** A Metra's catheter was inserted into $B^{1+2}a$ and the contrast medium was instilled. A "thumb print" indentation is visible at the bifurcation of $B^{1+2}a$ into i and ii. The wall of $B^{1+2}a$ is irregular in outline. This is considered to be due to infiltration by the tumor in that area.

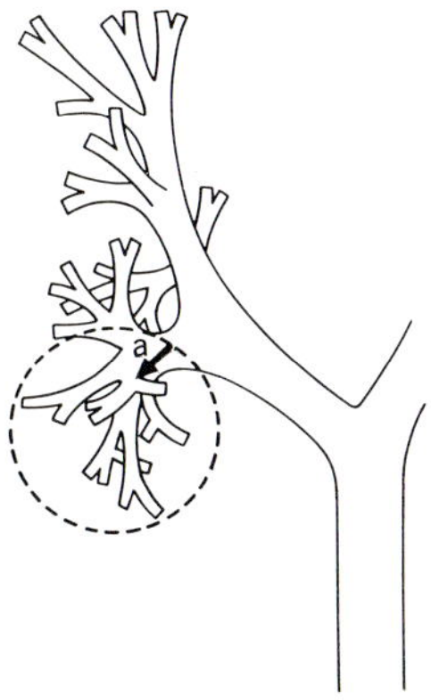


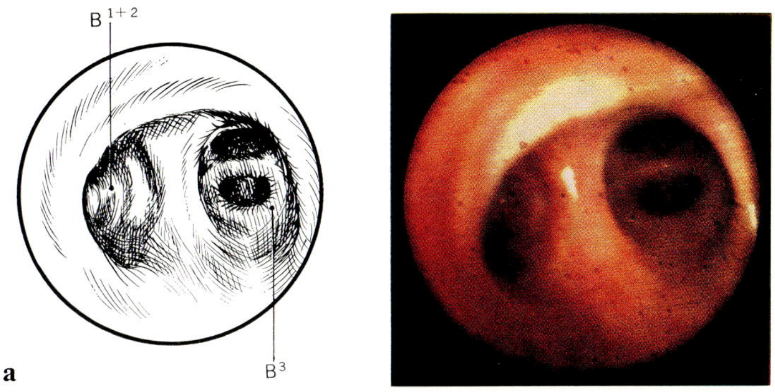


288 a

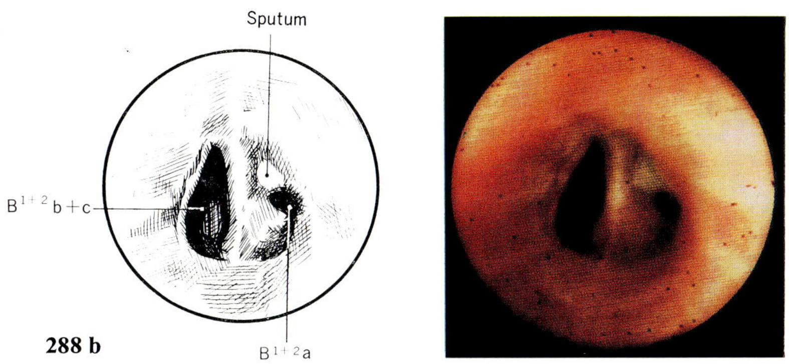


288 b

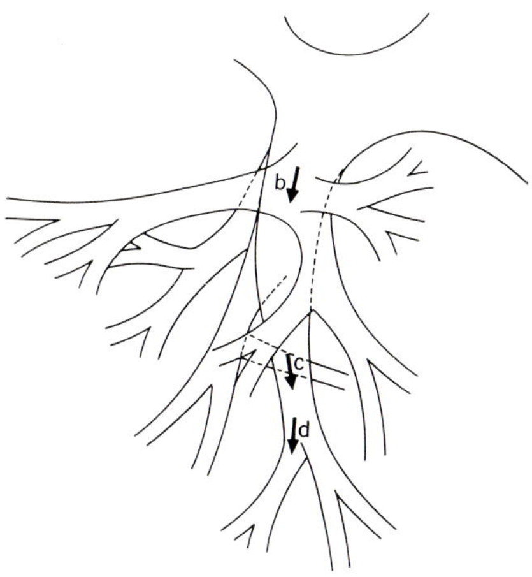


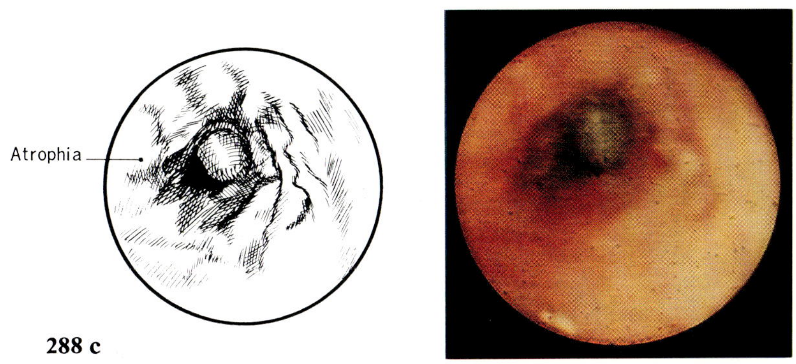


288 c

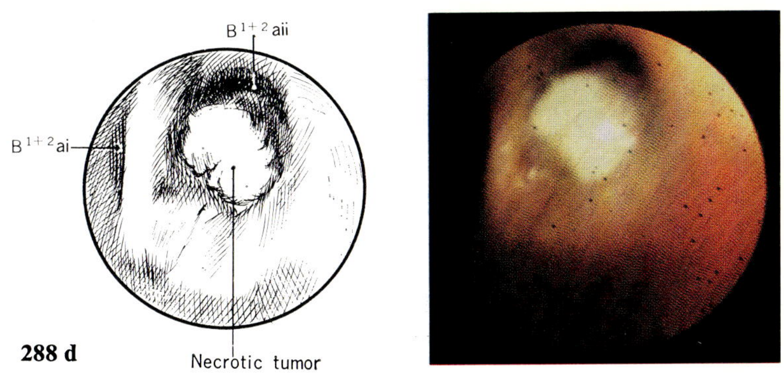


288 d

**Fig. 288 Fiberscopic findings:**

**a.** Each segmental bronchus of the upper division is normal.

**b.** The bifurcation of $B^{1+2}a$ and $B^{1+2}b+c$ is also normal.

**c.** $B^{1+2}a$ is atrophic and stenosed. The tumor is visualized just distally.

**d.** $B^{1+2}aii$ is practically obstructed by the necrotic tumor. Irregular-surfaced tumor is barely seen beyond this.

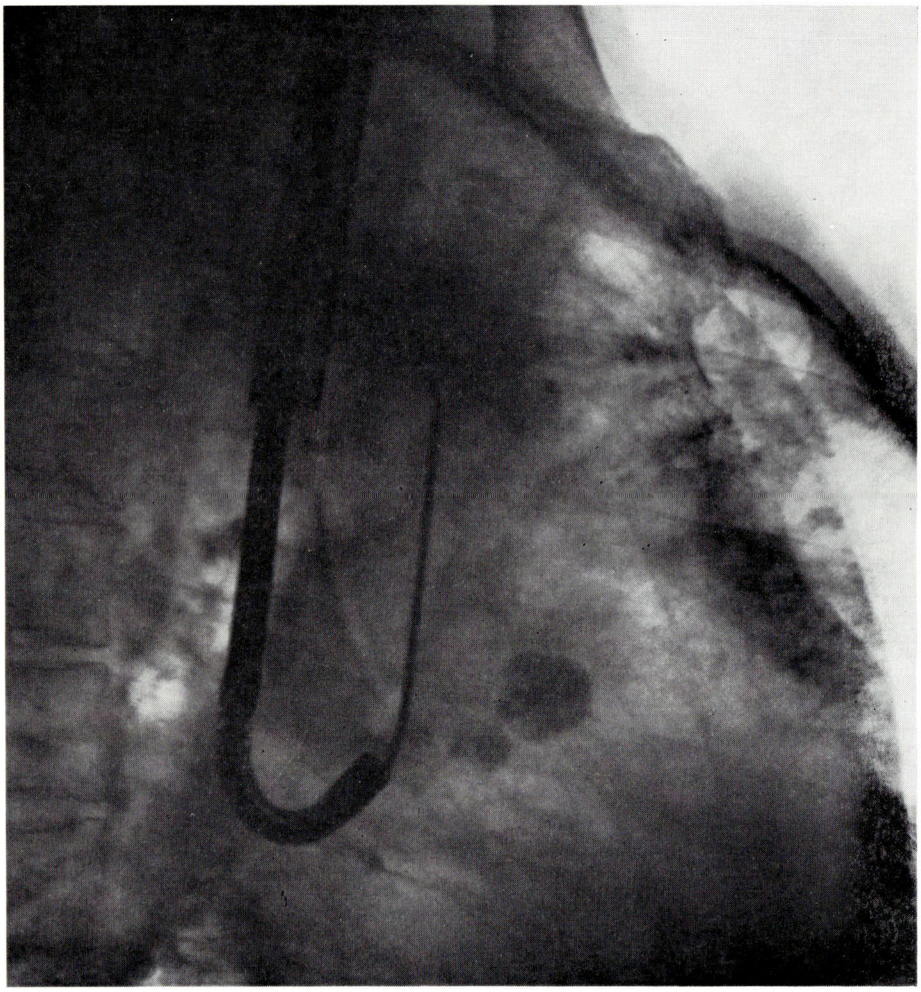

**Fig. 289 Curettage:** The curette just enters the tumor after having passing along $B^{1+2}a$.

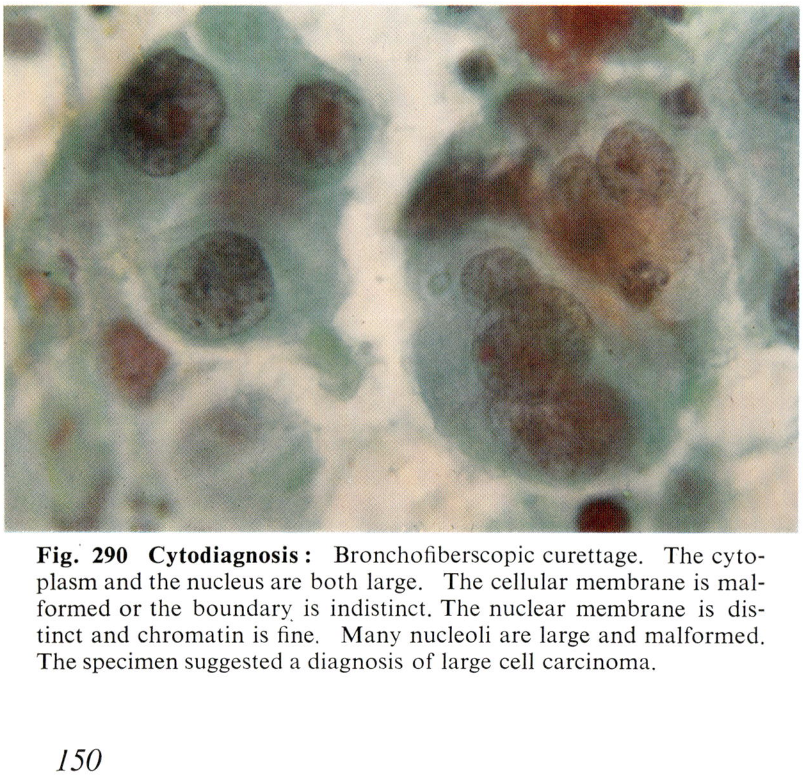

**Fig. 290 Cytodiagnosis:** Bronchofiberscopic curettage. The cytoplasm and the nucleus are both large. The cellular membrane is malformed or the boundary is indistinct. The nuclear membrane is distinct and chromatin is fine. Many nucleoli are large and malformed. The specimen suggested a diagnosis of large cell carcinoma.

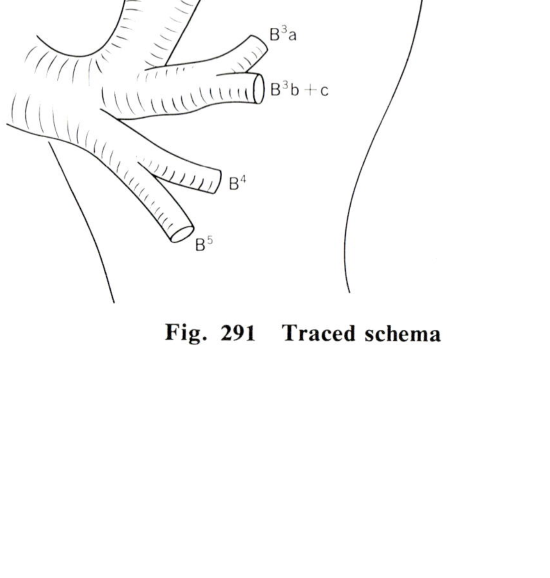


**Fig. 291 Traced schema**

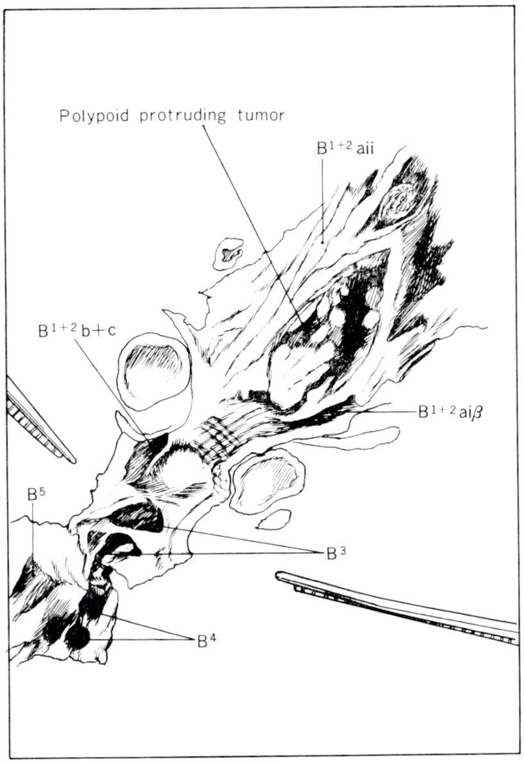


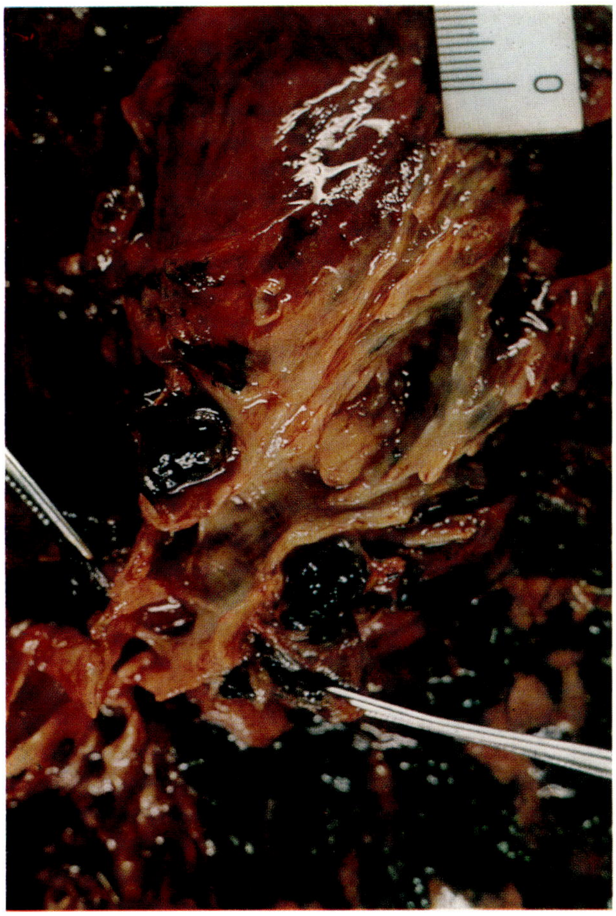

**Fig. 292 Macroscopic findings :** Fresh specimen cut open to expose change in the left upper division bronchus to $B^{1+2}a$. A small tumor projecting into the lumen of $B^{1+2}a$ in a polypoid fashion, protuberance being approximately 10mm, is a part of the cancer, 40×30mm.

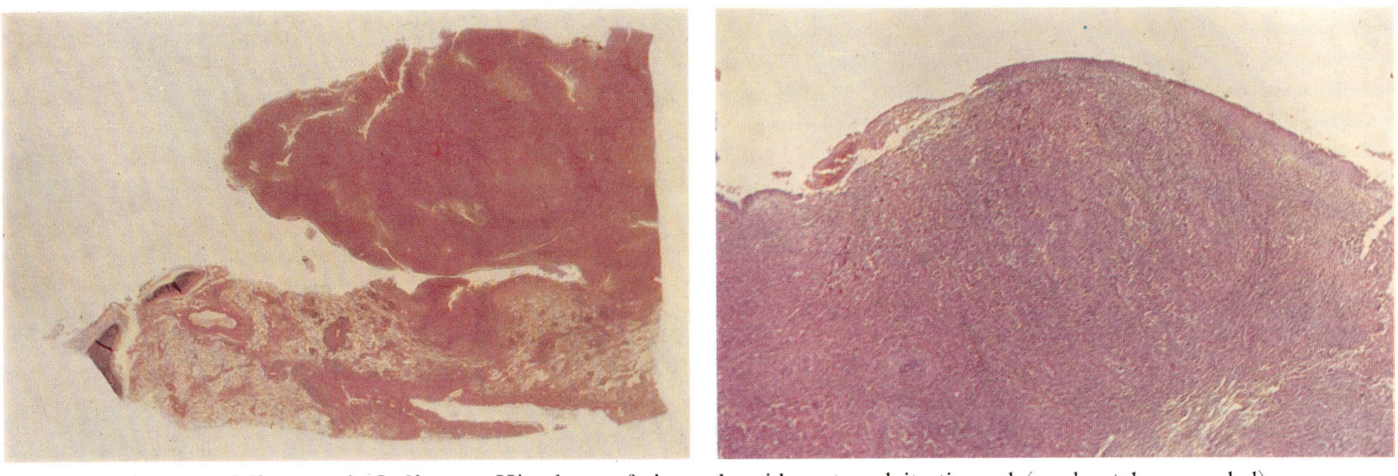

**Fig. 293 Microscopic findings :** Histology of the polypoid part and its tip end (moderately expanded). Diagnosis : Large cell carcinoma with squamous metaplasia at the tip.

## COMMENT :

On analysis, these plates are typical of large cell carcinoma. The polypoid protrusion in particular was confirmed by bronchofiberscopy. When a necrotic tumor is encountered bronchofiberscopically, the curette must be advanced as far as possible in order to obtain a satisfactory biopsy specimen. Obtaining a biopsy specimen of the necrotic area is obviously inadequate.

## Case 20 Large Cell Carcinoma (56, female)

**Chief complaint :** An abnormal shadow.
**Pathological diagnosis :** Large cell carcinoma based on resected lung.
**Case history :** For about a half year, the patient raised a small amount of sputum. Ten days before, the patient was hospitalized for severe back pains and received therapy for myocardial infarction. An abnormal shadow, however, was discovered on the chest X-ray film so the patient was referred to our hospital. The patient had never smoked. Fifteen years ago she underwent an operation for stomach cancer.

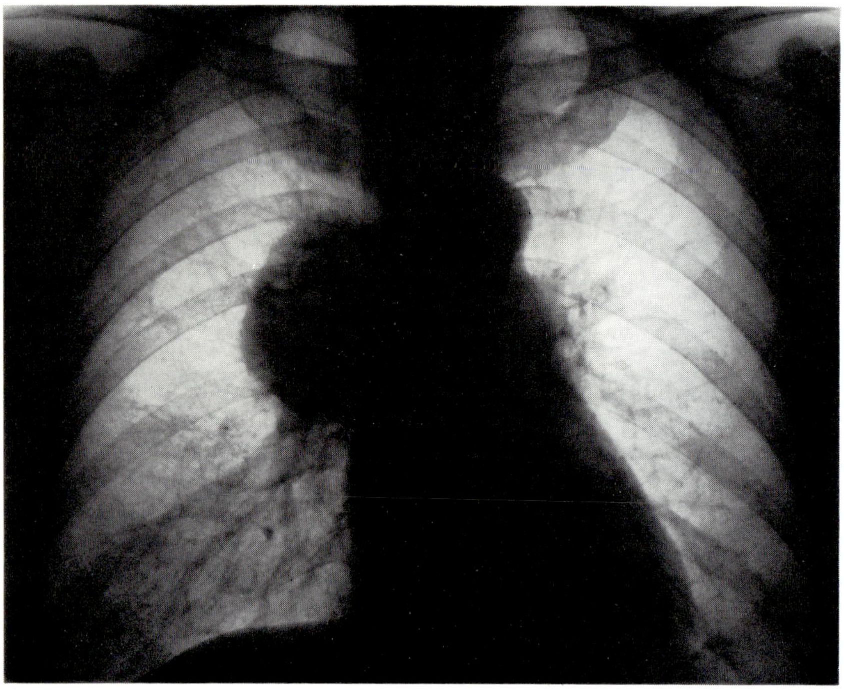

294

**Fig. 294 Chest X-ray, frontal :** A large tumor, 70×75 mm, having sharp borders, is located near the right lung hilum. The tumor is relatively uniform and contains a sac-like cavity.

**Fig. 295 Chest X-ray, lateral :** The tumor is anterior to the hilum. The anterior segment ($S^3$) is atelectatic and contains a sac-like ectasis.

**Fig. 296 Tomogram, lateral :** The previously described findings are more clearly defined.

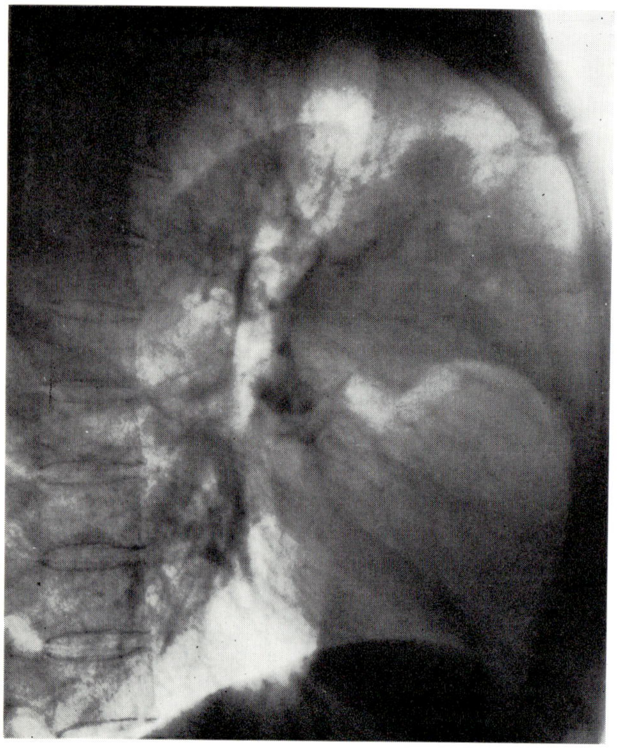

295

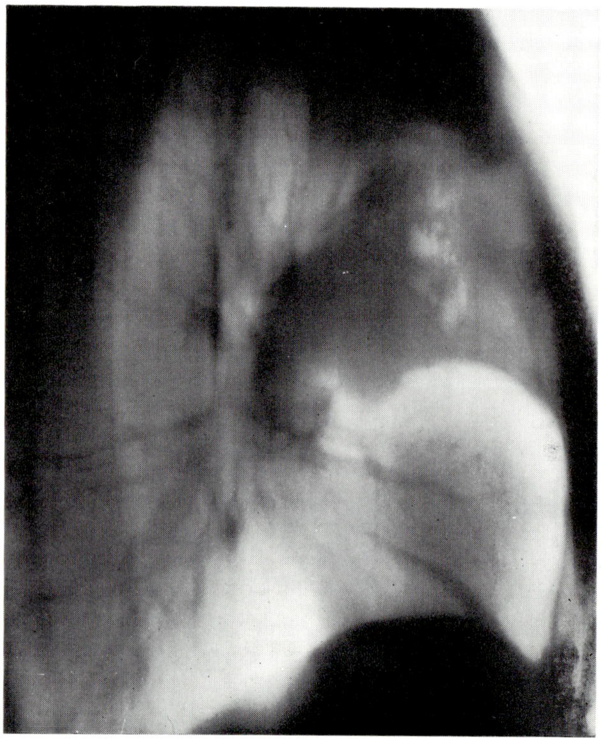

296

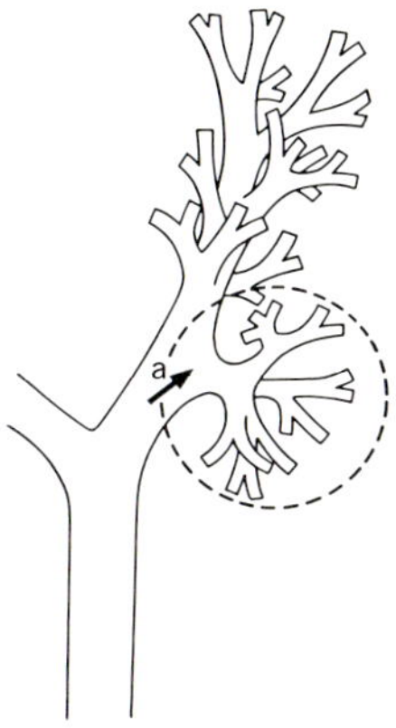


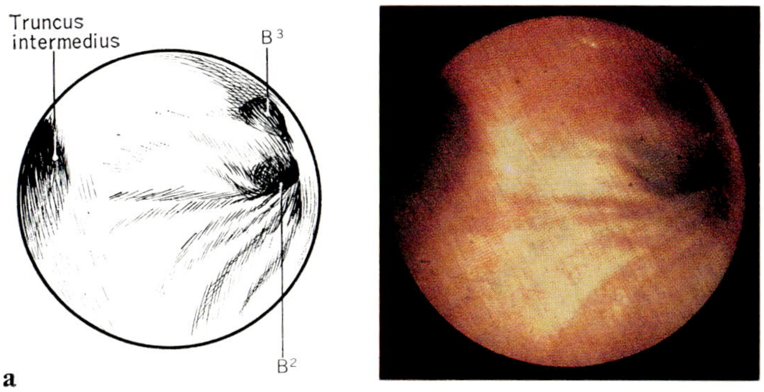


297 a

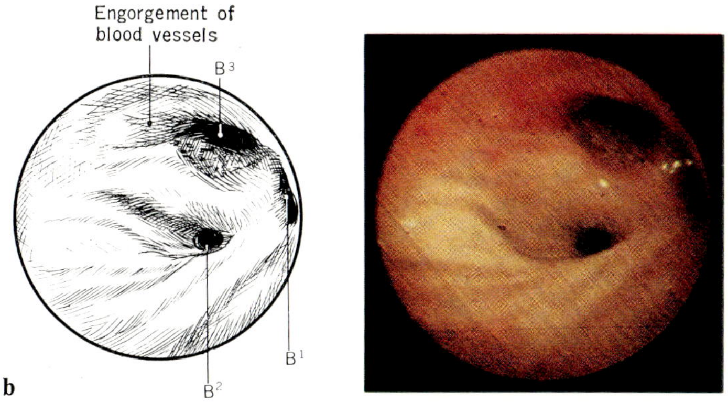


297 b

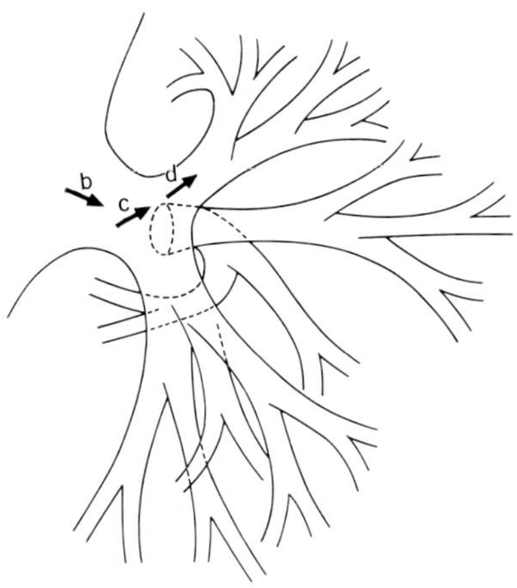


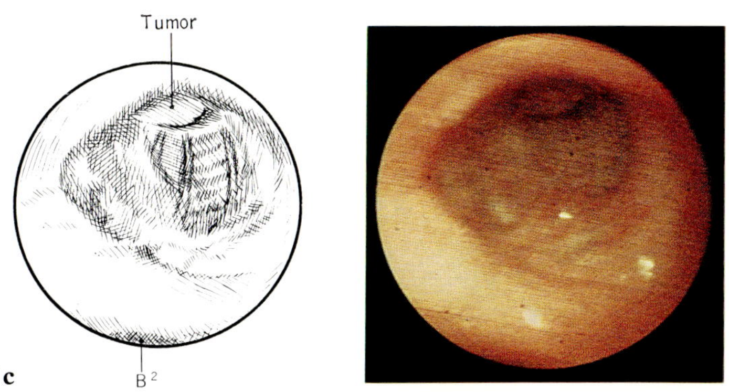


297 c

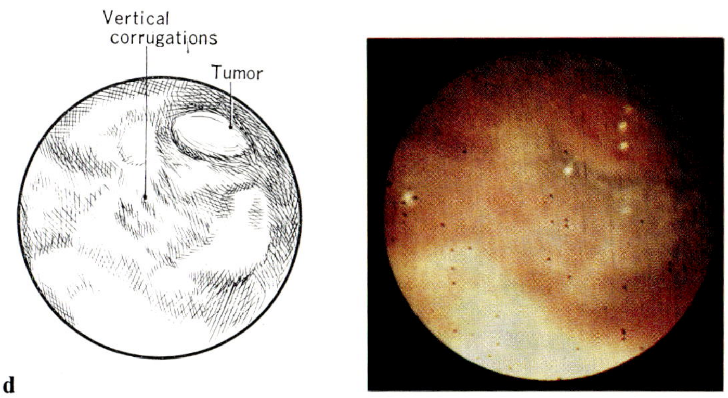


297 d

**Fig. 297 Fiberscopic findings:**

**a.** The orifice of the upper lobe bronchus is normal.

**b.** The anterior wall of $B^3$ presents vascular engorgement. $B^2$ is slightly stenotic.

**c.** A polypoid tumor is observed in $B^3$, obstructing the bronchus.

**d.** The $B^3$ lumen is corrugated vertically. The bronchus appears atrophic. The tumor obstructing $B^3$ is smooth-surfaced.

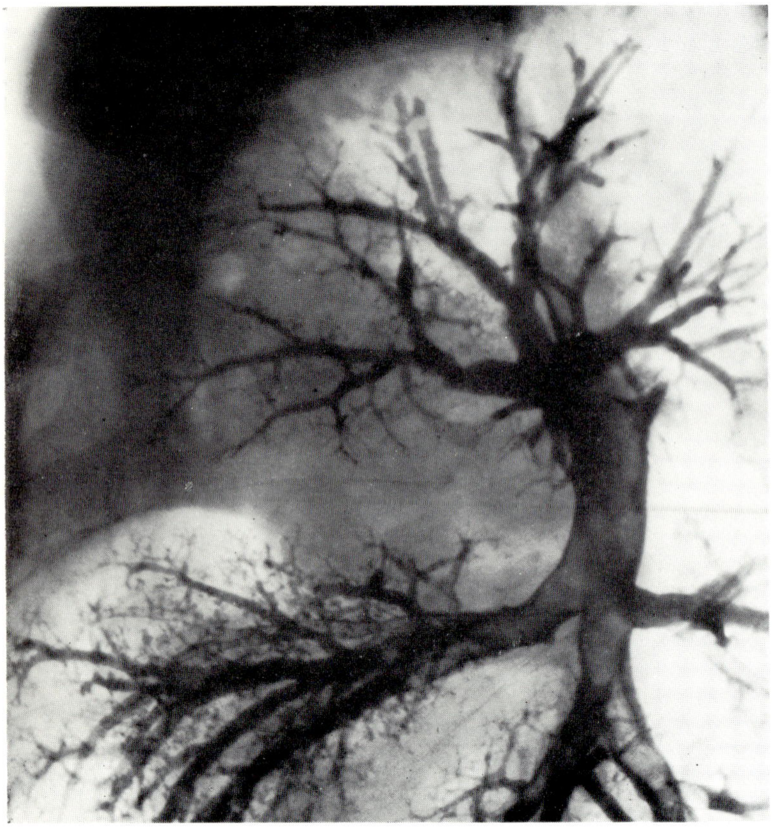

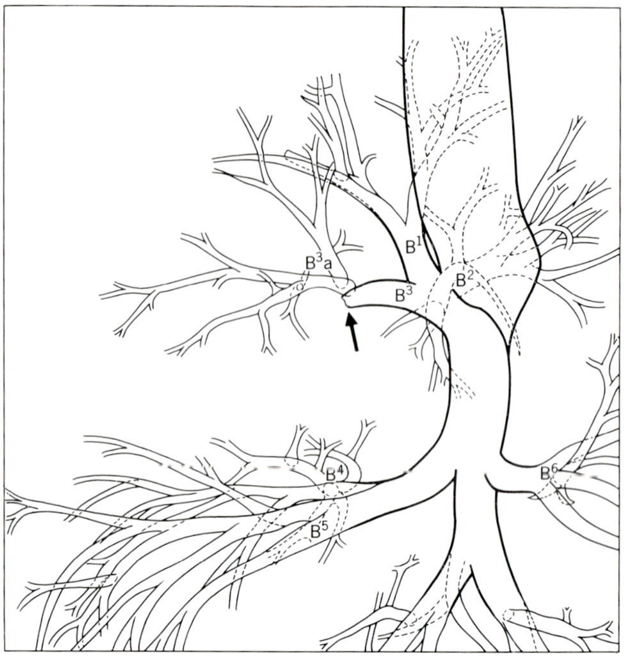


**Fig. 298 Bronchogram, highly oblique:** There is an obstruction at $B^3b$ (arrow). $B^3a$ is not stenotic, but the branches are widely separated. $B^2b$ is deviated because of the obstruction of $B^3b$.

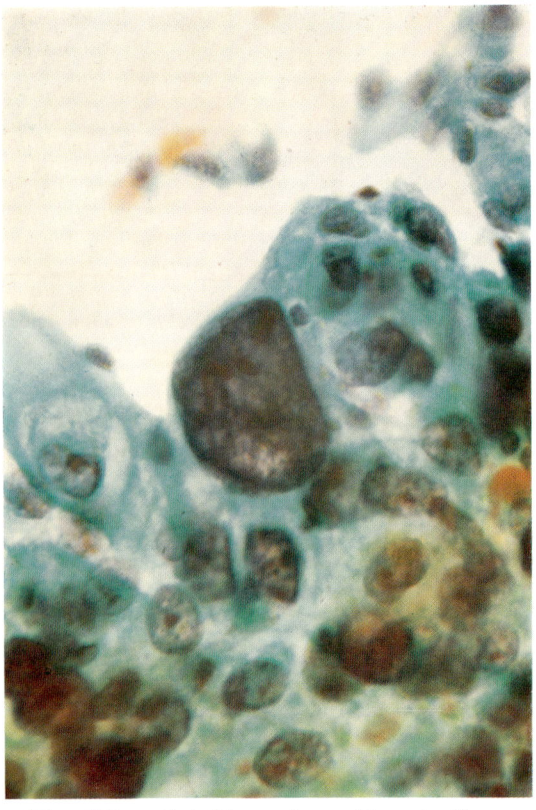

**Fig. 299 Cytodiagnosis:** Bronchofiberscopic curettage. Cell boundaries are indistinct. The nuclei are malformed. A cell with a huge nucleus is present in the cluster in which each cell differs markedly in size. Diagnosis from these findings: Large cell carcinoma.

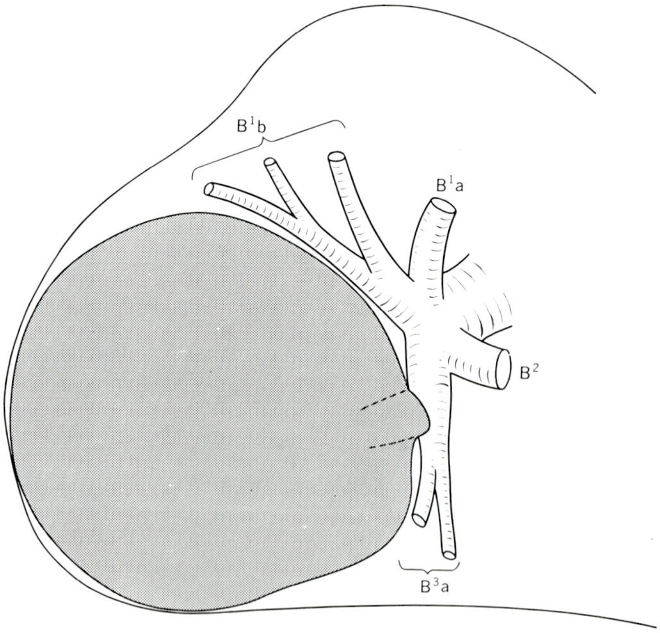


**Fig. 300 Traced schema:** Tumor, $80 \times 60$ mm, protrudes partly into $B^3$ from $B^3b$.

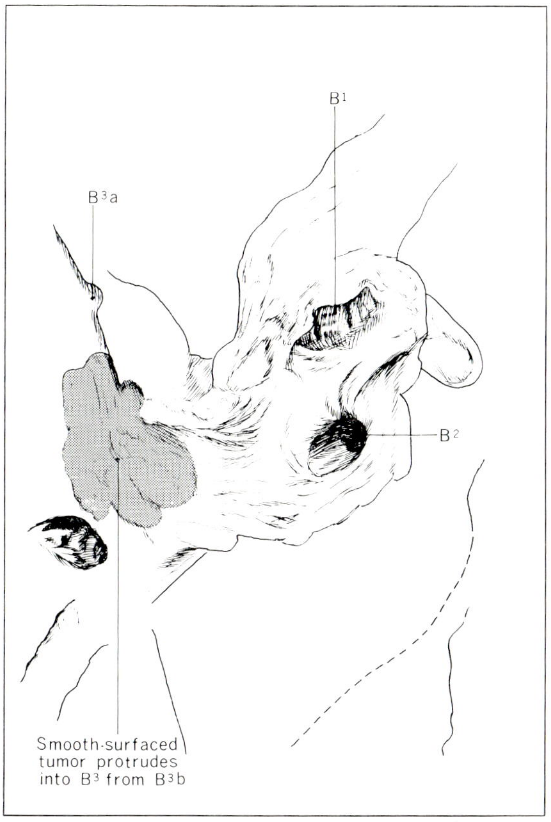


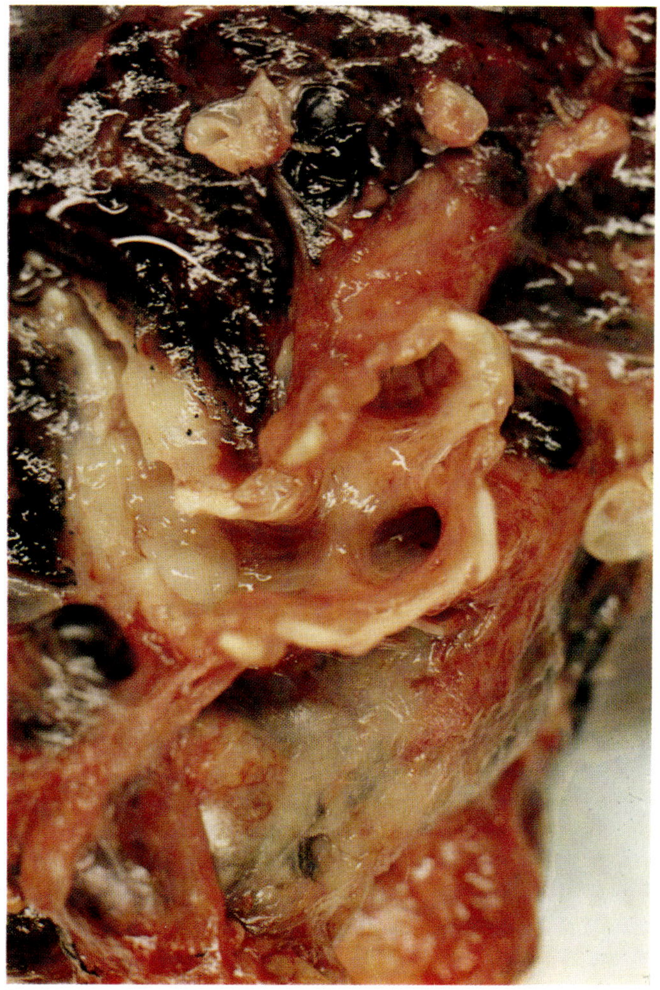

**Fig. 301 Macroscopic findings :** Fresh specimen of $B^3a$, slightly opened : contact print. A smooth-surfaced small tumor is visible at the site corresponding to $B^3b$.

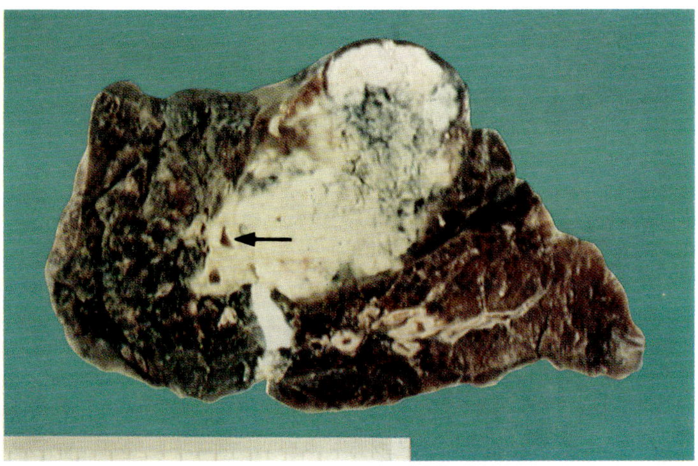

302

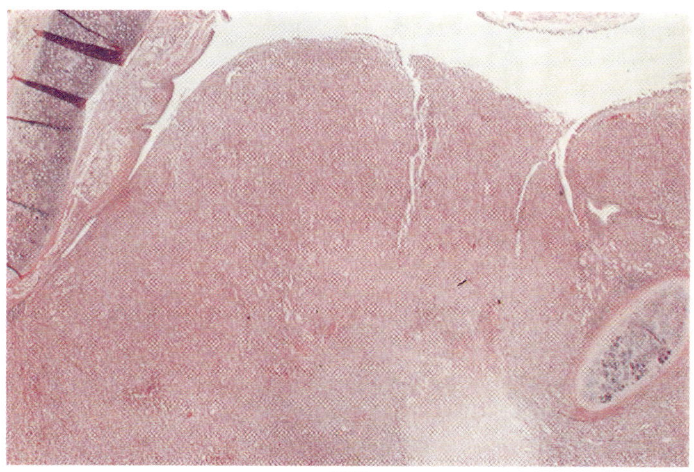

303

**Fig. 302 Macroscopic findings :** The tumor, 80×60mm, has distinct boundaries, accompanied by moderate anthracosis and central fibrosis. Part of the tumor is projecting into the lumen of $B^3$ (arrow).

**Fig. 303 Microscopic findings :** A poorly differentiated large cell carcinoma is demonstrated in the lumen of $B^3$.

## COMMENT :

Typical case of large cell carcinoma. Bronchofiberscopic findings and those from the fresh specimen correspond.

## Case 21 Large Cell Carcinoma (67, male)

**Case history :** The patient, a male and a heavy smoker, presented at our hospital complaining of sudden onset of sputum heavily streaked with blood. The chest X-ray revealed a tumor shadow 25×25 mm. Bronchofiberscopy revealed the site of the hemoptysis which led to a definite diagnosis.

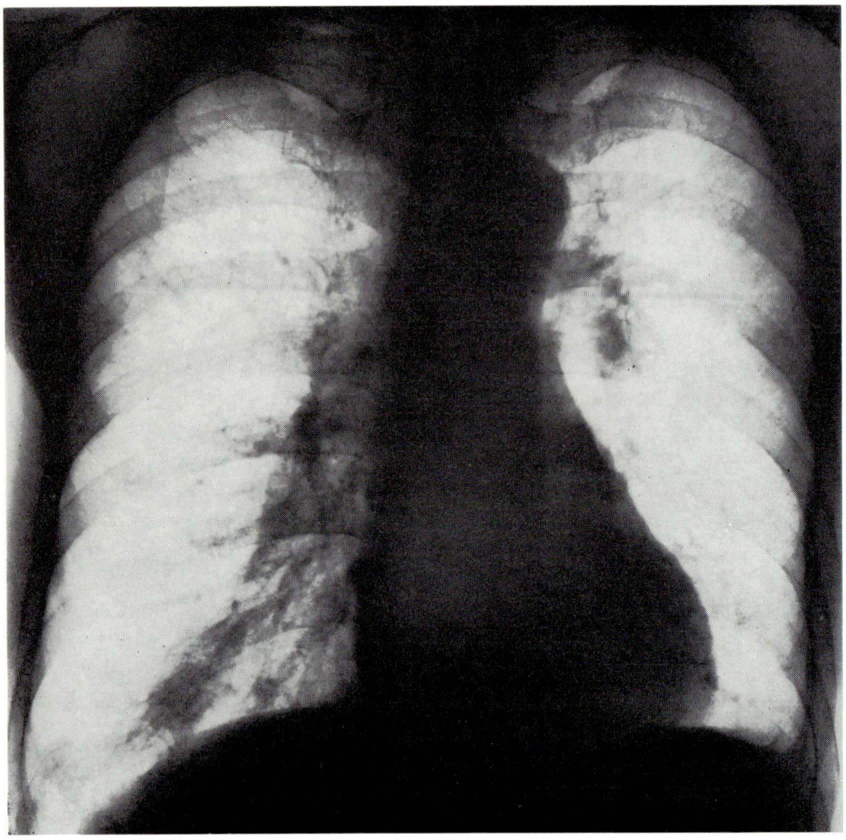

**Fig. 304 Chest X-ray, frontal :** A 24×24 mm density is visible in the right lower lung field, with cord-like strands between it and the hilum.

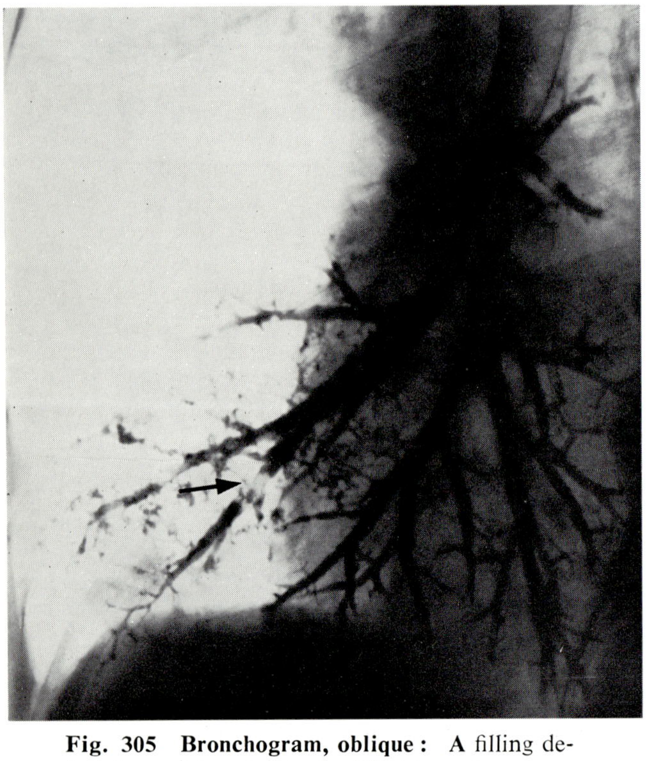

**Fig. 305 Bronchogram, oblique :** A filling defect (arrow) is noted in the $B^8$bii bronchus.

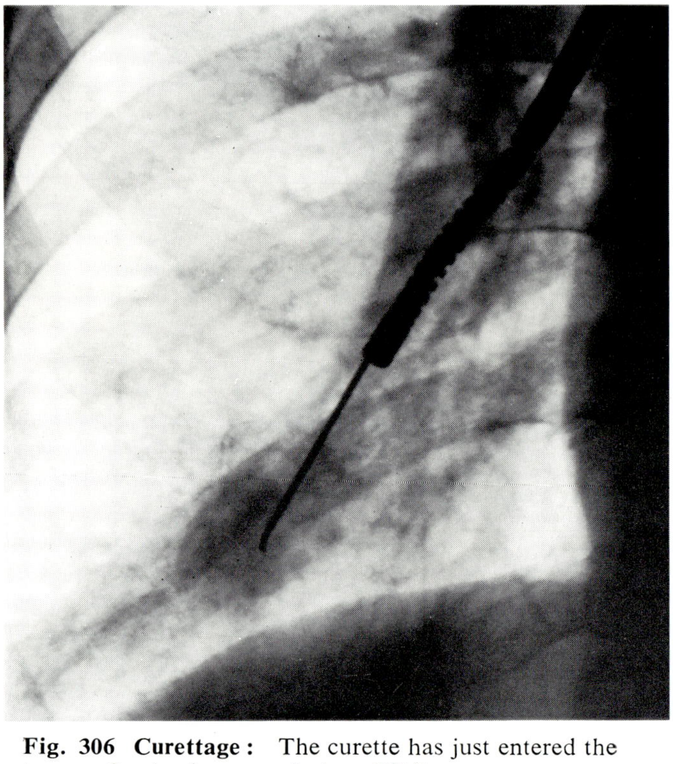

**Fig. 306 Curettage :** The curette has just entered the tumor after having passed along $B^8$bii.

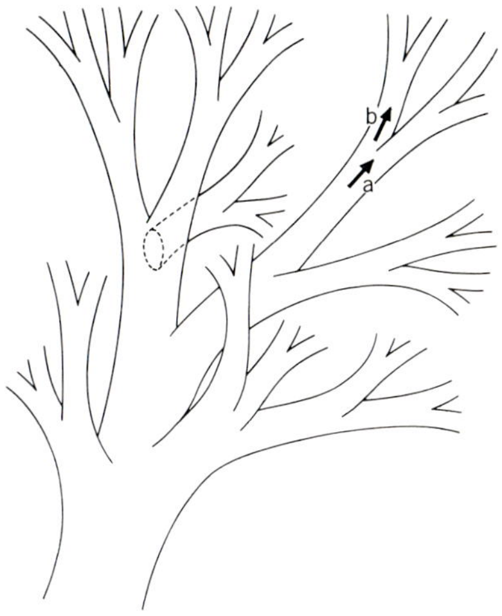


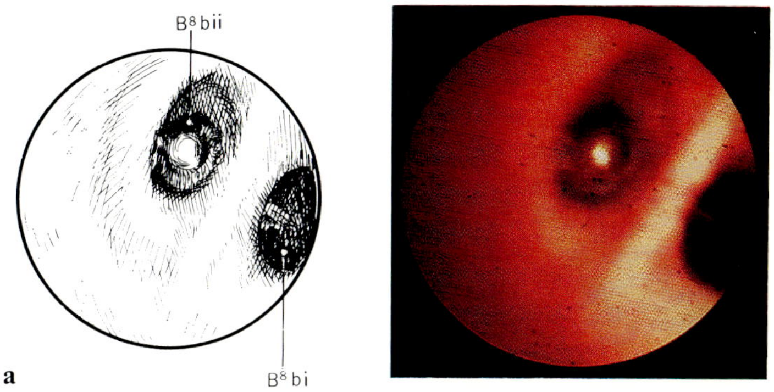


307 a

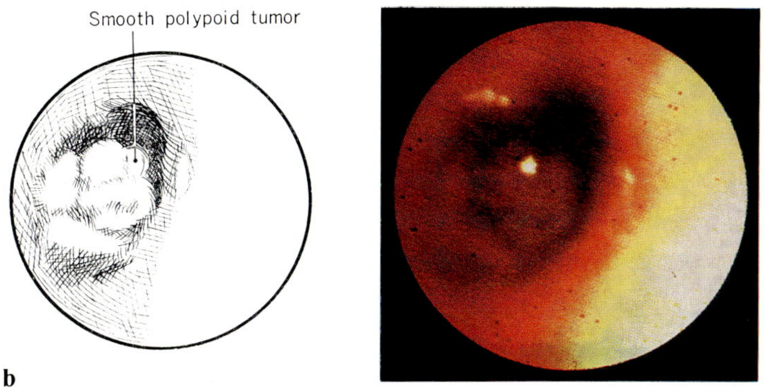


307 b

**Fig. 307 Fiberscopic findings :**

**a.** On introducing the bronchofiberscope, the hemorrhage was found to come from a left basal bronchus. Advancing the instrument further into $B^8b$, the site of bleeding from the peripheral portion of $B^8b$ was confirmed. After removal of the blood, a tumor was found in $B^8bii$ almost completely obstructing the bronchus.

**b.** The surface of the tumor is smooth and it is polypoid in shape. A small amount of blood oozes continuously from the region within the bronchus. This site was curetted. Diagnosis : Large cell carcinoma.

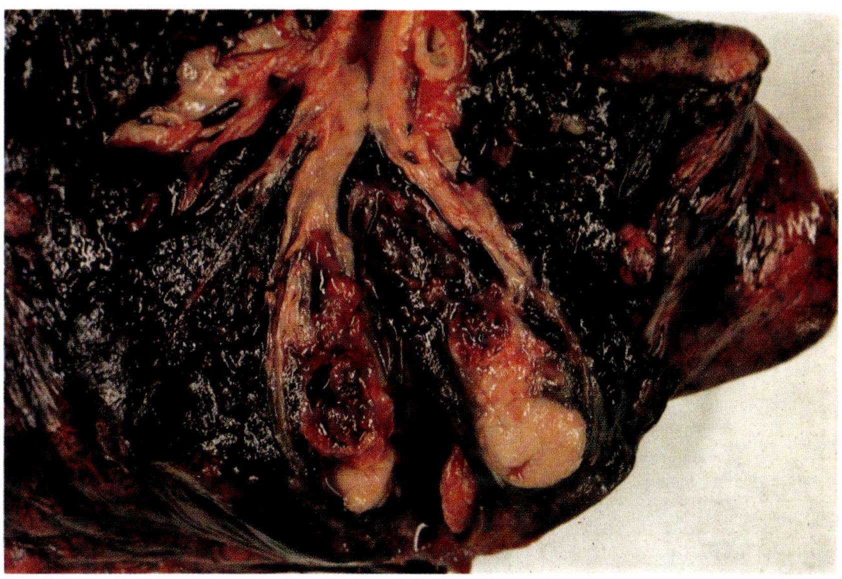

**Fig. 308 Macroscopic findings :** The fresh specimen shows that a tumor, 20×20 mm, is located atthe peripheral part of $B^8bii$, and is protruding polyplike toward the direction of $B^8b$ with blood coagulation.

**COMMENT :**

In most cases of undifferentiated large cell carcinoma, the tumor protrudes into the bronchial orifice like a polyp. This is a view of such protrusion observed through a flexible bronchofiberscope.

## Case 22 Large Cell Carcinoma (68, male)

**Case history :** The patient was told of the presence of a shadow in the left upper lung field on a chest X-ray one year ago, and was put under the doctor's observation. The lesion meanwhile increased in size and the patient was referred to our hospital. Based on the bronchogram and bronchofiberscopy at our hospital, the case was diagnosed as carcinoma. Surgical operation was performed, but the aorta was found to be adherent to the tumor, so radiation was administered.

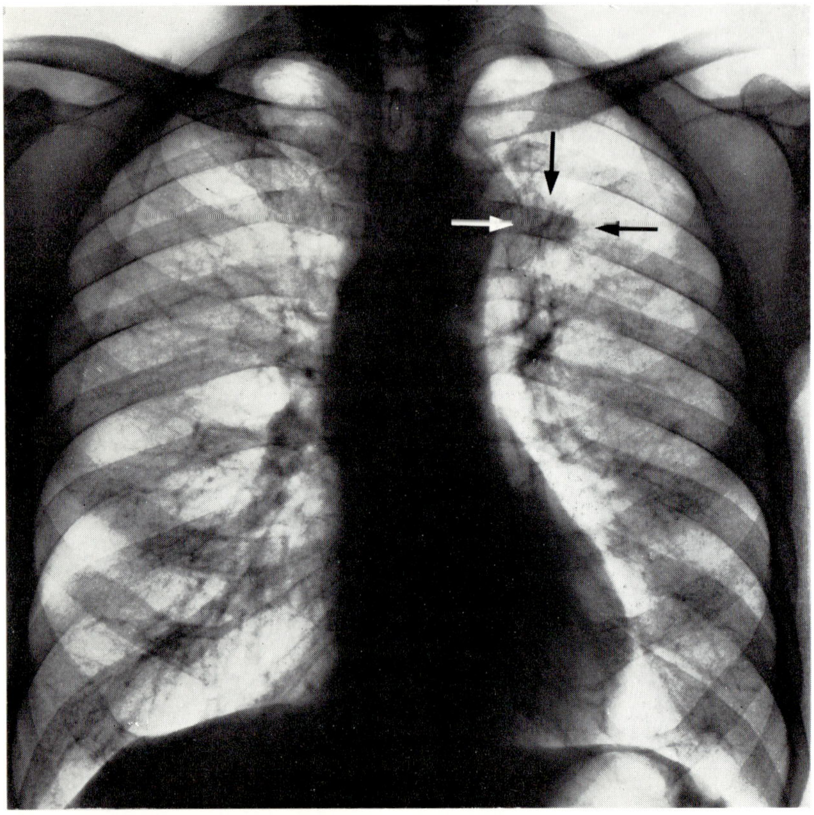

**Fig. 309 Chest X-ray, frontal :** An irregular tumor shadow, 20×30 mm in extent, is located in the medial aspect of the left $S^{1+2}$ (apico-posterior segment).

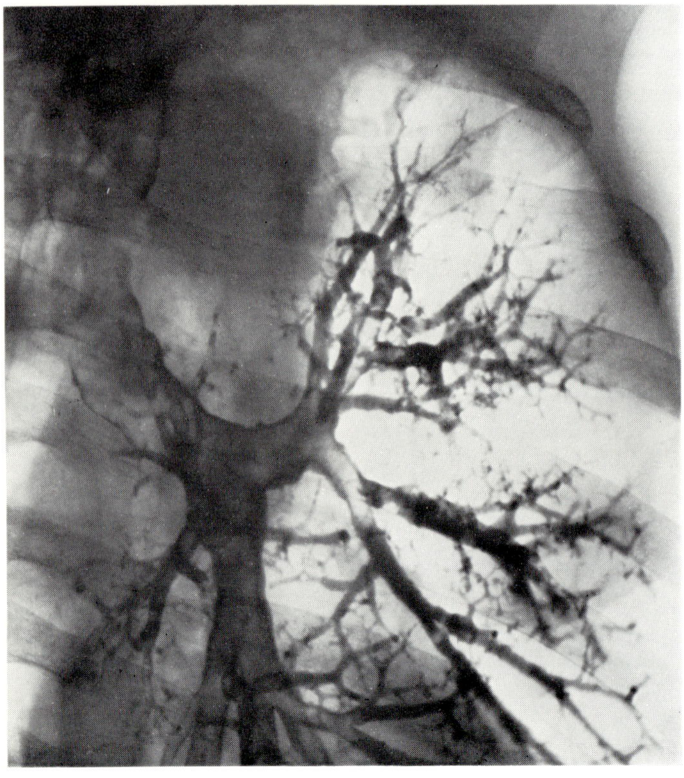

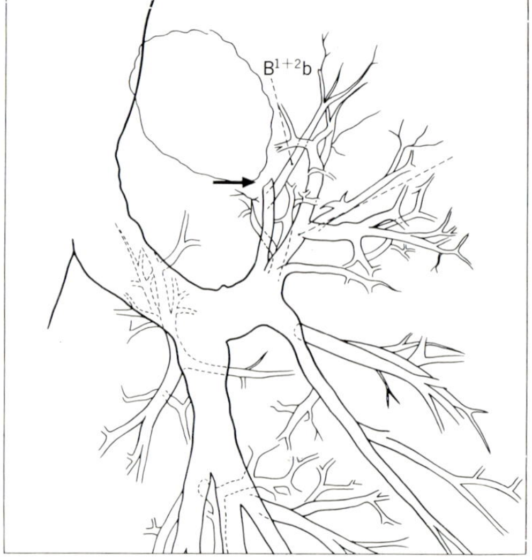


**Fig. 310 Bronchogram, oblique :** A stenotic interruption (arrow) is noted in $B^{1+2}a$. $B^{1+2}b$ is normal.

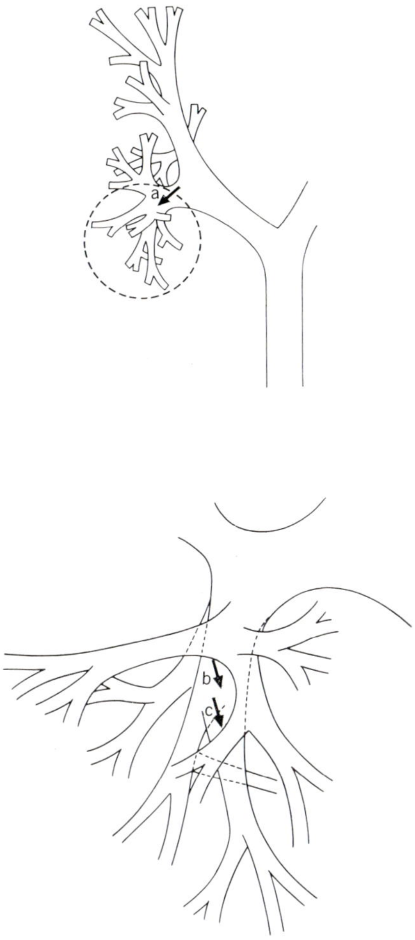


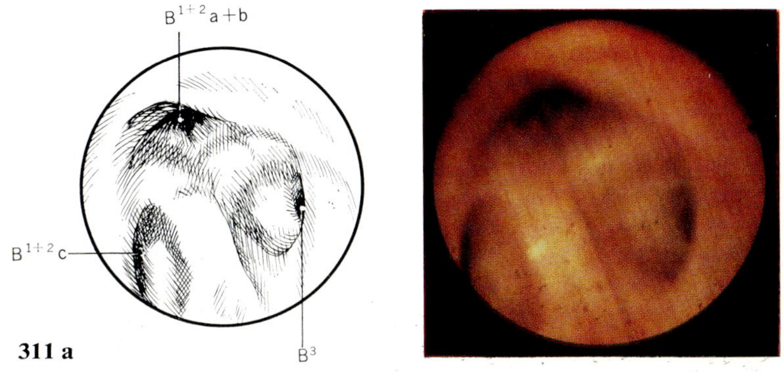


311 a

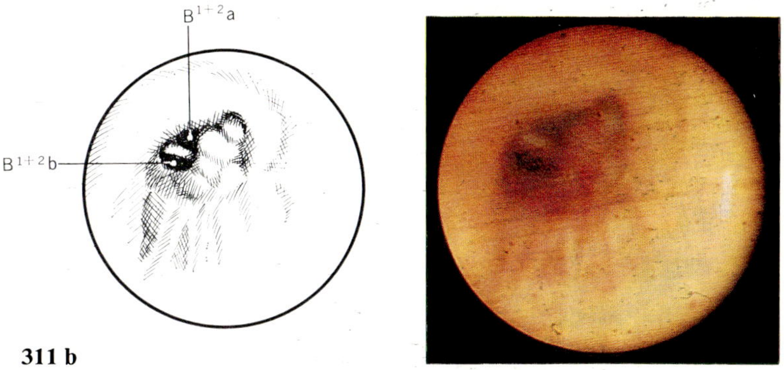


311 b

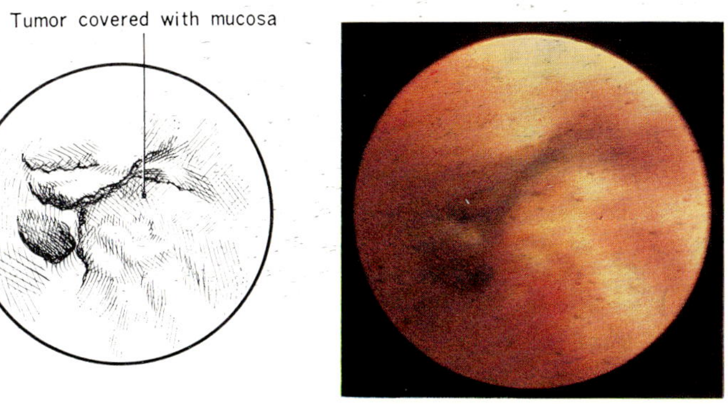


311 c

**Fig. 311 Fiberscopic findings:**

**a.** The upper division bronchus branches into three: $B^{1+2}a+b$, $B^{1+2}c$ and $B^3$, according to the present nomenclature. These sub-branches, the author suggests, may be called $B^1$, $B^2$ and $B^3$.

**b.** Deep in $B^{1+2}a+b$, the lumen becomes slightly flattened and stenosis is visualized at $B^{1+2}a$.

**c.** $B^{1+2}a$ is obstructed anteriorly and posteriorly by a tumor covered with mucosa. The posterior wall is slightly uneven. A small curette was inserted into this area. Cytological diagnosis: Large cell carcinoma.

## Case 23 Large Cell Carcinoma (79, male)

**Case history :** A large, dense shadow was found in the hilum of the left lung 3 months ago. The case was diagnosed at our hospital as anaplastic carcinoma based on bronchofiberscopy and fiberscopic cytology. Chemotherapy with Mitomycin® and irradiation were both instituted.

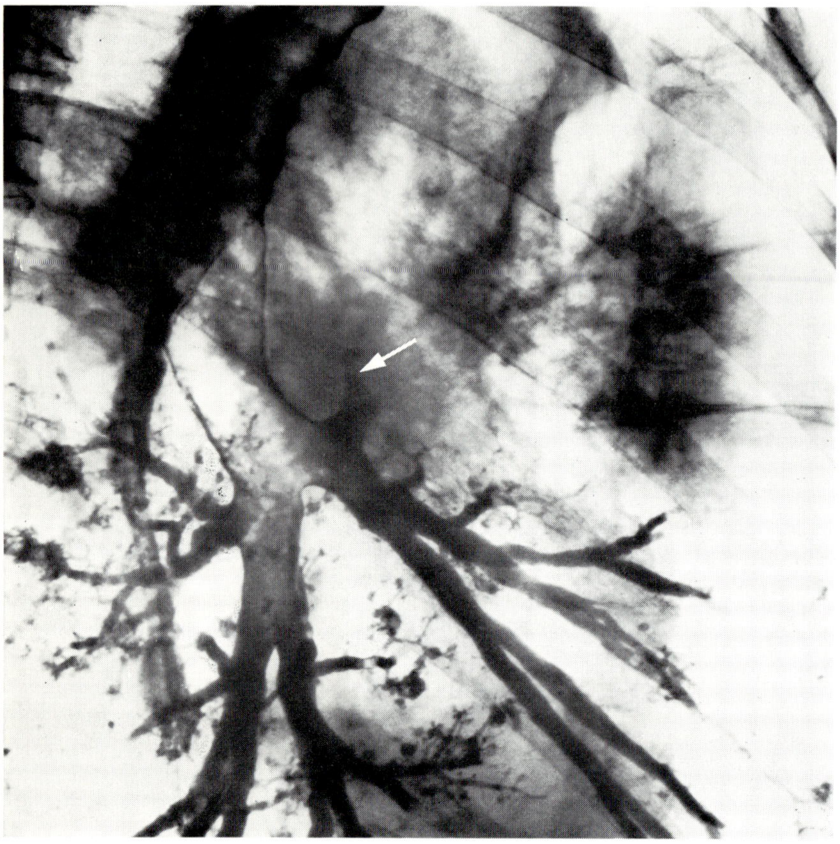

**Fig. 312 Bronchogram, oblique :** The upper division bronchus of the left upper lobe is stenosed at the point of branching into the upper division and the lingula (arrow).

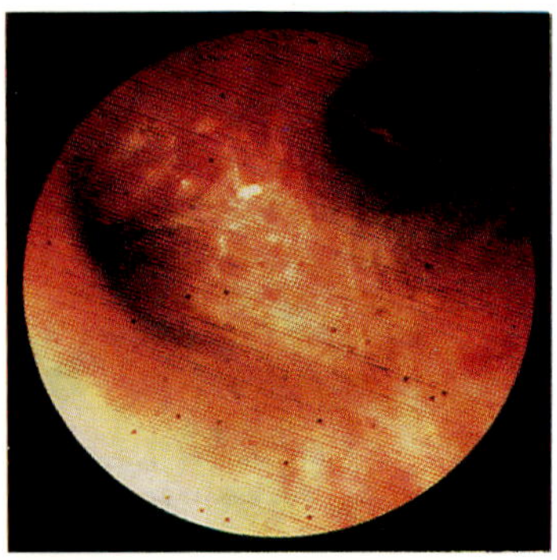

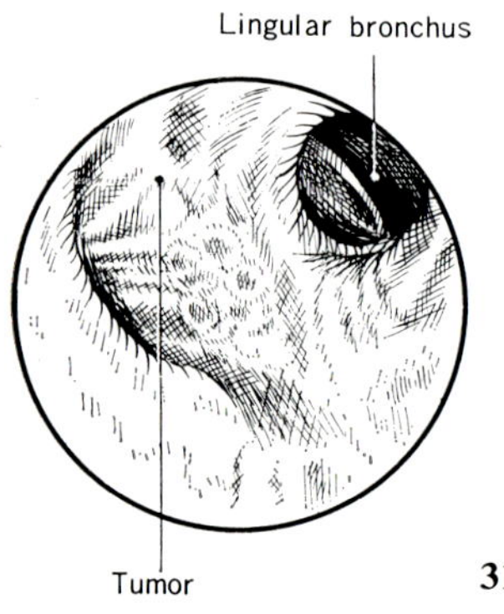


**313 a**

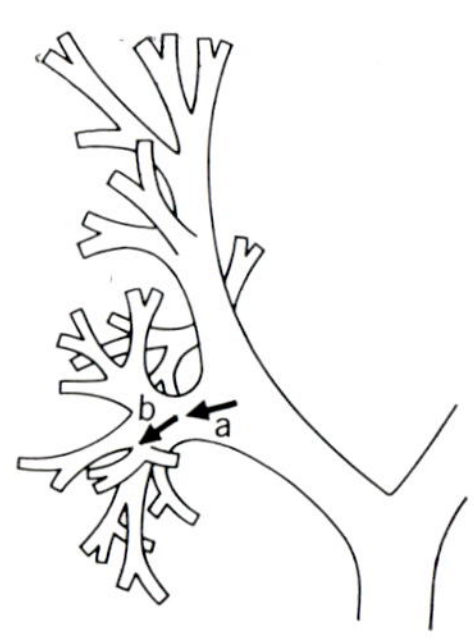


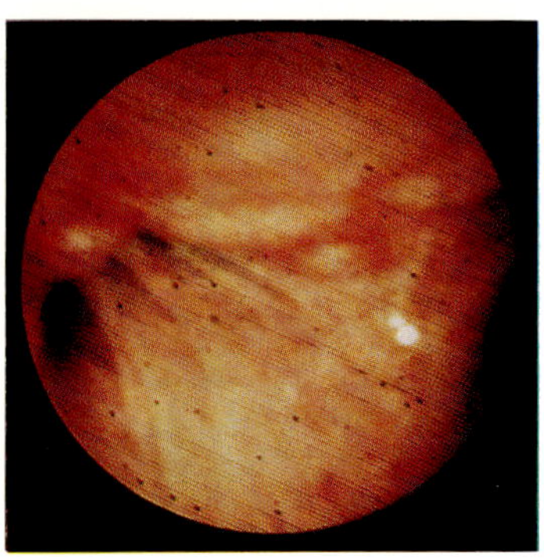

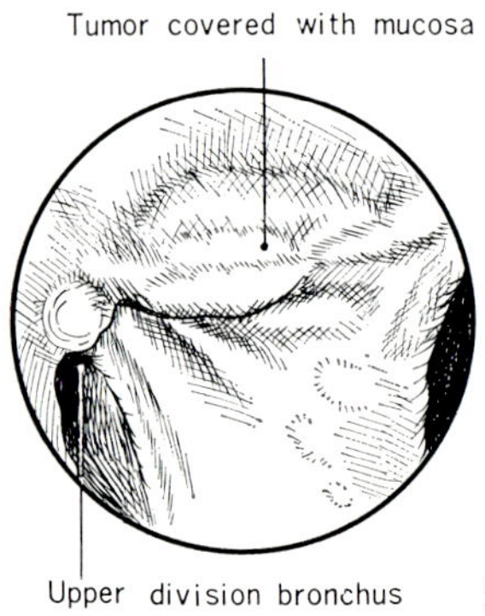


**313 b**

**Fig. 313 Fiberscopic findings :**

**a.** The septum between the upper division and the lingular bronchus is thickened, lacks cartilage rings, and slightly bleeding. Notice the presence of a tumor on the anterior wall.

**b.** Within the upper division bronchus, a tumor covered with mucosa is located on the anterior wall. Still deeper in the bronchus, part of the tumor has eroded through the mucosa. The membrane of $B^{1+2}$ and $B^3$ is contracted. This case was diagnosed as anaplastic carcinoma by biopsy of the tumor with a small curette at bronchofiberscopy.

# Case 24 Large Cell Carcinoma (57, female)

**Case history :** A chest X-ray taken because of a traffic accident one month ago revealed an abnormal shadow. The patient was asymptomatic. Bronchofiberscopy and bronchography at our hospital resulted in a diagnosis of a large cell carcinoma. Middle and lower lobectomy was performed.

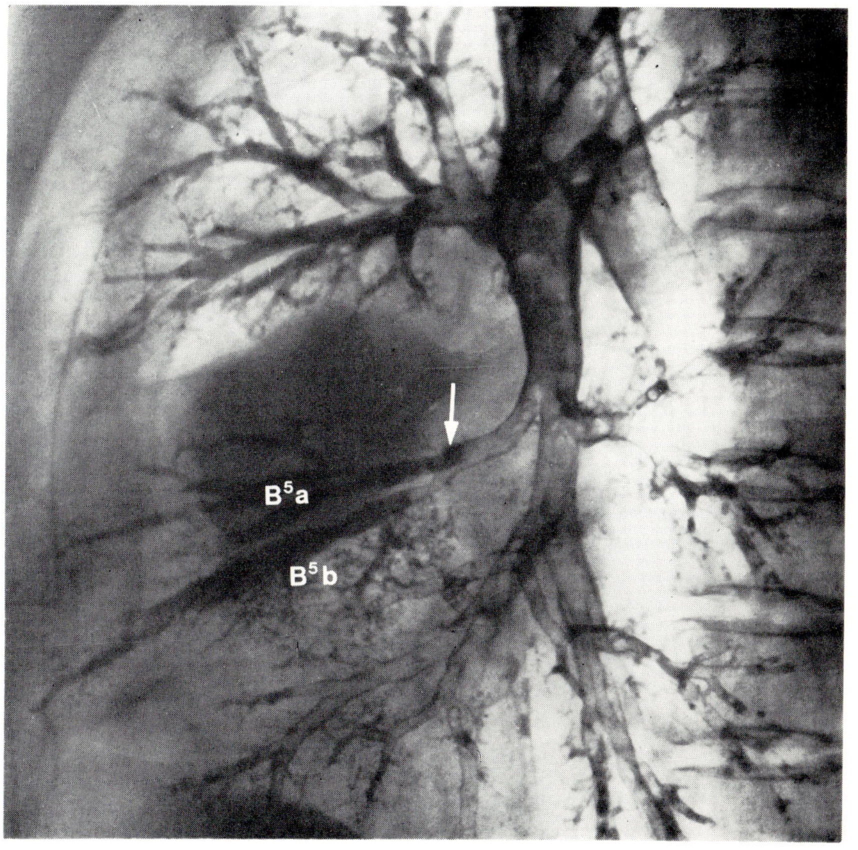


**Fig. 314 Bronchogram, marked oblique :** There is obstruction of $B^4a$ (arrow). The peripheral branches of $B^5$ are ectatic. The branches of $B^5$ are markedly coalesced.

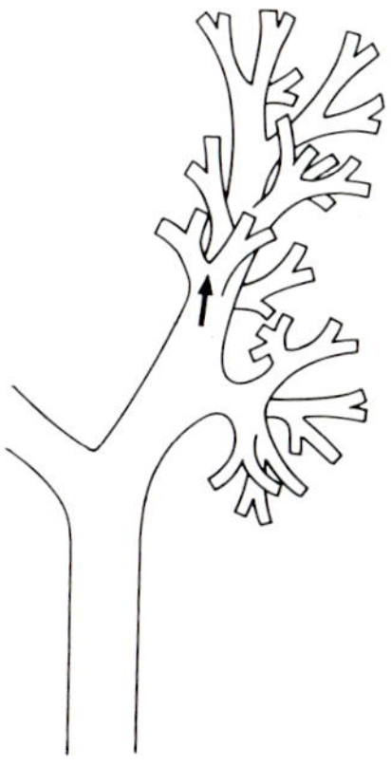

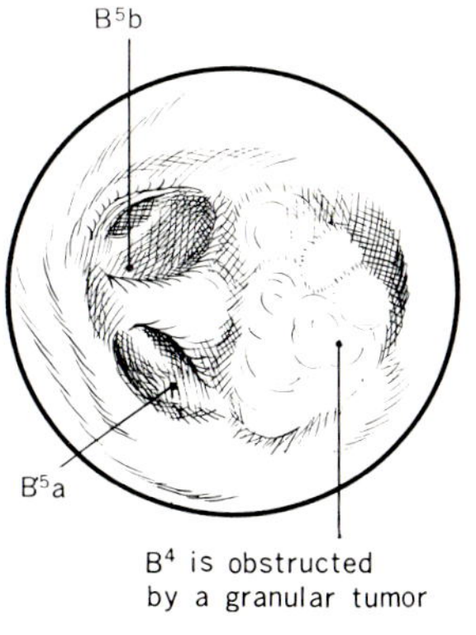


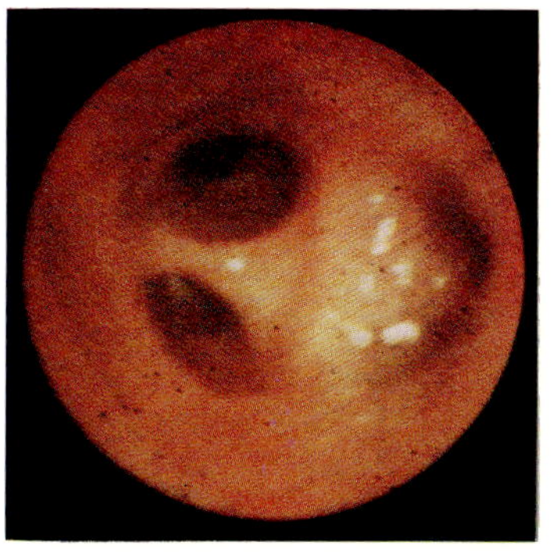

**Fig. 315 Fiberscopic findings :** $B^4$ is obstructed by a granular tumor. The obstruction here corroborates the findings in the bronchogram. The case was diagnosed as a large cell carcinoma by a biopsy obtained with a small curette from this area.

## Case 25 Large Cell Carcinoma (43, female)

**Case history :** The patient had a sore throat 5 months ago. Ten days ago she noticed her sputum was stained with blood. The chest X-ray disclosed an abnormal shadow. At our hospital the case was diagnosed as a large cell carcinoma by bronchofiberscopic biopsy. Metastatic tumor was found in a scalene lymph node. Mitomycin® and irradiation were administered concurrently, but the patient died.

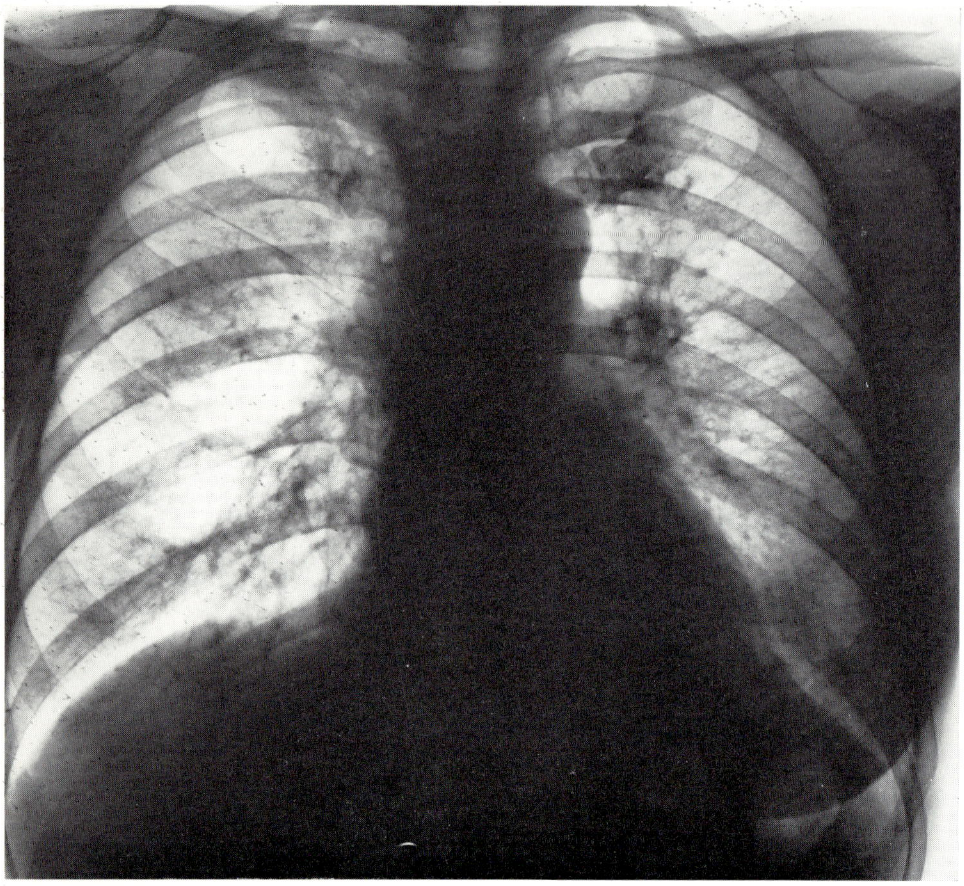

**Fig. 316 Chest X-ray, frontal :** A shadow is present due to a tumescence in the right hilum. The cord-like shadow in the right $S^1$ (apical segment) is thought to be due to fibrosis.

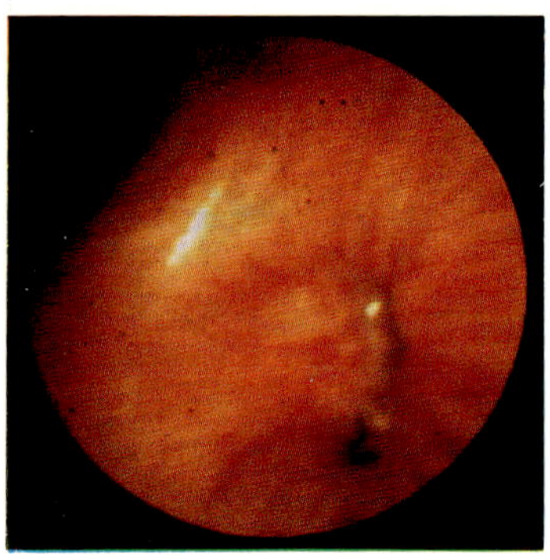

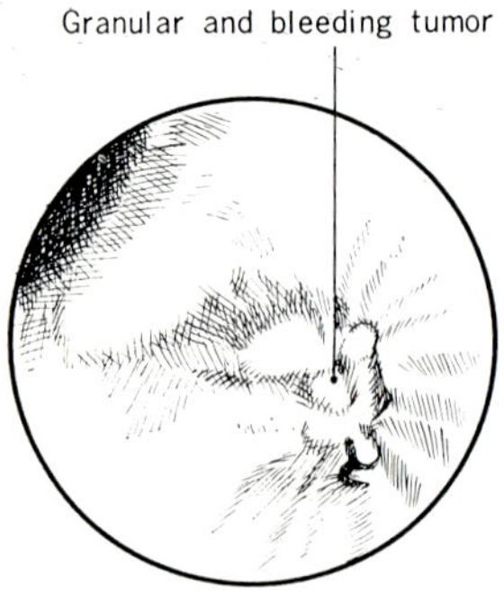


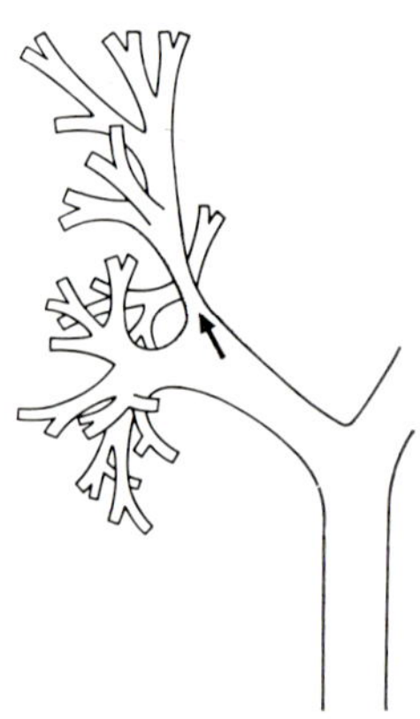

**Fig. 317 Fiberscopic findings :** The left truncus inferior lacks normal mucosal structure, and is almost completely stenotic with a tumor that is granular and bleeding.

# Case 26 Large Cell Carcinoma (48, male)

**Chief complaint :** Persistent cough.

**Case history :** The patient suffered from a persistent cough for two months. He had a fever of 39°C a month ago, was diagnosed as a pneumonia and then referred to our hospital. Chest X-ray film indicates a large tumor shadow within the lower part of the right hilum.

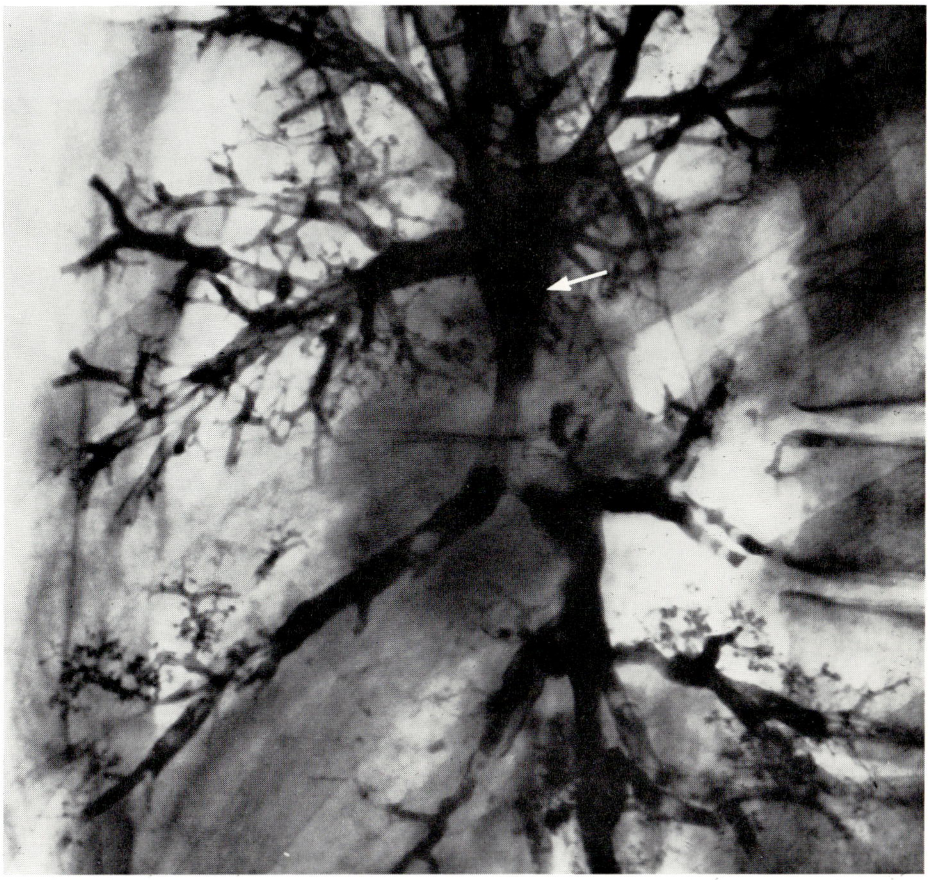

**Fig. 318 Bronchogram, markedly oblique, almost lateral view :** Marked stenosis (arrow) is present in the right main bronchus down to the middle lobe orifice, considered to be tractional. The middle lobe, as well as the lower lobe bronchi are markedly stenotic.

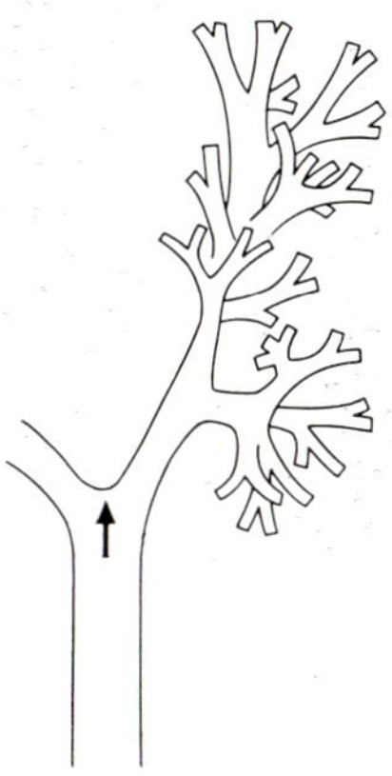

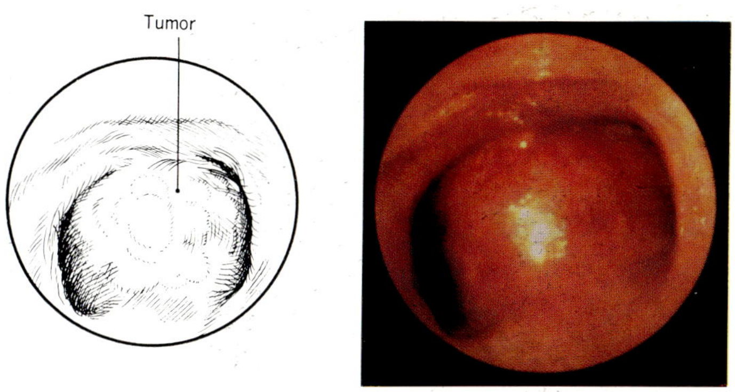


**Fig. 319 Fiberscopic findings :** Notice the tumor within the carina, markedly obstructing both the right and left main bronchi. The case was diagnosed as large cell carcinoma based on biopsy of this part. Caution : Biopsy in such a case may cause severe bleeding.

## Case 27 Adenocarcinoma (52, male)

**Chief complaint :** An abnormal shadow.
**Definitive clinical diagnosis :** Adenocarcinoma by curettage at bronchofiberscopy.
**Pathological diagnosis :** Papillary adenocarcinoma.
**Case history :** A $10 \times 10$ mm lesion was discovered in the left lung by mass survey four years previously. Examination followed, which were negative for cancer. He therefore received treatment for pulmonary tuberculosis. However, since the lesion increased in size under treatment, he was referred to our hospital for further studies.

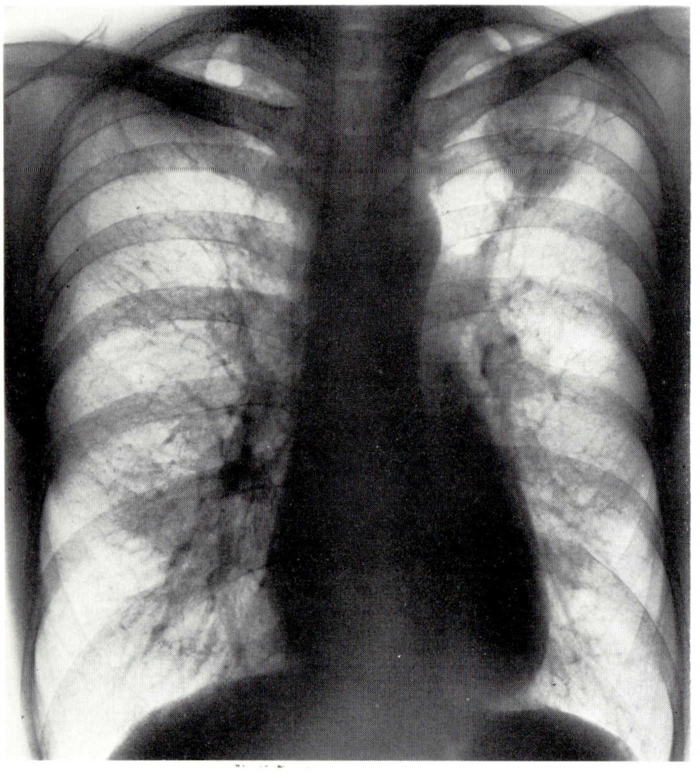

**Fig. 320 Chest X-ray, frontal :** A shadow $30 \times 30$ mm is present in the left lung field, with indistinct borders and not solid. No satellite lesions are recognized around the shadow. Two pleural indentations are noted and in one, linear markings are seen between the lesion and the pleura. As for the relationship between the lesion and the pulmonary hilum, the vessel shadow at the hilum is retracted upward. Elevation of the hilum and the pleural indentations indicate contraction of the lesion. These findings are compatible with a diagnosis of pulmonary tuberculosis.

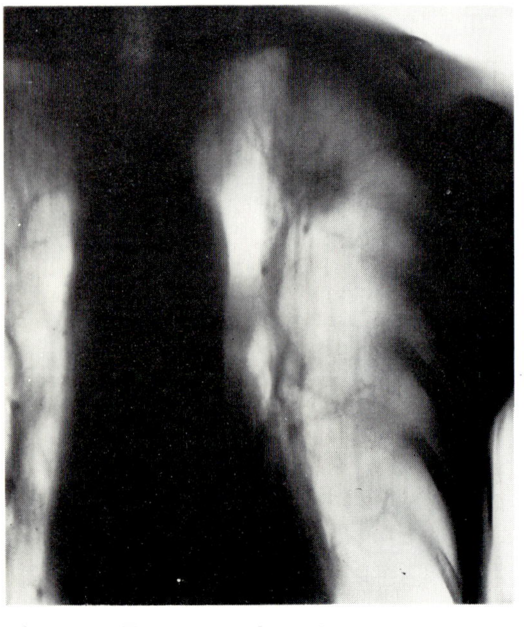

**321 a**

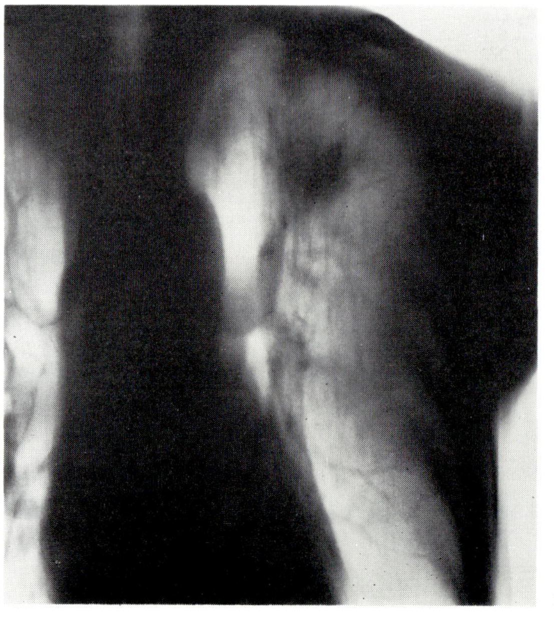

**321 b**

**Fig. 321 Tomogram, frontal :**
**a.** The tomogram 7 cm from the back reveals the relationship between the tumor and the blood vessel shadows which run around the tumor. Posterior to the tumor is present a linear pleural indentation.
**b.** Another tomogram 9 cm from the back shows clearly the relationship of the tumor to the air bronchogram of $B^{1+2}a$ and $B^{1+2}b$. A pleural indentation is present.

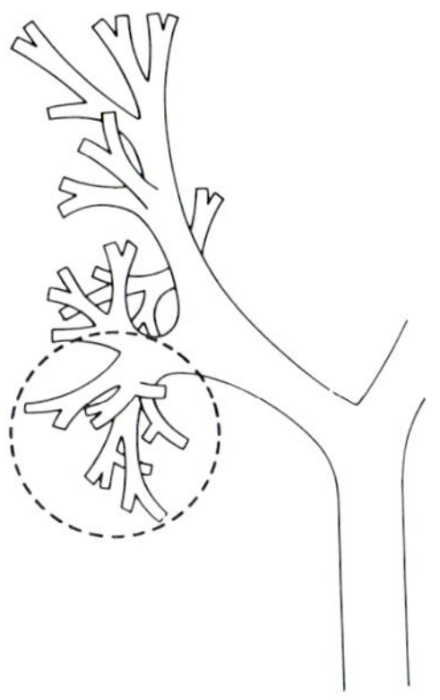

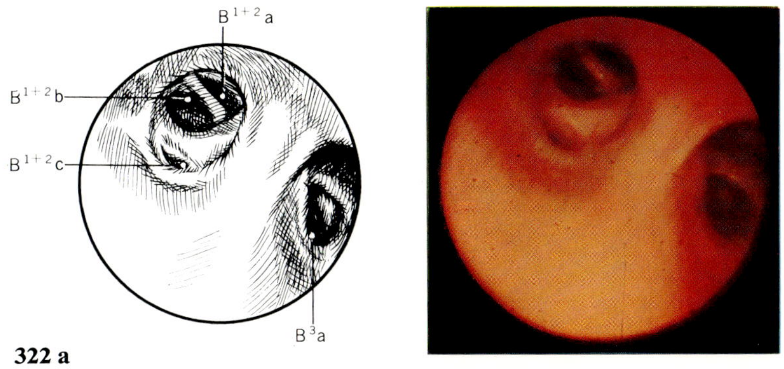


322 a

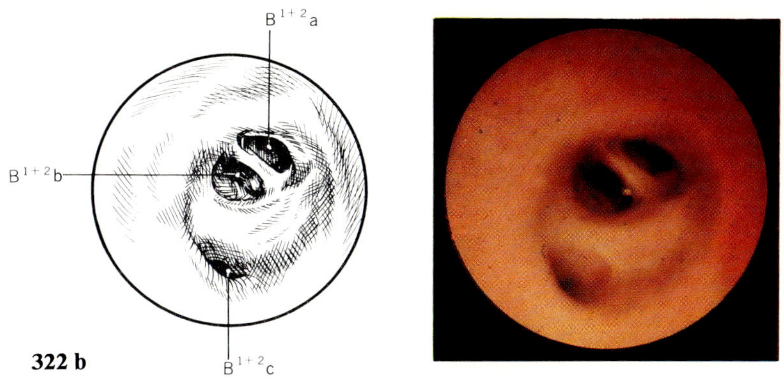


322 b

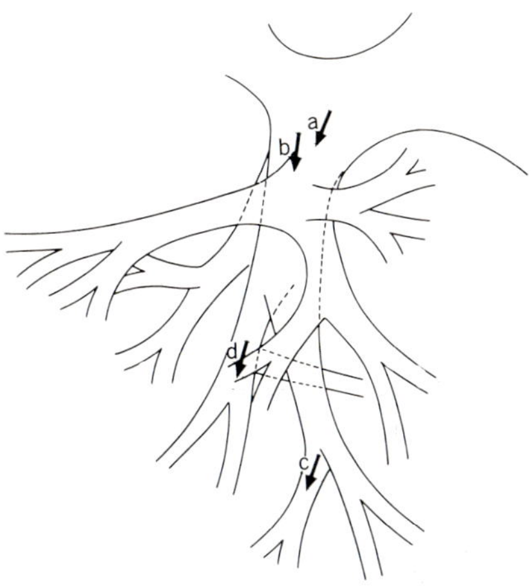


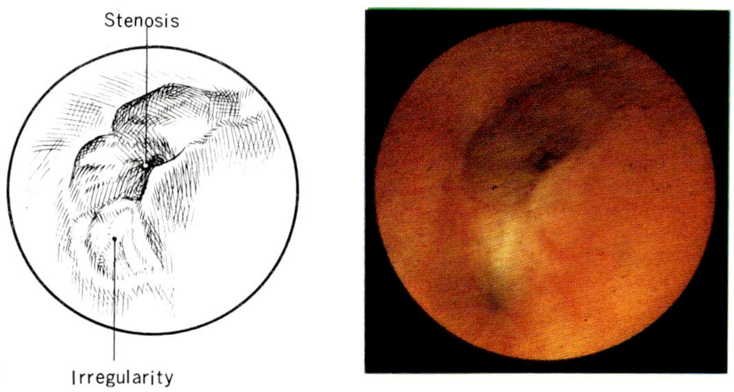


322 c

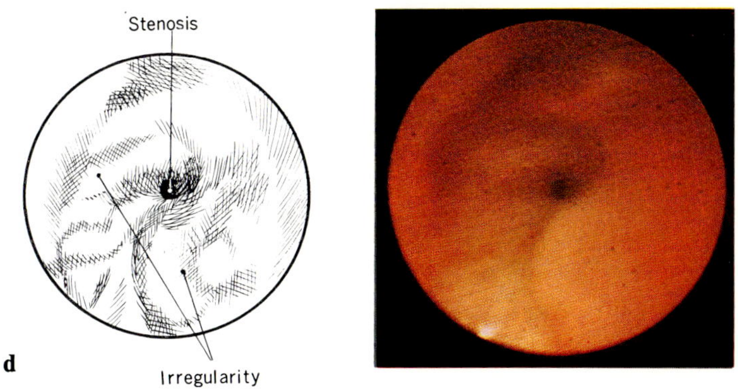


322 d

**Fig. 322 Fiberscopic findings :**

**a.** Upper division bronchus is normal.

**b.** Each of $B^{1+2}$ subsegmental bronchi is normal.

**c.** In $B^{1+2}ai$, the bronchial mucosa is irregular, the cartilage is unclear, and the lumen is stenosed. The picture shows $B^{1+2}ai$ entering the tumor with the lumen narrowed to a slit.

**d.** Stenosed part of $B^{1+2}bii$ and irregularity of the mucosa. Here also the bronchus entering the tumor is stenosed.

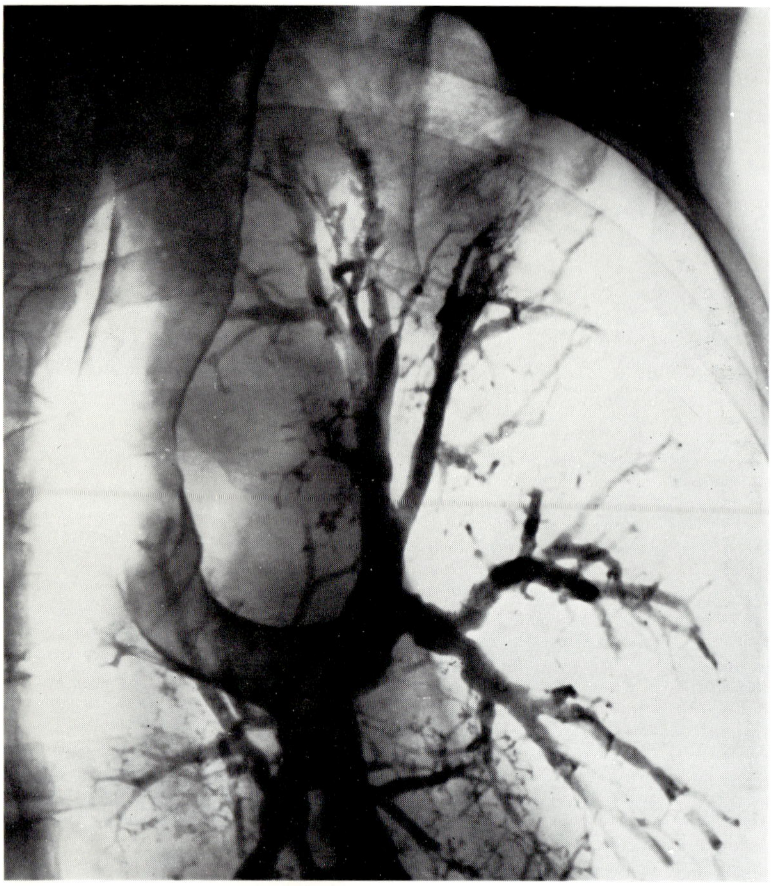

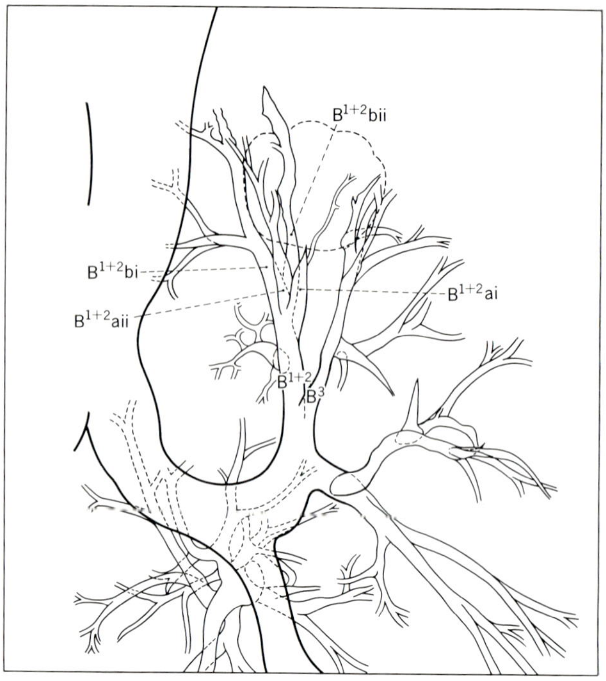


**Fig. 323 Bronchogram :** Tapered stenosis is present at $B^{1+2}$ai which is the principal bronchus. $B^{1+2}$bii is partly stenosed forming a point and is ectatic as if to surround the lesion. $B^{1+2}$a and $B^{1+2}$b are markedly coalesced. The branches of $B^3$ converge. These findings are present in pulmonary tuberculosis. X-ray film manifestations alone are not sufficient to diagnose lung cancer.

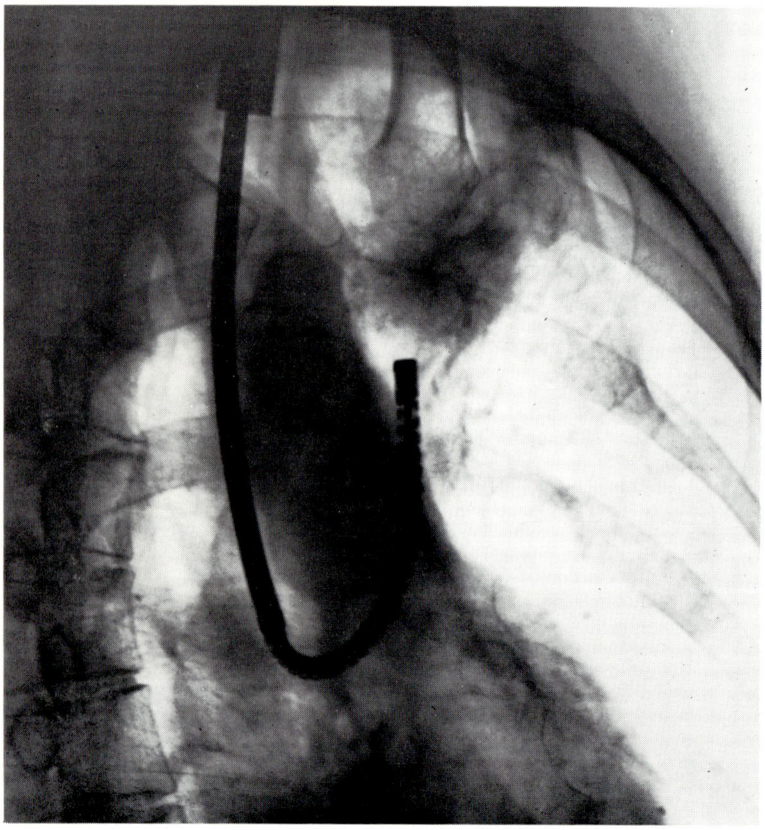

**Fig. 324 Bronchofiberscopy :** X-ray film showing a bronchofiberscope inserted into the $B^{1+2}$a bronchus.

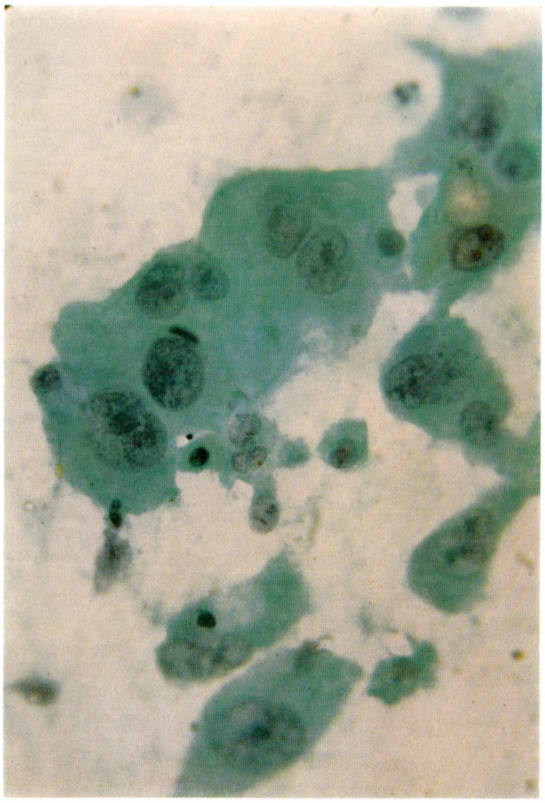

**Fig. 325 Cytodiagnosis :** Bronchofiberscopic curettage. The cytoplasm has distinct boundaries but occupies a broad area. Mucous vacuoles are present. Diagnosis : Adenocarcinoma.

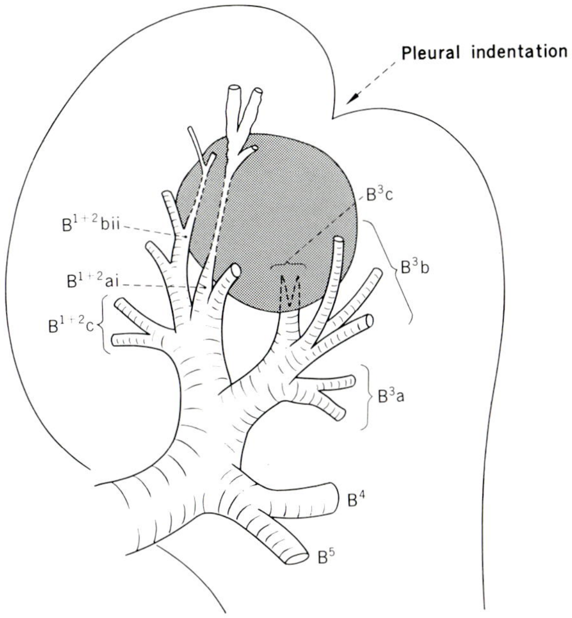


**Fig. 326 Traced schema :** Four bronchi, $B^{1+2}ai$, $B^{1+2}bii$, $B^3ai$ and $B^3aii$, enter the tumor of 35×30 mm.

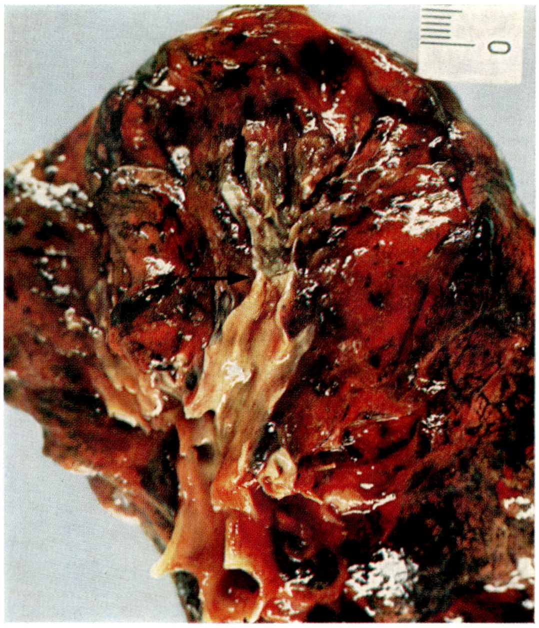

**Fig. 327 Macroscopic findings :** Fresh specimen showing the upper division bronchus to $B^{1+2}a$ (photo trimmed). One of the affected bronchi, $B^{1+2}ai$, enters the peripheral lesion markedly narrowed, with its periphery slightly ectatic.

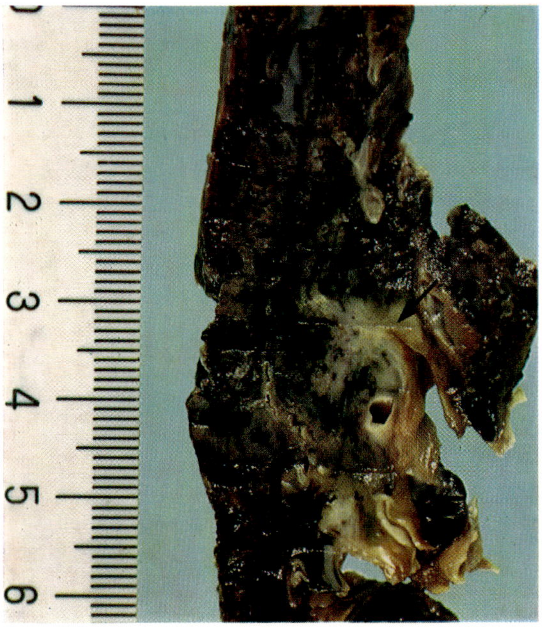

**Fig. 328 Macroscopic findings :** Fixed specimen. The lesion reveals intense anthracosis and indistinct boundaries on the cut surface. $B^{1+2}ai$ (arrow) passes through the inner side and the relatively ivory white part of the tumor.

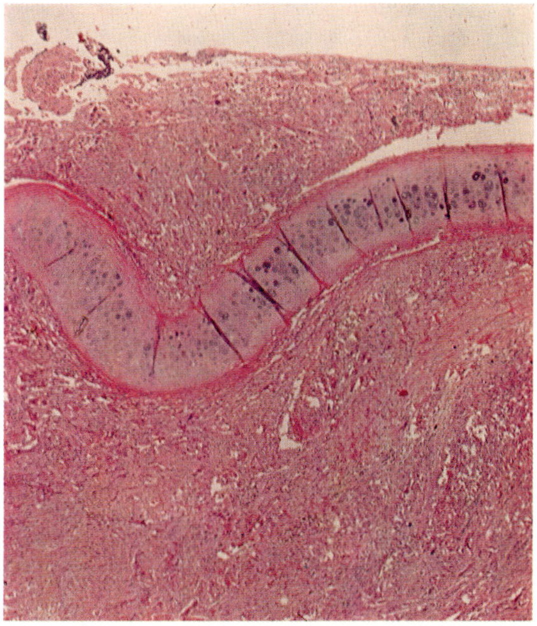

**Fig. 329 Microscopic findings :** Histological picture of $B^{1+2}ai$ nearly stenosed by the tumor. The tumor infiltrates the bronchial wall and has destroyed the mucosa(upper left). The epithelium has desquamated but the basal membrane remains (upper right).

## COMMENT :

This case was first misdiagnosed as pulmonary tuberculosis and after the tumor grew a definitive diagnosis of papillary adenocarcinoma was established. Bronchographic findings were also misdiagnosed as pulmonary tuberculosis because of an abnormal coalescence of bronchi. Bronchofiberscopic findings, on the contrary, revealed findings obviously different from those of any inflammatory disease. Bronchofiberscopic curettage in such a case is a powerful and efficient weapon. A bronchogram, especially an accurately prepared one, is essential for the exact location of the bronchial focus.

## Case 28 Adenocarcinoma (67, male)

**Chief complaint :** Abnormal shadow on the chest X-ray film.

**Definitive clinical diagnosis :** Adenocarcinoma by cytology of the second bronchofiberscopic curettage.

**Pathological diagnosis :** Adenocarcinoma, moderately differentiated.

**Case history :** The patient had a severe cough for about two months. An abnormality was found on the chest X-ray film, and he was referred to our hospital. He smoked about ten cigarettes a day from age 20 to 41.

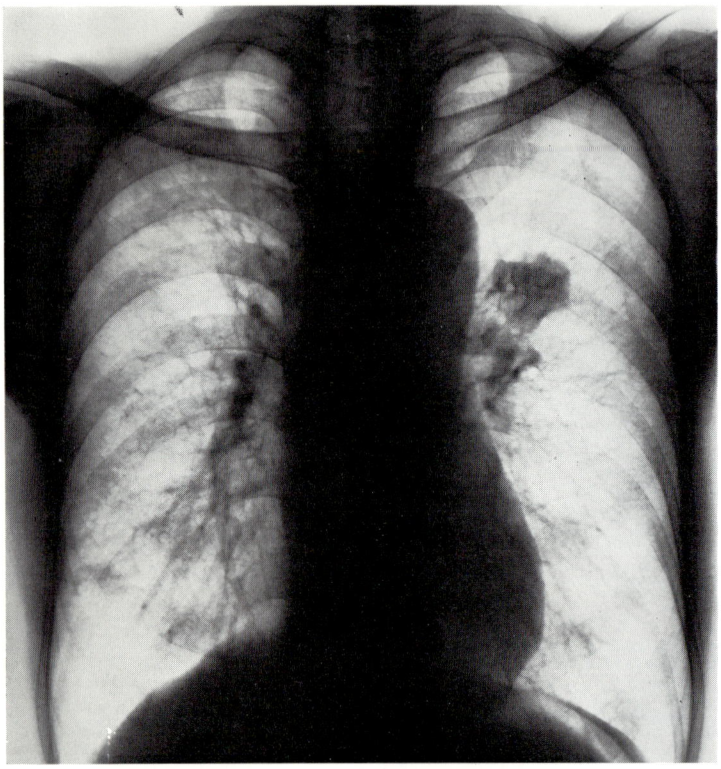

**Fig. 330 Chest X-ray, frontal :** An irregular tumor with sharp borders is visible near the hilum in the mid-left lung. No enlarged lymph nodes are seen in the hilum.

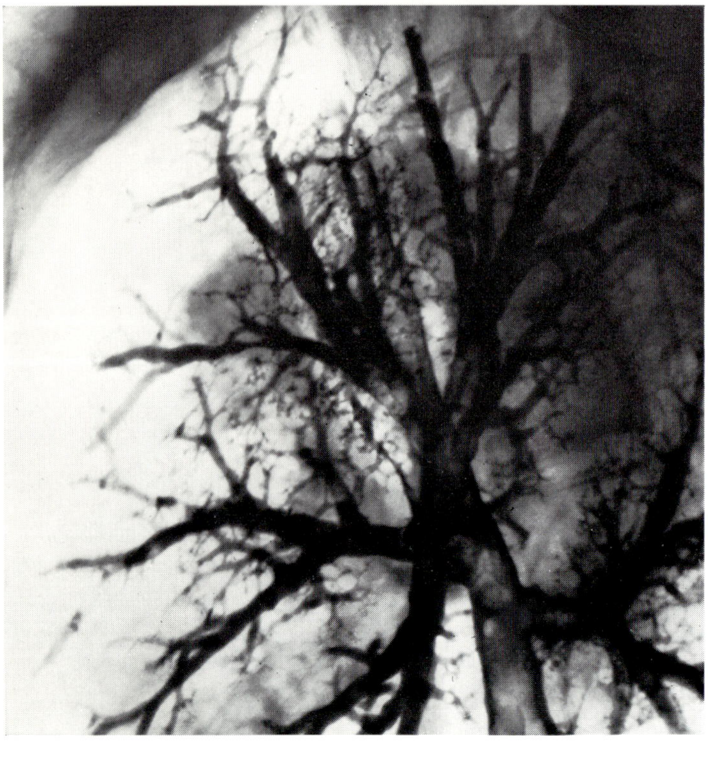

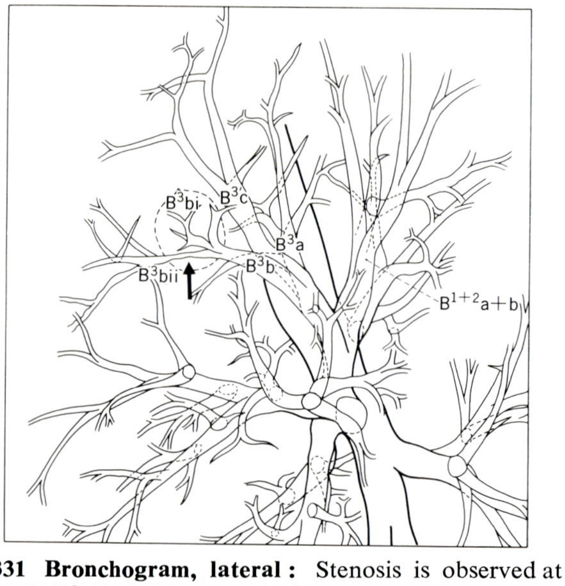


**Fig. 331 Bronchogram, lateral :** Stenosis is observed at the origin of $B^3bii$ (IVth bronchus) and ectasis is seen further peripherally. Another stenosis, pointed in shape, is present on a peripheral branch of $B^3bi$, and the branches are stenosed entering the tumor.

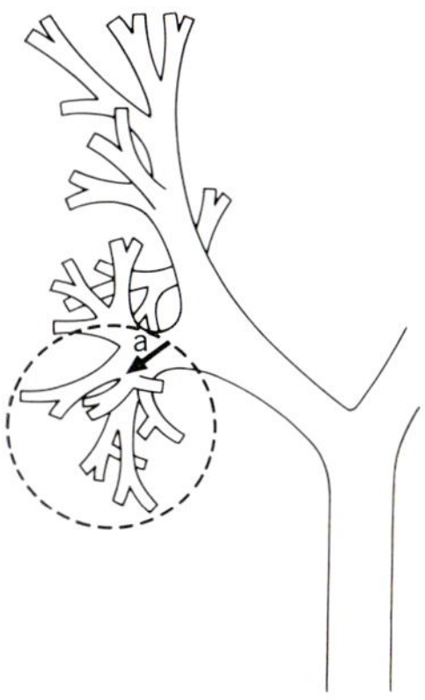


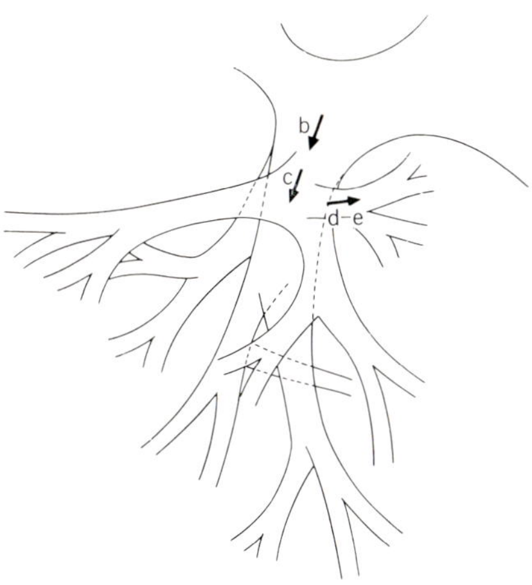


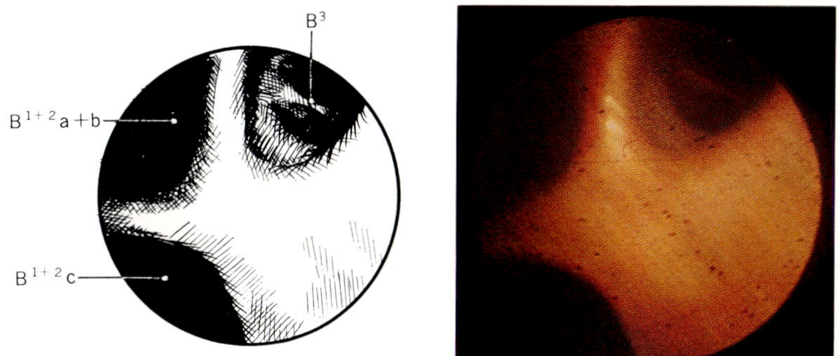


332 a

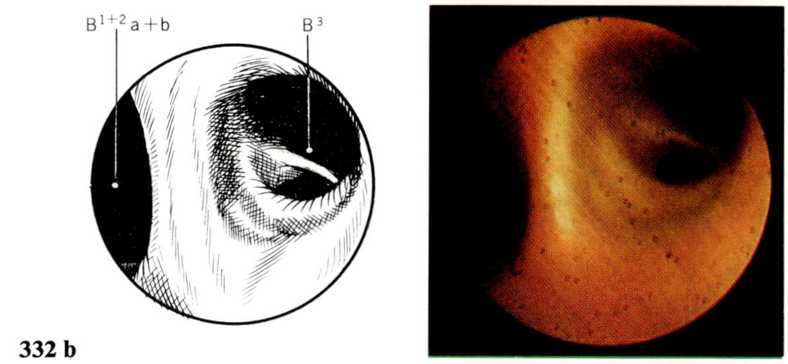


332 b

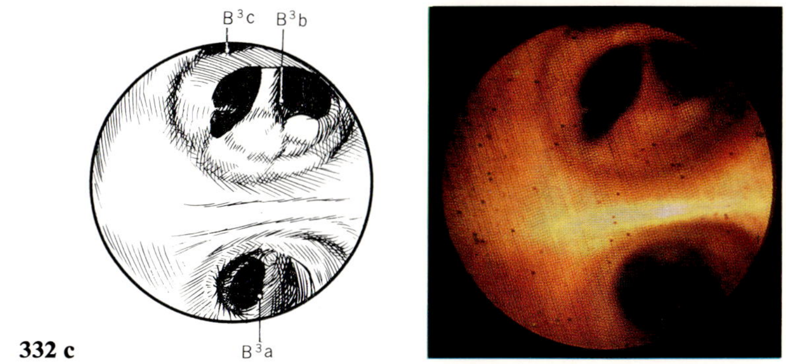


332 c

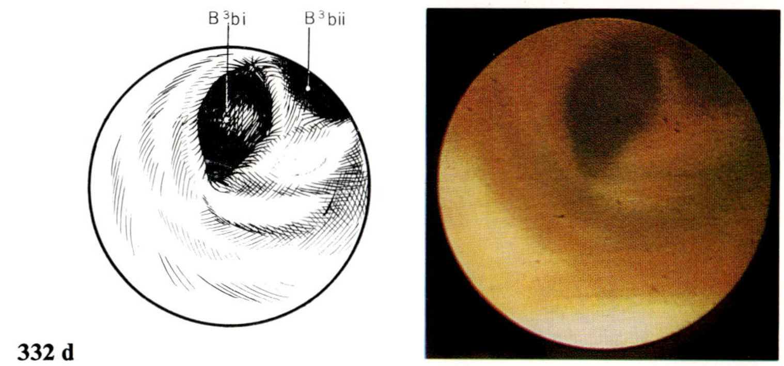


332 d

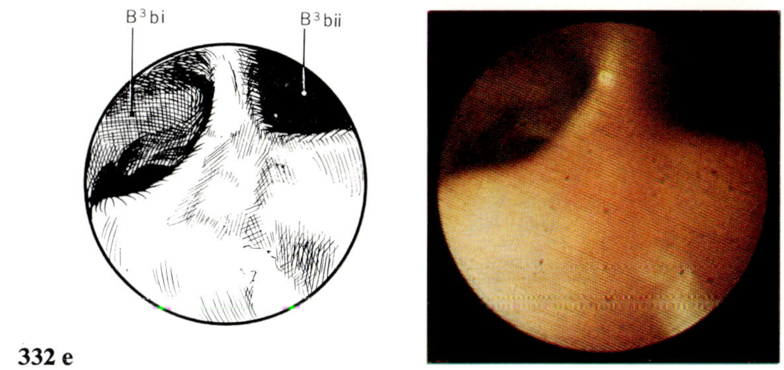


332 e

**Fig. 332 Fiberscopic findings:**

**a.** The upper division bronchus trifurcates into $B^{1+2}a+b$ ($B^1$), $B^{1+2}c$ ($B^2$) and $B^3$.

**b.** The bifurcation of $B^3$ and $B^{1+2}a+b$ is normal.

**c.** $B^3$ trifurcates into $B^3a$, $B^3b$ and $B^3c$.

**d.** Fiberscope in $B^3b$.

**e.** The bifurcation of $B^3bi$ and $B^3bii$.

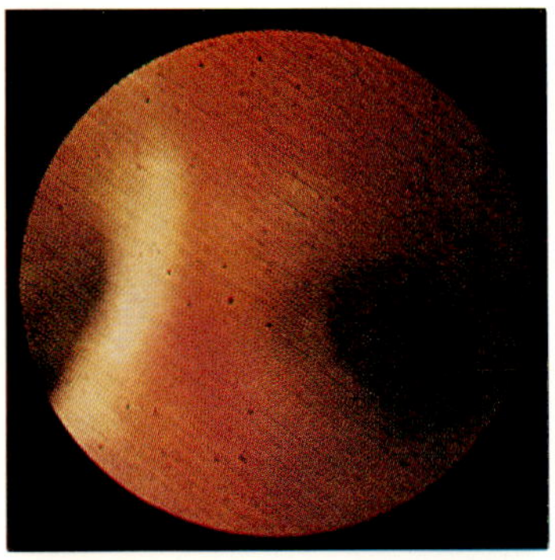

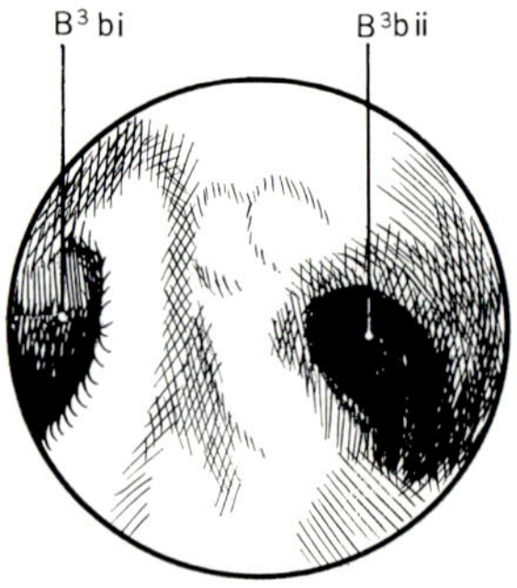


332 f

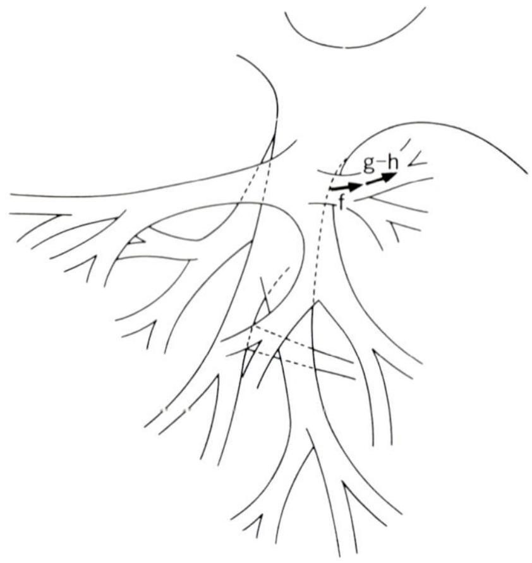

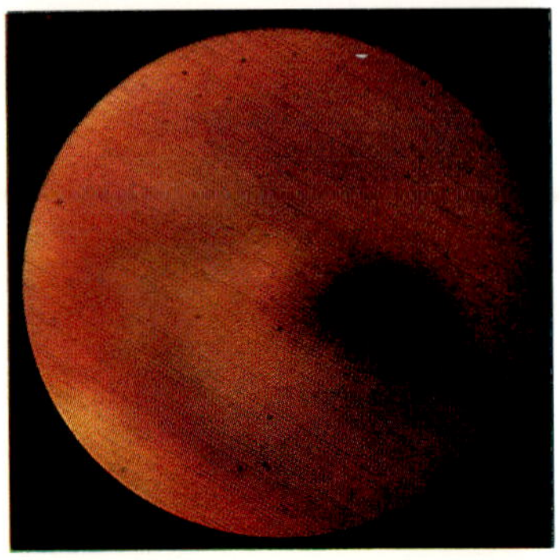

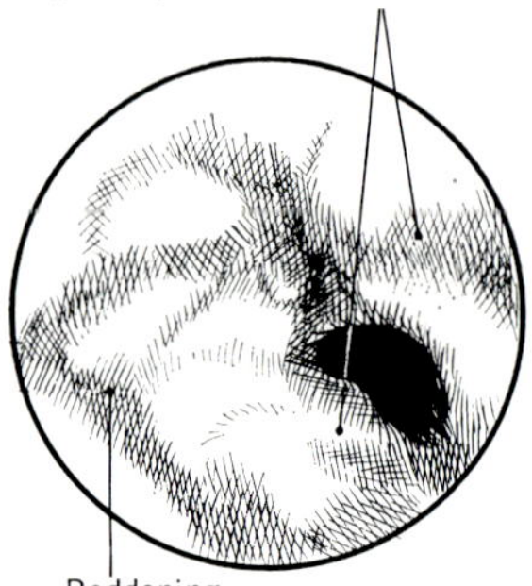


332 g

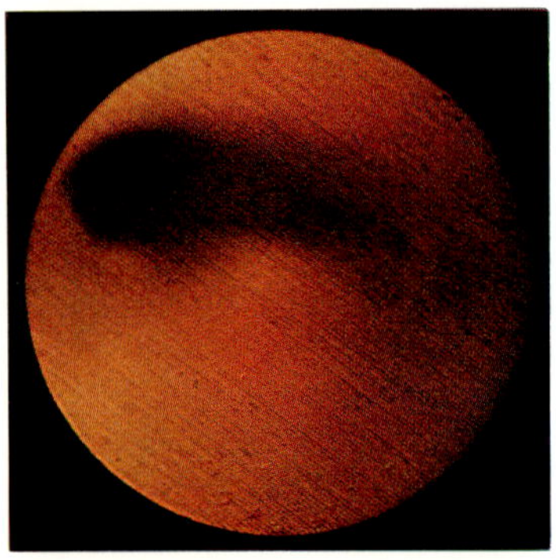

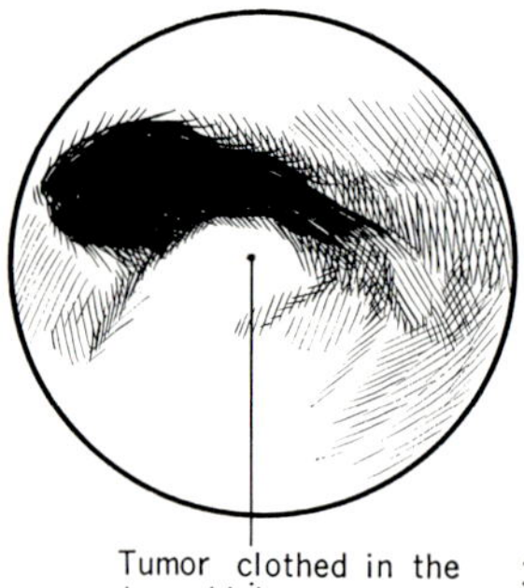


332 h

**f.** The posterior wall of B³bii : Note irregularity of the mucosa and obscured cartilages.

**g.** In B³bii, slight redness prominent, irregularity of the mucosa and stenosis are present. The bronchographic findings showing B³bii entering the tumor and being stenosed well coincide with the bronchofiberscopic findings.

**h.** Farther in the bronchus, the mucosa is quite irregular and carcinoma covered with mucosa is noted. In adenocarcinoma the mucosa of the draining bronchus is frequently intact. In such cases, the tumor can be visualized through the epithelium or the submucosal.

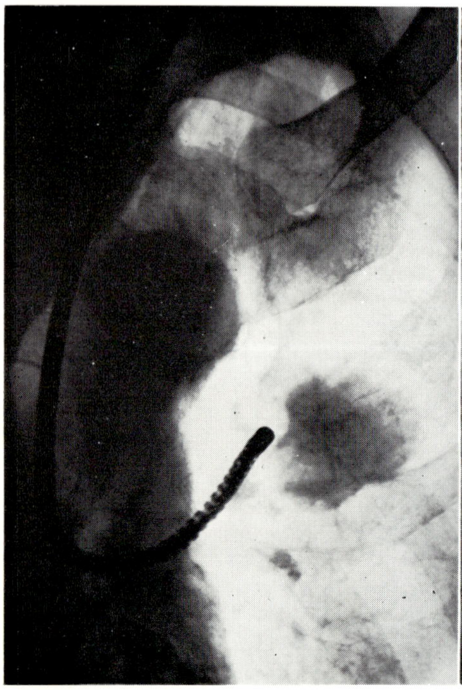

333

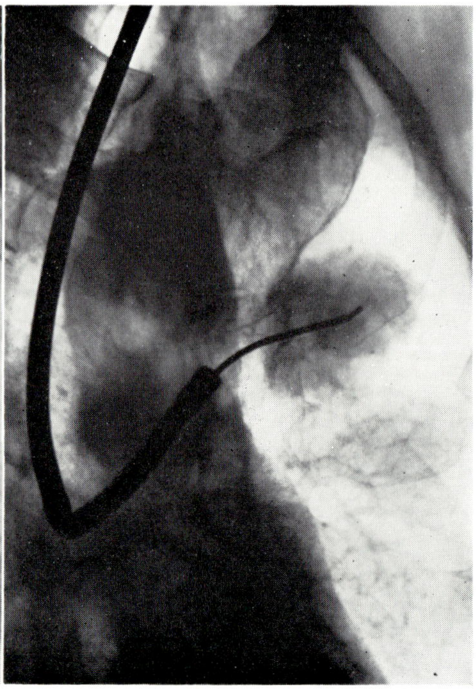

334

**Fig. 333 Bronchofiberscopy :** X-ray film of a bronchofiberscope, 4 mm, Machida make, inserted into B³bii.

**Fig. 334 Curettage :** Histological diagnosis under bronchofiberscopy. The tip of the bronchofiberscope has entered B³b and a small curette has passed through B³bii into the tumor.

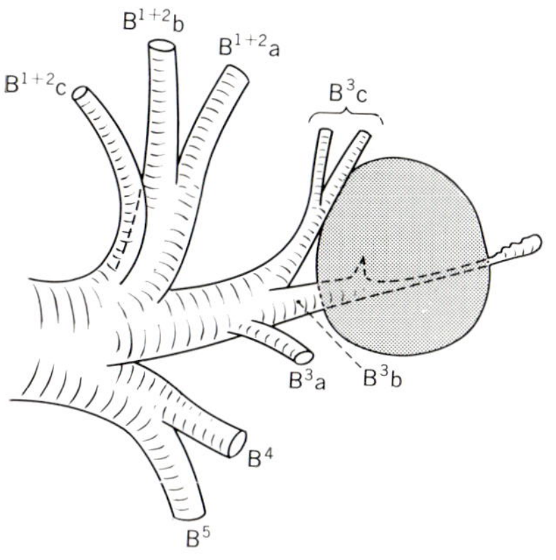


**Fig. 335 Traced schema:** $B^3b$ goes through carcinoma but it is stenosed. The bronchial mucosa here is involved by tumor. Occasionally the bronchial adventitial coat or submucosal tissues are involved; and, when advanced, the tumor may involve the mucosa.

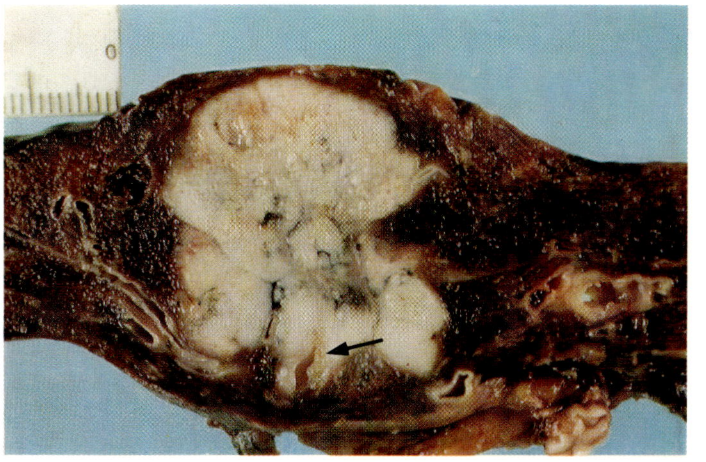

**Fig. 336 Macroscopic findings:** The cut surface of the tumor is irregularly circular, ivory white, homogeneous, and the center is slightly fibrosed. The obliquely sectioned affected bronchus, $B^3b$ (arrow), is infiltrated by tumor from outside of the bronchial wall.

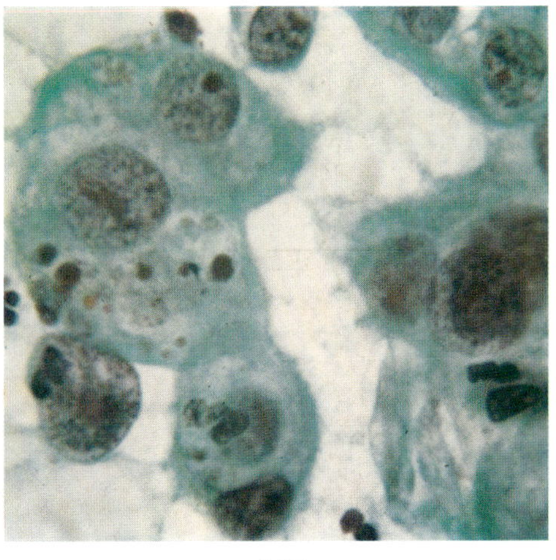

**337**

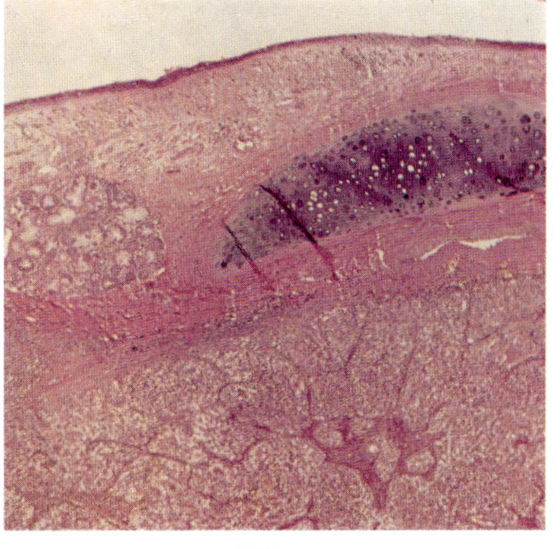

**338 a**

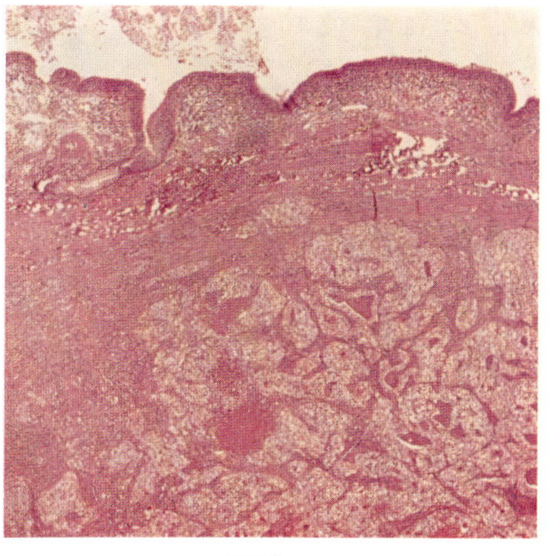

**338 b**

**Fig. 337 Cytodiagnosis:** Bronchofiberscopic currettage. The cytoplasm is pale-stained and indistinct in boundaries. The nuclei are elliptical and the nuclear membrane is thickened. A single detached nucleolus is prominent. The specimen suggested a diagnosis of adenocarcinoma.

**Fig. 338 Microscopic findings:** Cancer infiltration into the affected bronchus is limited to the outer bronchial membrane in (a), but in (b) reaches the submucous tissue. These findings reveal stenosis (b) and the pathological histology of (b) the stenotic portion and (a) slightly proximal to (b) obtained bronchofiberscopically.

**COMMENT**:

This is a typical case of adenocarcinoma in which bronchofiberscopic findings provide characteristic information. In adenocarcinoma, the tumor occasionally presents itself in the bronchial lumen but more often the carcinoma can be seen through the mucosa. In the peripheral bronchi, however, the bronchial mucosa is so thin that the lumen present findings of mucosal irregularity, tortuous engorgement of blood vessels, and unclearness of the cartilages. It is important that bronchofiberscopic photography in a peripheral bronchus should, as in this case, be taken in good serial order; otherwise the arrangement of photographs at a later date will be difficult.

## Case 29 Adenocarcinoma (38, male)

**Chief complaint :** Bloody sputum.
**Definitive clinical diagnosis :** Adenocarcinoma, histologically diagnosed by curettage under broncho-fiberscopy.
**Pathological diagnosis :** Papillary adenocarcinoma moderately differentiated.
**Case history :** Bloody sputum was noticed by the patient. The chest X-ray film revealed an abnormal shadow. At the time the patient visited our hospital, the hemoptysis had ceased. Smoking habit, 20 to 30 cigarrettes a day, inhaled deeply, since 21 years of age.

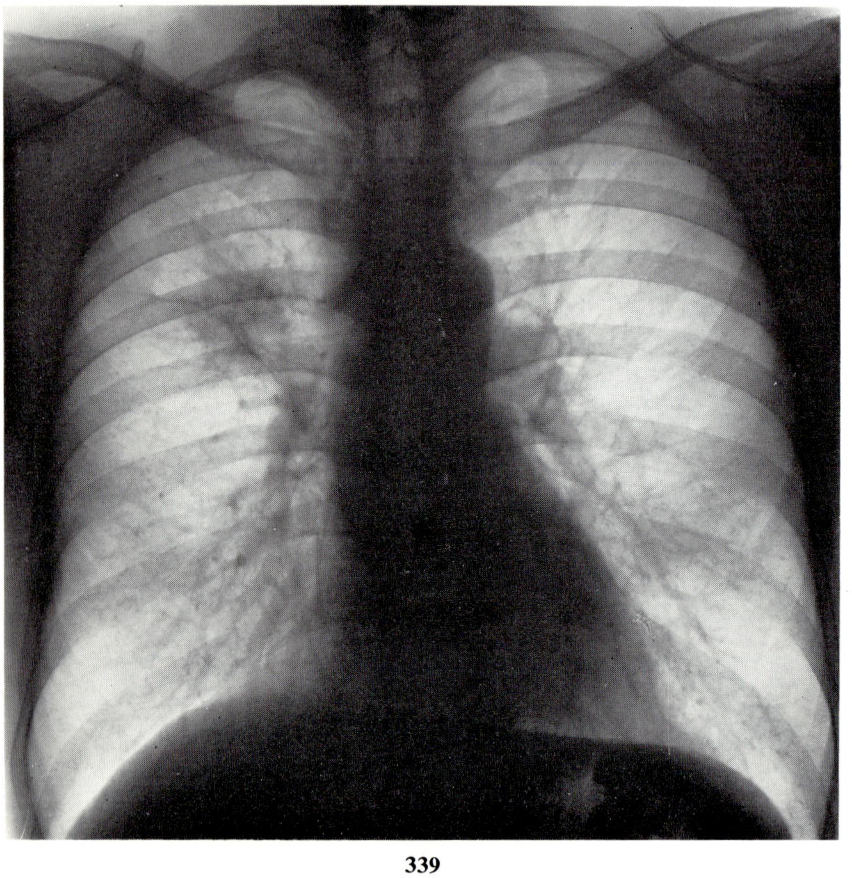

339

**Fig. 339 Chest X-ray, frontal :** A tumor shadow, with indistinct margins and a number of notches, is present, and near the outside of the tumor a pleural indentation is seen.

**Fig. 340 Tomogram :**
**a.** The tomogram 14 cm from the posterior shows the markedly radiating tumor and the notches.
**b.** Another tomogram 15 cm from the posterior reveals radiolucency.

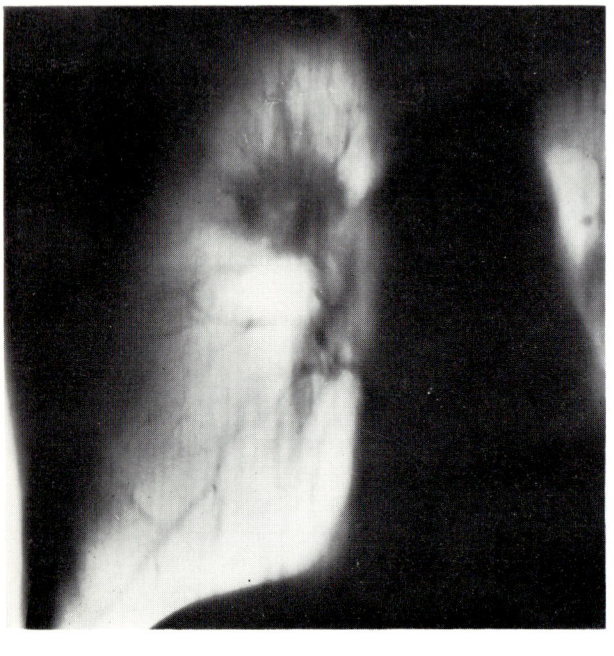

340 a

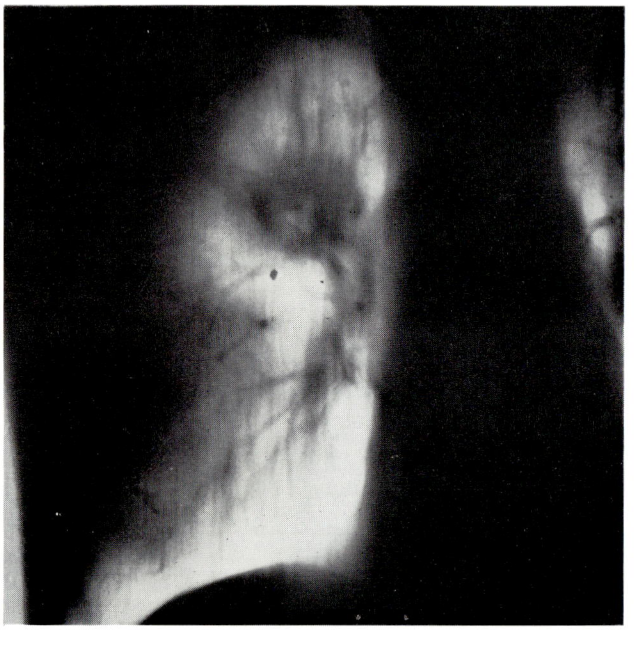

340 b

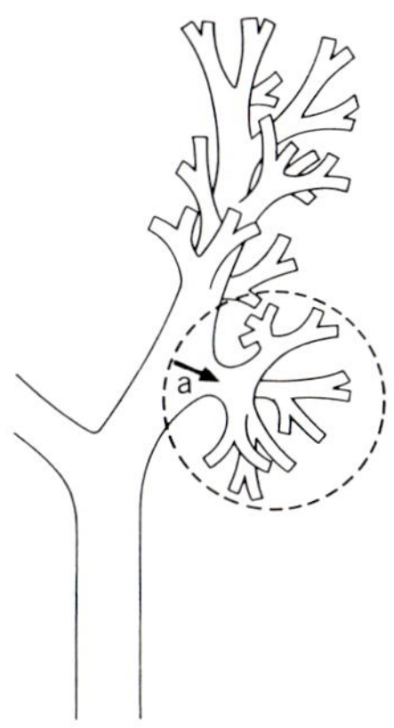


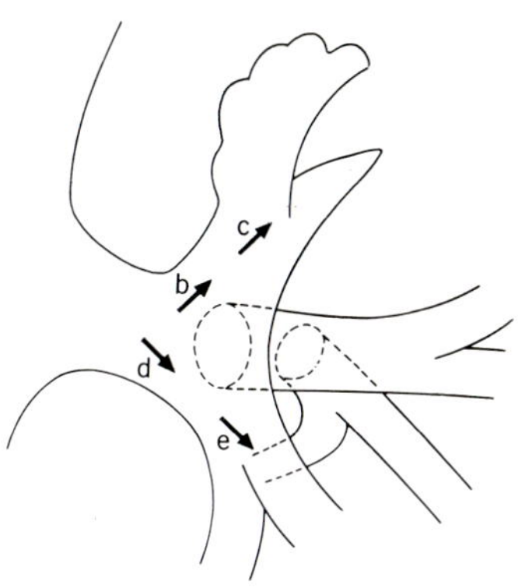


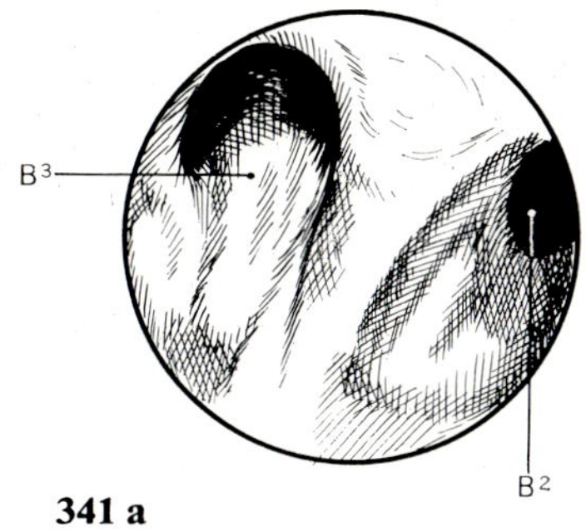


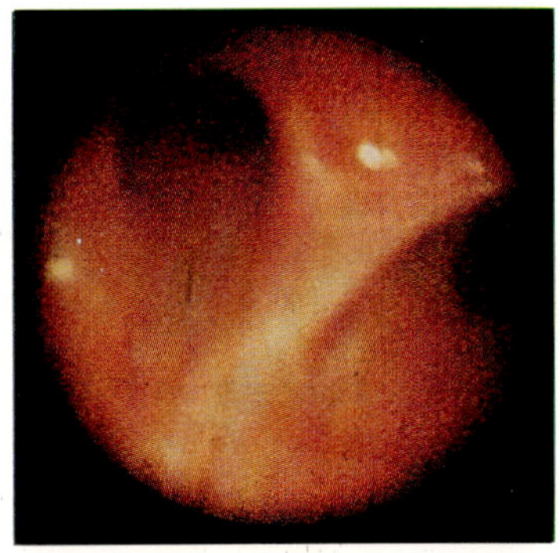

341 a

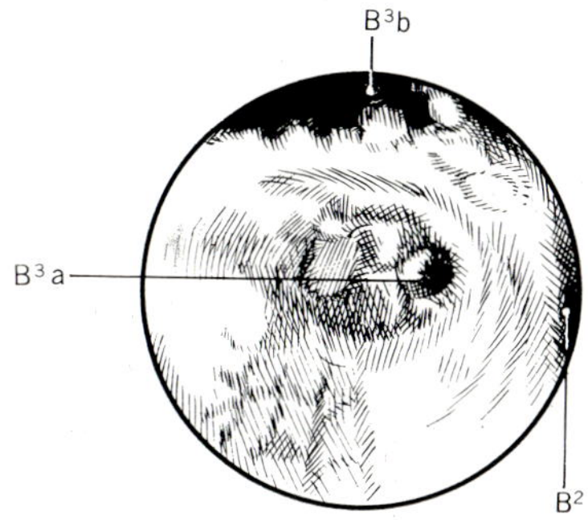


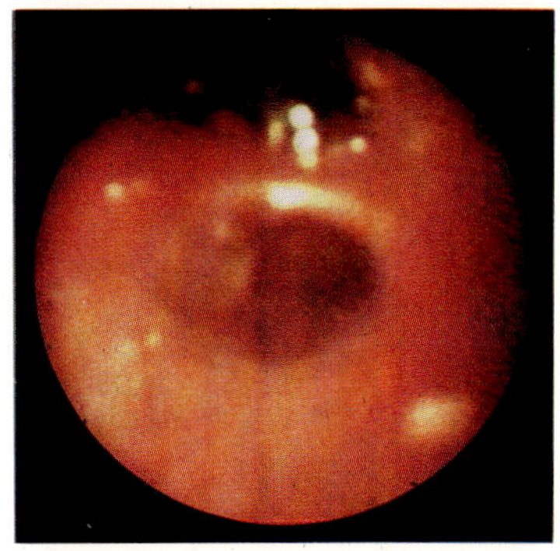

341 b

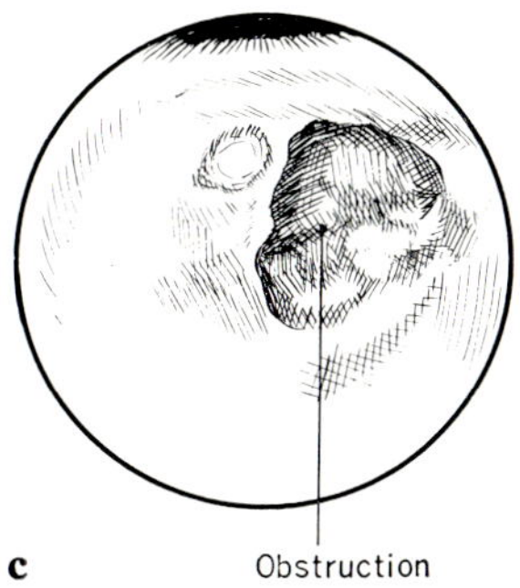


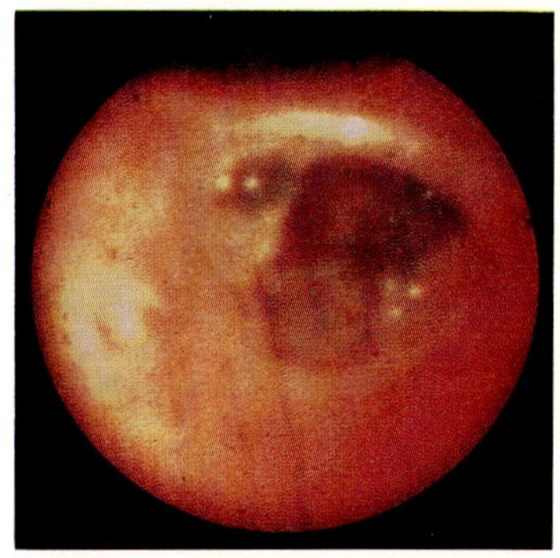

341 c

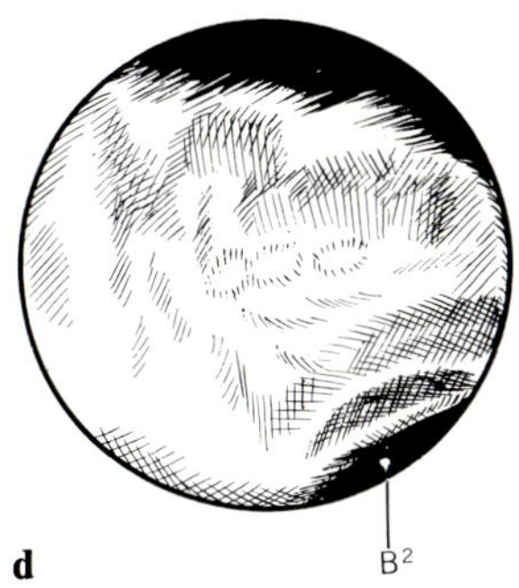


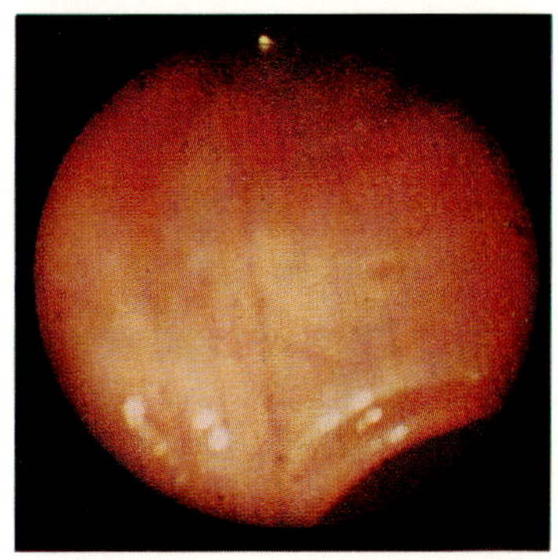

341 d

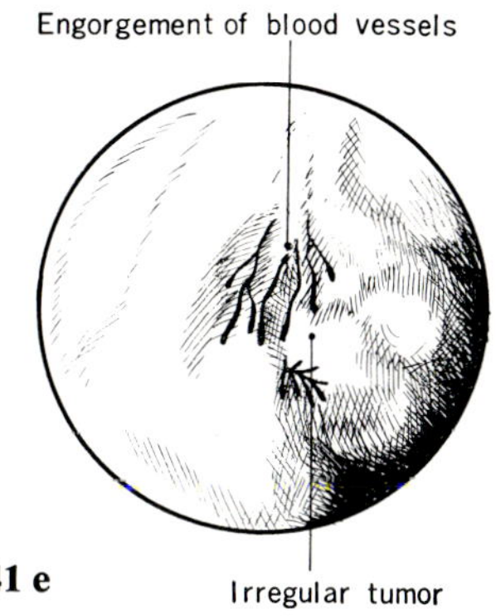


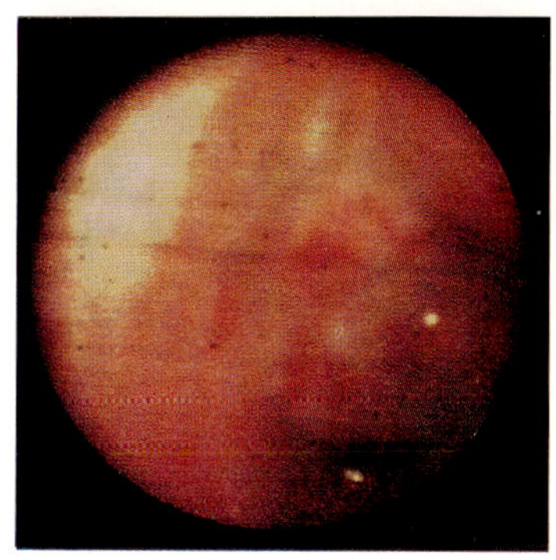

341 e

**Fig. 341 Fiberscopic findings :**

**a.** The bifurcation of $B^2$ and $B^3$ is normal.

**b.** $B^3$a and $B^3$b are both normal at the bifurcation, but just distally, $B^3$b is filled with blood and the orifice of $B^3$a is slightly irregular.

**c.** $B^3$a is obstructed just within the orifice. The mucosa of the obstructed bronchus is irregular.

**d.** The mucosa of the posterior wall in $B^1$ is slightly irregular.

**e.** The distal part of $B^1$ presents irregularity of the mucosa, vascular engorgement and lack of cartilages. Irregular mucosa is apparently caused by protrusion of the carcinoma.

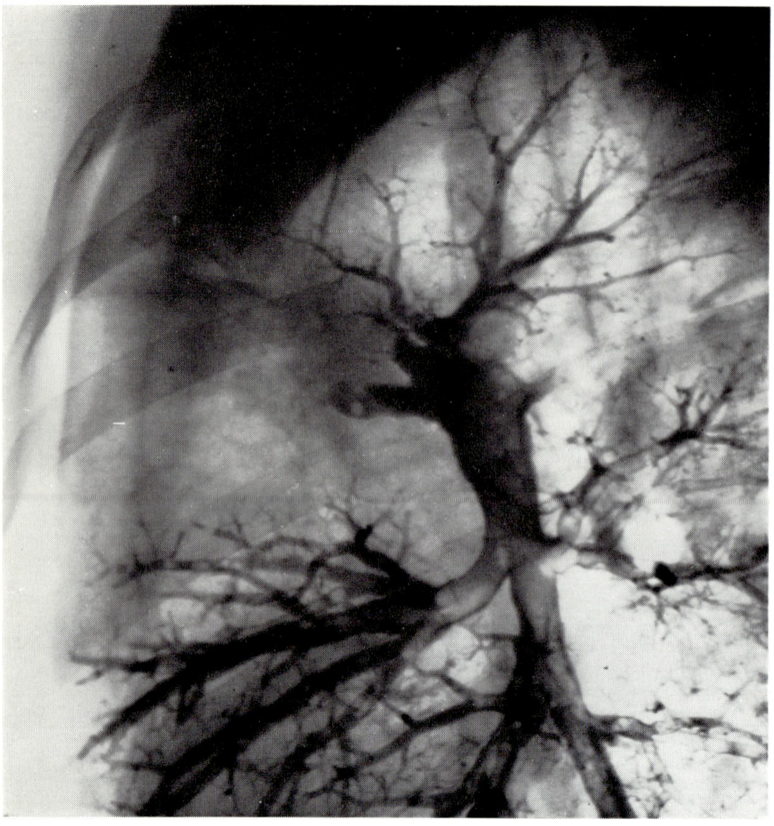

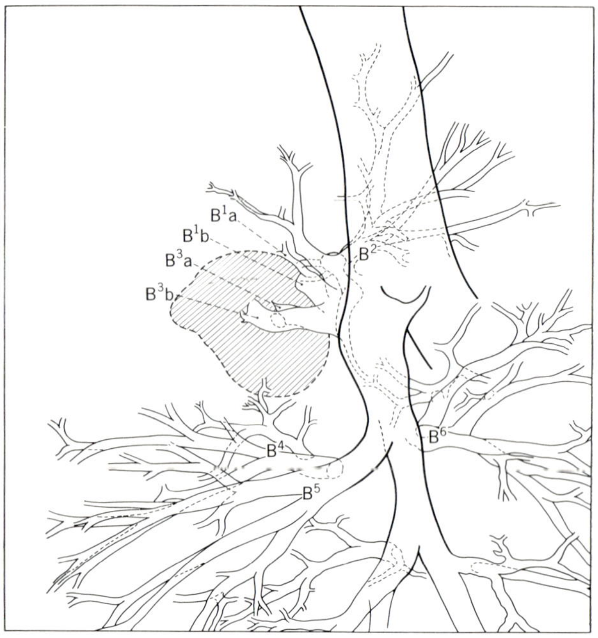


**Fig. 342 Bronchogram, oblique :** There is seen an irregular stenosis caused by the tumor in $B^1b$, and a conspicuous stenosis with smaller branches originating from it in $B^1a$. $B^3a$ is pointed and stenosed, and $B^3b$ ectatic to the anterior periphery of the tumor and then stenosed.

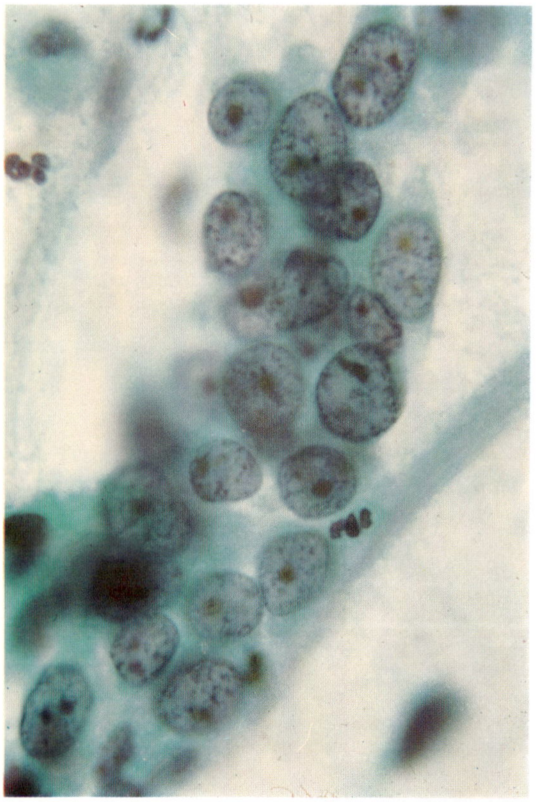

**Fig. 343 Cytodiagnosis:** Bronchofiberscopic curettage, demonstrating a large cluster of tumor cells. The nuclear membrane is slightly thickened. Chromatin is reticular and pale staining. These findings lead to a diagnosis of adenocarcinoma.

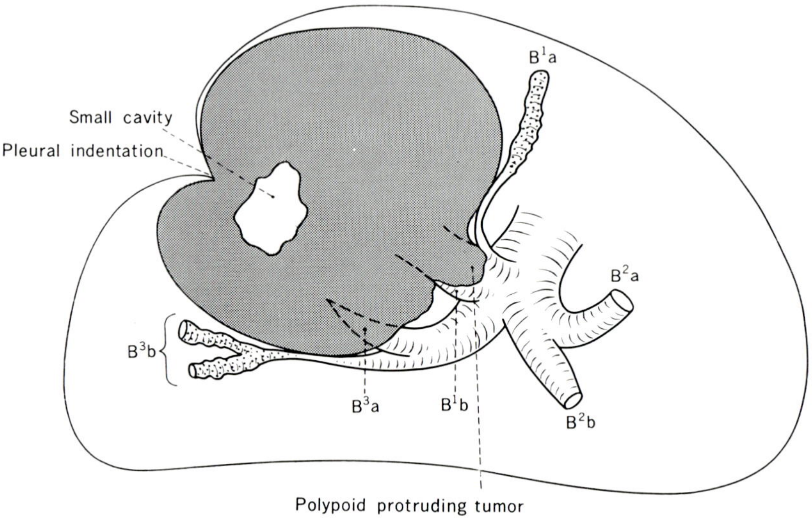


**Fig. 344 Traced schema :** Adenocarcinoma, with a small cavity near a marked pleural indentation, is situated around the lateral subsegment of the anterior segment ($S^3a$). The $B^3a$ bronchus, which is within the center of the tumor, is retracted, stenosed to a point, and infiltrated by tumor. $B^1b$ is also stenosed with a polypoid projection (part of the tumor) in the lumen.

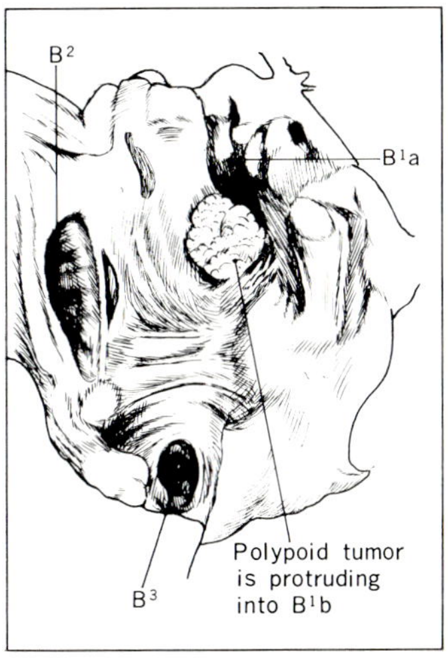


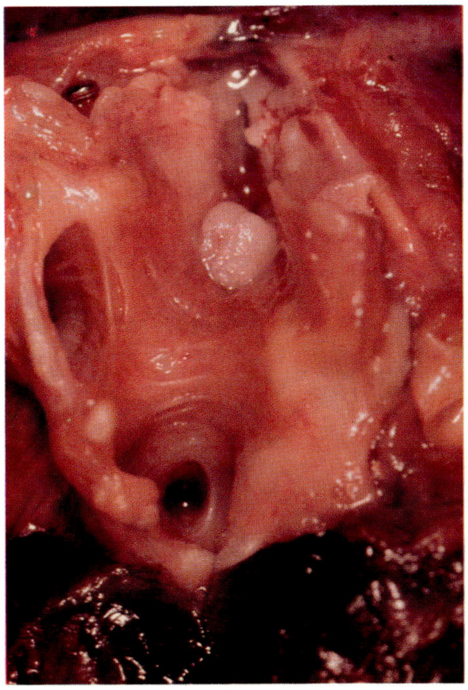

345 a

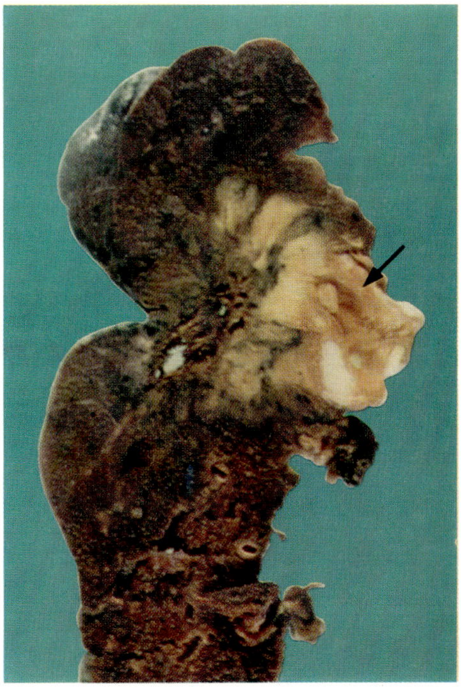

345 b

**Fig. 345 Macroscopic findings :**
**a.** Fresh specimen. The tumor is protruding into $B^1b$ and occludes the brochus.
**b.** Trimmed. The cut surface of the tumor is rich in coarse fibrous components, contains a small cavity, and its boundaries are indistinct. $B^1b$ (arrow) is obliterated at the periphery of the tumor, and a small tumor is protruding into the lumen.

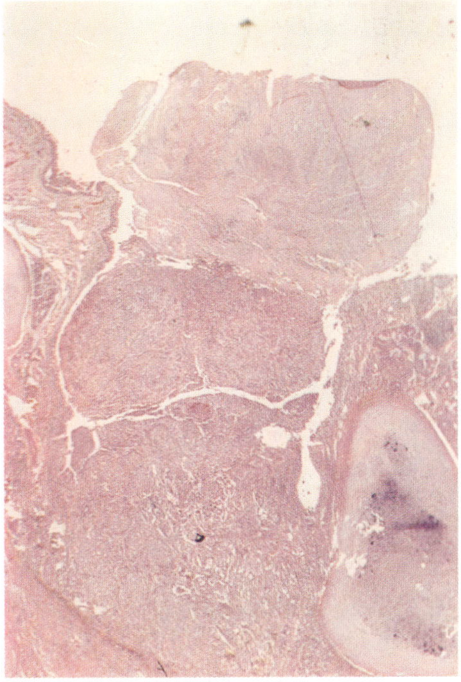

346 a

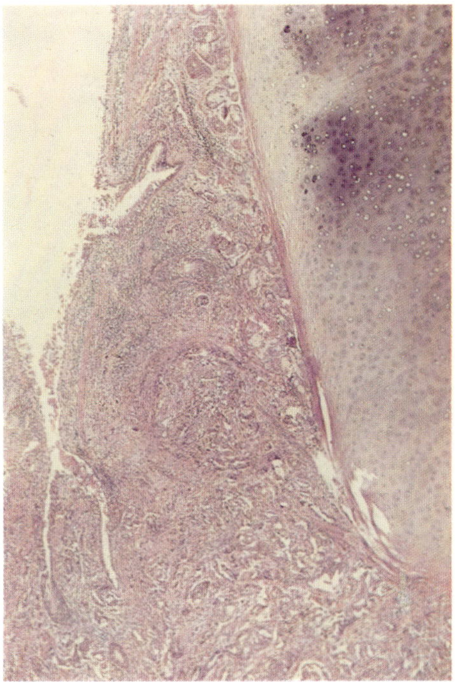

346 b

**Fig. 346 Microscopic findings:**
**a.** Histological picture of a polypoid projection into $B^1b$. The polypoid part is composed of the necrotic tip. The part near the root where cancer cells are solidly arranged, shows just the root portion of the papillary structure.
**b.** Histology of the tapered stenosis of $B^3a$. Cancer infiltration surrounds the bronchial cartilage and reaches the submucous tissue. Part of the bronchial epithelium has desquamated.

## COMMENT :

In this case, the bronchographic and bronchofiberscopic findings as described above, agree completely. Protruding polypoid adenocarcinoma is quite unusual.

## Case 30 Adenocarcinoma (68, female)

**Case history :** This patient had received annual mass survey chest X-rays. Three years ago a 20 mm shadow was found in the right lung. It was diagnosed as pulmonary tuberculosis and chemotherapy was instituted. Recently the shadow had grown larger so she visited our hospital. Bronchography and bronchofiberscopy were performed. Cytology by means of a small curette introduced through the bronchofiberscope diagnosed the case as an adenocarcinoma.

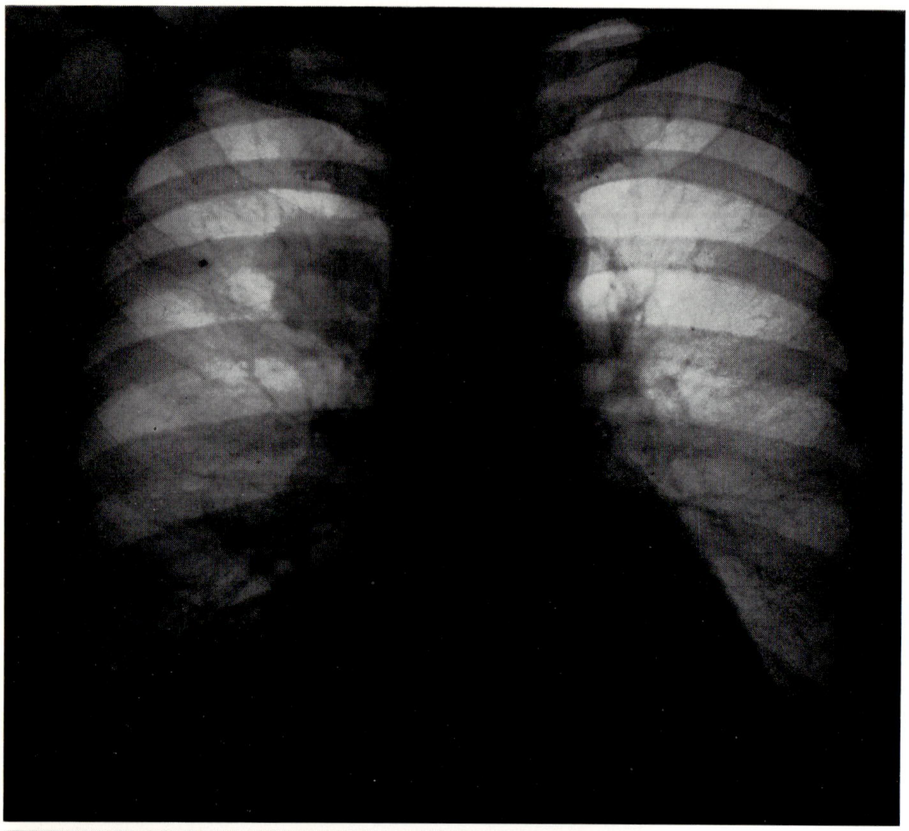

**Fig. 347 Chest X-ray, frontal :** A tumor, 40×40mm, with indistinct borders is located in the $S^1b$ subsegment of the right lung.

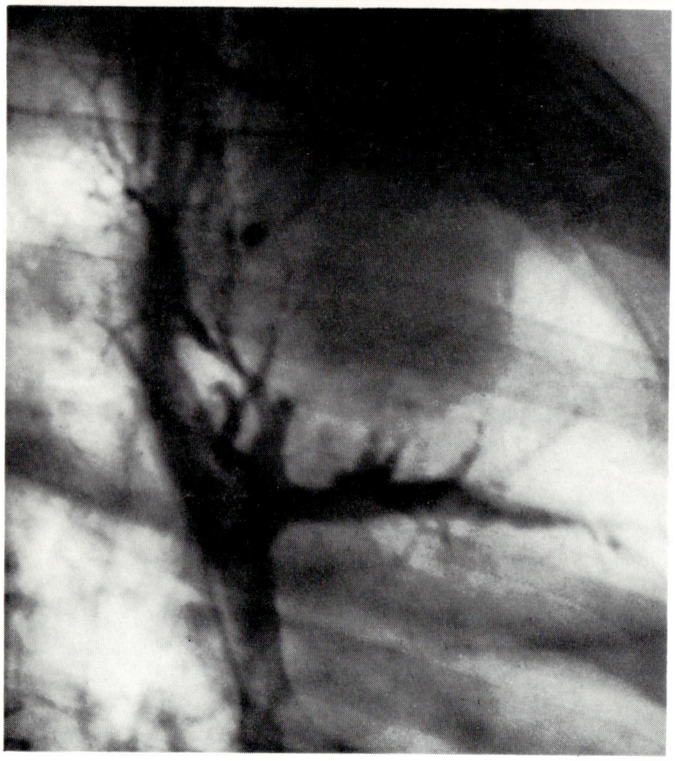

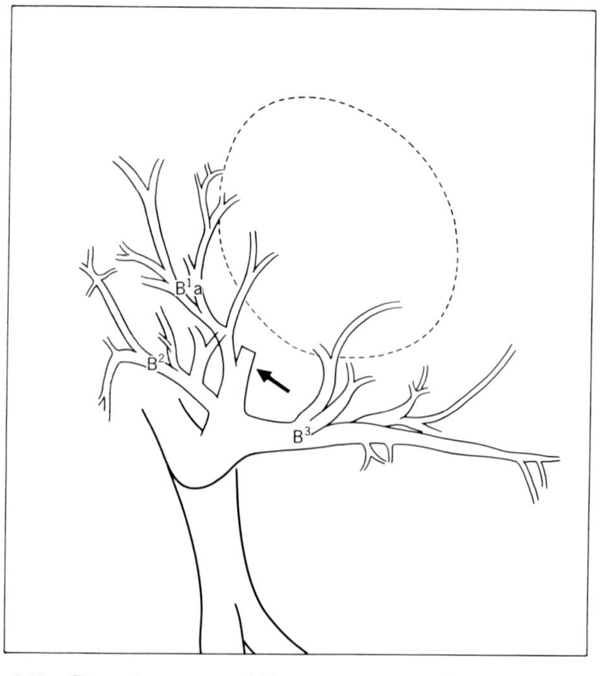


**Fig. 348 Bronchogram, oblique :** A stenosis due to a tumor is present at $B^1b$ (arrow).

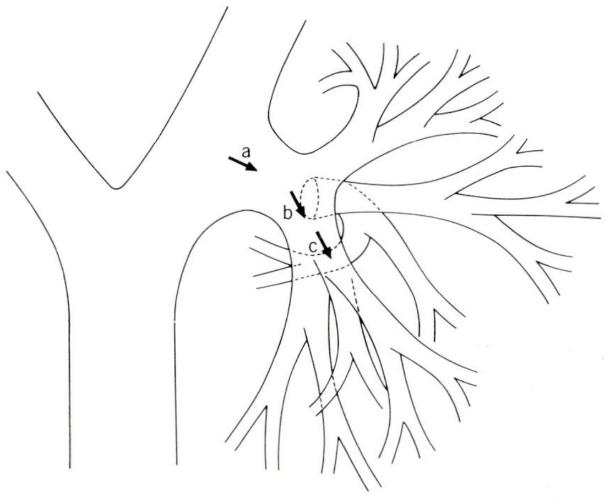


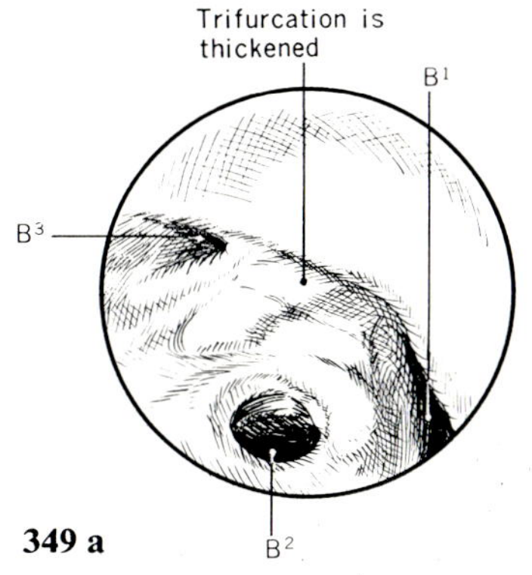


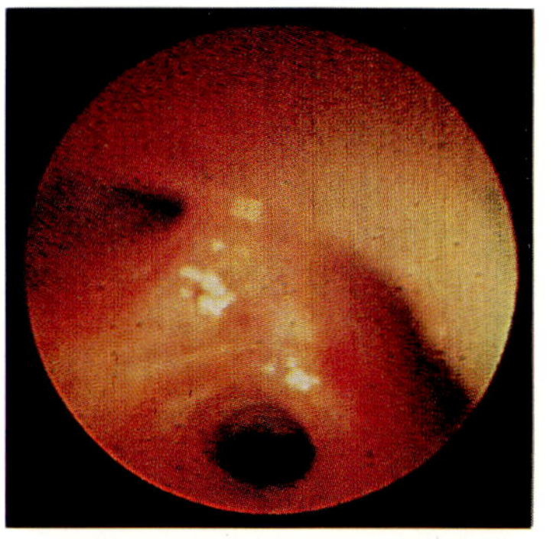

349 a

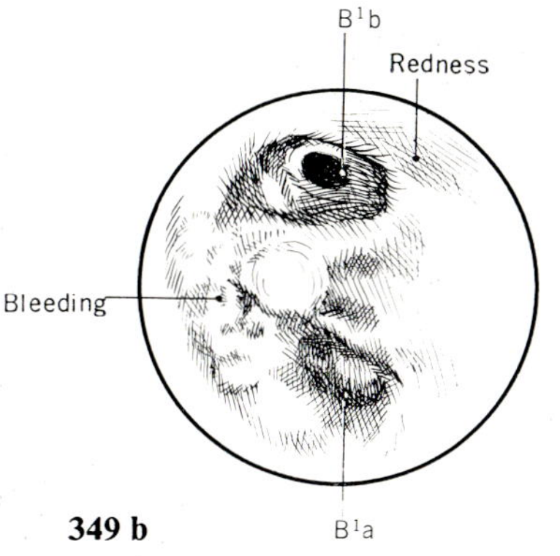


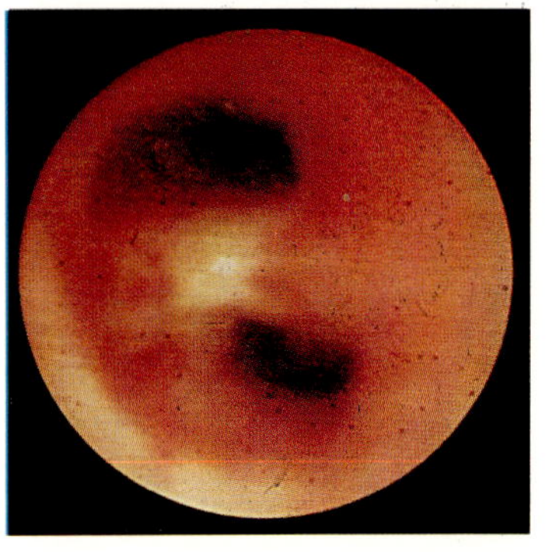

349 b

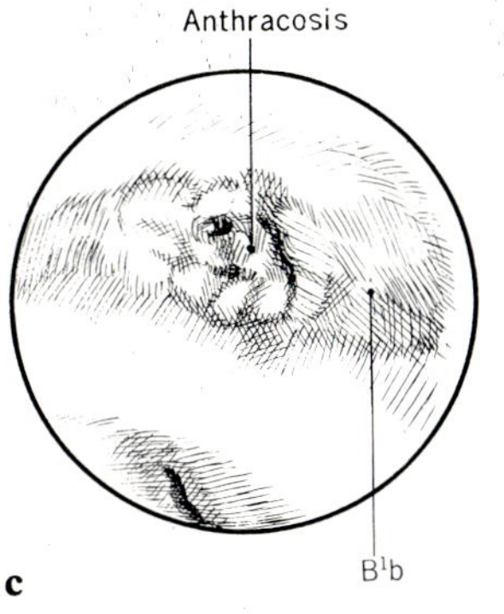


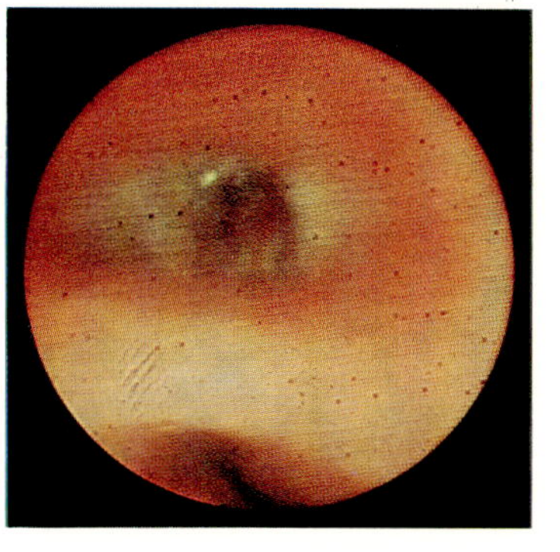

349 c

**Fig. 349 Fiberscopic findings:**

**a.** The trifurcation into $B^1$, $B^2$ and $B^3$ is thickened.

**b.** The septum of $B^1a$ and $B^1b$ is thickened and slightly bleeding. The bifurcation of $B^1b$ is reddened.

**c.** $B^1b$ is gradually stenosed and the mucosa is anthracotic. The periphery is obstructed. Curettage of this $B^1b$ bronchus established the diagnosis: adenocarcinoma.

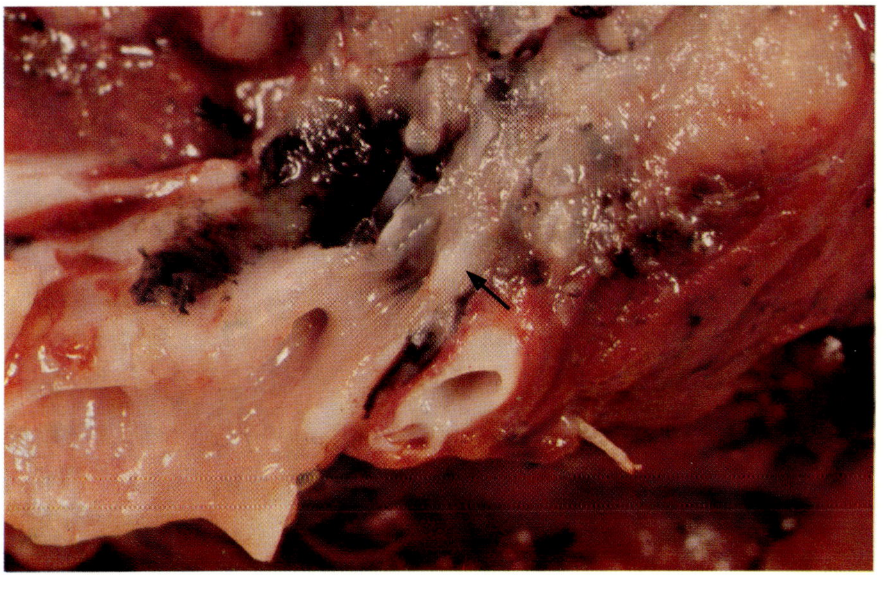

**Fig. 350 Macroscopic findings:** The resected lung shows the affected bronchus with anthracoses submucosally, and that the periphery of the bronchus ($B^1b$) entering the lesion is stenosed (arrow). Findings well correspond with those obtained bronchofiberscopically.

## Case 31 Adenocarcinoma (47, male)

**Case history :** One month ago an abnormal shadow was detected by a mass survey conducted at the patient's firm.
Bronchofiberscopy and cytology at that time resulted in a diagnosis of adenocarcinoma, for which an upper lobectomy was performed.

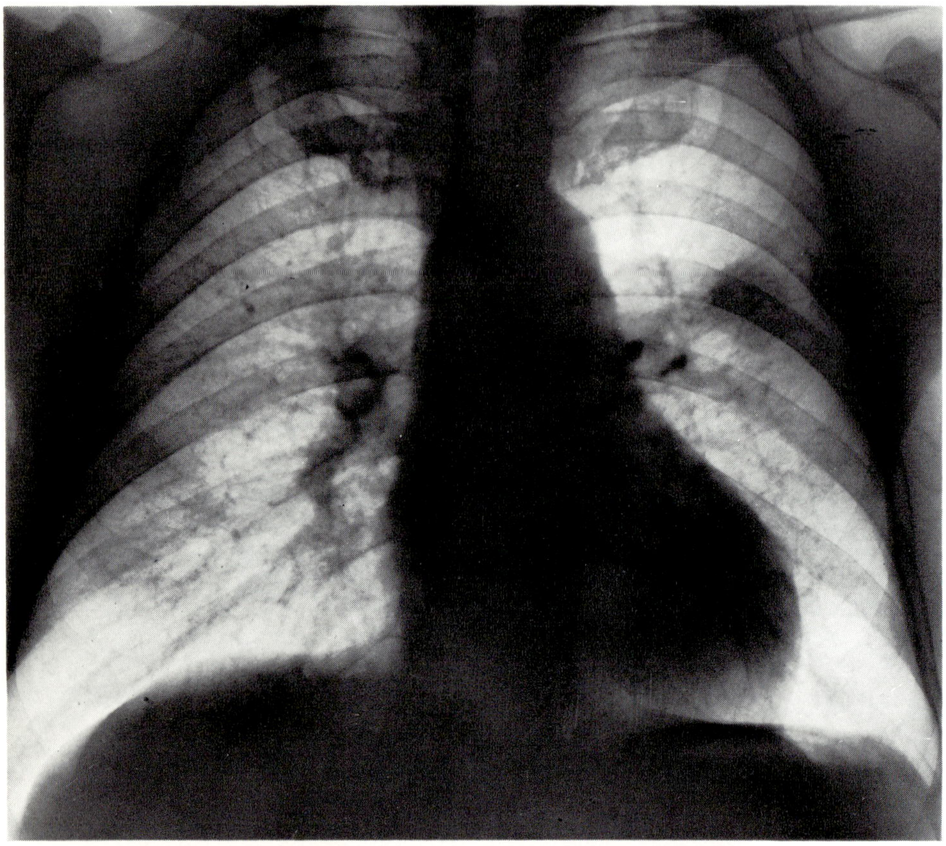

**Fig. 351 Chest X-ray, frontal :** A notched tumor shadow, 25×26 mm, is located in $S^{1+2}c$ of the left upper lobe.

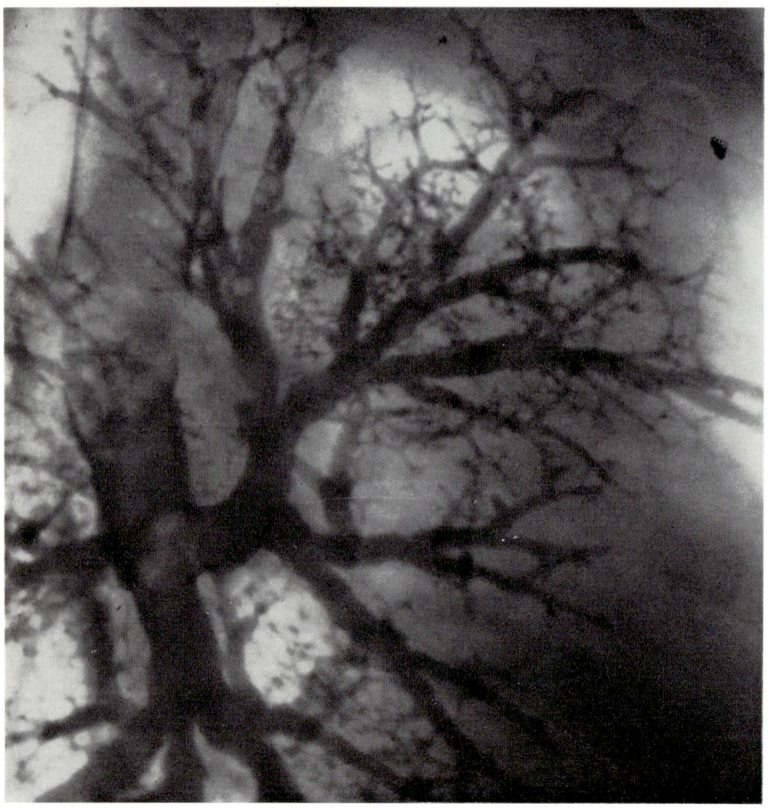

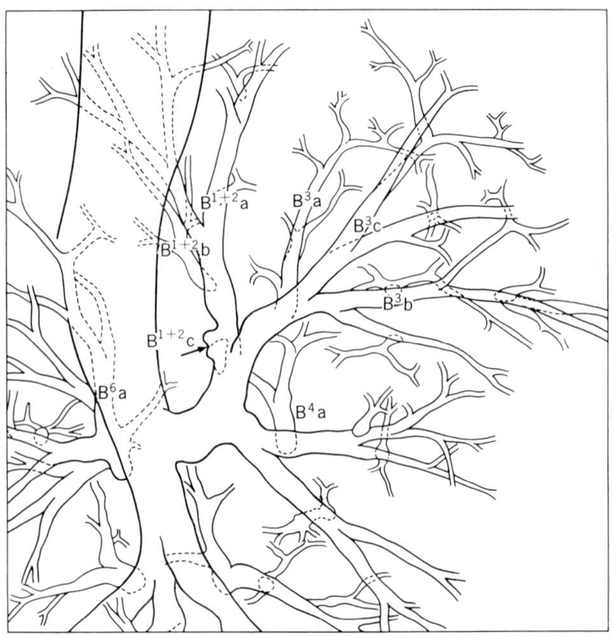


**Fig. 352 Bronchogram, oblique :** An ectatic obstruction is noted at $B^{1+2}c$ (arrow), but the bronchus is normal in other respects. As this picture shows, the affected is $B^{1+2}c$, so that a bronchofiberscope should be guided into this bronchus.

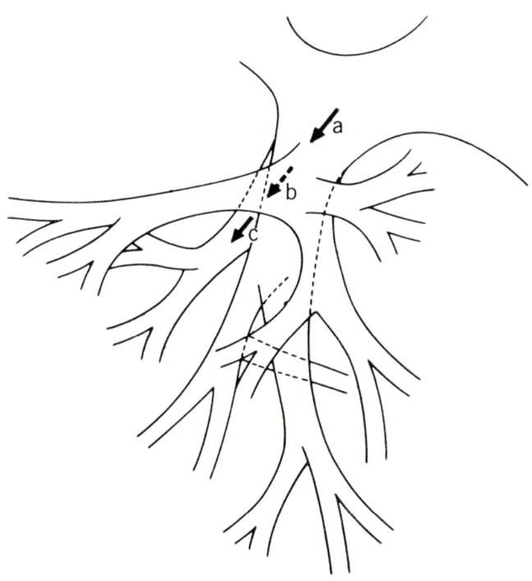


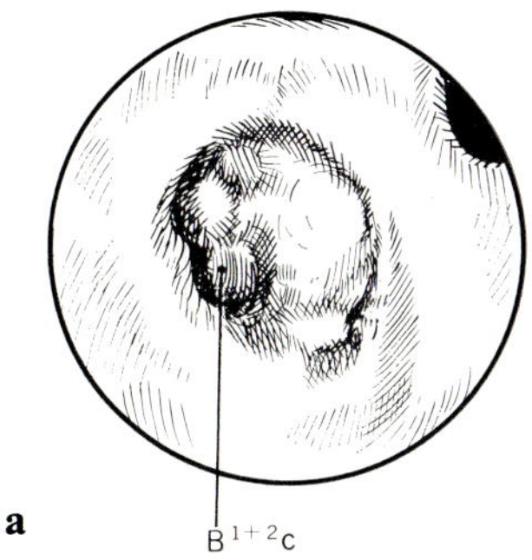


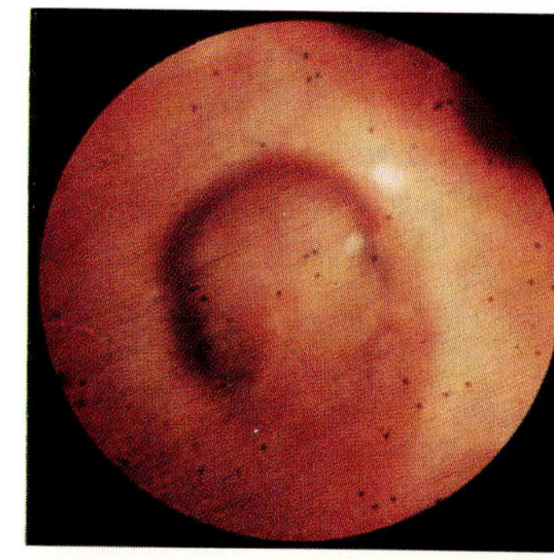

353 a

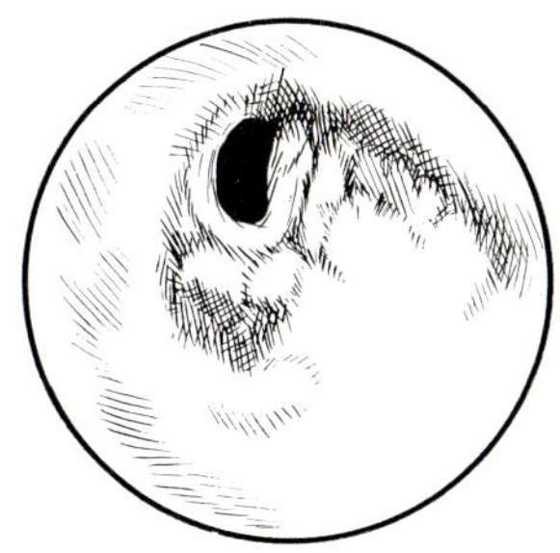

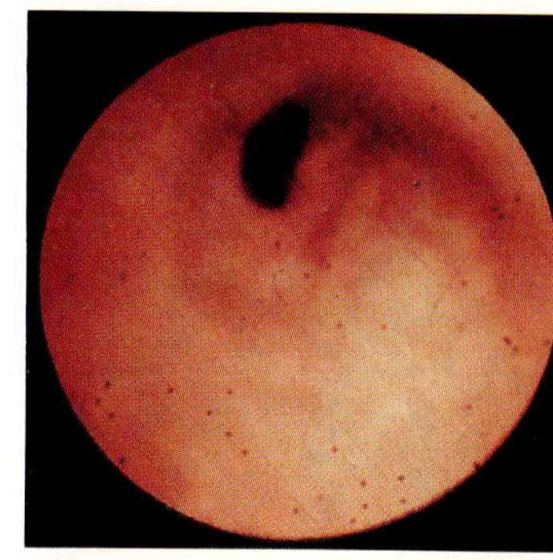

353 b

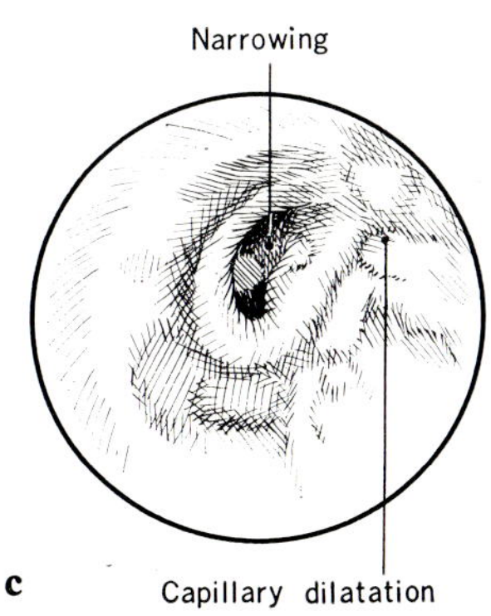


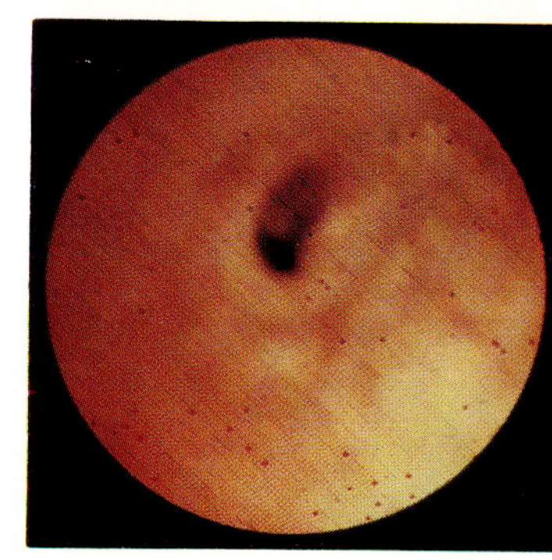

353 c

**Fig. 353 Fiberscopic findings :**

**a.** The orifice of B$^{1+2}$c is shown here, which is narrowed like a staircase.

**b.** When the fiberscope is advanced vascular engorgement is visualized and also lack of normal cartilage structure.

**c.** When it is advanced slightly farther, extreme narrowing of B$^{1+2}$c is disclosed. Insertion of a small curette into this area resulted in the diagnosis of adenocarcinoma.

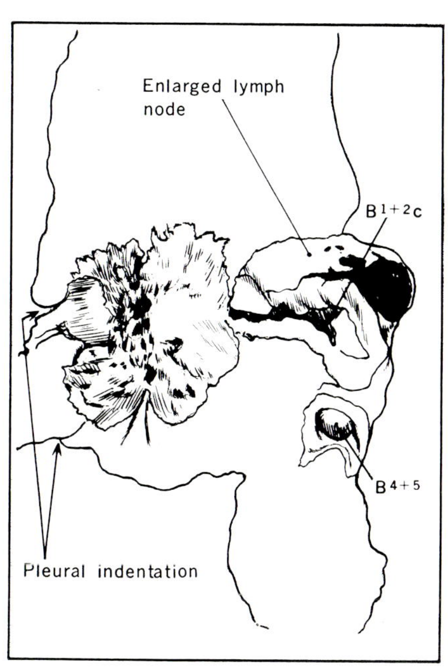


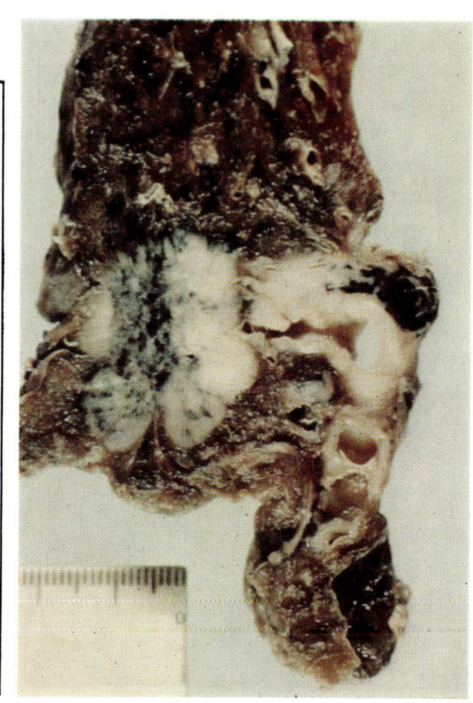

**Fig. 354 Macroscopic findings :** As the resected lung shows, a lymph node is enlarged around B$^{1+2}$c, which is stenosed because of tumescence. The adenocarcinoma is located slightly distal to this part.

## Case 32 Adenocarcinoma (70, female)

**Case history:** This patient had blood-stained sputum five months ago, but it was left untreated. An abnormal shadow was found on the chest X-ray film in a local mass survey. Diagnosis in our hospital: adenocarcinoma by bronchofiberscopic cytology. The right upper lobe was resected.

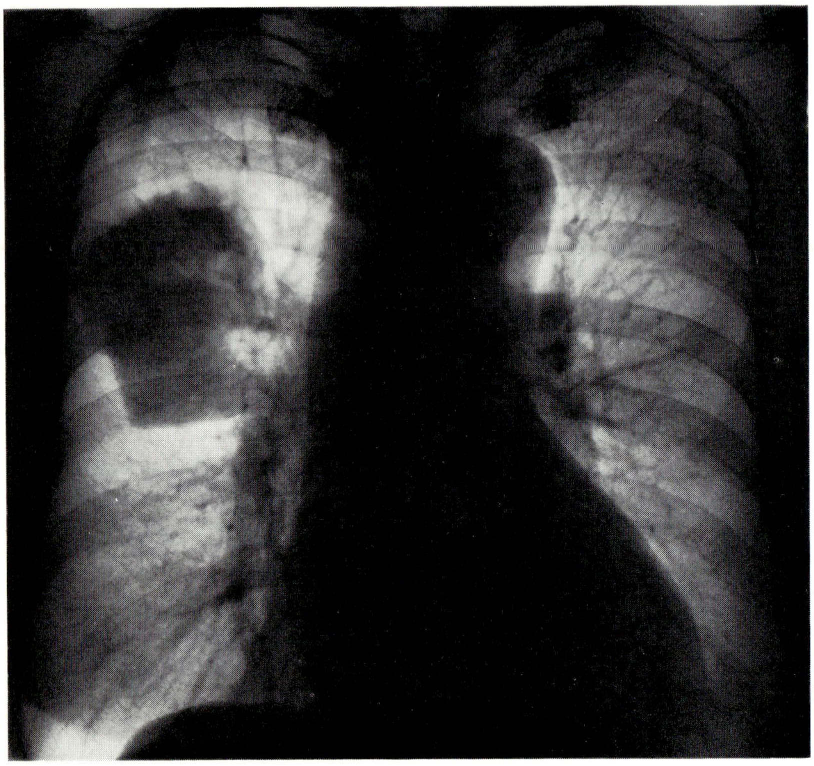

355

**Fig. 355 Chest X-ray, frontal:** A gigantic tumor, 60×80 mm, is located at the anterior segment ($S^3$) and contains a cavity.

**Fig. 356 a Tomogram, frontal** (11 cm from the back): The bronchus, $B^3ai$, is seen as if it has entered the tumor.

**Fig. 356 b Chest X-ray, lateral:** The tumor is located in $S^3$.

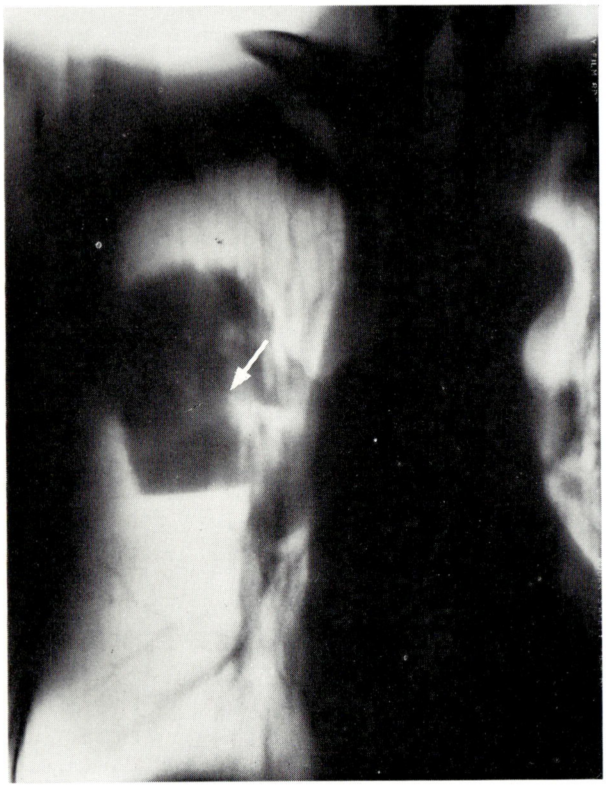

356 a

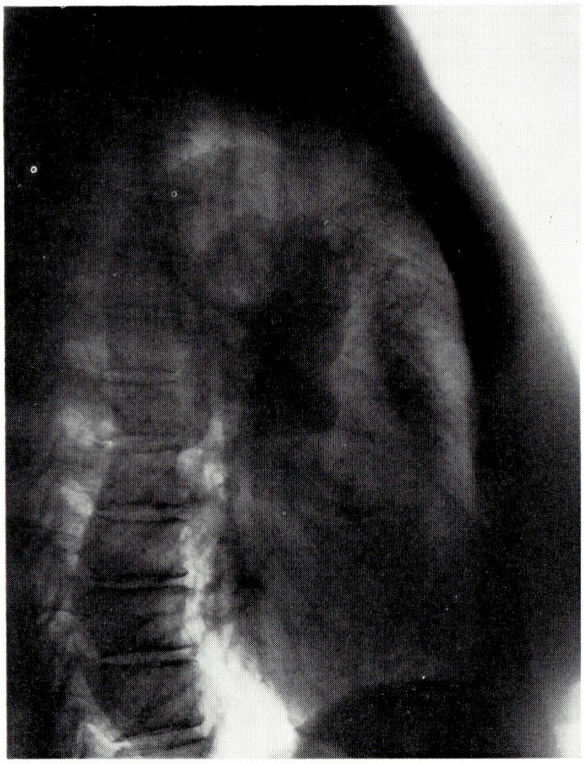

356 b

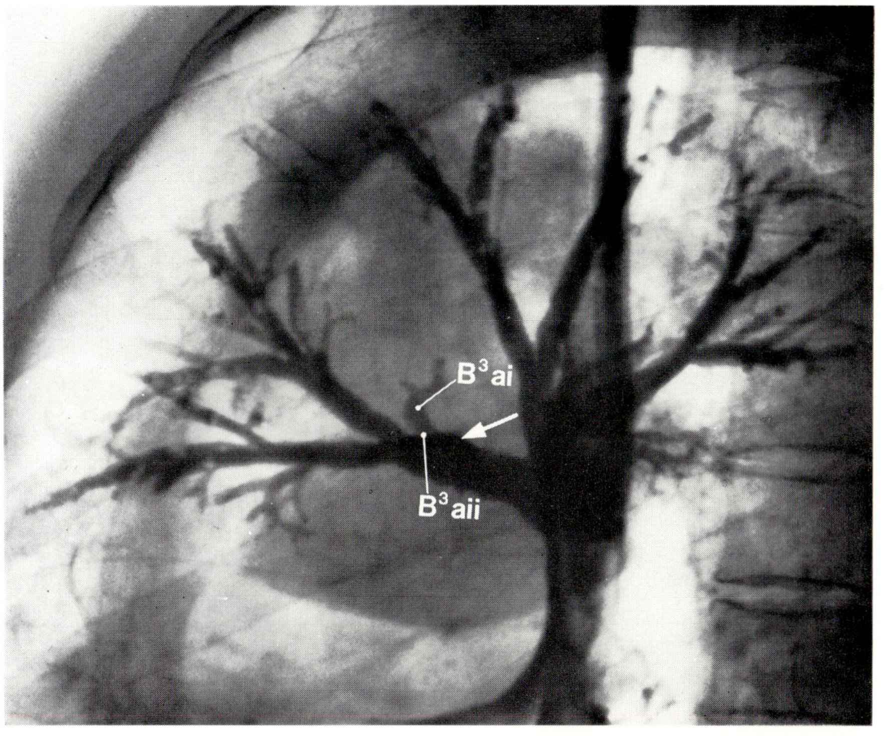


**Fig. 357 Bronchogram, highly oblique:** Stenosis is found at the entrance of $B^3a$ (arrow). $B^3ai\alpha$ and $B^3ai\beta$, which have branched from $B^3ai$, enter the tumor.

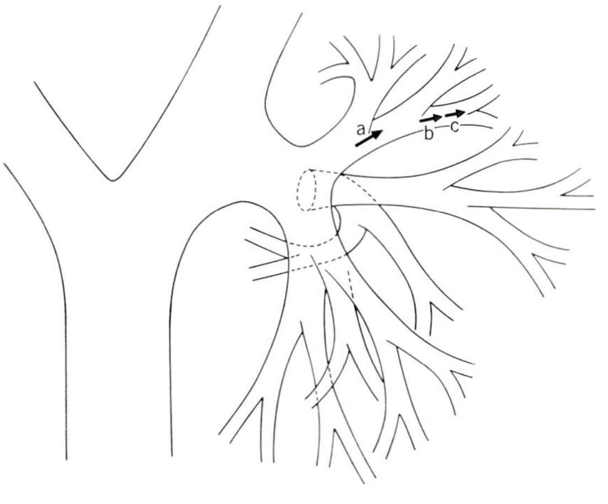


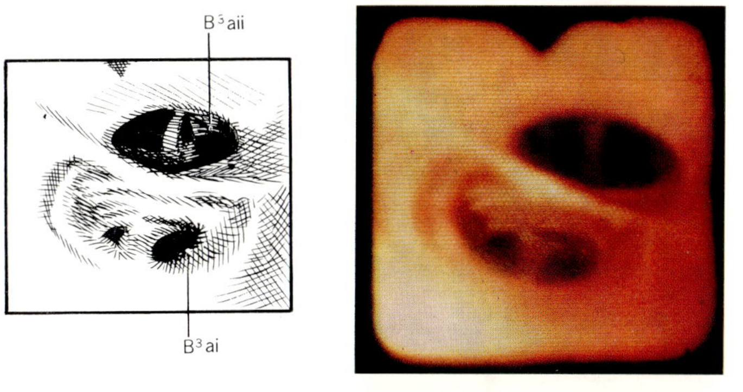


358 a

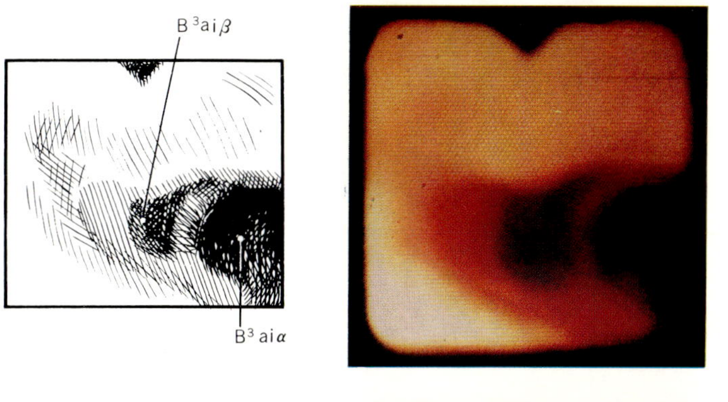


358 b

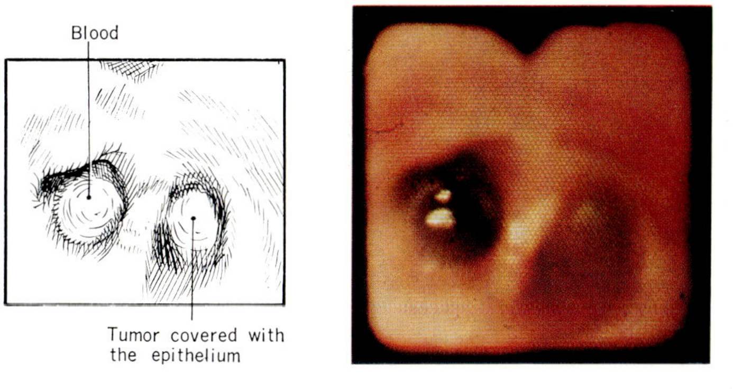


358 c

**Fig. 358 Fiberscopic findings:**
**a.** The orifice to $B^3a$ remains normal, while that to $B^3ai$ is slightly stenotic.
**b.** The orifices to $B^3ai\alpha$ and $B^3ai\beta$ are visualized. There is a protrusion of the mucosa at the latter orifice. The resected lung revealed that the carcinomatous infiltration had reached the bronchial adventitia at this portion.
**c.** $B^3ai\alpha$ is stenosed with a tumor covered with the epithelium. $B^3ai\beta$ is obstructed with blood.

## Case 33 Adenocarcinoma (69, female)

**Chief complaint :** Bloody sputum.

**Case history :** This patient had a cough with frequent blood stained sputum for one and a half years, but did not consult a doctor. In our hospital the case was diagnosed as adenocarcinoma based on sputum cytology. Surgical excision was not possible in this case, as the tumor involved the pulmonary blood vessels by pulmonary angiogram and also extended into the chest wall.

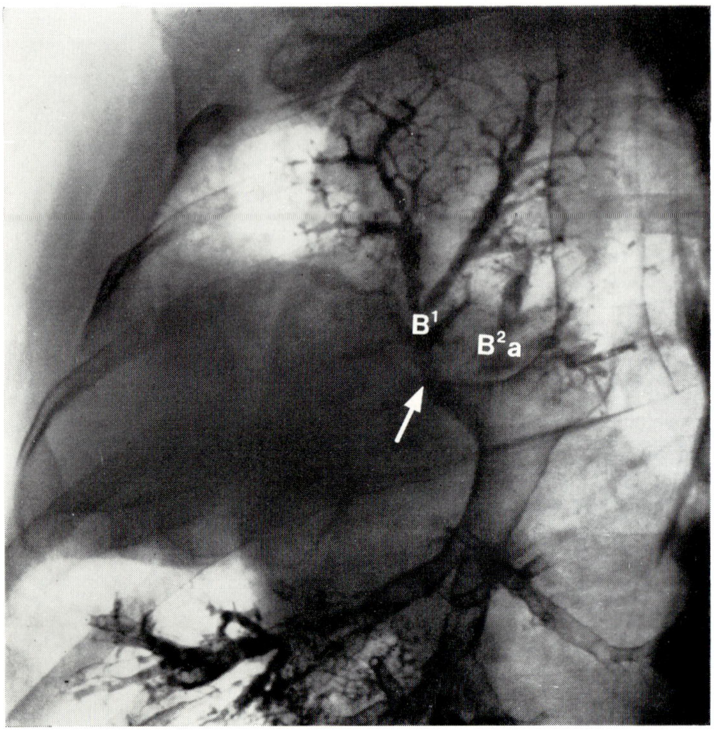


**Fig. 359 Bronchogram, oblique :** The right upper lobe bronchus is stenosed like a staircase. The entrance of $B^3$ is completely obstructed (arrow), with the entrance of $B^2$ stenosed and cylindrical bronchiectases in its peripheral bronchi. $B^1$ entrance is also obstructed but its peripheral bronchi are not ectatic. The tumor which originated in the periphery of $B^3$ has infiltrated its segmental and the upper lobe bronchi.

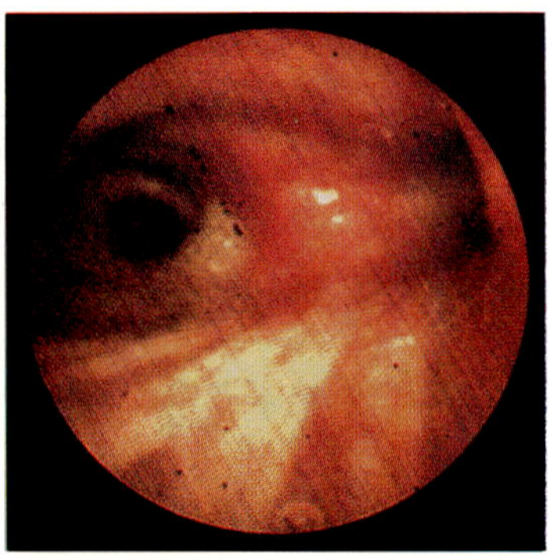

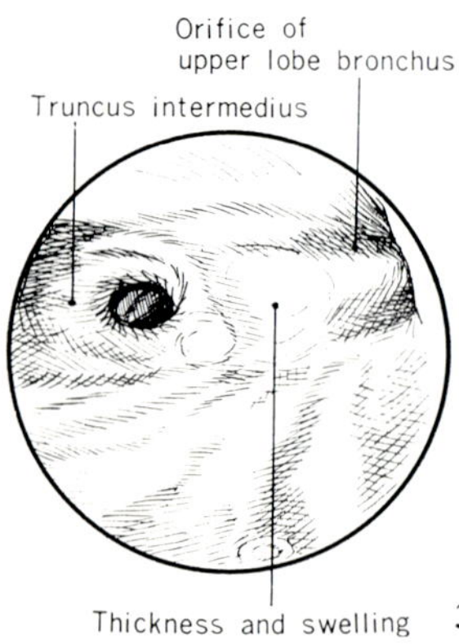


**360 a**

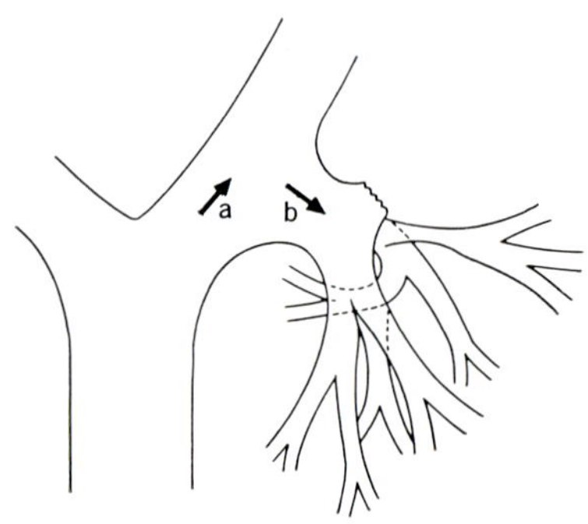


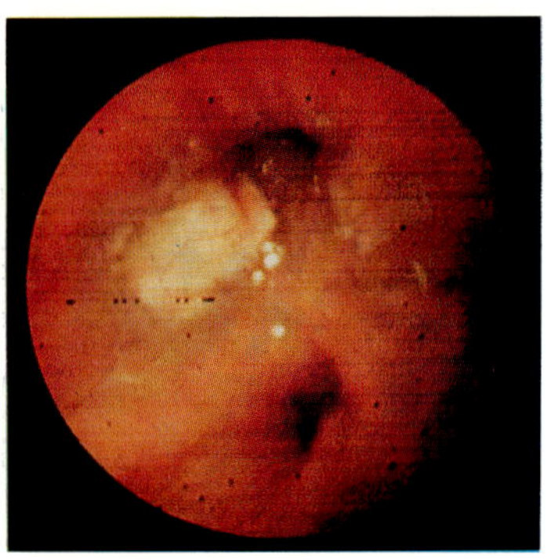

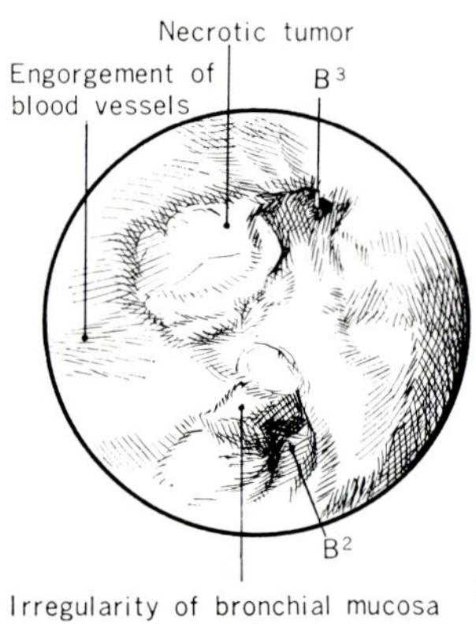


**360 b**

**Fig. 360 Fiberscopic findings :**

**a.** The bifurcation into the upper lobe bronchus and truncus intermedius is thickened and the mucosa is reddened, swollen and involved in vascular engorgement. The orifice of the upper lobe bronchus is stenosed. These findings are due to compression by the swollen lymph node immediately below the bifurcation.

**b.** $B^3$ is obstructed by a white, necrotic tumor. The stenosis of $B^1$ and $B^2$ is conspicuous. The orifice of $B^2$ particularly is uneven and infiltrated by carcinoma. The mucosa is uneven and the cartilagenous rings are not visible around the lumen of the upper lobe bronchus. At the bifurcation of $B^3$ and $B^2$ the blood vessels are engorged. These findings well coincide with those of the bronchogram.

## Case 34 Poorly differentiated adenocarcinoma (large cell type) (67, male)

**Chief complaint :** Bloody sputum.
**Case history :** The patient had cough, sputum and dyspnea during the past one year, and had bloody sputa since 7 months ago. Chest X-ray film at an other hospital revealed no abnormality. Two months ago when he again had bloody sputum, atelectasis was found in the left lung, and the patient was transferred to our hospital.

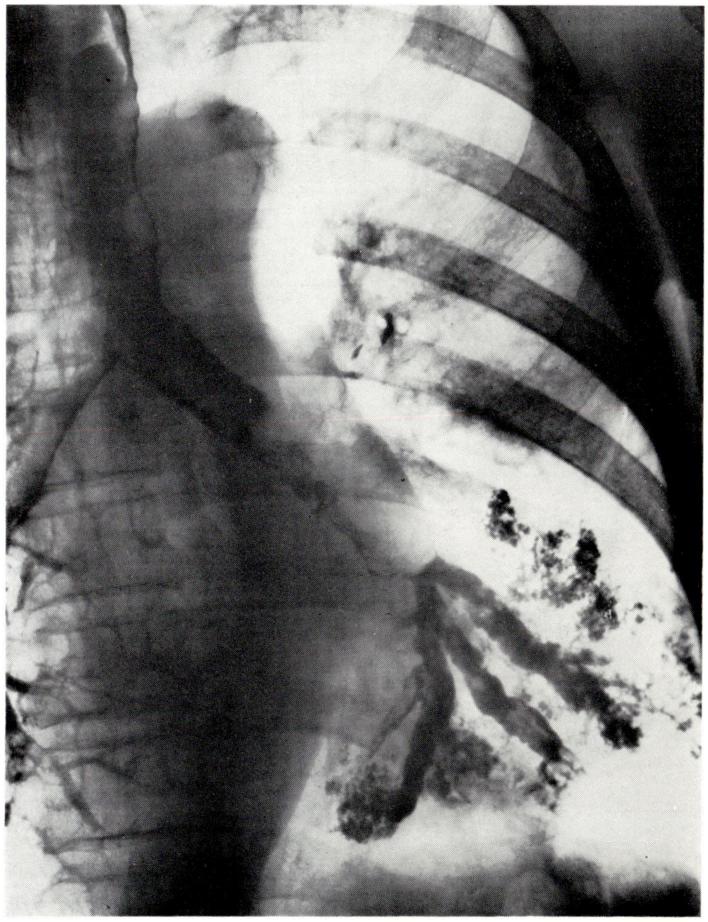

**Fig. 361 Bronchogram, slightly oblique :** A thumb print indentation due to a tumor is seen at the lower portion of the left main bronchus. Contrast medium entering this area reveals an irregular stenosis. Lower lobe bronchi are markedly ectatic.

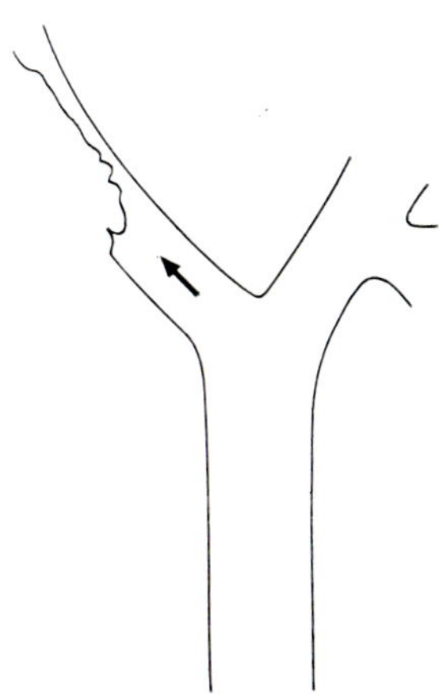

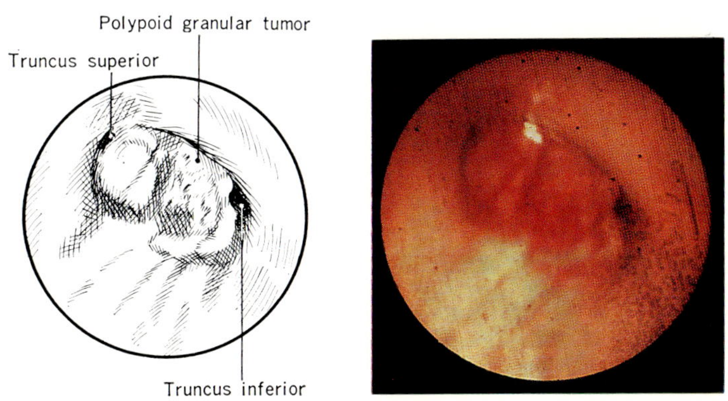


**Fig. 362 Fiberscopic findings:** The left main bronchus is obstructed by a tumor projecting from the posterior wall, having a polypoid granular and uneven surface. Thc biopsy spicimen of the tumor resulted in diagnosis of anaplastic carcinoma. Surgical operation performed; diagnosis was poorly differentiated adenocarcinoma (large cell type), 65×30 mm in size.

## Case 35 Small Cell Carcinoma (37, male)

**Case history:** One month ago, the patient had a pain in the anterior part of his right chest. The chest X-ray revealed an abnormal shadow. He was referred to our hospital. Bronchography and bronchofiberscopy were performed. Bronchofiberscopic cytology revealed a small cell carcinoma. Chemotherapy (Mitomycin® and others) and radiation therapy resulted in a remarkable improvement.

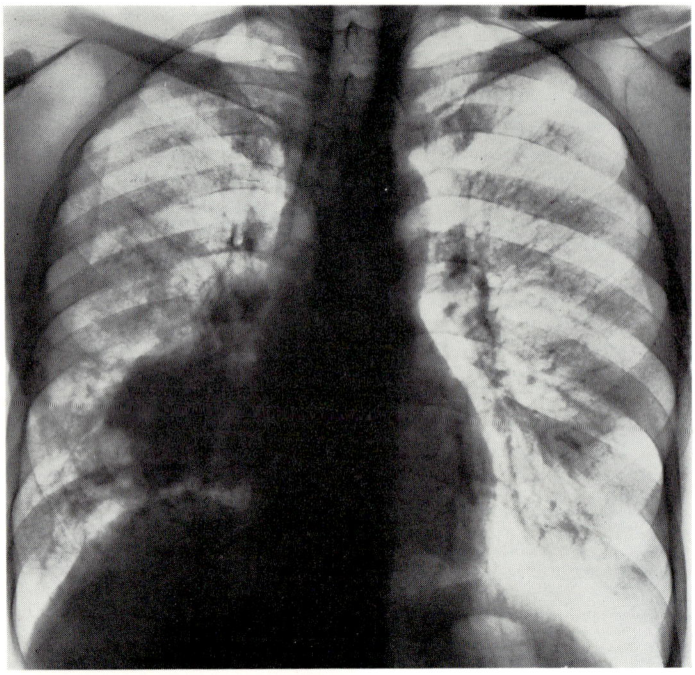

*Pre-chemotherapy*

**Fig. 363 Chest X-ray, frontal:** A tumor, 50×50 mm, is present involving the middle and lower lobe bronchi. Pneumonic infiltration was in the adjacent peripheral lung.

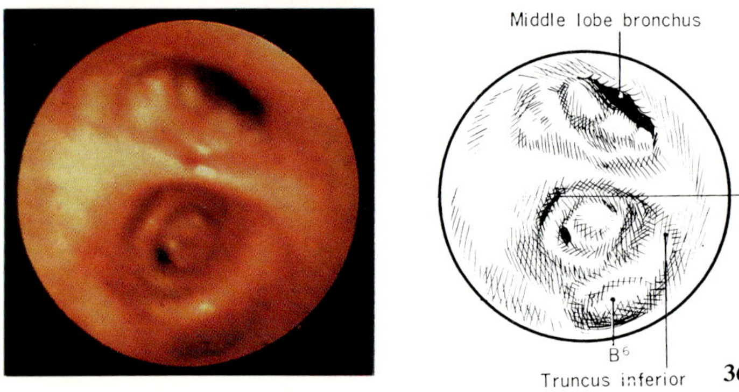


364 a

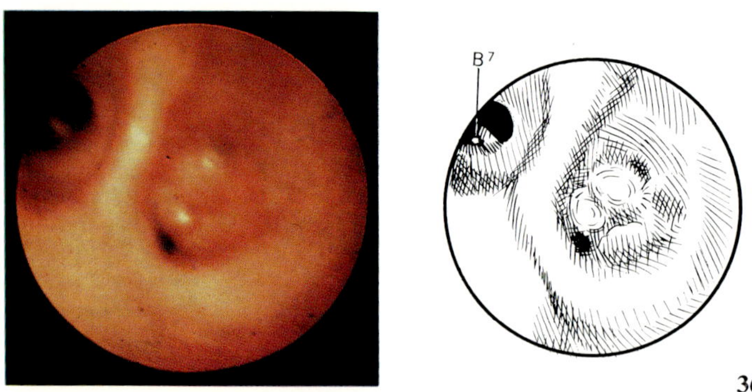


364 b

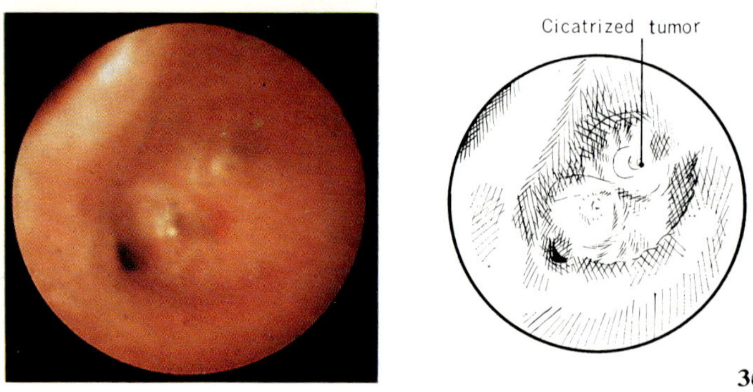


364 c

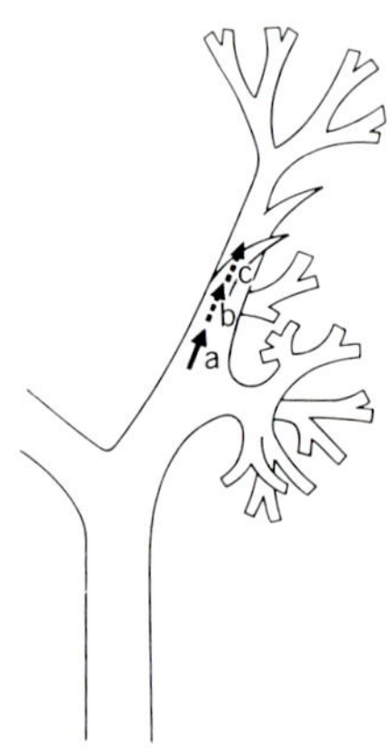


**Fig. 364 Fiberscopic findings:**

a. The main bronchus to the orifice of the truncus intermedius remains normal.
b. The posterior wall of the truncus intermedius is reddened. The mucosa of the orifice to the truncus inferior is irregular and obstructed with sputum.
c. When the sputum is aspirated, the truncus inferior is seen to be completely obstructed with an irregular tumor covered with the mucous membrane. Tumor is partly exposed.

*Post-chemotherapy*

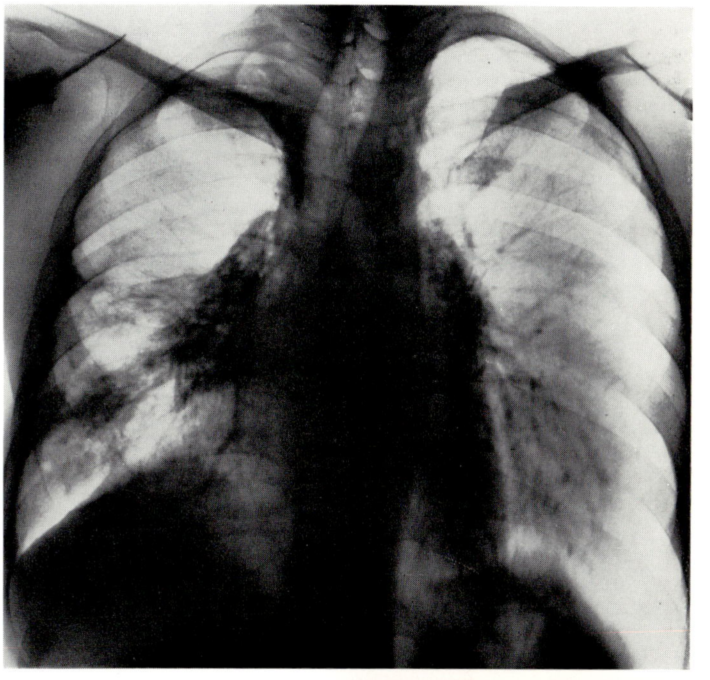

**Fig. 365 Chest X-ray, frontal:** At the right hilum, there is prominent irradiation fibrosis, and the tumor shadow is obscure.

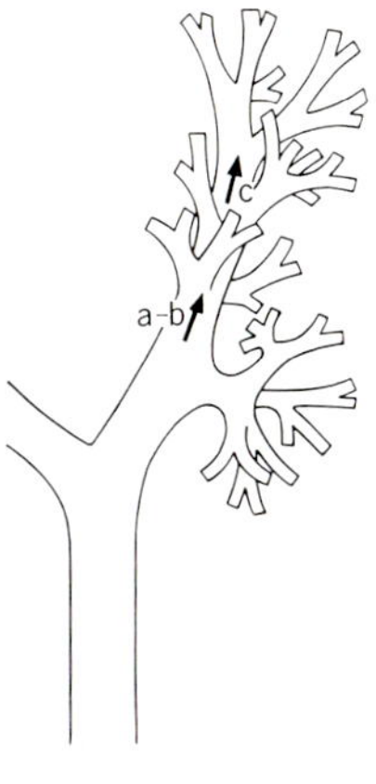


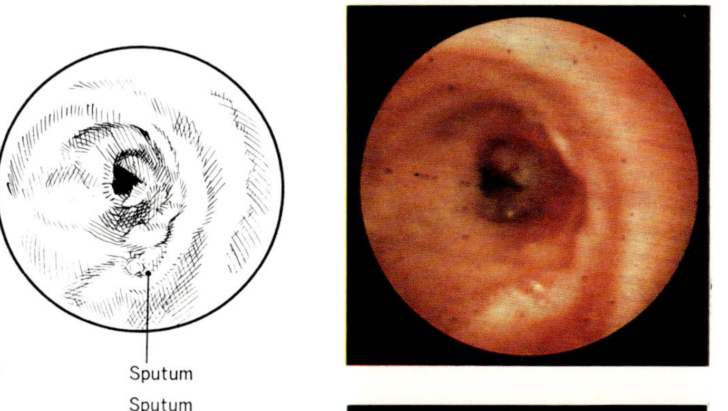


366 a

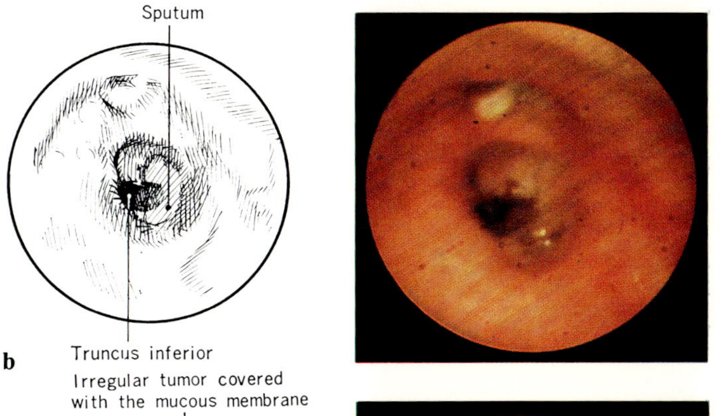


366 b

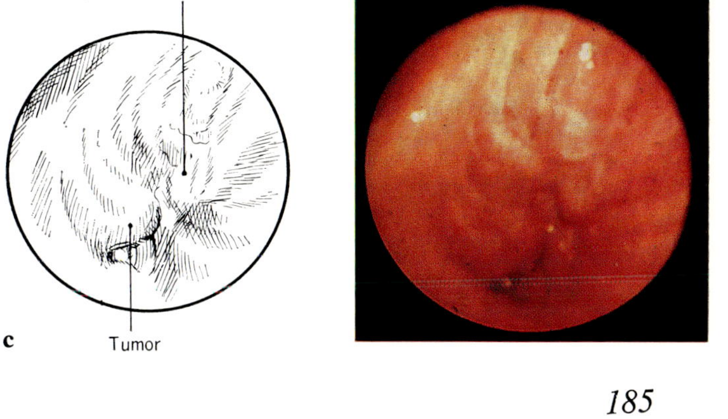


366 c

**Fig. 366 Fiberscopic findings:**

**a.** The tumor previously seen at the orifice of the truncus inferior has disappeared entirely and slight edema now visualized of the mucosa. The orifices of $B^6$, $B^7$ and $B^{8+9+10}$ can be seen beyond.

**b.** Edema noted at the orifice $B^{8+9+10}$, with unclear cartilages.

**c.** More peripherally, the bronchus ($B^{8+9+10}$) is practically occluded. The surface of the tumor is not irregular nor bleeding as noted previously, but is cicatrized.

## Case 36 Small Cell Carcinoma (49, female)

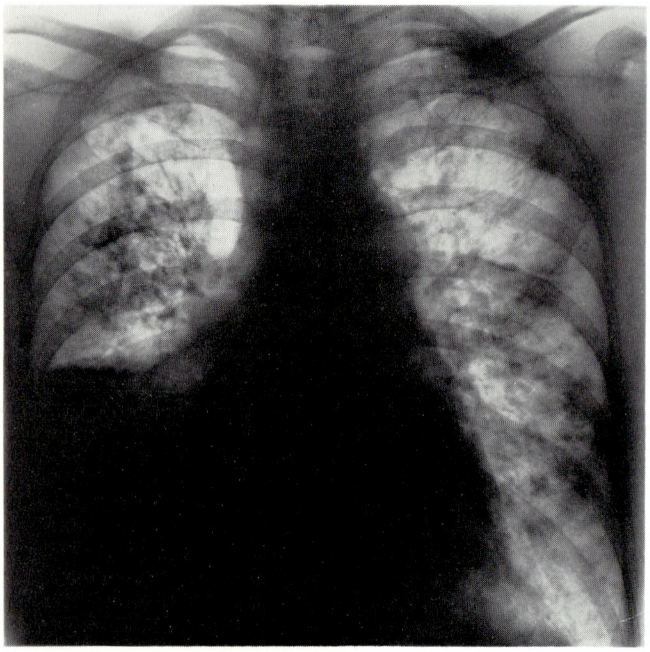

**Case history :** This patient had bloody sputum half year ago, and a chronic cough with sputum for several years. She was diagnosed as bronchial asthma. A month ago, her voice became hoarse so she came to our hospital. Biopsy with the bronchofiberscope resulted in a diagnosis of a small cell carcinoma. Mitomycin® and Urokinase® were administered, together with irradiation (4,000R). The patient died after 7 months.

*Pre-chemotherapy*

**Fig. 367 Chest X-ray, frontal :** Pre-chemotherapy and pre-irradiation.

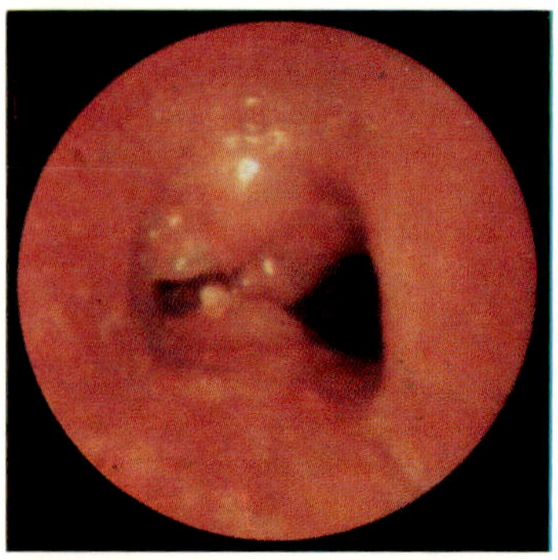

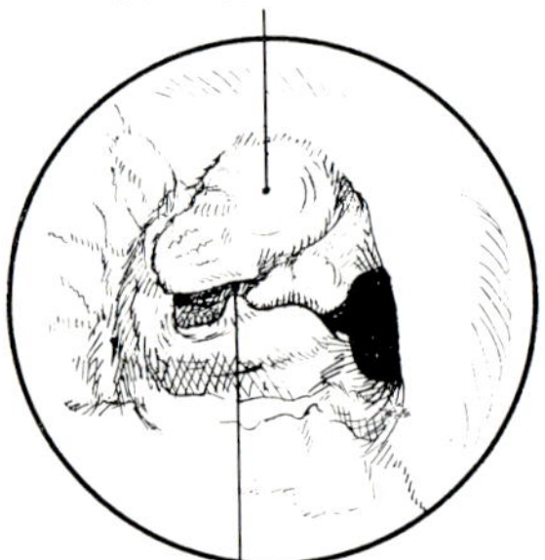


**368 a**

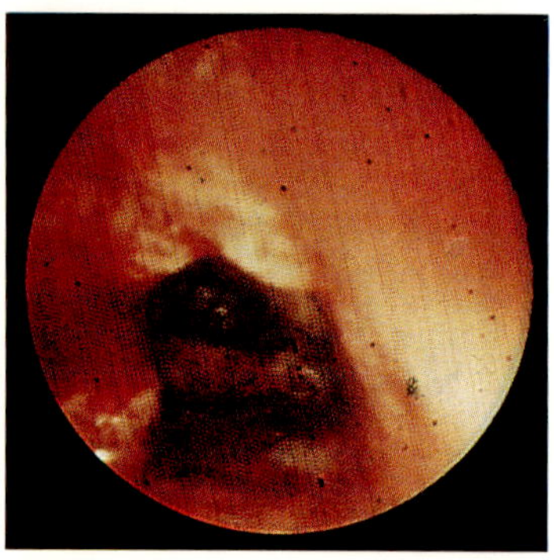

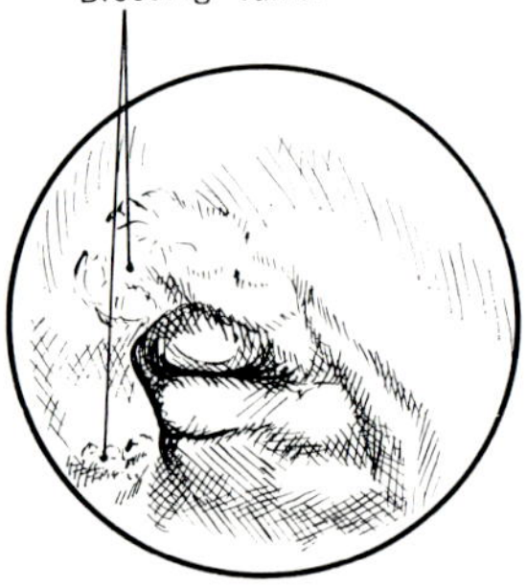


**368 b**

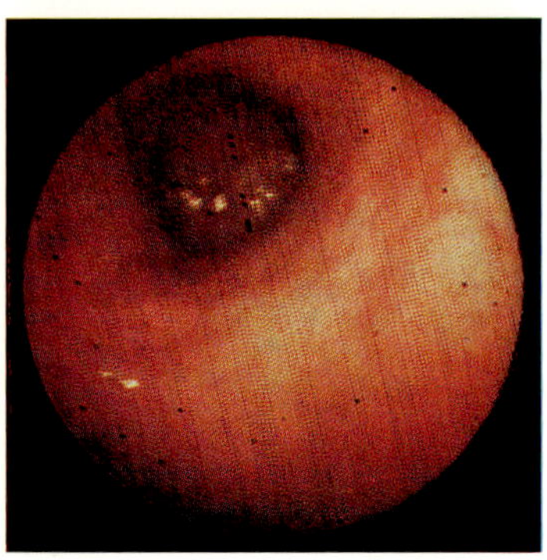

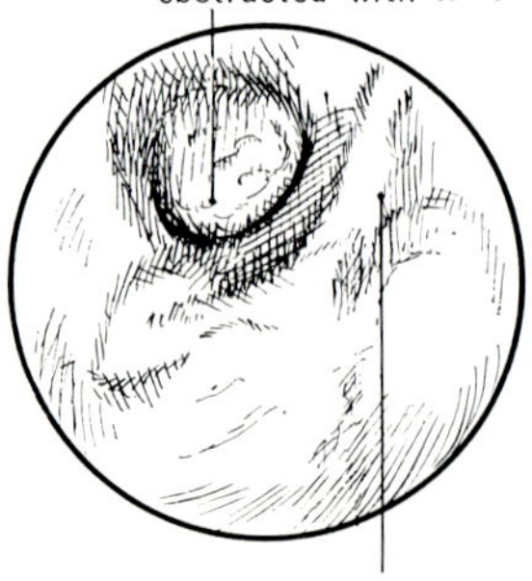


**368 c**

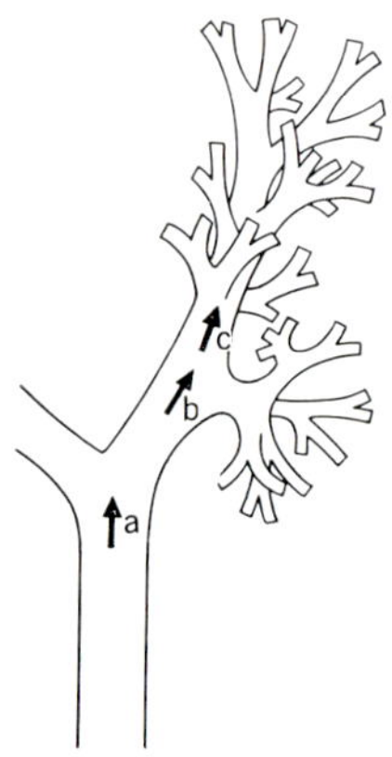


**Fig. 368 Fiberscopic findings :** The tumor severely infiltrated the lower part of the trachea to the tracheal bifurcation. There is obviously infiltration in the main bronchus accompanied by stenosis. Deeper, the truncus intermedius is markedly infiltrated, with bleeding. The middle lobe bronchus is obstructed by the tumor.
**a.** Tracheal bifurcation
**b.** Truncus intermedius
**c.** Middle lobe bronchus

*Post-chemotherapy*

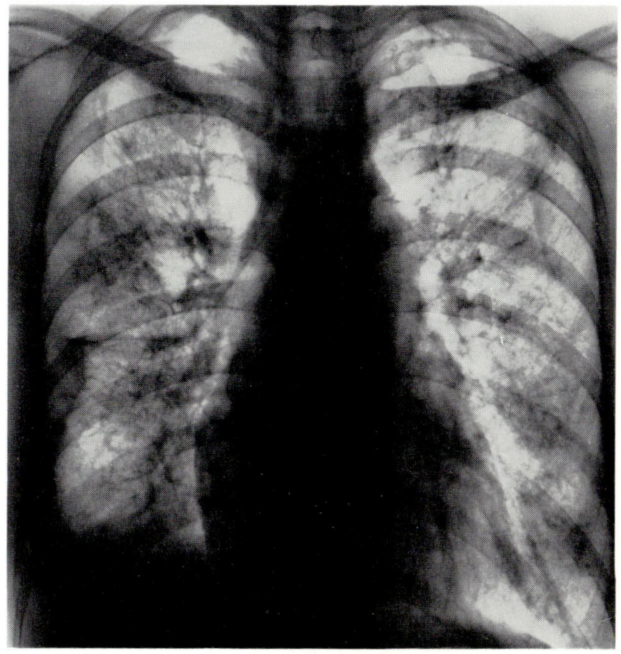

**Fig. 369 Chest X-ray, frontal:** Post-chemotherapy and post-irradiation.

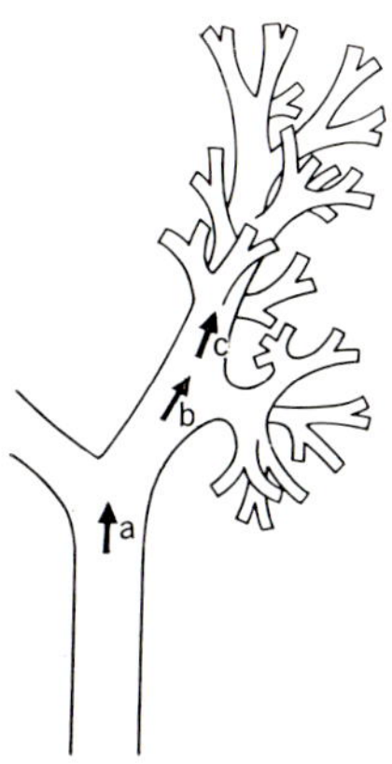


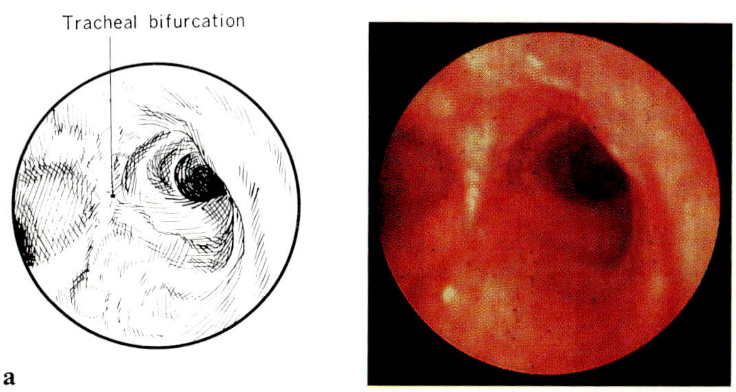


**370 a**

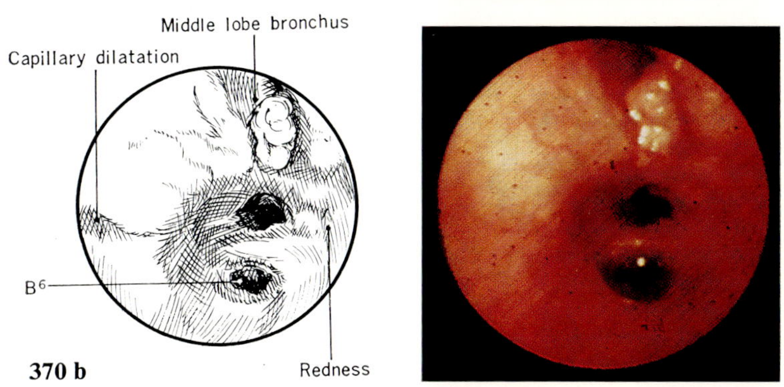


**370 b**

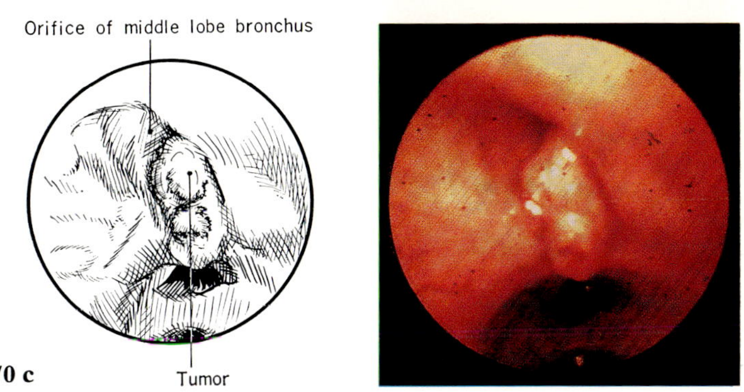


**370 c**

**Fig. 370 Fiberscopic findings:** Some improvement is noted in the major bronchi by the combined application of chemotherapy and irradiation. Principal tumor situated in the middle lobe bronchus, however, was still present.
**a.** Tracheal bifurcation
**b.** Truncus intermedius
**c.** Middle lobe bronchus

## Case 37 Small Cell Carcinoma (56, male)

**Case history :** A year ago the patient's chronic cough was diagnosed as bronchial asthma at some clinic. A month ago he had a fever of 39°C and was admitted to a hospital with the diagnosis of pneumonia. On bronchography, obstruction was found in the left upper lobe. He was referred to our hospital as a possible lung cancer case. At our hospital, sputum cytology repeated three times were negative. Bronchofiberscopic cytology resulted in the diagnosis of small cell carcinoma. The therapy was initially two injections of Mitomycin® (10 mg), introduced into the bronchial artery, followed by irradiation.

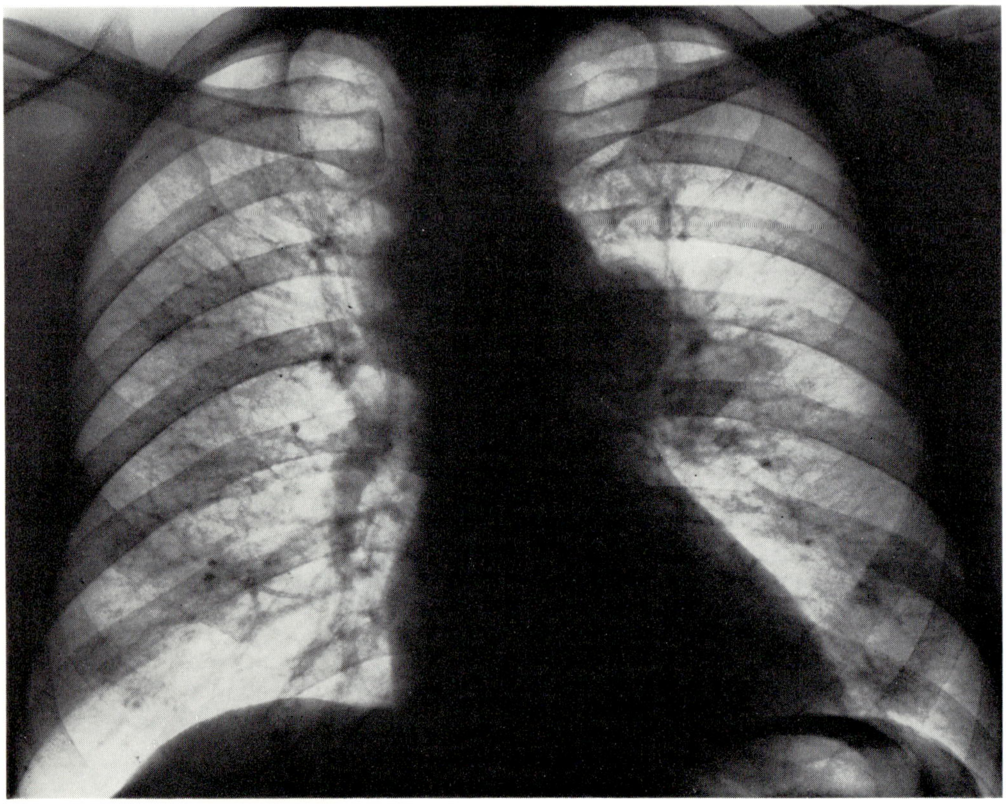

**Fig. 371 Chest X-ray, frontal :** There is a tumor mass in the left hilum with a small adjacent area of pneumonitis. An enlarged lymph node is present near the right mediastinum.

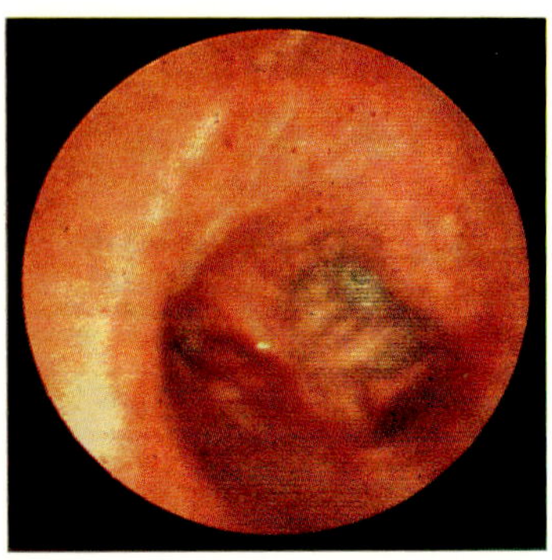

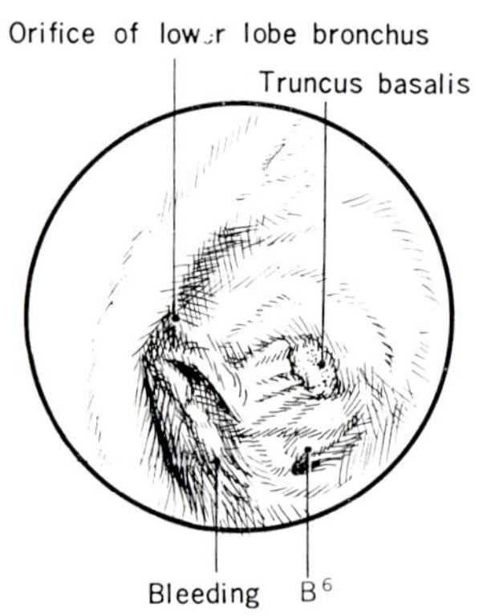


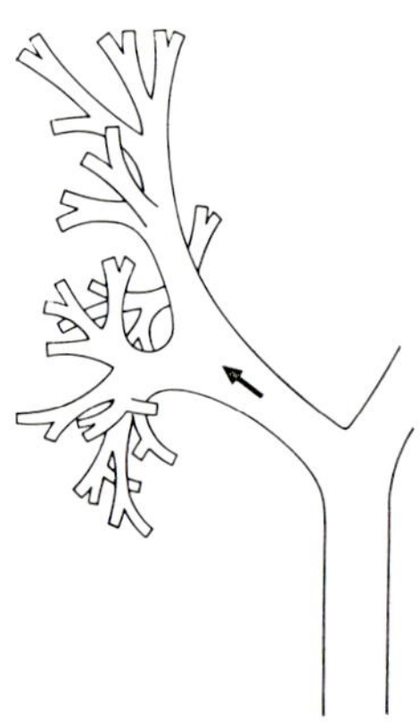

**Fig. 372 Fiberscopic findings :** The left truncus superior is obstructed with a tumor and the lingular bronchus is slightly stenosed. The entire mucosa of the truncus superior is very irregular, lacking cartilage rings and accompanied by bleeding. In small cell carcinoma one often finds malignant infiltration surrounding the tumor focus in the bronchus.

# Case 38 Small Cell Carcinoma (35, male)

**Case history :** The patient was warned two years previously of an abnormal shadow on his chest X-ray film, which was suspicious of lung cancer. He finally came to our hospital and on bronchofiberscopy, a tumor was found in the left truncus inferior. Cytology at that time revealed a small cell carcinoma. He was irradiated, the total dosage being 4,000 R. Recently his cough and sputum increased, suggesting recrudescence. Bronchofiberscopy was again performed.

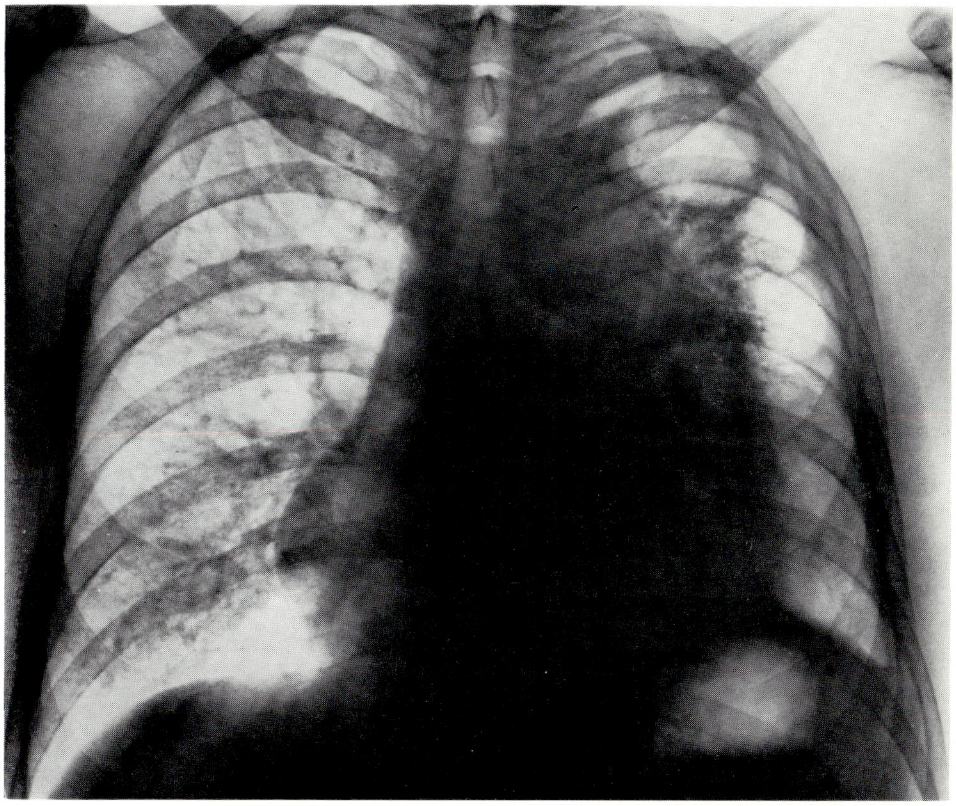

**Fig. 373 Chest X-ray, frontal :** The film is one taken post-irradiation. The mediastinum is thickened. Irradiation fibrosis is marked over the area from the left upper to the lower lung field. The tumor remains indistinct since it is obscured by fibrosis.

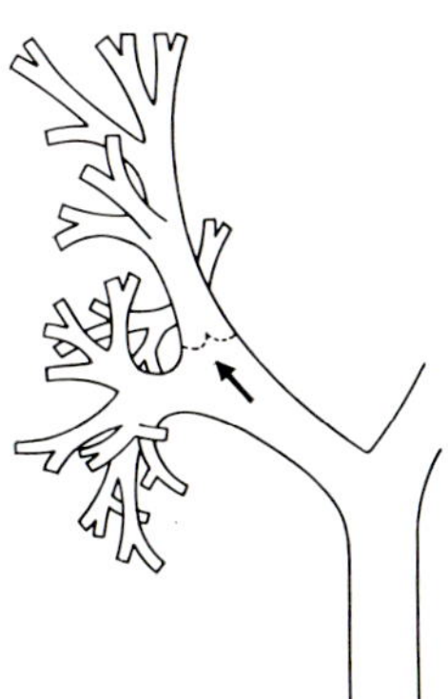

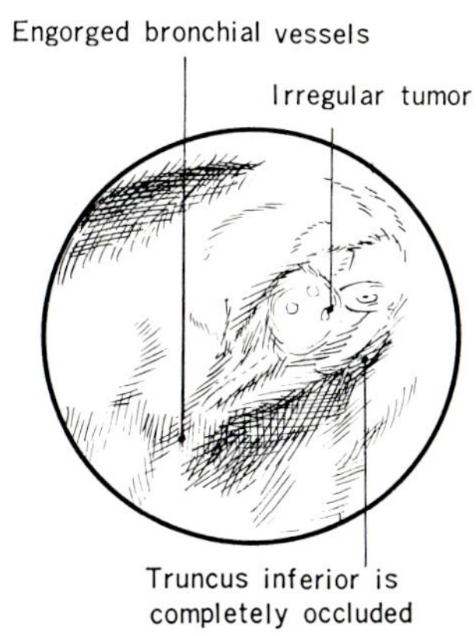


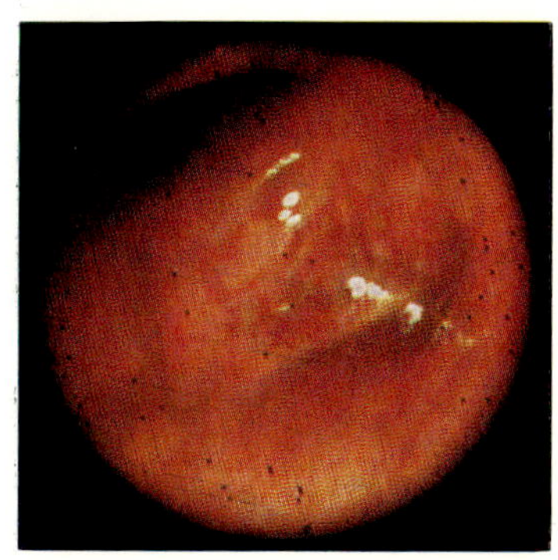

**Fig. 374 Fiberscopic findings :** The left truncus inferior is completely obstructed. The spur therein is slightly irregular and uneven. This is considered to be the site of the tumor. The upper lobe septum is also thickened. The infiltration extends from the orifice of the lower lobe bronchus to the lower part of the left main bronchus. Small cell carcinoma was re-confirmed in the specimen obtained with a small curette from the lower lobe bronchus. Diagnosis : Recrudescence of small cell carcinoma.

## Case 39 Alveolar Cell Carcinoma (33, male)

**Case history :** The patient had paroxysms of cough for three months and was referred to our hospital as a lung cancer suspicious. Cytologic examination of the sputum revealed malignant cells and bronchofiberscopy followed immediately. Curettage diagnosed the case as a well differentiated adenocarcinoma. Chemotherapy and radiation were given but the patient died after a year. Autopsy diagnosed as alveolar cell carcinoma.

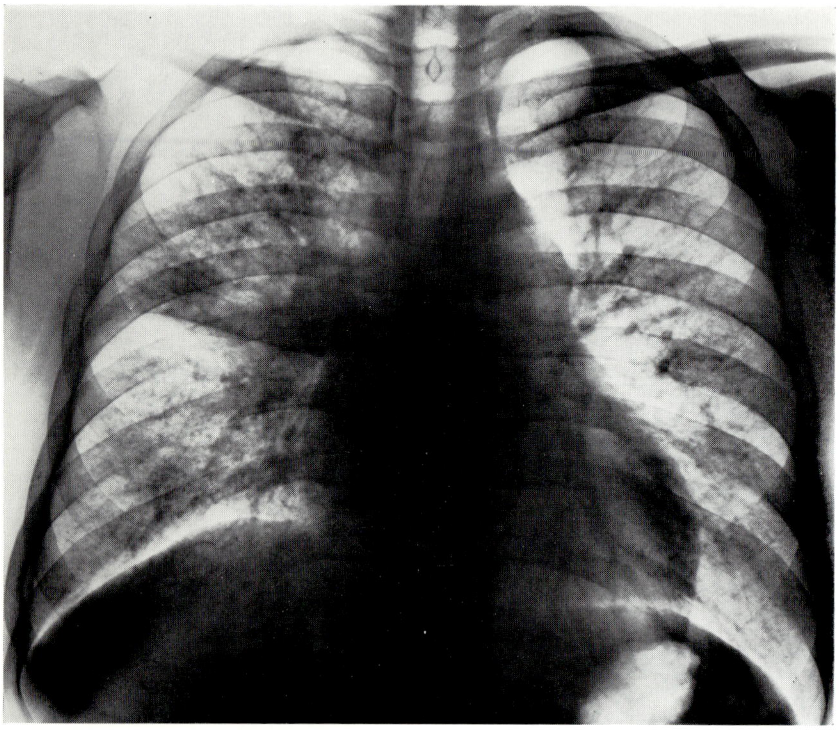

**Fig. 375 Chest X-ray, frontal :** A dense shadow indicative of infiltration is located in the right upper lobe. Atelectasis is observed in the anterior segment ($S^3$) in particular. Infiltrative shadow is also present in the middle lobe.

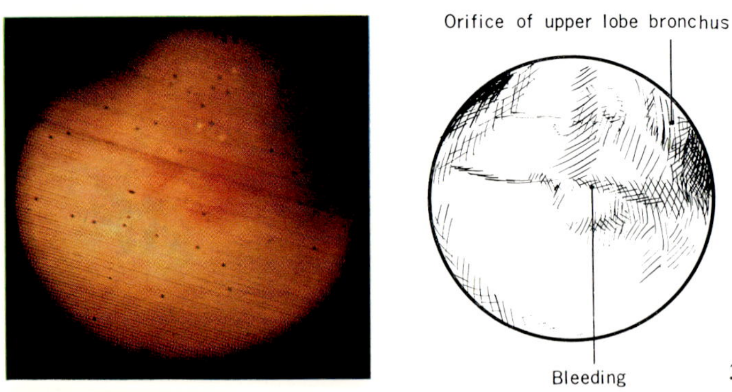


376a

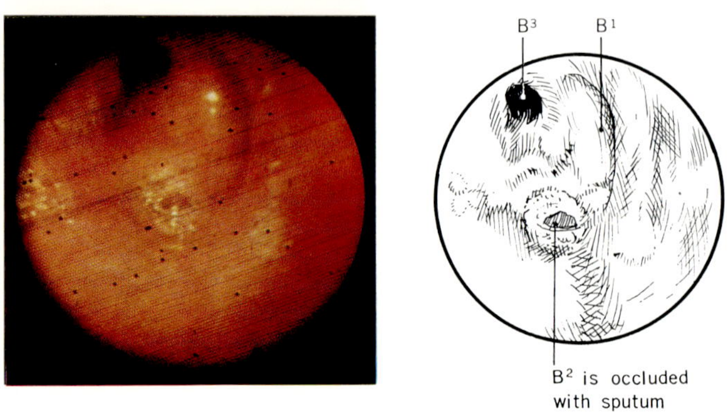


376 b

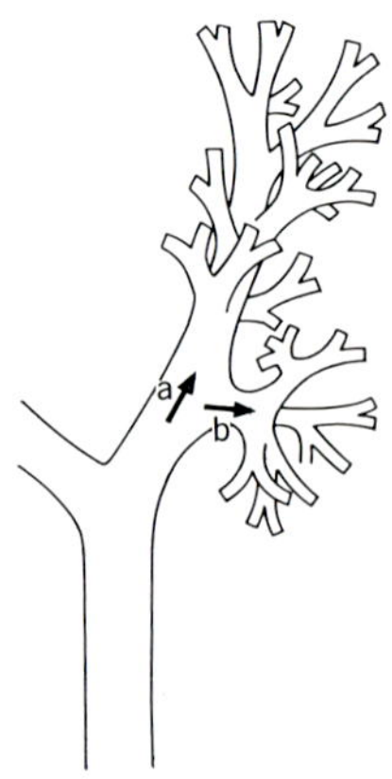


**Fig. 376 Fiberscopic findings :**

**a.** Bleeding site at the orifice of the right upper lobe bronchus. The orifice of the upper lobe is markedly swollen, obscuring the cartilage rings.

**b.** The right upper lobe bronchus and the orifices of the segmental bronchi are reddened and swollen markedly. Each of these orifices provides similar findings. The orifice of $B^3$ is slightly uneven and irregular. $B^2$ is occluded with sputum. These findings are hardly distinguishable from those of an inflammation.

## Case 40 Metastasis of Seminoma (41, male)

**Case history :** Five years ago the patient had a testicular neoplasm, which was resected. Pathological diagnosis was seminoma. An abnormal shadow was detected in the right lung a month after orchidectomy. Chemotherapy with Mitomycin® was given. As the tumor continued to grow, radiation with $^{60}Co$ was given two years ago, with the tumor practically disappearing. A year ago, another tumor grew at the same location and the right upper lobe became obstructed. The patient then came to our hospital and bronchofiberscopy was performed. Cytology by means of a curette passed through the bronchofiberscope resulted in a diagnosis of metastatic seminoma. Radiation therapy was given by means of a linear accelerator.

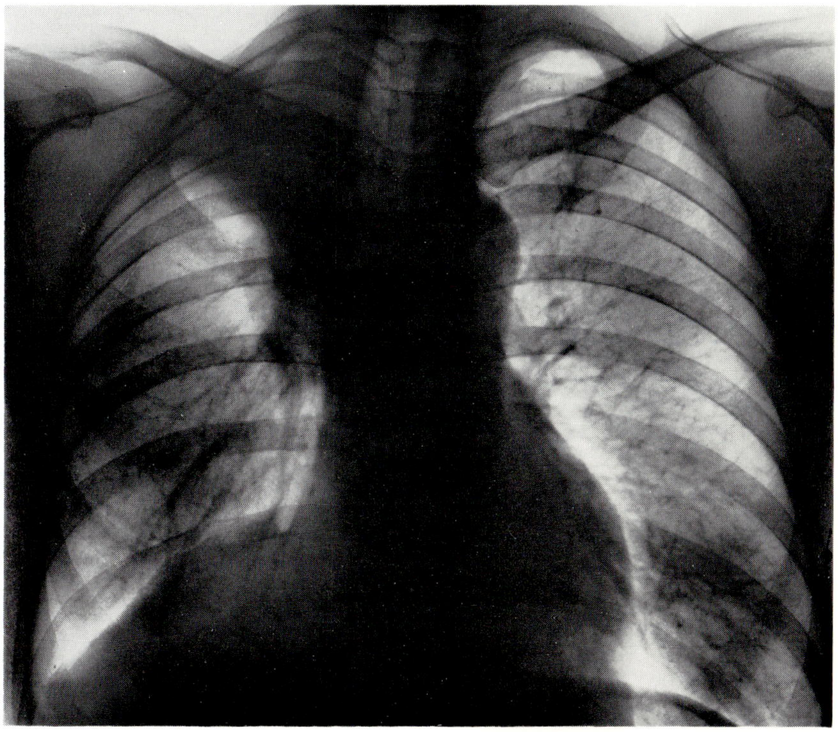

**Fig. 377 Chest X-ray, frontal :** A tumor-like shadow and an atelectasis due to the neoplasm are present at the hilum of the right upper lobe.

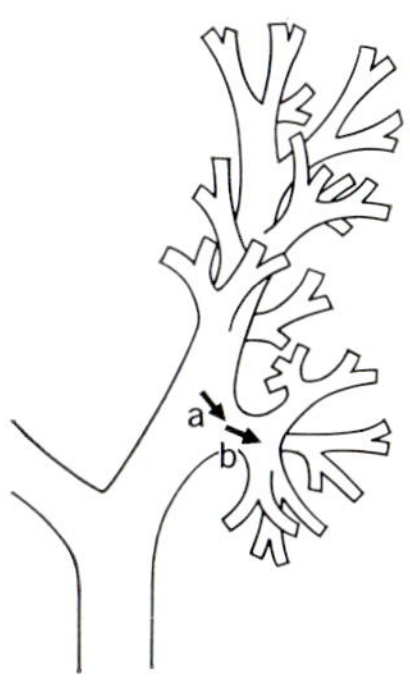


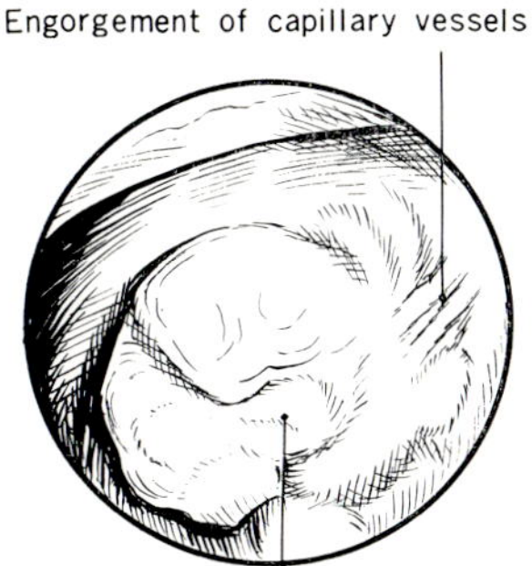


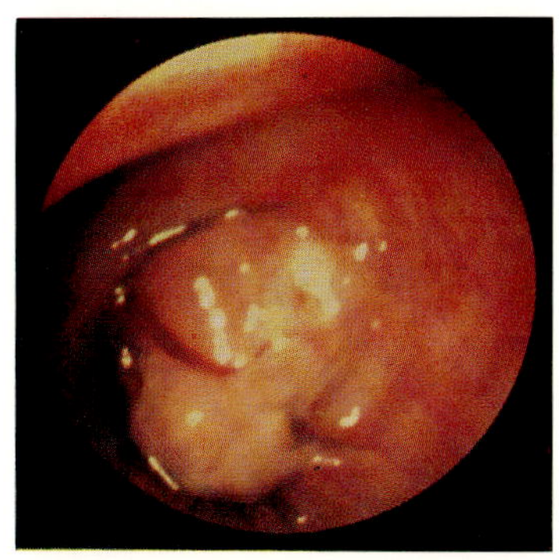

378 a

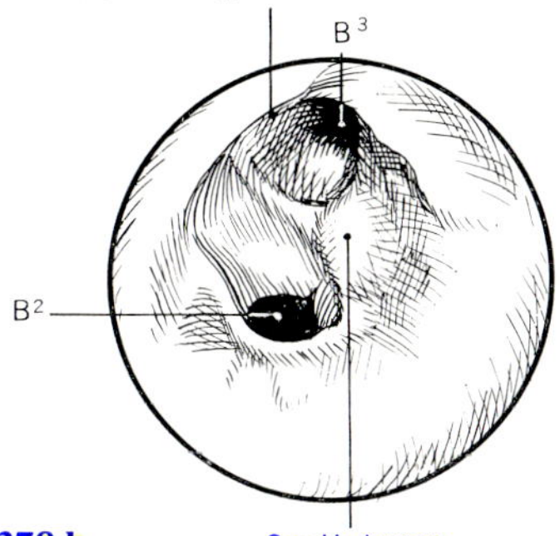


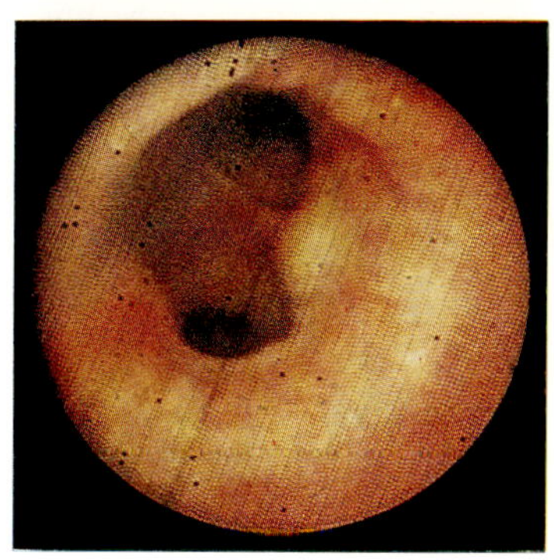

378 b

**Fig. 378 Bronchoscopic findings :**

**a.** A lateral-viewing telescope discloses obstruction of the upper lobe bronchus by a polypoid tumor, engorgement of capillary vessels on the surrounding bronchial wall and irregularity of the wall; all of these findings suggesting an infiltration of carcinoma.

**b.** Bronchofiberscopic findings after irradiation therapy: The large tumor has decreased considerably in size by irradiation (4,500 R), with only small residual tumors remaining. As compared to pre-irradiation findings, the therapy has resulted in marked improvement.

# Case 41 Adenoid Cystic Carcinoma (41, female)

**Case history :** For six months, this patient underwent treatment for pulmonary tuberculosis, which appeared in the form of atelectasis of the right lung. After admission to our hospital she underwent bronchoscopy and the case was diagnosed as adenoid cystic carcinoma by biopsy. Right pneumonectomy was performed.

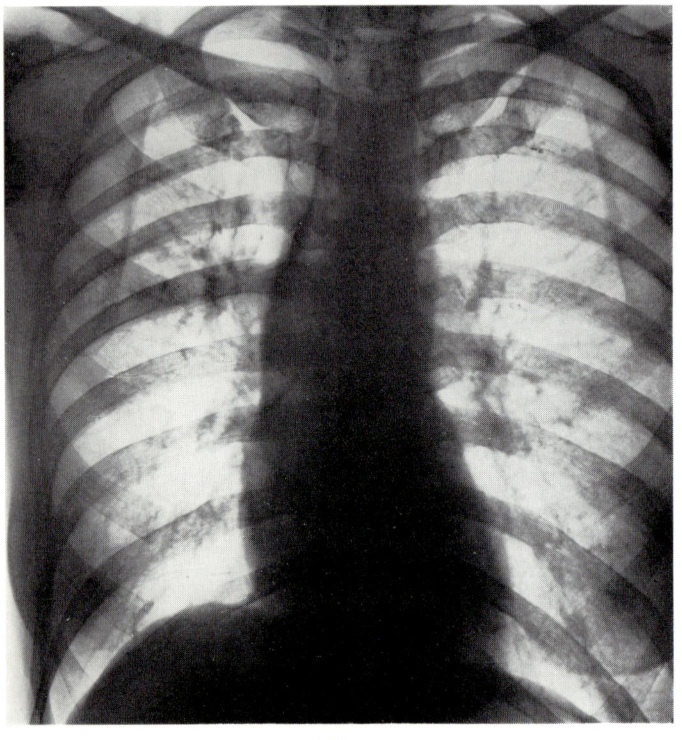

379 a

**Fig. 379 Chest X-ray, frontal :**
**a.** This was taken two years before in the mass survey. Notice retrospectively that a shadow at the right hilum was overlooked.
**b.** The film shows the time when atelectasis was developed in the right lung. The heart is displaced to the right thorax. The right lower lobe is slightly pneumatized.
**c.** A 40×40 mm tumor is located at the right main bronchus. The middle and lower lobes are atelectatic. The trachea is deviated to the right with air retained in the upper lobe.

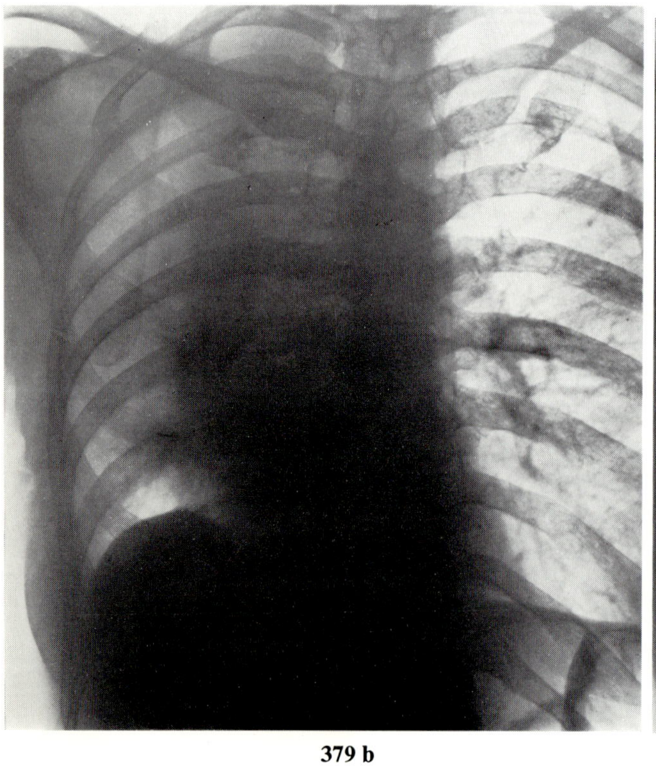

379 b

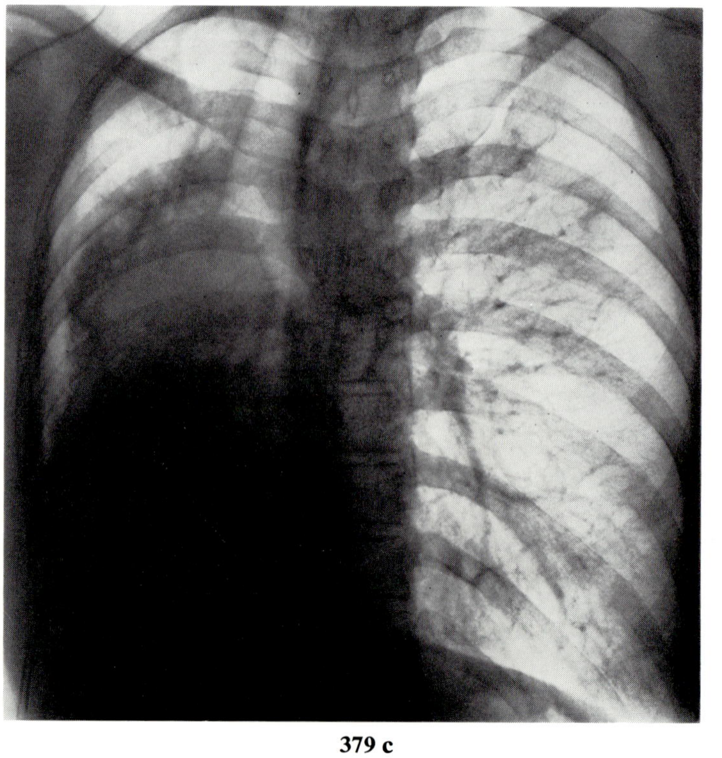

379 c

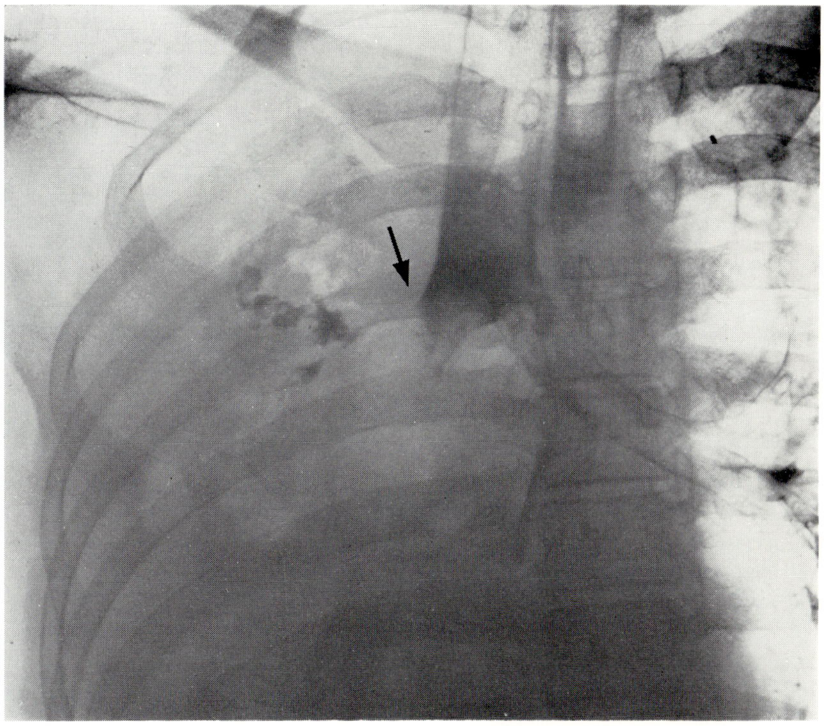

**Fig. 380 Bronchogram, oblique :** The right main bronchus is irregularly obstructed. The upper bronchus is slightly stenosed (arrow). $B^3$ has a sac-like ectasis.

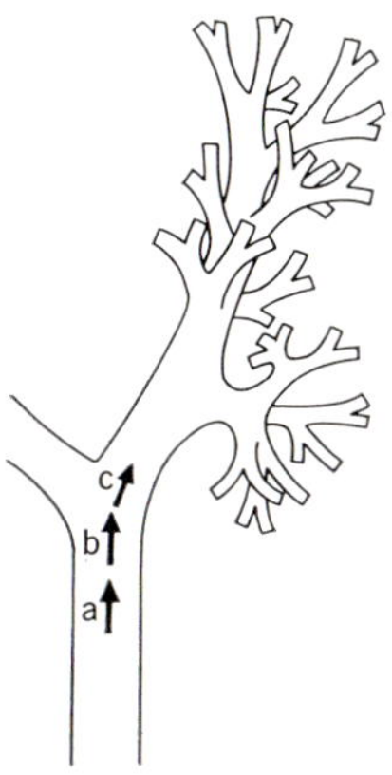


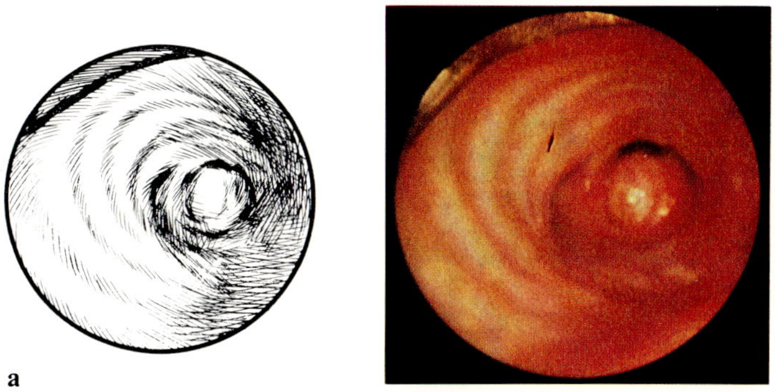

381 a

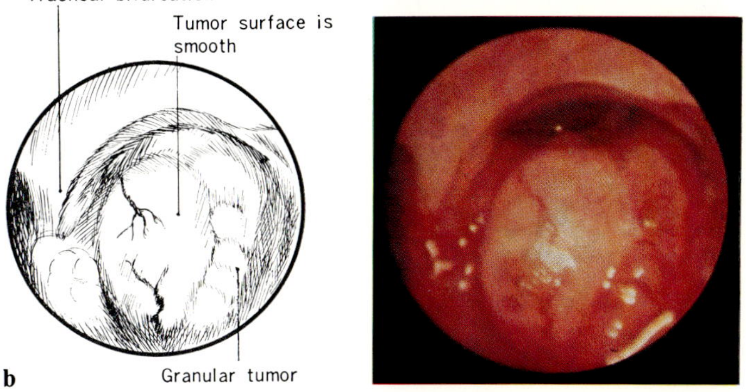


381 b

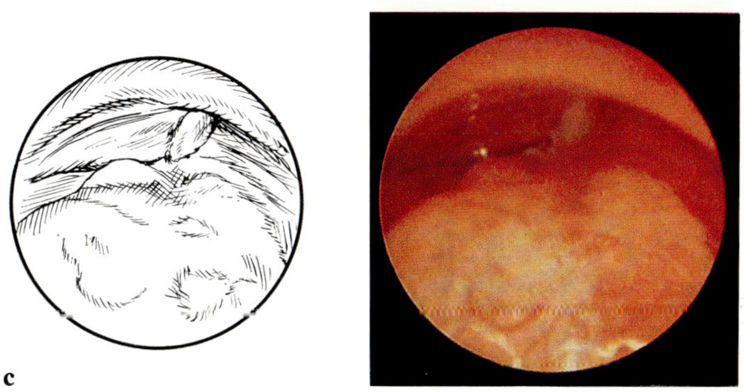

381 c

**Fig. 381 Fiberscopic findings :**

**a.** The lower part of the trachea is normal. The tumor obstructing the right main bronchus is seen in the distance.

**b.** Tumor is located on the posterior wall of the right main bronchus, obstructing the lumen. The tumor surface is smooth, blood vessels are tortuous, and the basal part of the tumor is granular. Such findings of the surface are quite unlike that of a carcinomatous tumor.

**c.** Tortuous blood vessels are clearly visualized in the main bronchus.

## Case 42 Adenoid Cystic Carcinoma (42, female)

**Case history :** The patient had been informed of an abnormal shadow in a mass survey, and underwent treatment for pulmonary tuberculosis. A month ago, she visited our hospital for further examinations. Bronchofiberscopy revealed a tumor. Cytology by means of a small curette diagnosed the case as an anaplastic carcinoma. Left upper lobectomy was performed. The resected specimen disclosed that a 55×49 mm tumor was an adenoid cystic carcinoma.

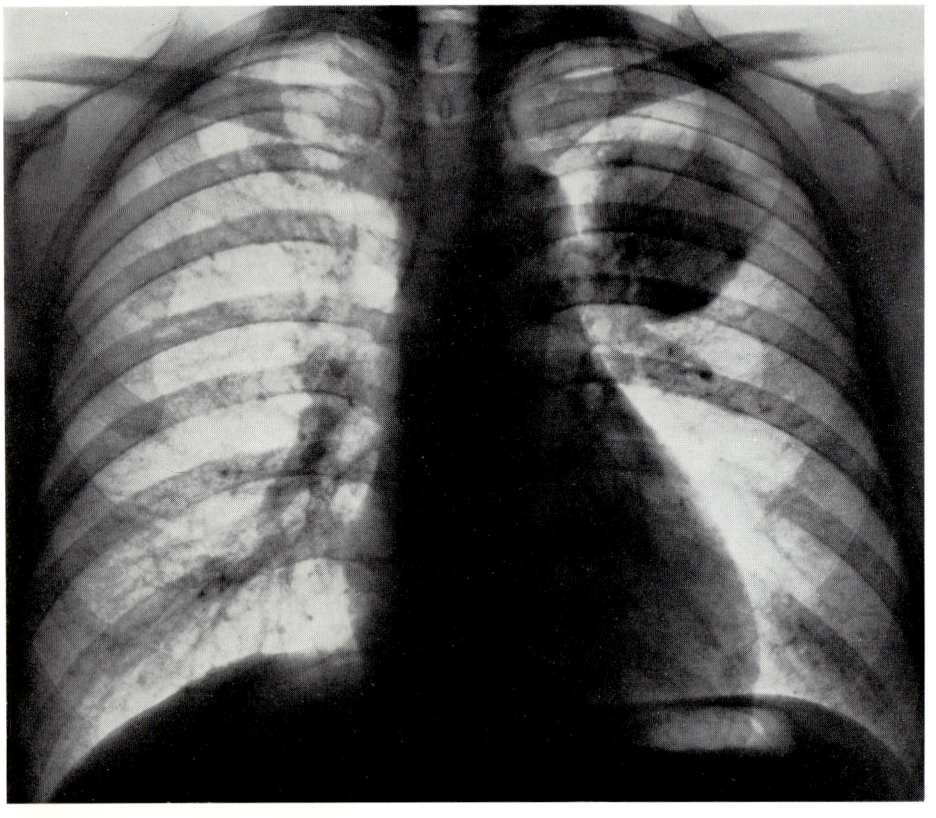

**Fig. 382 Chest X-ray, frontal :** A large tumor-like shadow, 50×50 mm, with indistinct boundaries, is located in the left upper lobe.

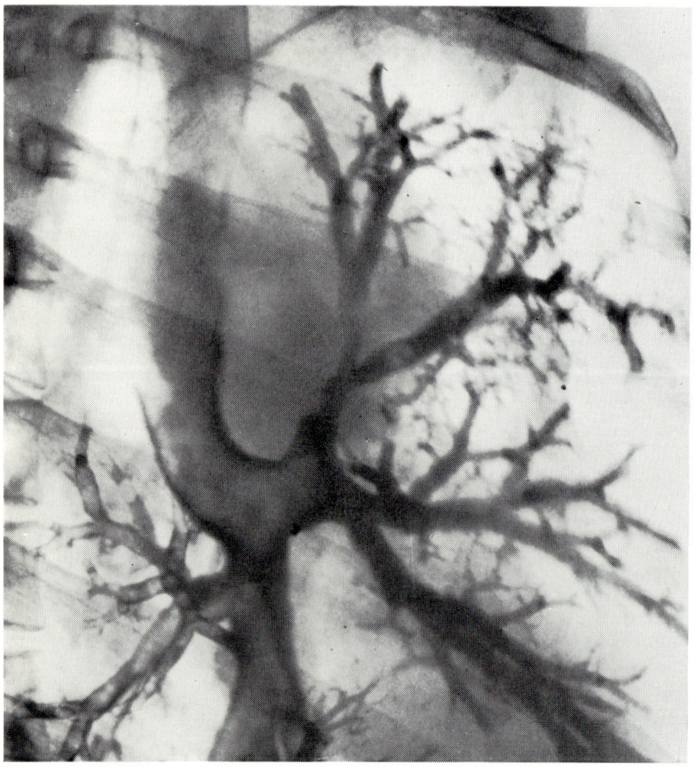

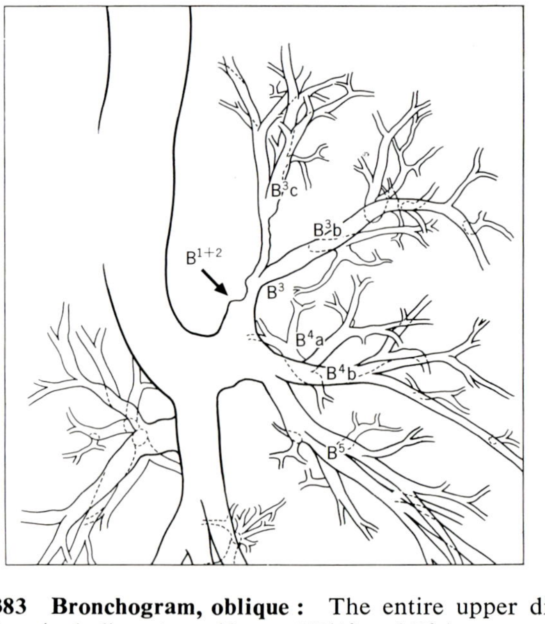


**Fig. 383 Bronchogram, oblique :** The entire upper division bronchus including the orifices of $B^{1+2}$ and $B^3$ is stenosed by a tumor. $B^{1+2}$ is almost completely obstructed (arrow).

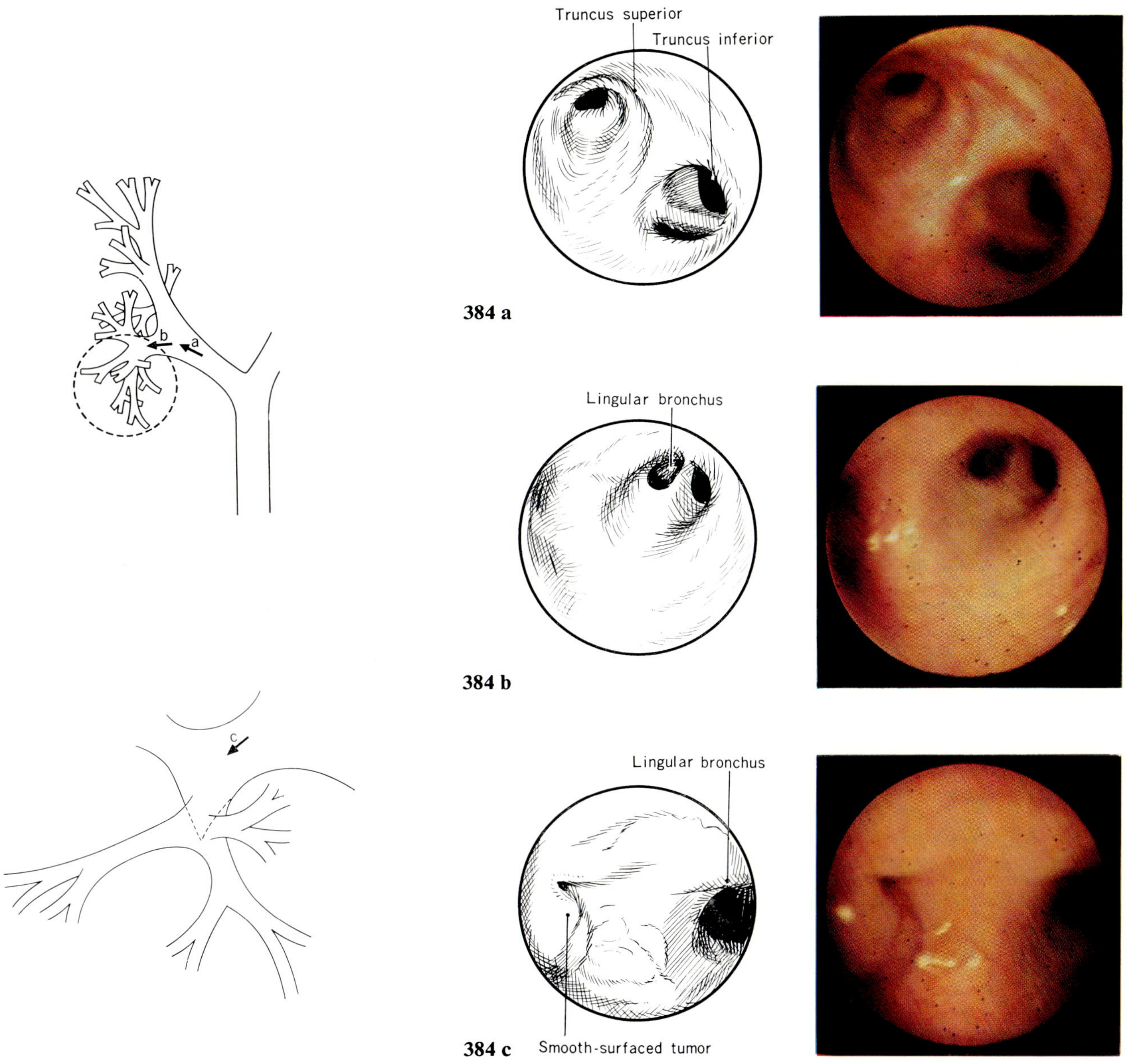


**Fig. 384 Fiberscopic findings :**

**a.** The left upper and lower bronchi are normal.

**b.** The orifice of the left upper bronchus is normal. The septum between the upper division bronchus and the lingular bronchus is thickened.

**c.** The orifice of the upper division bronchus is slightly edematous, with engorged blood vessels. The upper division bronchus is nearly obstructed by a smooth-surfaced tumor, and a very small cleft is left at the right lower corner. Cytology of the curetted specimen was interpreted as a case of anaplastic carcinoma. Histodiagnosis, however, revealed an adenoid cystic carcinoma.

## COMMENT :

It is often difficult to discriminate bronchoscopically between adenoid cystic carcinoma or the adenocarcinoma originating from the bronchial gland as observed in this case. The criterion is that in adenoid cystic carcinoma the tumor is generally smooth on the surface with capillary dilatation, and is usually found in a relatively large bronchus.

# II. Inflammatory Diseases of the Lung

## Case 43 Pulmonary Tuberculosis and Silicosis (61, male)

**Case history :** The patient has been a stone cutter for 45 years. He has had difficulty in breathing for 2 months, so visited a certain hospital. Diagnosis : Silicosis. But since a tumor-like shadow was found on the chest X-ray film, he came to our hospital for further examination. Bronchofiberscopic cytodiagnosis was negative but there was insufficient evidence to exclude carcinoma. Operation was performed. Diagnosis from the resected lung was pulmonary tuberculosis and silicosis.

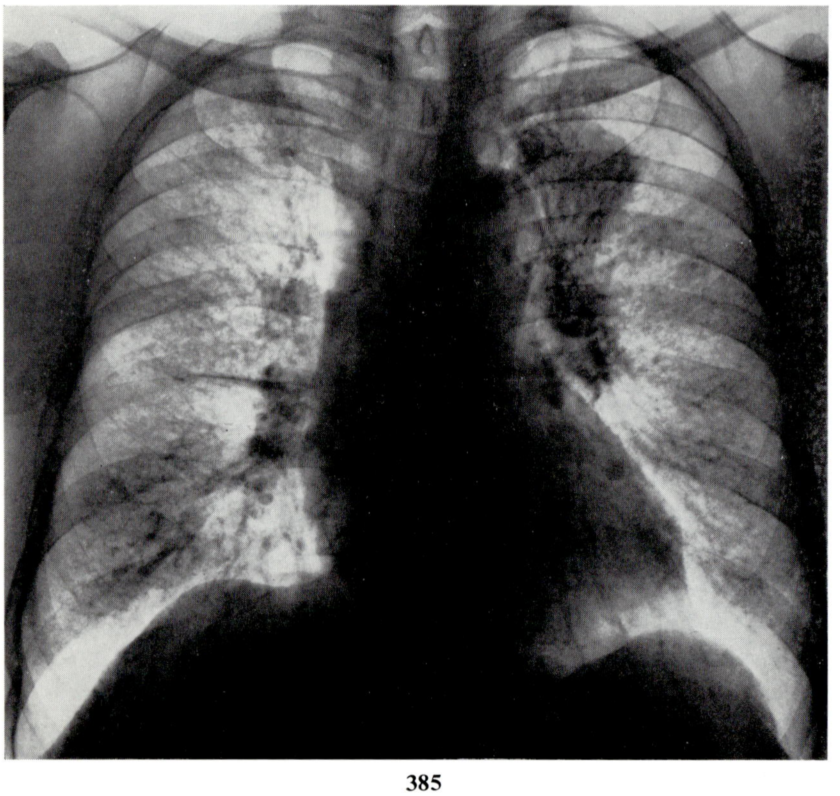

385

**Fig. 385 Chest X-ray, frontal :** A number of millet-sized nodules are scattered throughout both lung fields. An irregular-shaped shadow 35×40mm with indistinct boundaries is seen in the left upper lung field. A lymph node near the hilum is enlarged.

**Fig. 386 Bronchogram, marked oblique :** The orifice of $B^{1+2}$ is stenosed (arrow). $B^{1+2}$ and its branches are abnormally coalesced and converge. $B^{1+2}$b and $B^{1+2}$c, which enter the lesion, are not definitely ectatic nor obstructed. These findings suggest inflammation, but still suspicious of carcinoma.

**Fig. 387 Curettage :** Oblique X-ray film showing a small curette within the lesion. The tip of the curette is just at the point of the lesion passing through $B^{1+2}$ cii. Cytodiagnosis at this site was negative and neither were tubercle bacilli found.

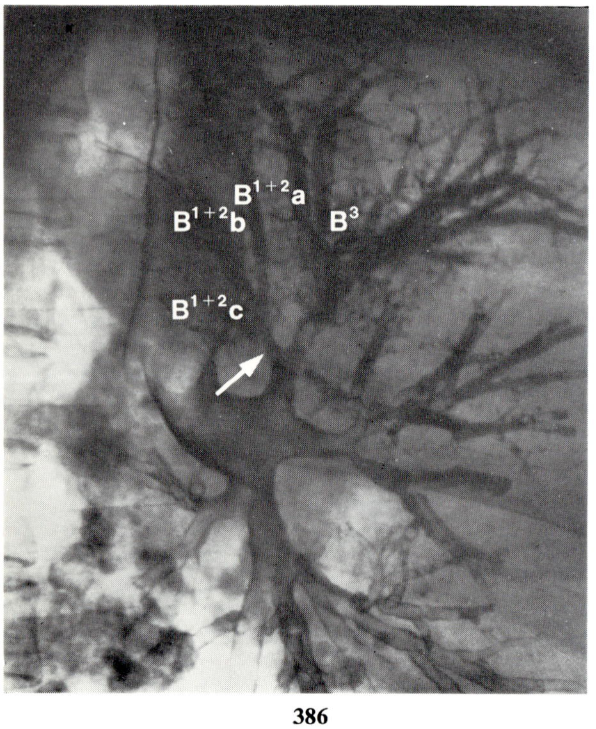


386

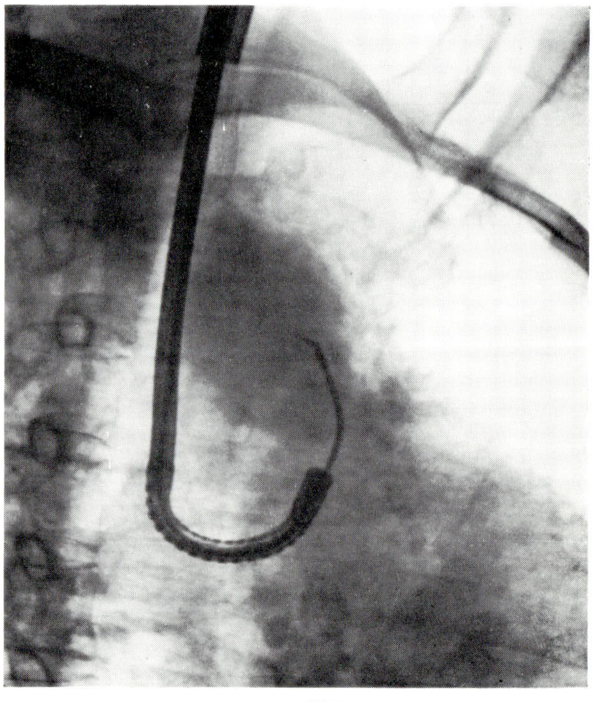

387

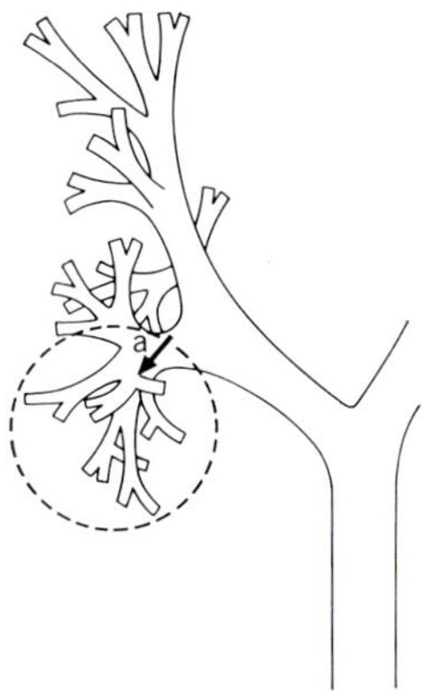

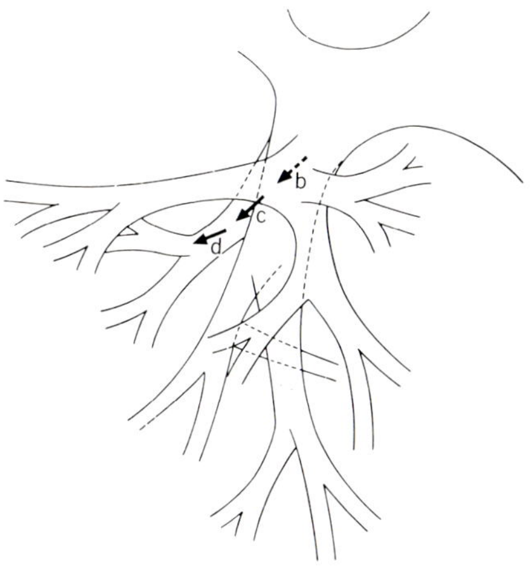


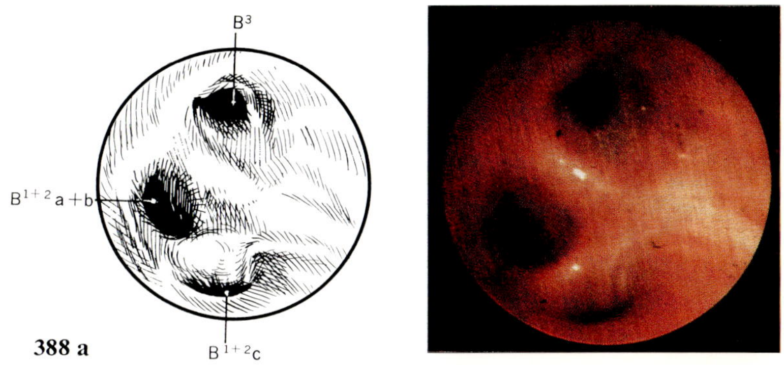


388 a

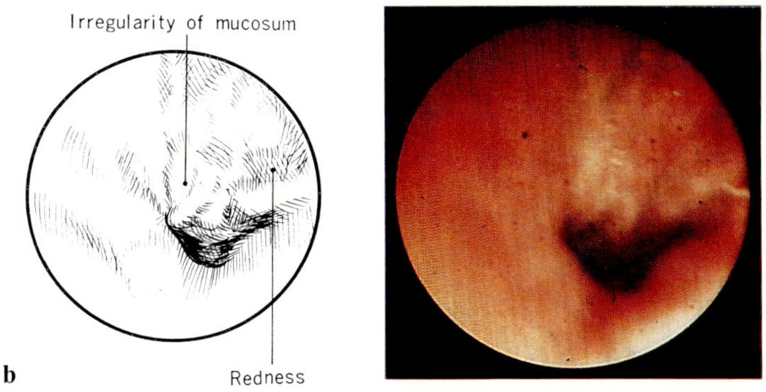


388 b

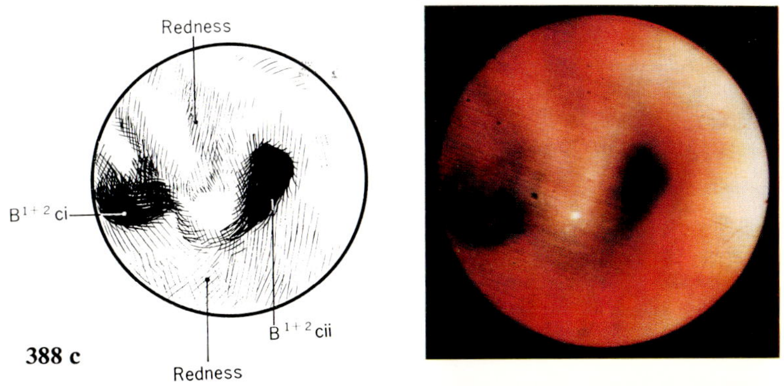


388 c

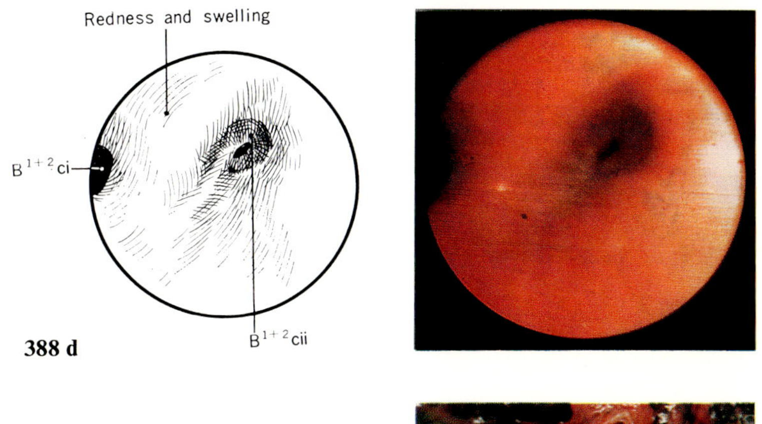


388 d

**Fig. 388 Fiberscopic findings :**

**a.** $B^{1+2}a+b$, $B^{1+2}c$ and $B^3$ are visualized by the fiberscope. The bifurcation of $B^{1+2}$ and $B^3$ is thickened and edematous. The orifice of $B^{1+2}a+b$ is edematous and stenosed. $B^{1+2}c$ is more stenosed.

**b.** The orifice of $B^{1+2}c$ is reddened, swollen and irregularly stenosed. Converging longitudinal folds are seen in the bronchial lumen.

**c.** Furtherin, $B^{1+2}c$ bifurcates into i and ii. $B^{1+2}c$ is stenosed and $B^{1+2}cii$ is reddened, bleeding and irregularly.

**d.** The orifice of $B^{1+2}cii$ is markedly reddened and stenosed peripherally. A curette inserted more peripherally into this branch caused severe bleeding.

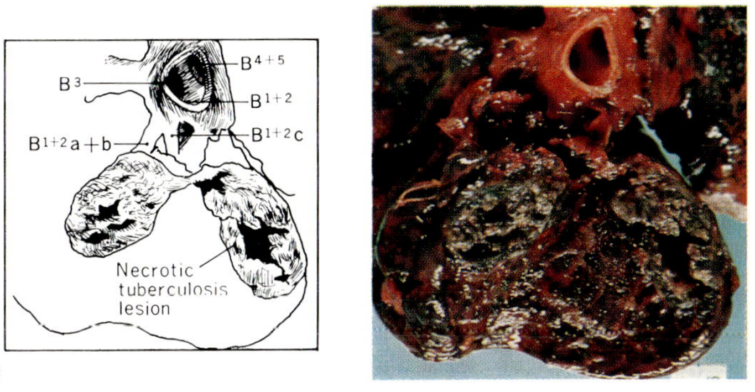


389

**Fig. 389 Macroscopic findings :** Fresh specimen showing the opened lesion at horizontal subsegment of apico-posterior segment ($S^{1+2}c$). The focus is 30× 40mm with a necrotic central part. On the surface of visceral pleura a number of nodules 1 to 3 mm in size were present.

## Case 44 Pulmonary Tuberculosis – Draining Bronchus from a Cavernous Tuberculosis
(33, female)

**Case history :** One month ago, when the patient had a tubal pregnancy, an abnormal shadow was detected on the chest X-ray film. The patient visited our hospital, suspected of chorisonic-epithelioma. Bronchogram disclosed a cavity in $B^6$. Bronchial washing performed during bronchofiberscopy revealed tubercle bacilli, Gaffky III.

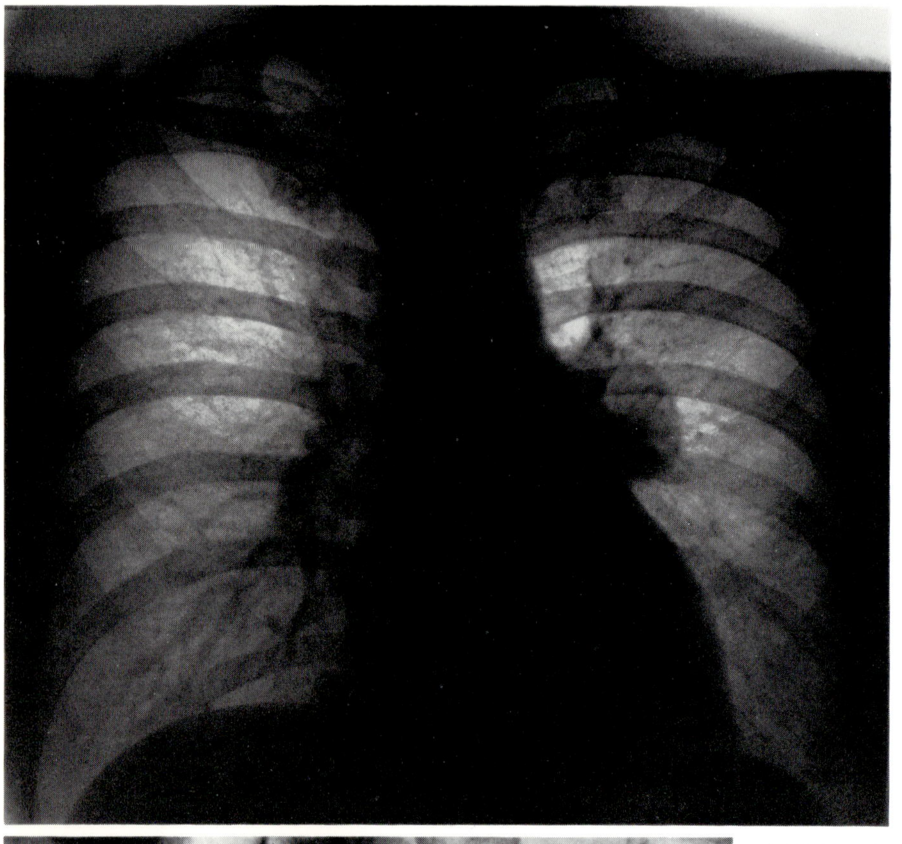

**Fig. 390 Chest X-ray, frontal :** A tumor-like shadow of 40×40mm with distinct borders is present in the superior segment of left lower lobe ($S^6$). No abnormality is found in the remaining lung fields.

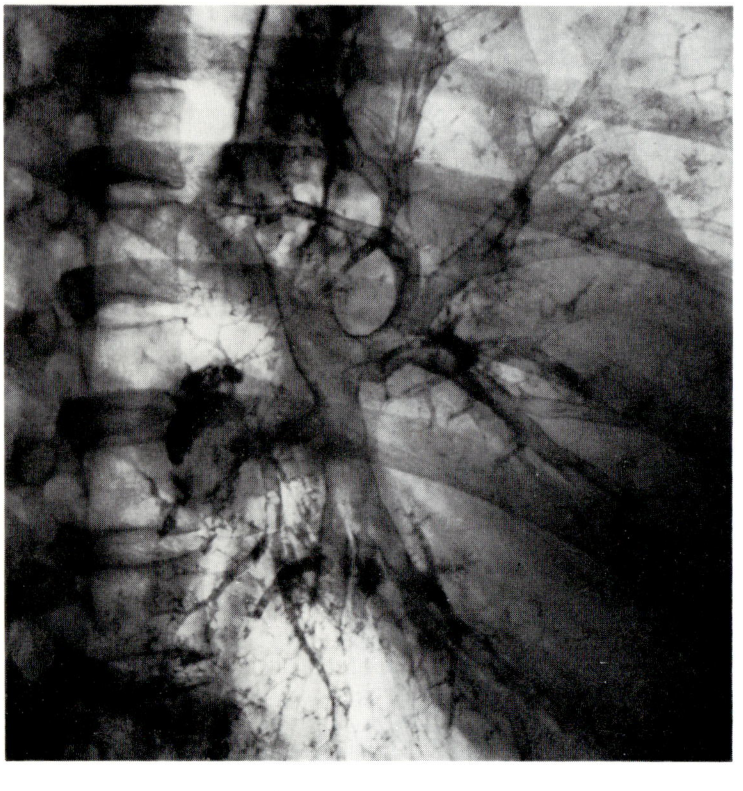

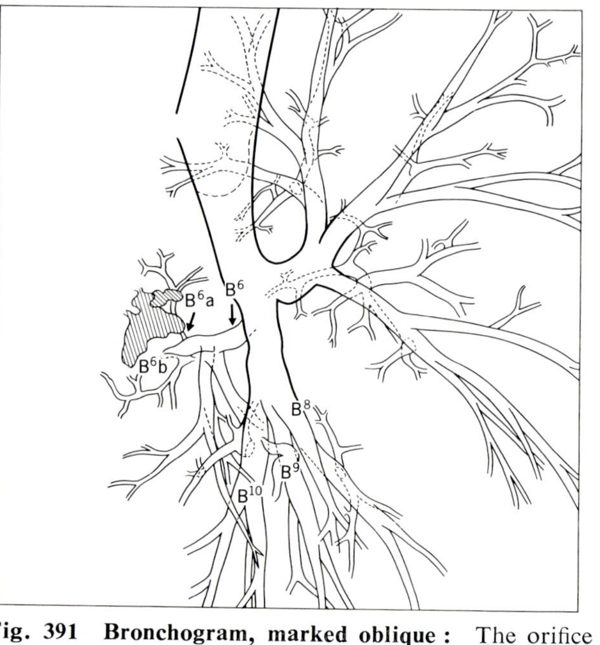


**Fig. 391 Bronchogram, marked oblique :** The orifice of $B^6$ is smooth and gradually narrowed (arrow), apparently due to edema. $B^6a$ and $B^6b$ are both stenosed (arrow), but become ectatic peripherally within the tumor-like shadow, forming a cavity.

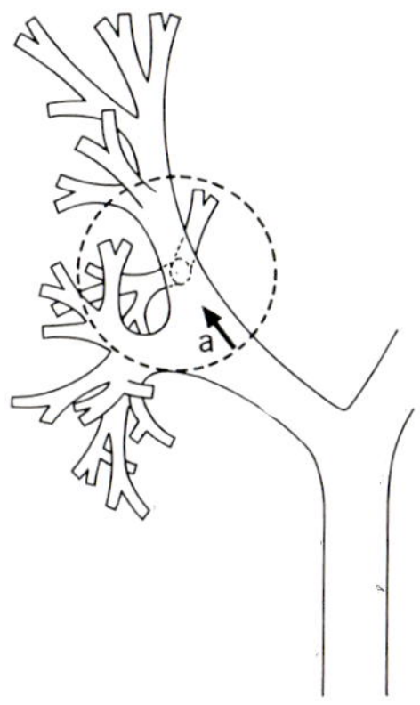


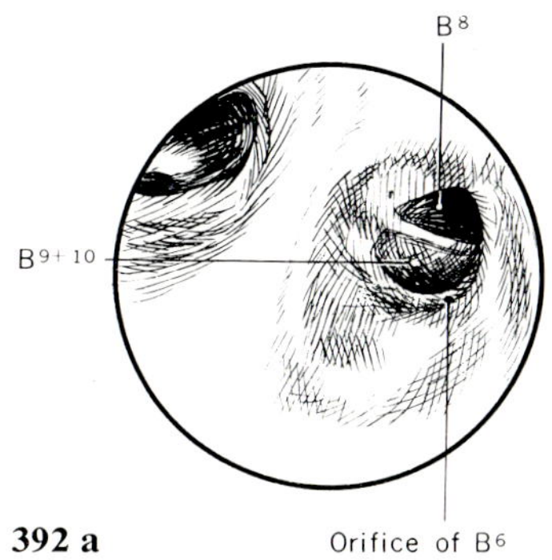


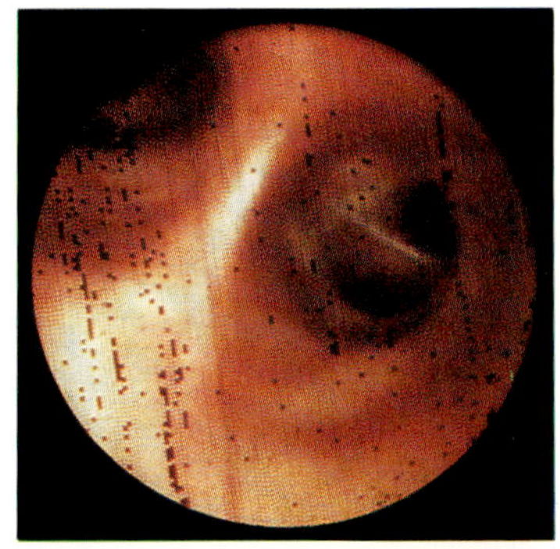

392 a

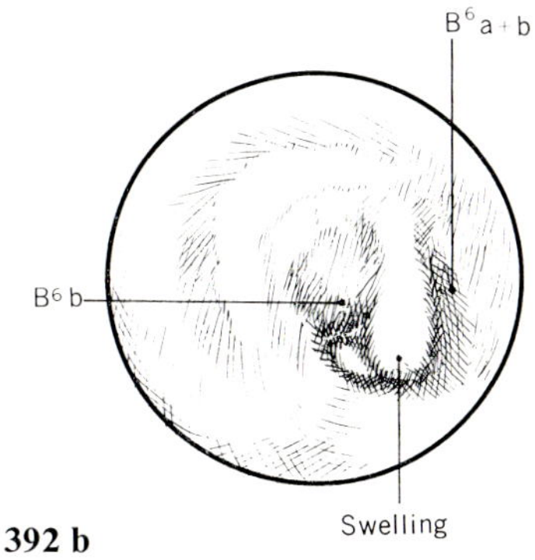


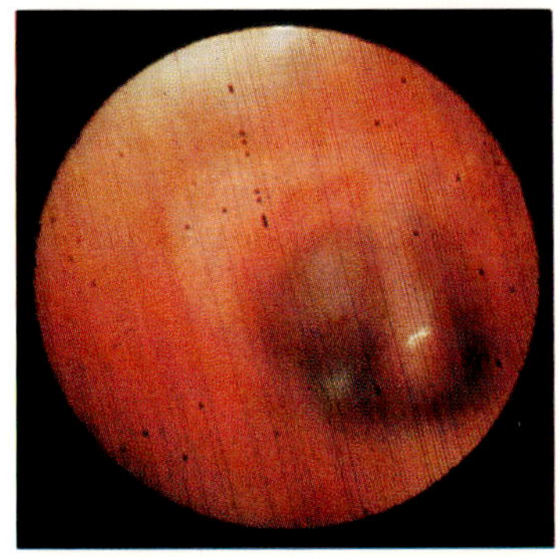

392 b

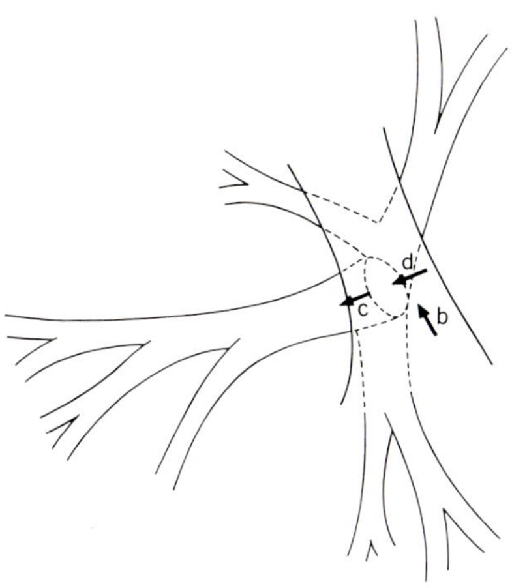


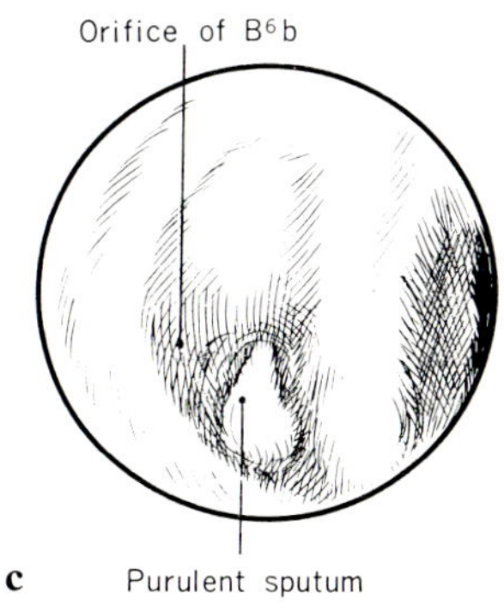


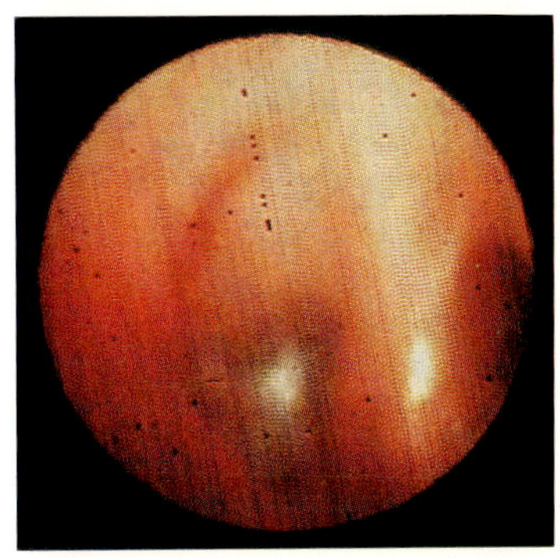

392 c

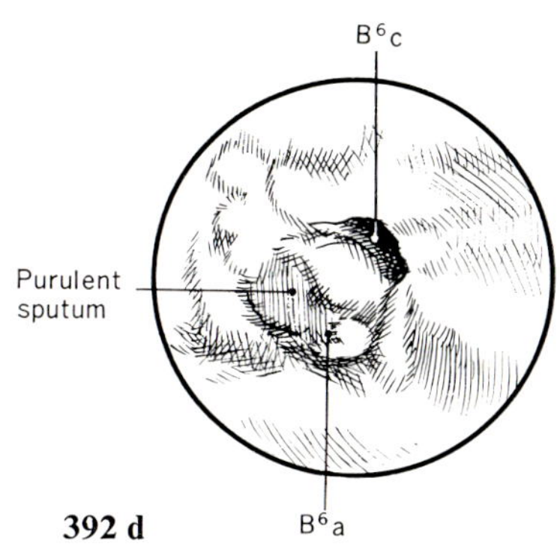


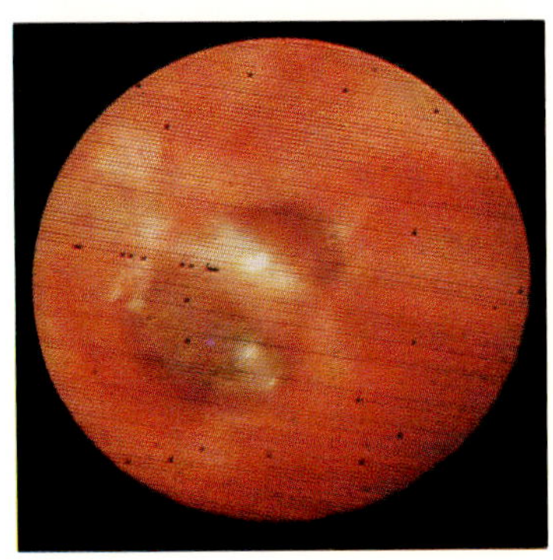

392 d

**Fig. 392 Fiberscopic findings :**

**a.** Marked redness and swelling noted on the posterior wall of the entrance to the lower lobe bronchus, especially near the orifice of $B^6$.

**b.** Redness and swelling are present at the orifice of $B^6$. The bifurcation of $B^6a+c$ and $B^6b$ are thickened due to the edema.

**c.** The orifice to $B^6b$ is gradually stenosed with reddening and swelling, and its peripheral part is clogged with purulent sputum.

**d.** The orifice to $B^6a+c$ is markedly reddened and swollen and the orifice of $B^6a$ and $B^6c$ is thickened. The peripheral part of $B^6a$, like that of $B^6b$, is obstructed with purulent sputum. There is marked reddening and obstruction of the orifice of $B^6c$.

These findings are due to inflammatory changes. The bronchial washing of $B^6a$, b revealed the presence of tubercle bacilli.

## Case 45 Pulmonary Tuberculosis – Post-chemotherapy Stenosis (46, female)

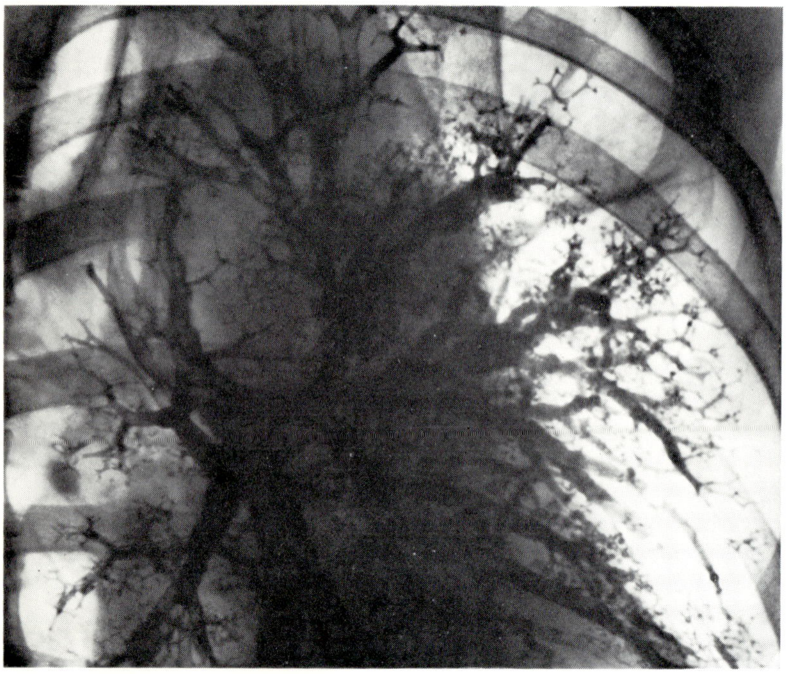

**Chief complaint :** Cough and sputum.
**Case history :** The patient had chronic cough with sputum for the past 6 months. Diagnosis at a certain hospital was bronchitis, but the therapy there showed no improvement. At our hospital the diagnosis by bronchogram was bronchitis tuberculosa. At bronchofiberscopy performed later, Gaffky VIII was detected from the bronchial washings. Prednisolone and Streptomycin were administered. Four months later when bronchoscopic examination was repeated, the marked granulation tissue previously seen had healed, resulting in bronchostenosis.

### *Pre-chemotherapy*

**Fig. 393 Bronchogram, oblique :** There is irregularity of the wall of the left upper lobe bronchus with stenosis, and distention of the peripheral bronchi. Slight crowding of the bronchi is noted. Diagnosis reached was bronchitis tuberculosa from these and routine X-ray film findings.

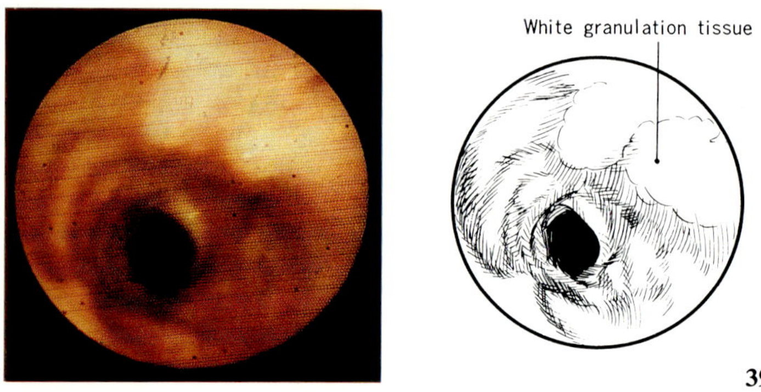


**394 a**

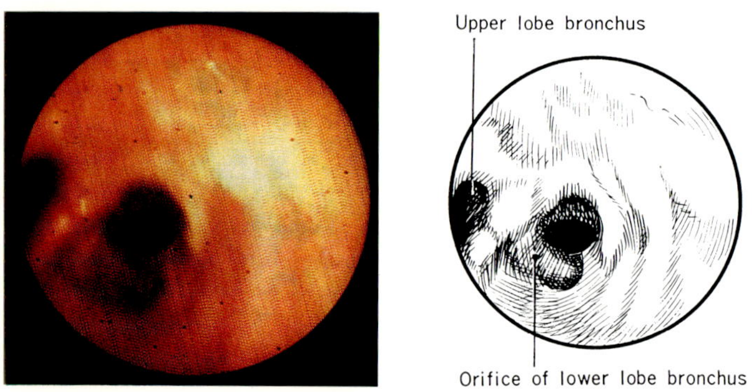


**394 b**

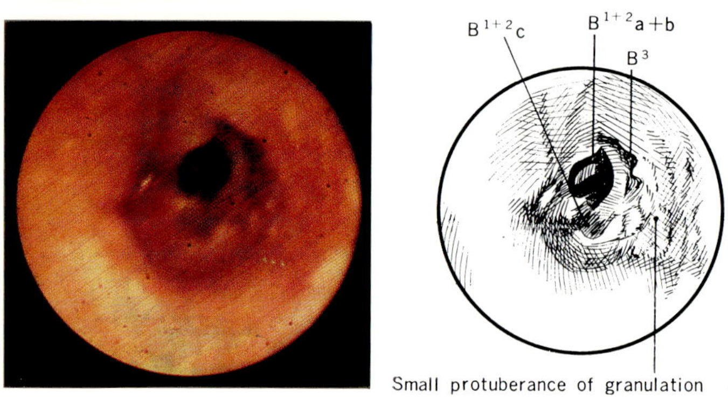


**394 c**

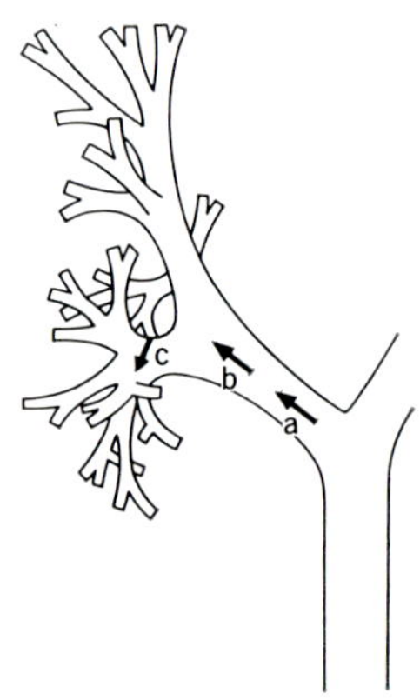


**Fig. 394 Fiberscopic findings :**
**a.** There is irregularity, white granulation tissue and hyperemia in the left main bronchus.
**b.** Protruding red granulations noted at the entrance of the upper lobe bronchus, with intense redness and obscured cartilages.
**c.** The upper division bronchus reveals marked swelling, redness, edema and protuberance of granulations.

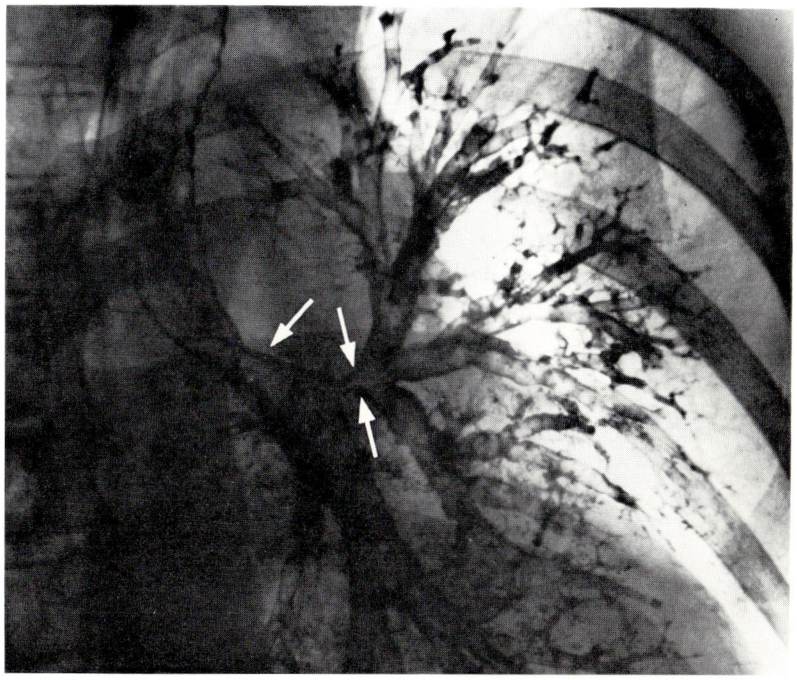

## *Post-chemotherapy*

**Fig. 395 Bronchogram, oblique :** The left main bronchus now reveals a stenosis which was not visualized in the previous examination (arrow). The entrance to the left upper lobe bronchi is markedly stenosed(arrow). The peripheral branch bronchi show bronchiectasis more clearly.

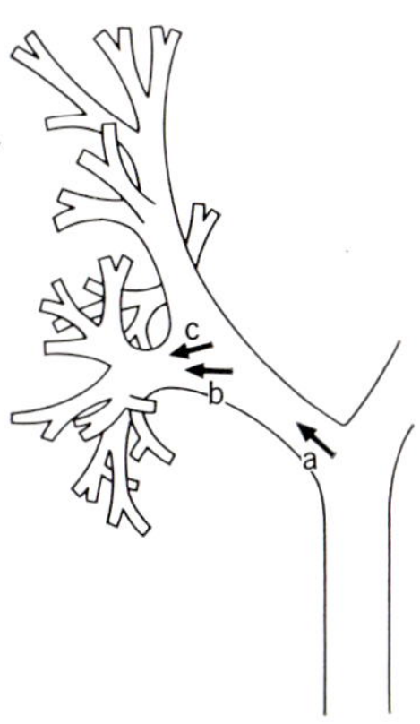


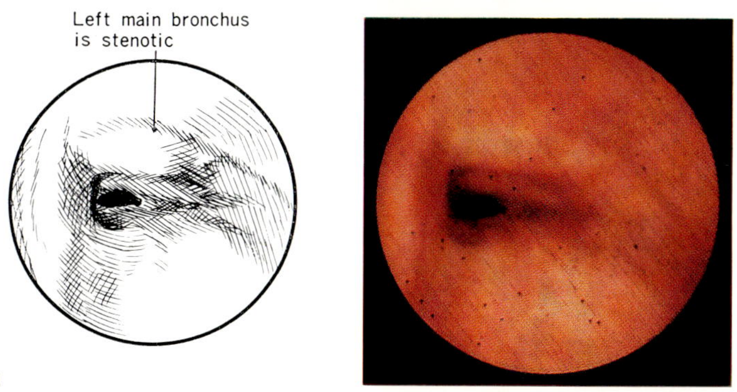


**396 a**

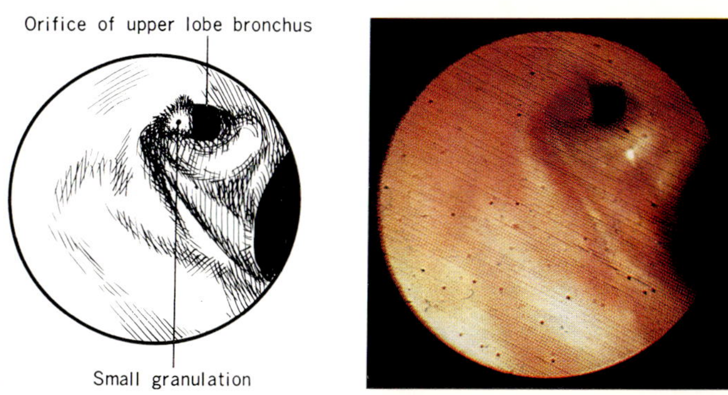


**396 b**

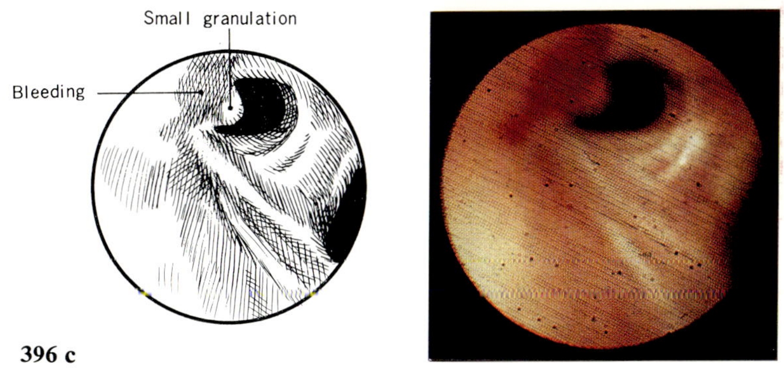


**396 c**

**Fig. 396 Fiberscopic findings :**

**a.** The left main bronchus shows less redness and irregularity, although capillaries are engorged. The cartilage rings are barely visible. The acute inflammation due to bronchitis tuberculosa has subsided, but there is now present generalized concentric stenosis.

**b.** Granulation tissue still remains at the entrance of the upper lobe bronchus and the obstruction there is more marked.

**c.** Overall, the granulation tissue and inflammatory changes are less recognizable. With the healing of the bronchial tuberculosis, stenosis has resulted.

## Case 46 Pulmonary Tuberculosis – Stenosis of the Major Bronchus (52, male)

**Chief complaint :** Chest pain.

**Case history :** Artificial pneumothorax had been administered for two years pulmonary tuberculosis 20 years ago. Recently, left chest wall pain led the patient to visit our hospital. Bronchofiberscopy revealed a conspicuous stenosis of the left main bronchus, but tubercle baccilli were not found.

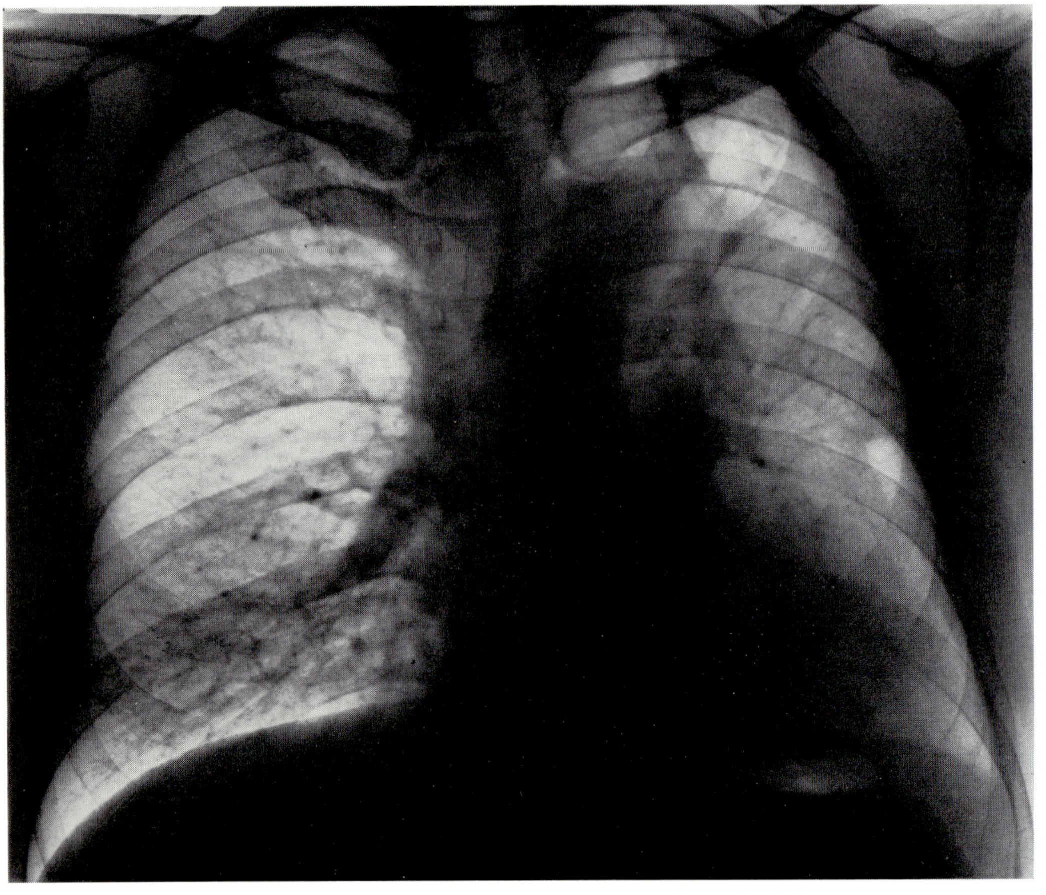

**Fig. 397 Chest X-ray, frontal :** A tumor shadow is located at the left hilum. Mediastinal thickening is present and the left main bronchus is retracted upward.

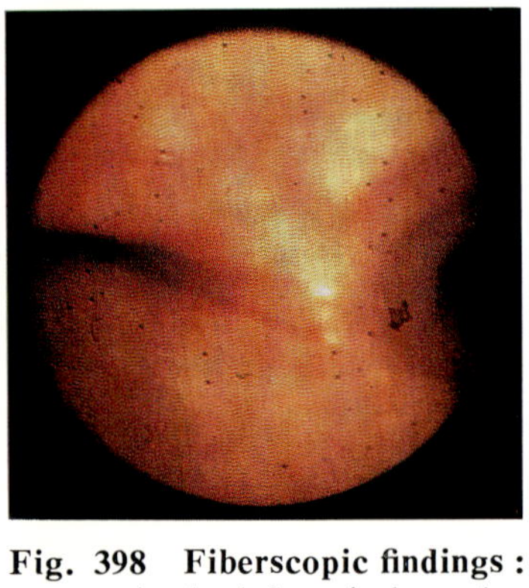

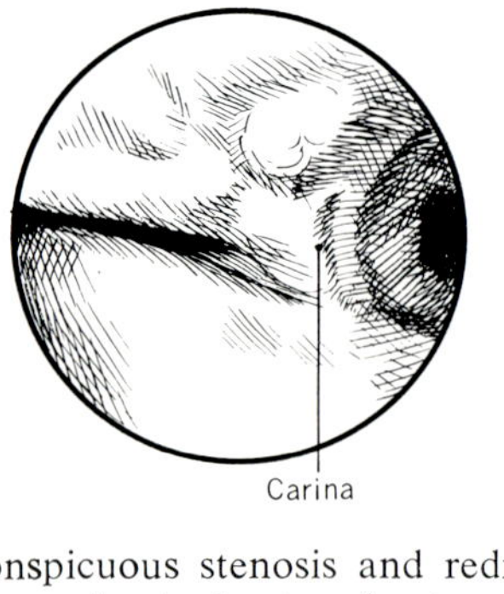


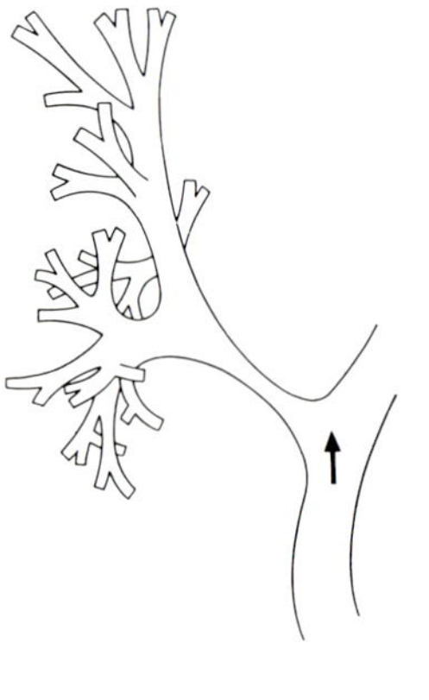

**Fig. 398 Fiberscopic findings :** Conspicuous stenosis and redness are present in the left main bronchus. The carina is shortened antero-posteriorly, and broadened.

# Case 47 Pulmonary Tuberculosis – Obstruction of the Major Bronchus (39, female)

**Chief complaint :** Cough, persisting for the past 3 months.
**Case history :** Chest X-ray revealed atelectasis of the left lower lobe and an inflammatory change in the upper lobe. Bacteriological examination of sputum proved the presence of tubercle bacilli, Gaffky III. Bronchofiberscopy was performed.

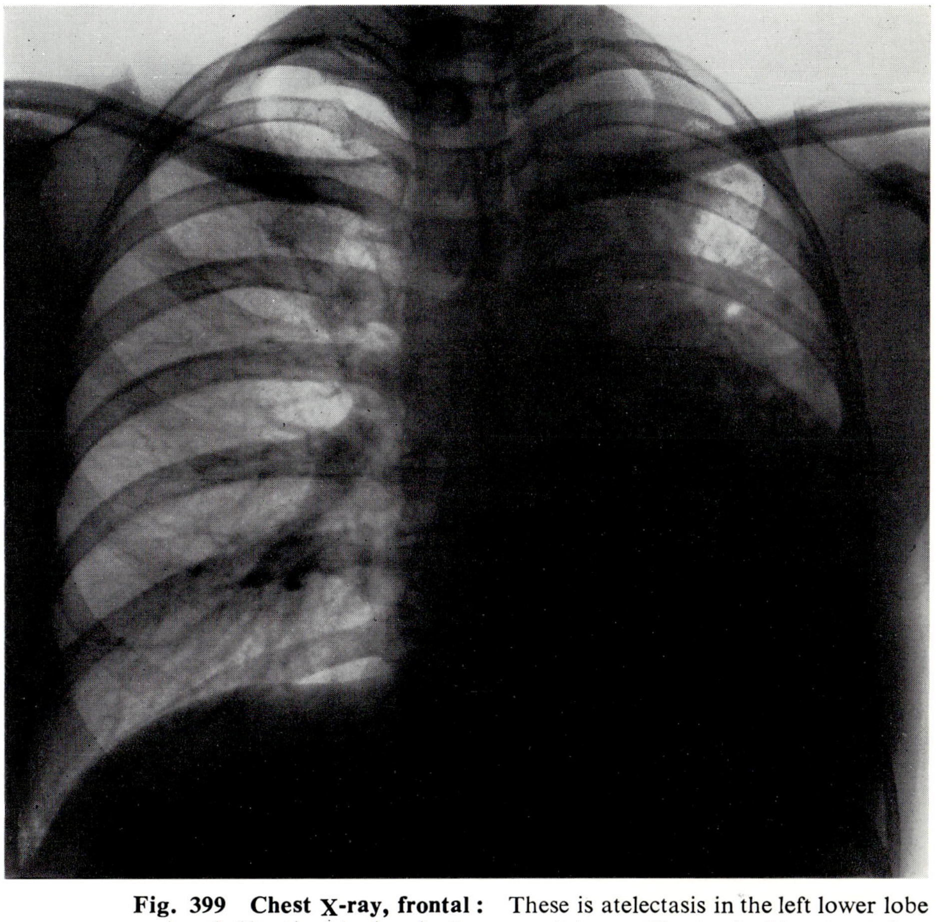

**Fig. 399 Chest X-ray, frontal :** These is atelectasis in the left lower lobe and an infiltrative shadow in the upper lobe. The trached is retracted to the left.

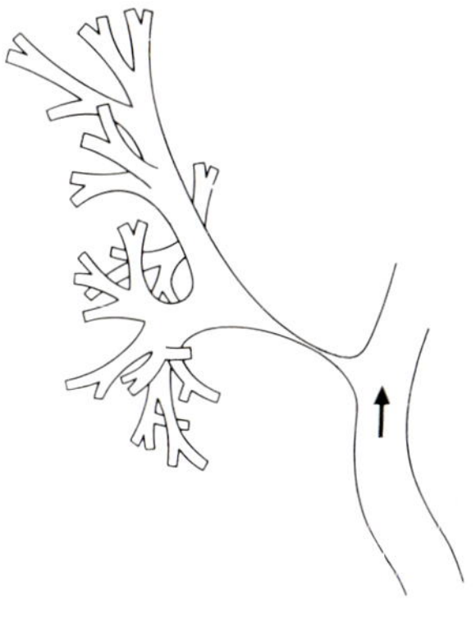

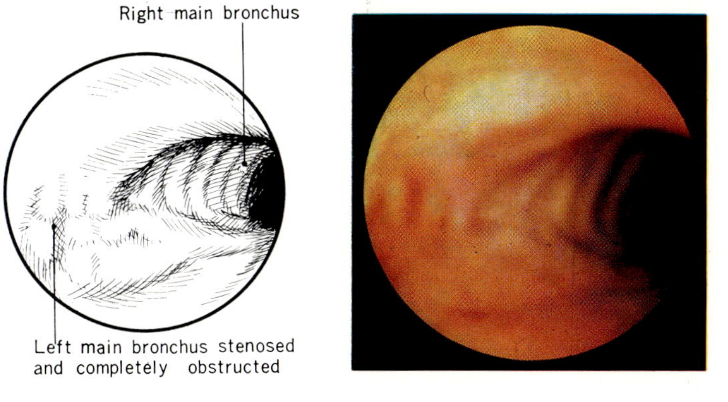


**Fig. 400 Bronchoscopic findings :** Rigid bronchoscopy disclosed the left main bronchus to be completely obliterated. No redness nor swelling is seen here.

## Case 48 Pulmonary Tuberculosis – Tuberculous Fibricaseous Granuloma (27, male)

**Case history :** About 5 months ago the patient had a fever of 39°C. The chest X-ray revealed an abnormal shadow in the apical segment ($S^1$) of the right upper lobe. While administrating antituberculosis agents, bronchography and bronchofiberscopy were performed. Bronchofiberscopic curettage was negative cytologically. Operation was performed on the right lung. Pathologic diagnosis based on the resected lung : Tuberculous fibrocaseous granuloma.

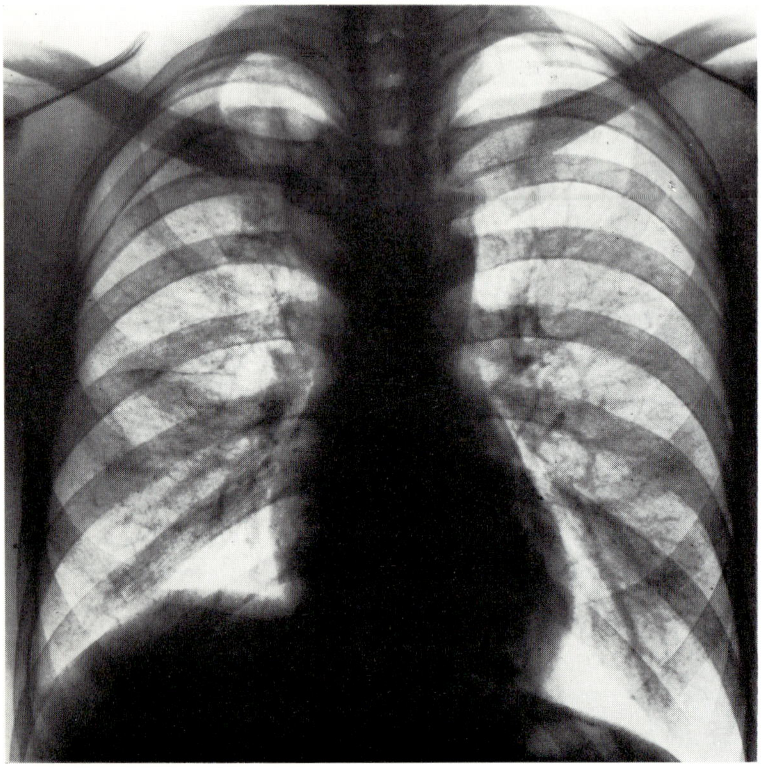

**Fig. 401 Chest X-ray, frontal :** An abnormal shadow with a relatively distinct border is located near the mediastinum. Fibrotic strands are noted in the peripheral part.

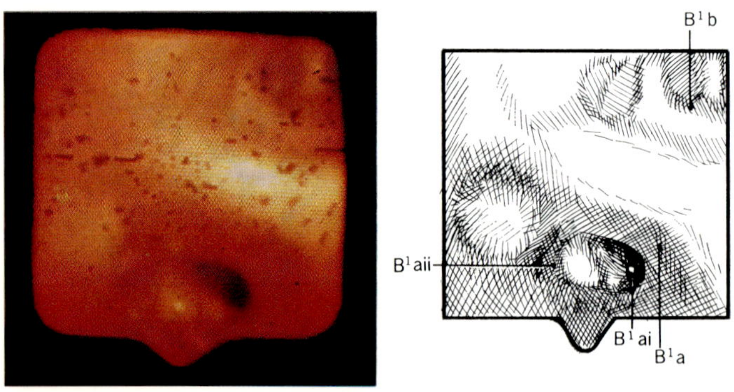


**402 a**

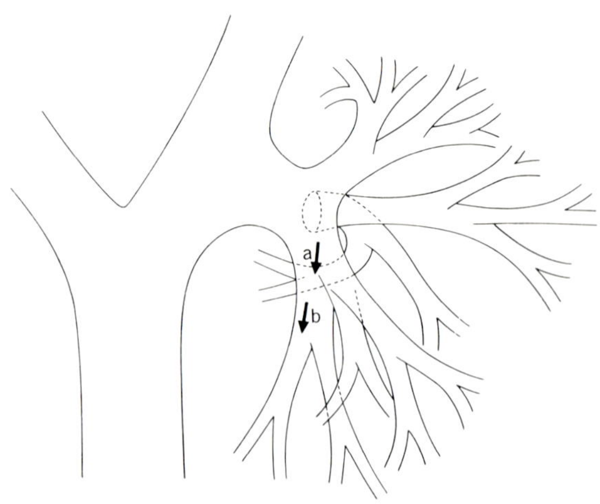


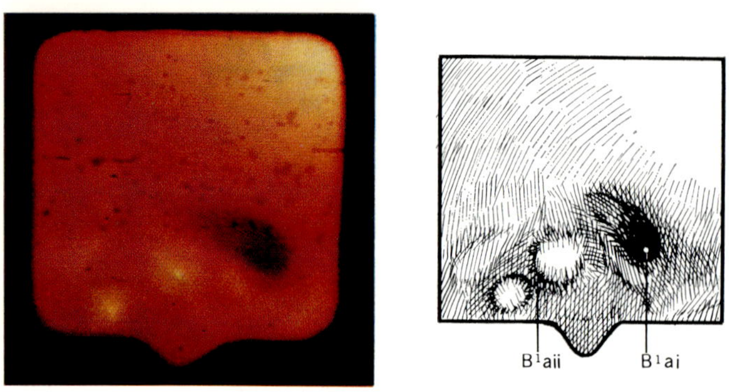


**402 b**

**Fig. 402 Fiberscopic findings :**
- **a.** The orifice of $B^1$ai is reddened and stenosed markedly. The septum between $B^1$ai and $B^1$aii is edematous.
- **b.** A closer view of $B^1$ai reveals more reddening and stenosis. These findings are not characteristic of any type of lung cancer.

## Case 49 Pulmonary Tuberculosis – Cavernous Drainage Bronchus of a Cavity (30, male)

**Case history :** A month ago the patient had a fever of 40°C. A chest X-ray revealed an infiltration containing a cavity in the superior segment of the left lower lobe ($S^6$). Bronchogram showed $B^6a+b$ to form the drainage bronchus. Bronchial washings performed at bronchofiberscopy proved the presence of Tubercle bacilli, Gaffky V.

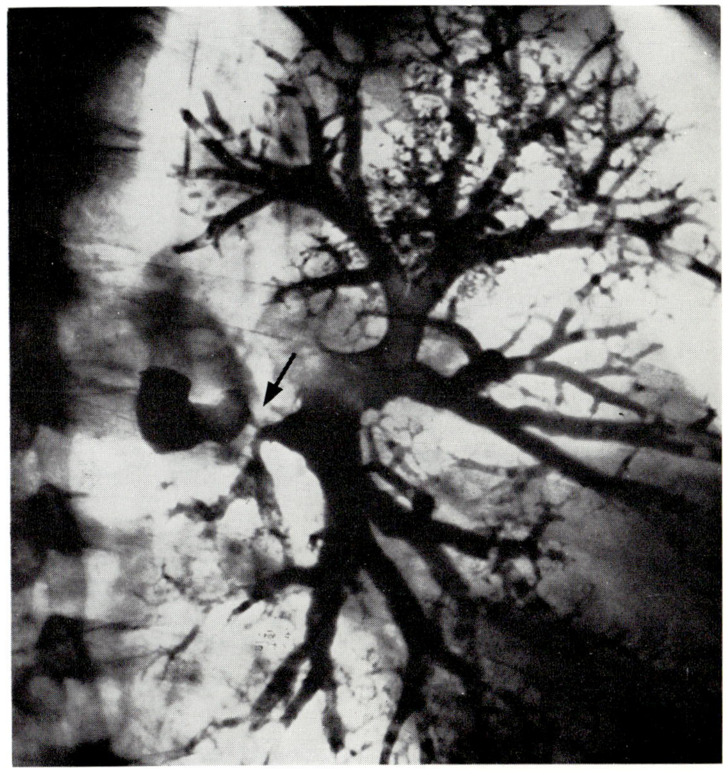

**Fig. 403 Bronchogram, oblique :** $B^6$ is gradually narrowed. The entrance into $B^6a+b$ is stenosed (arrow) as narrow as a thread and distally, a cavernous shadow is seen.

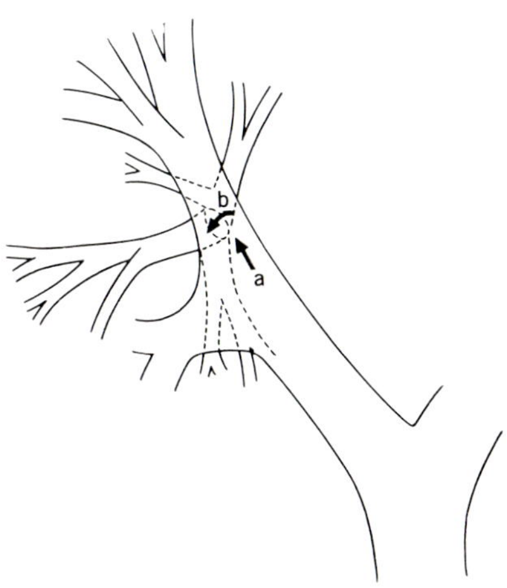


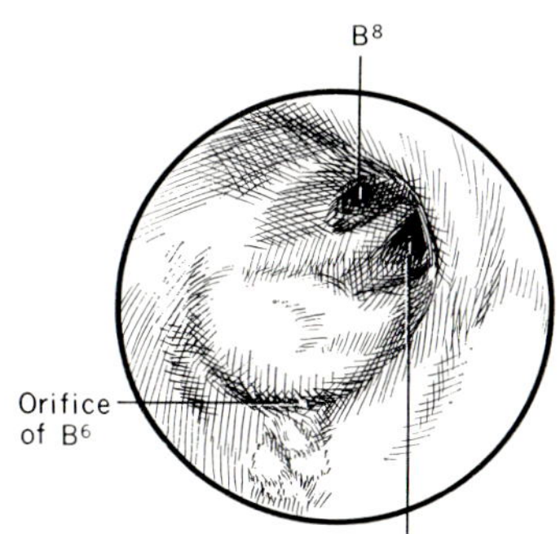


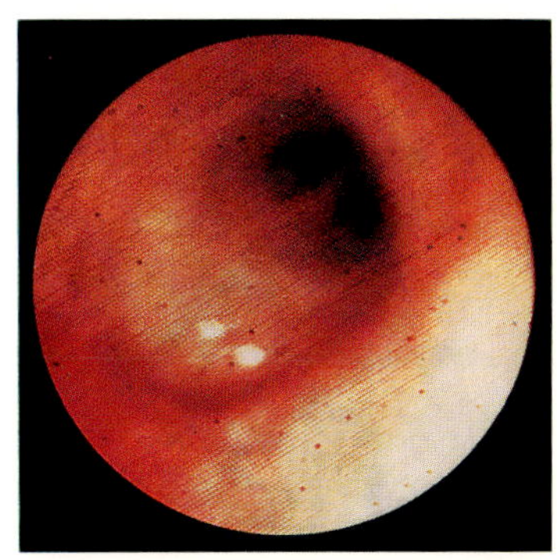

**404 a**

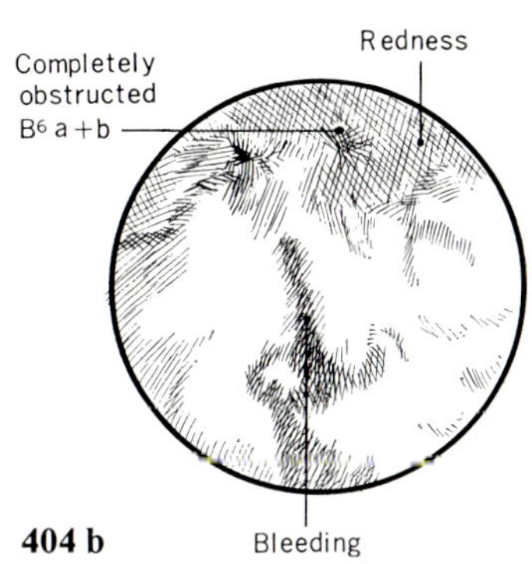


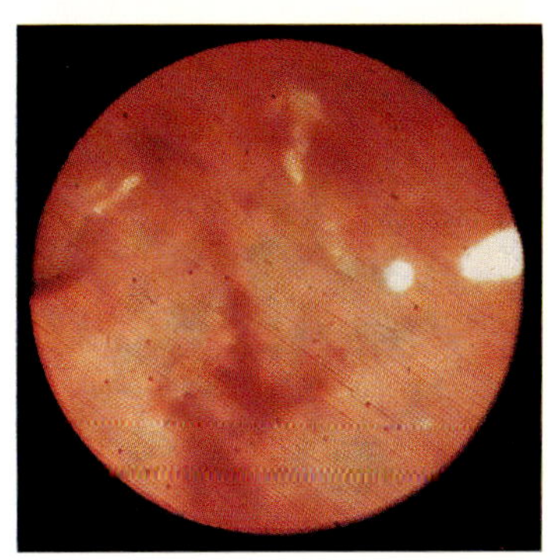

**404 b**

**Fig. 404 Fiberscopic findings :**

**a.** Swelling at the $B^6$ orifice is conspicuous. Bronchial washings here proved the presence of M. tuberculosis.

**b.** Near the entrance to $B^6a+b$ there is capillary engorgement and swelling. The entrance of $B^6a+b$ is completely obstructed. The narrow thread-like passage seen on the bronchogram is not visualized.

## Case 50 Bronchitis (39, female)

**Chief complaint :** Persistent coughing.

**Case history :** The patient had a persistent cough for 4 months. During the past 2 months, she had more sputum and difficult breathing. On bronchography, marked stenosis was found. The case was diagnosed as bronchitis bronchofiberscopically. Prednisolone, tetracycline and I. N. H. (isoniazid) were administered for 2 months. Subjective symptoms have improved considerably.

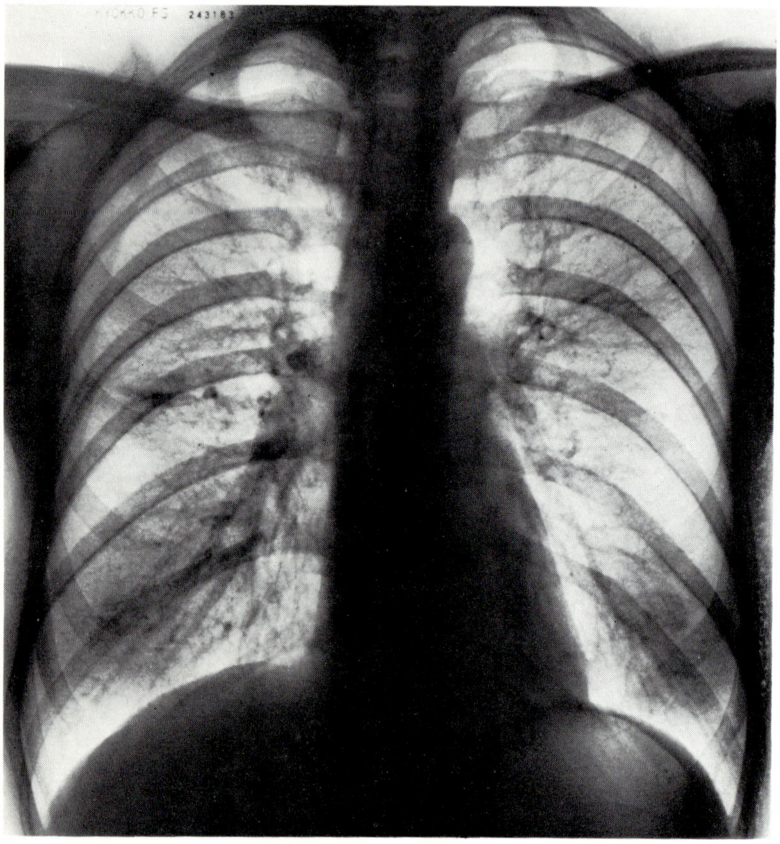

**Fig. 405 Chest X-ray, frontal, before chemotherapy :** Except for a small calcified lymph node in the right hilum, no particular abnormality is in the lung fields.

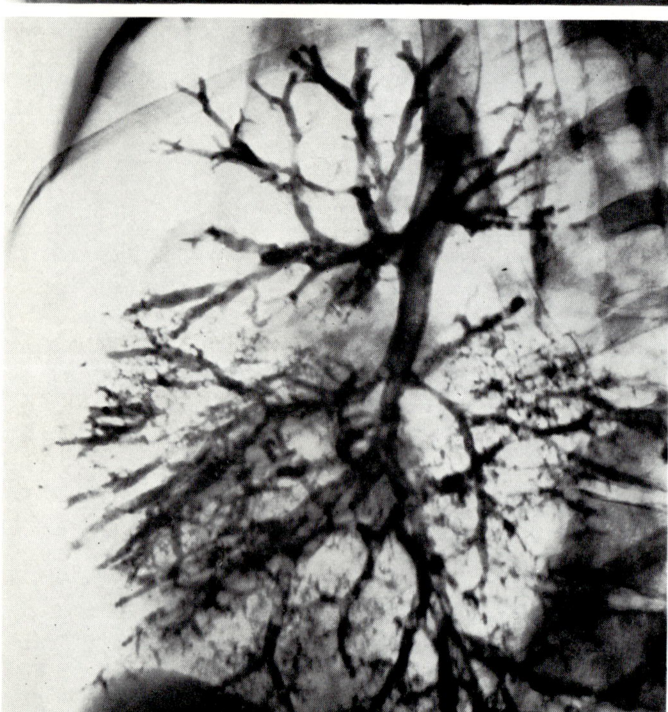

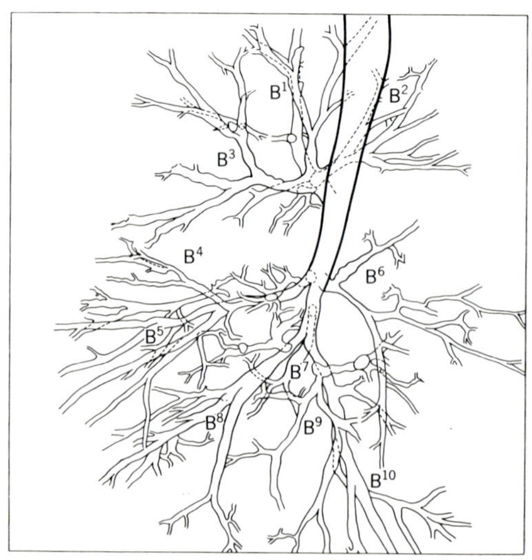


**Fig. 406 Bronchogram, markedly oblique :** Almost all the right bronchi from the major bronchus to subsegmensal ones are stenosed. Marked stenosis is seen particularly in the upper and middle lobe bronchi.

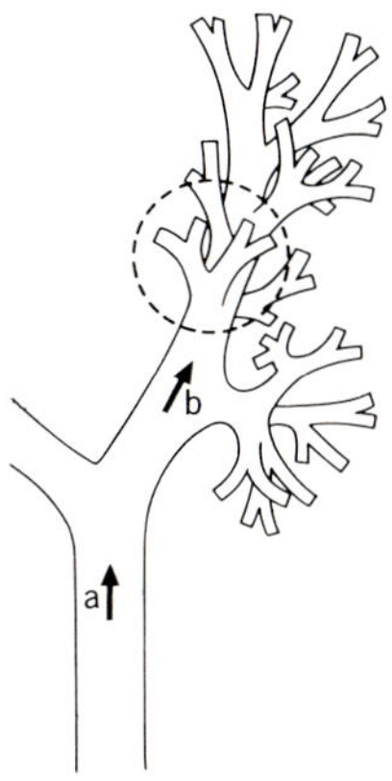


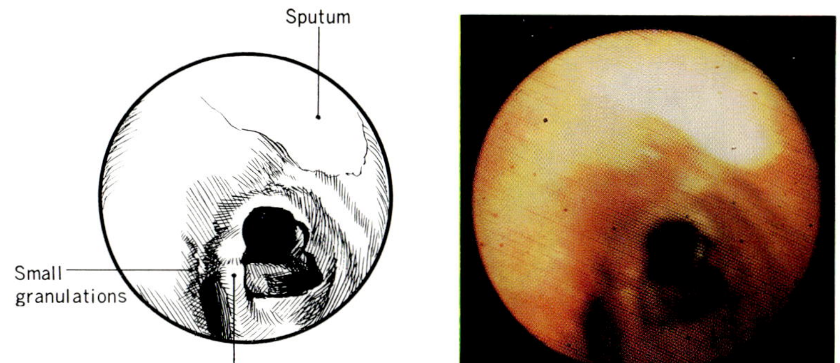

407 a

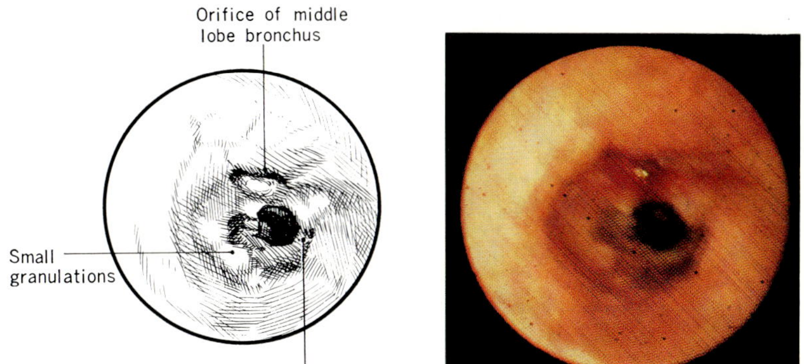


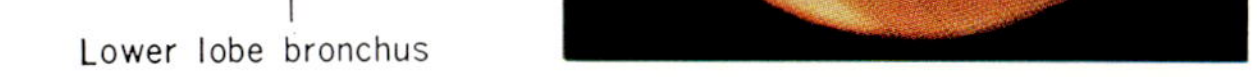


407 b

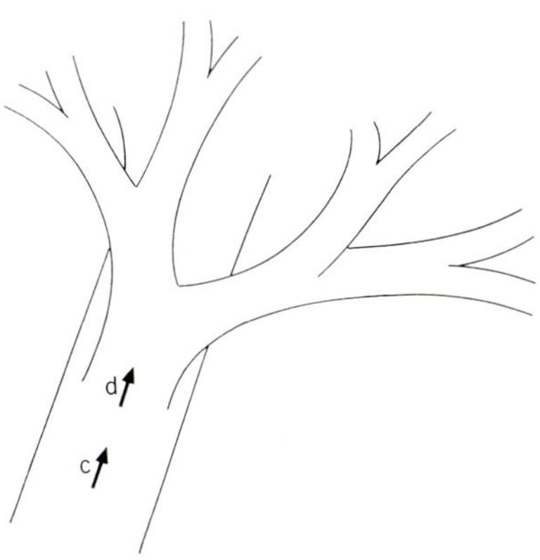


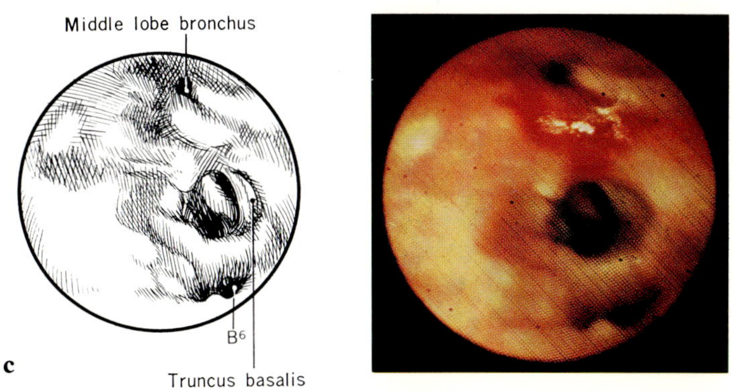


407 c

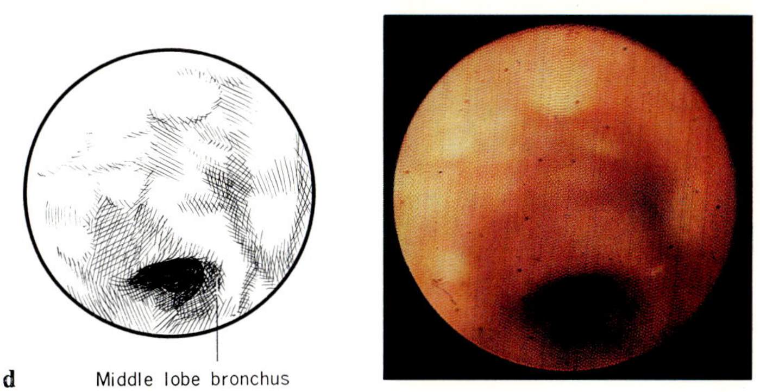


407 d

**Fig. 407 Fiberscopic findings:**

**a.** A number of small granulations with redness are seen protruding from the left wall of the trachea. White substance observed on the anterior wall is purulent secretions.

**b.** The right main bronchus and the truncus intermedius are swollen and irregular. Granulations similar to those on the tracheal wall are protruding from these walls, with some bleeding.

**c.** The entrance of the middle lobe bronchus is covered with irregular granulation tissue and stenosed. Some bleeding is noted. The bronchus is discharging purulent secretions. Irregularity the lower lobe bronchus but it is covered with mucosa and the irregularity is coarse, unlike that due to carcinoma.

**d.** Enlarged view of irregularity found in the orifice of the middle lobe bronchus.

## Case 51 Bronchitis (59, female)

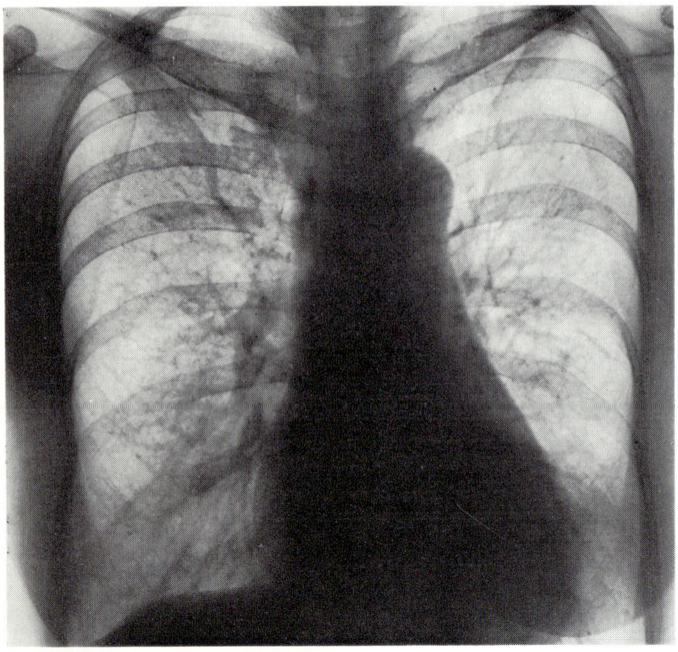

**Chief complaint :** Bloody sputum.
**Case history :** Bloody sputum was expectorated a year and a half ago. A month ago bloody sputum was again produced, before coming to our hospital.

**Fig. 408 Chest X-ray, frontal :** No special change is observed.

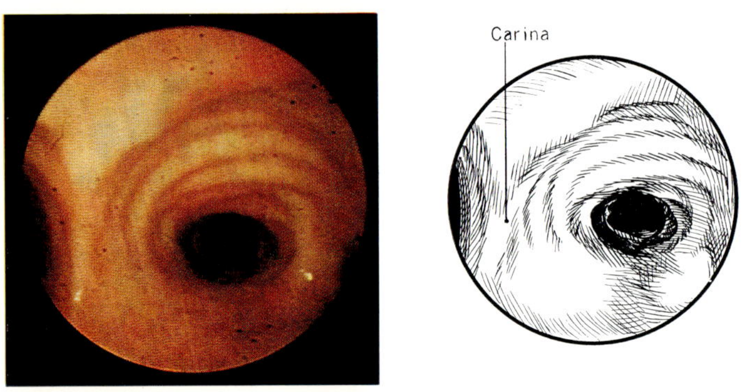


**409 a**

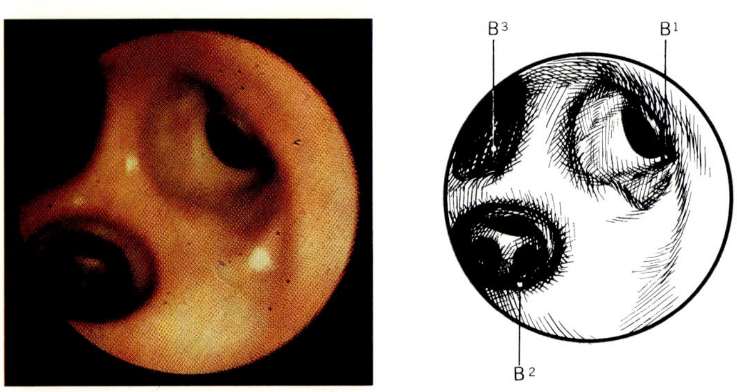


**409 b**

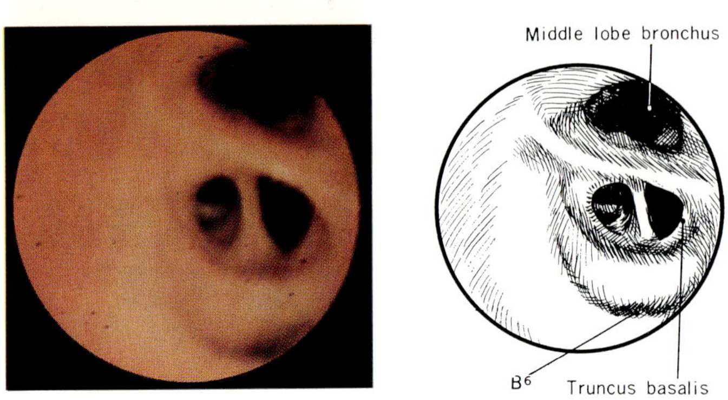


**409 c**

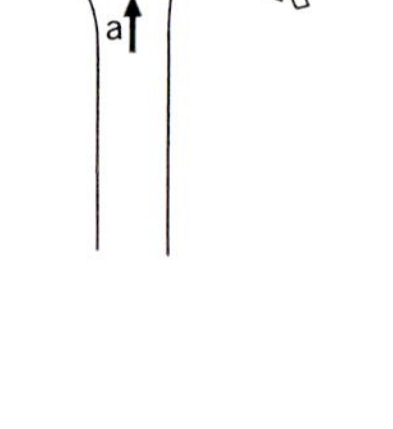


**Fig. 409 Fiberscopic findings :**

- **a.** Cartilage rings in the right main bronchus are clearly recognized.
- **b.** Cartilage rings are observed in the upper lobe bronchus. Bronchi ahead are well seen. The mucosa is pale.
- **c.** The same findings are present in the lower lobe bronchi.

# Case 52 Bronchitis Atrophicans (72, female)

**Chief complaint :** Hemoptysis.
**Case history :** Two months ago the patient had a hemoptysis of 50 ml. Chest X-ray did not reveal any specific change. Bronchofiberscopy did not reveal any evidence of a tumor after a thorough examination of all subsegmental bronchi bilaterally. Findings compatible with bronchitis atrophicans were noted in the right upper lobe.

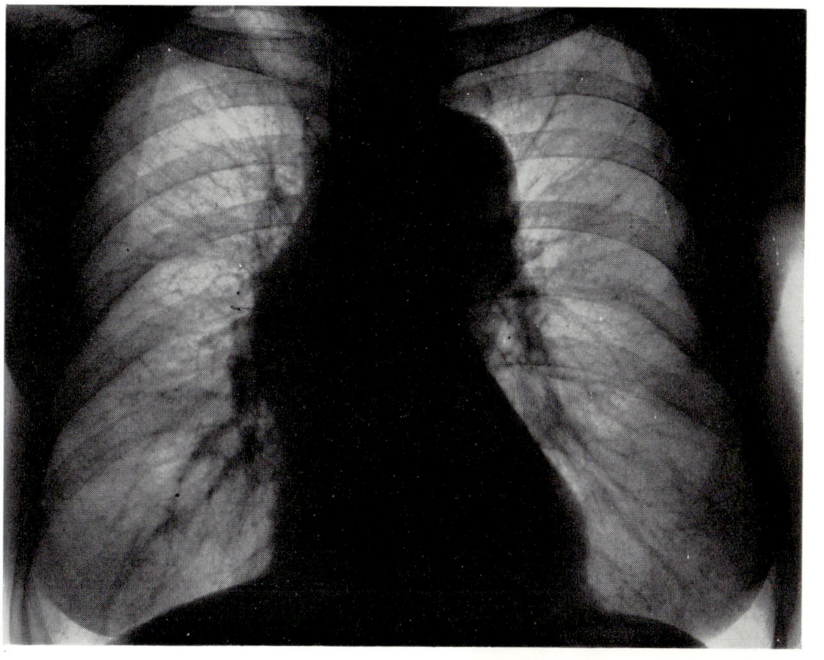

**Fig. 410 Chest X-ray, frontal :** Cartilages of the trachea are conspicuous. Both lung fields are emphysematous, with no evidence of a tumor shadow. Cordlike shadows are noted in the right upper field.

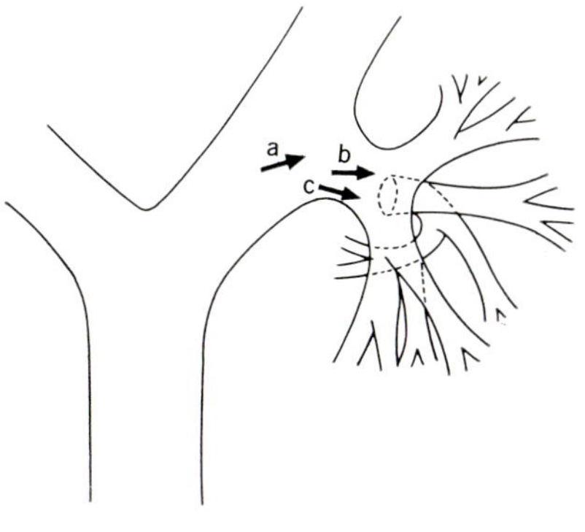


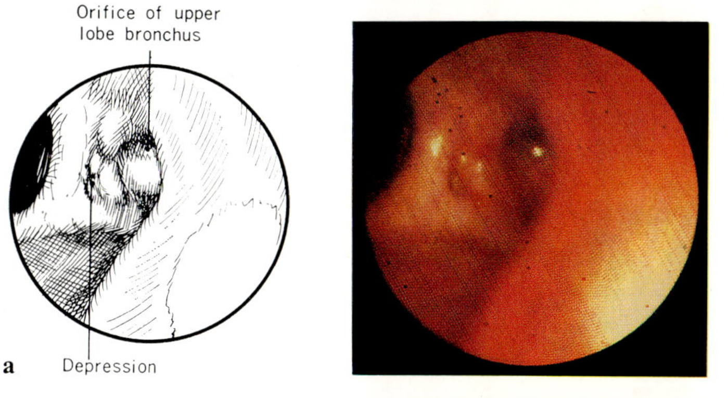


411 a

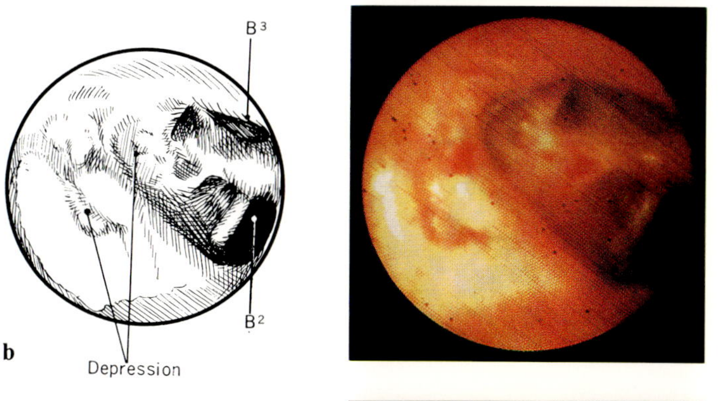


411 b

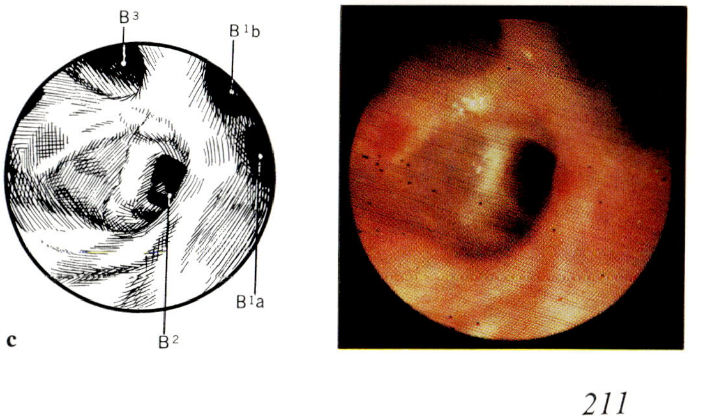


411 c

**Fig. 411 Fiberscopic findings :**
**a.** There is a depression in the entrance to the right upper lobe bronchus.
**b.** At the entrance to $B^3$, a depression is observed. Slight bleeding is visible and capillary vessels are engorged.
**c.** At the entrance of $B^2$, a depression is noted. This is caused by mucosal atrophy.

Thus : in each segmental and subsegmental bronchus, there appear conspicuous cartillaginous rings, depressions, or occasionally transverse striations between the longitudinal corrugations. These are characteristic changes of bronchitis atrophicans.

## Case 53 Bronchial Cyst (29, female)

**Case history :** An abnormal shadow was found in a mass survey two years ago. During the following two years therapy was given for tuberculosis but the shadow increased in size. Further examinations were conducted in our hospital. Bronchograms suggested the diagnosis of pulmonary tuberculosis, and bronchofiberscopy also suggested the same disease. Histology by curettage at bronchofiberscopy was attempted, but the curette did not enter the tumor-like shadow. Cytological examination was negative for tumor cells. No definite proof was obtained to rule out malignant tumor. Lobectomy was performed. Pathological diagnosis : Bronchial cyst 40 × 30 × 50 mm found in $S^3c$.

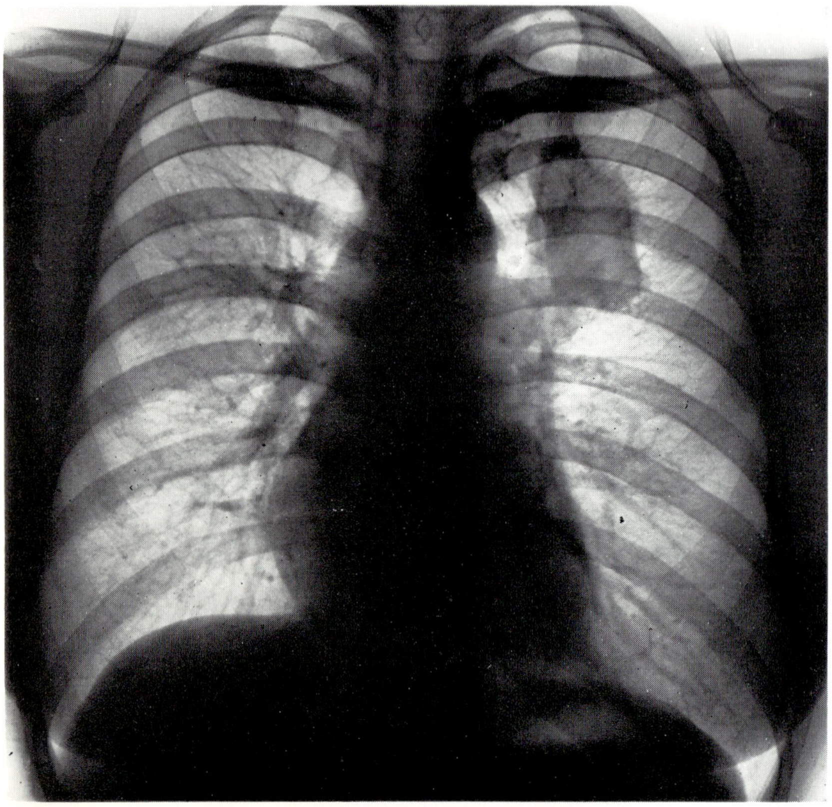

**Fig. 412 Chest X-ray, frontal :** In the left upper lung field an irregularly shaped tumor-like shadow with indistinct boundaries is seen. No cord-like bronchial shadows are present and the surrounding lung is perfectly normal.

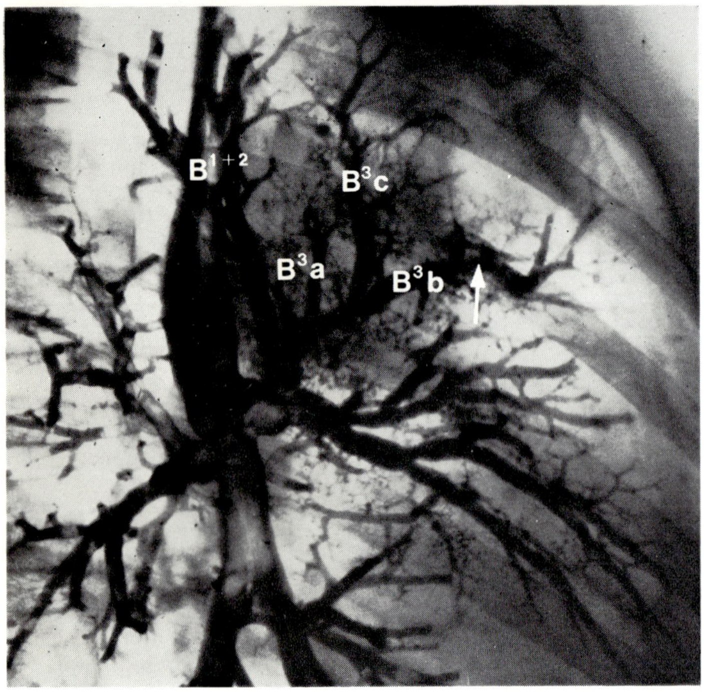


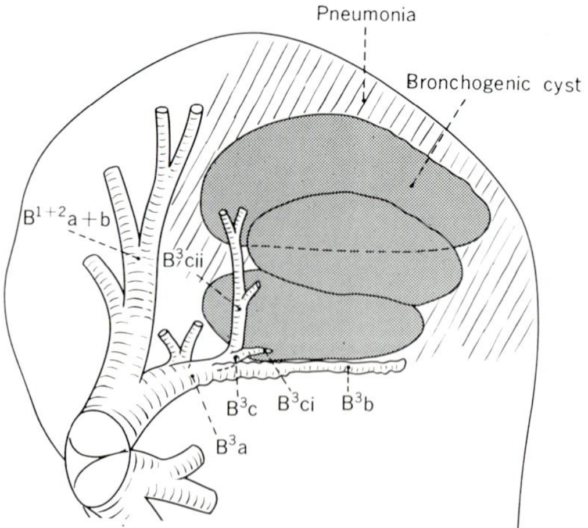


**Fig. 414 Traced schema**

**Fig. 413 Bronchogram, highly oblique :** $B^{1+2}$ presents a marked convergence of fibrosis. A tumor-like lesion is at the periphery of $B^3b$ (arrow), $B^3b$ itself is angulated. No distinct obstruction can be demonstrated, and it seems that part of $B^3b$ passes through the lesion. $B^3c$ is filled with the contrast medium and its peripheral bronchi are not stenosed.

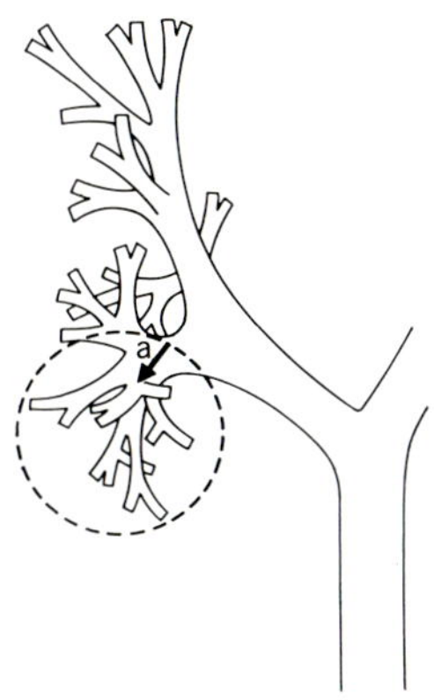


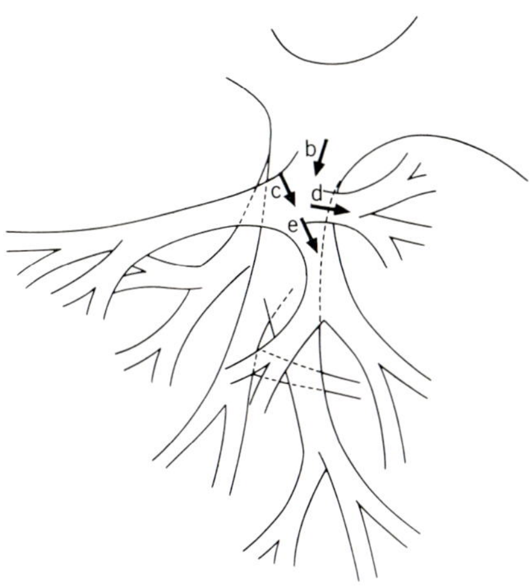


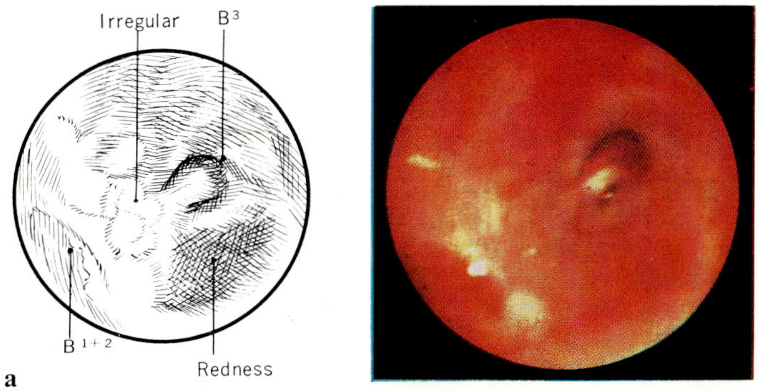


415 a

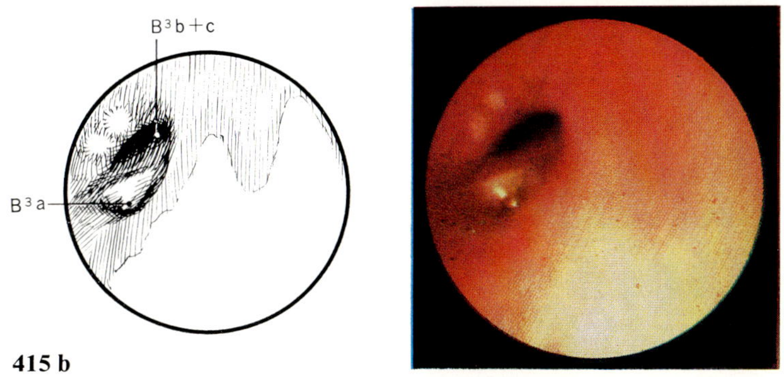


415 b

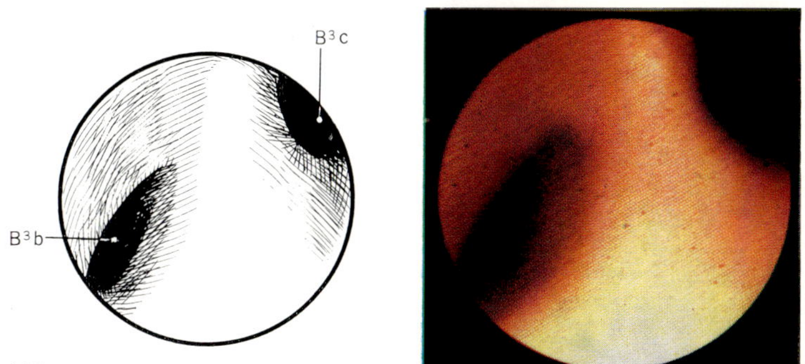


415 c

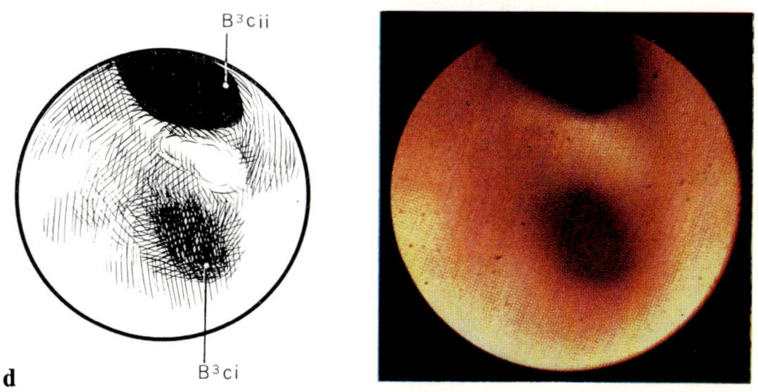


415 d

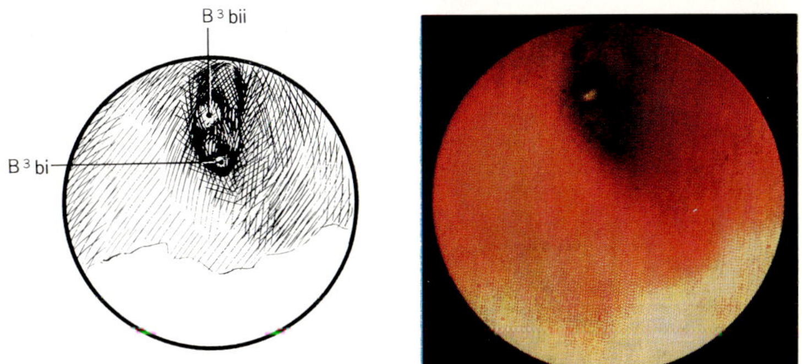


415 e

**Fig. 415 Fiberscopic findings:**

**a.** The entrance and the bifurcation into $B^{1+2}$ and $B^3$ are markedly inflamed, irregular, and the cartilage rings are unclear.

**b.** $B^3$ is slightly stenosed, inflamed and swollen. Swelling is intense at the bifurcation of $B^3$a and $B^3$b+c.

**c.** This is a view of $B^3$b and $B^3$c as seen through the 4 mm bronchofiberscope. Swelling is marked. The bronchial walls are not irregular.

**d.** This is i and ii of $B^3$b. They are practically normal.

**e.** This is i and ii of $B^3$c. $B^3$b is markedly inflamed and elliptically stenosed.

When the bronchofiberscope is advanced into $B^3$bi and observed under X-ray TV fluoroscopy, the tip of the fiberscope is near but not in the lesion. A 5 mm bronchofiberscope with curette was then used. The curette passed through the 5 mm bronchoscope could be introduced near but not into the lesion. Biopsy: Negative for cancer. Bronchial washings: Negative for tubercle bacilli.

## Case 54 Pulmonary Abscess (32, male)

**Chief complaint :** Chronic cough.

**Case history :** Cough, continuing since two years ago, became severe recently. The patient was referred to our hospital. Examination with the flexible bronchofiberscope revealed an inflammatory stenosis at $B^6$. The atelectasis of superior segment of the right lower lobe ($S^6$) improved with chemotherapy.

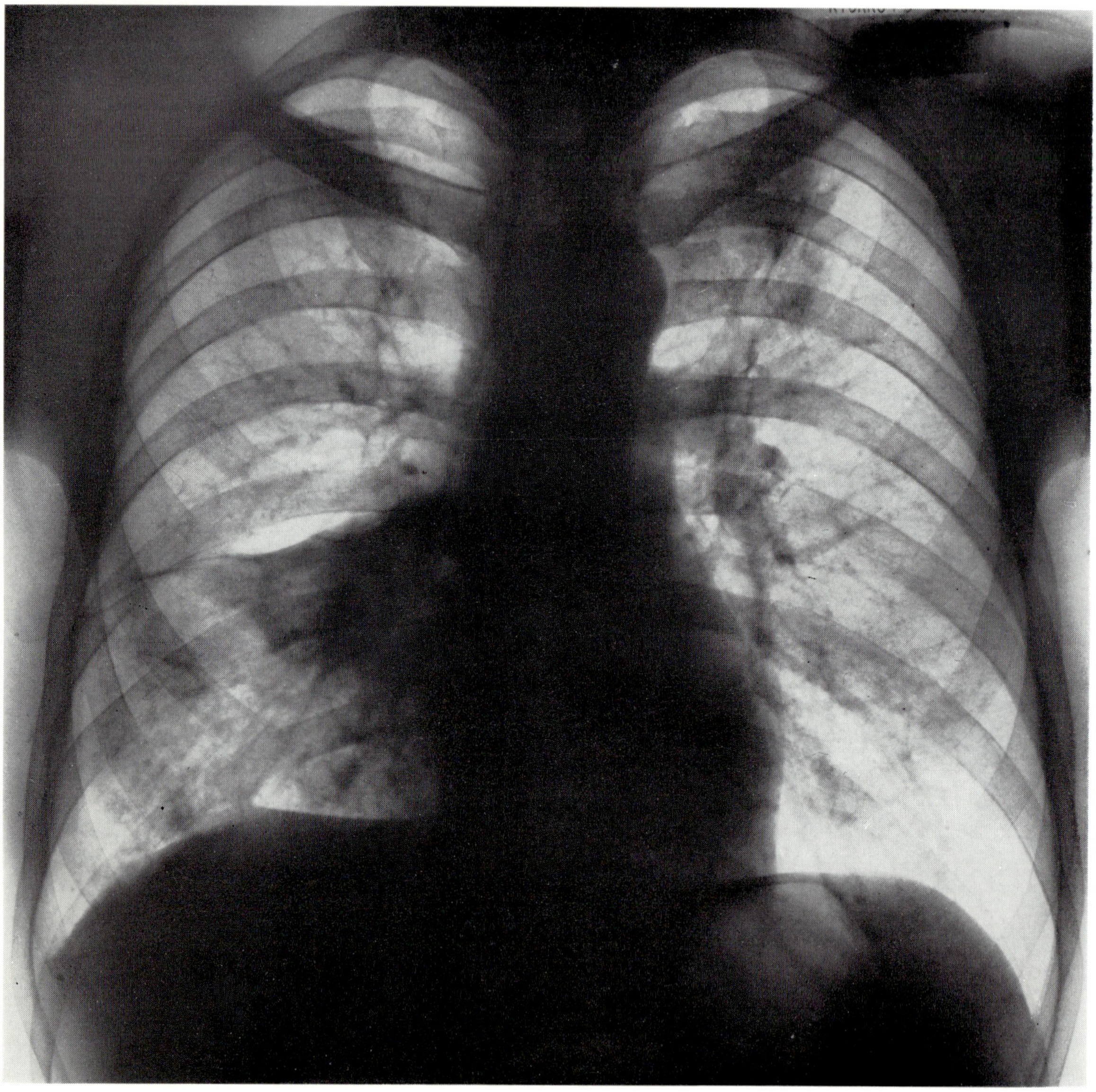

**Fig. 416 Chest X-ray, frontal :** An atelectatic shadow is located in the superior segment of the right lower lobe ($S^6$) and a moderate ectasis in the basal segment.

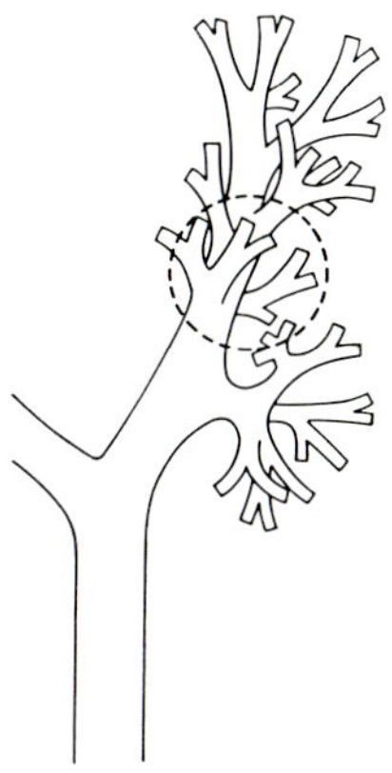

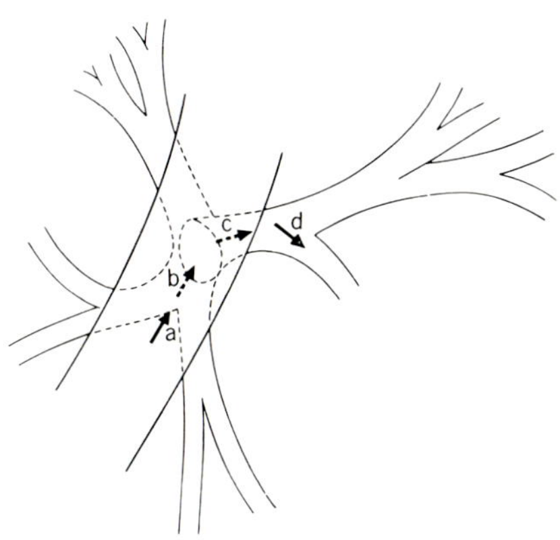


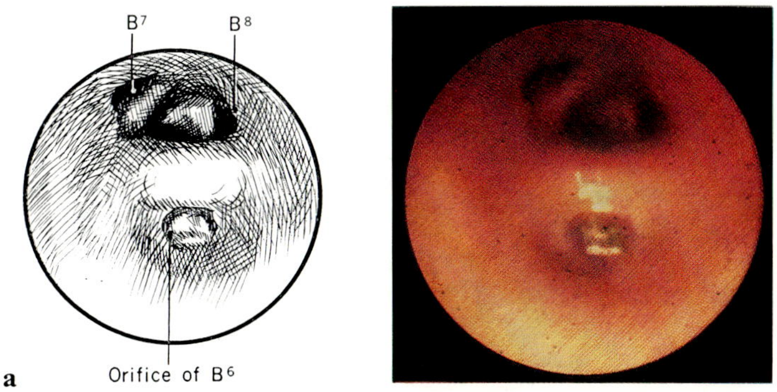


417 a

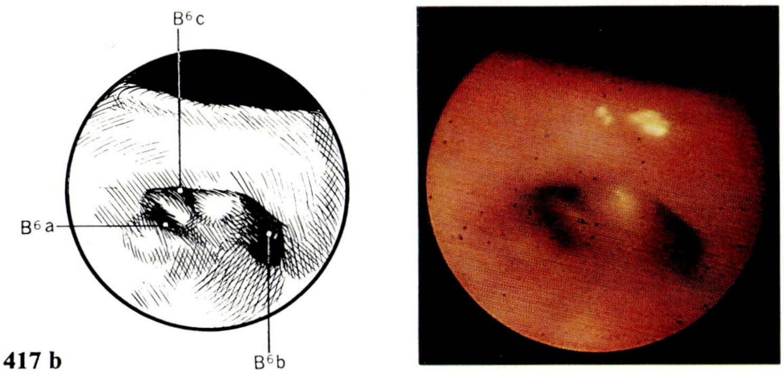


417 b

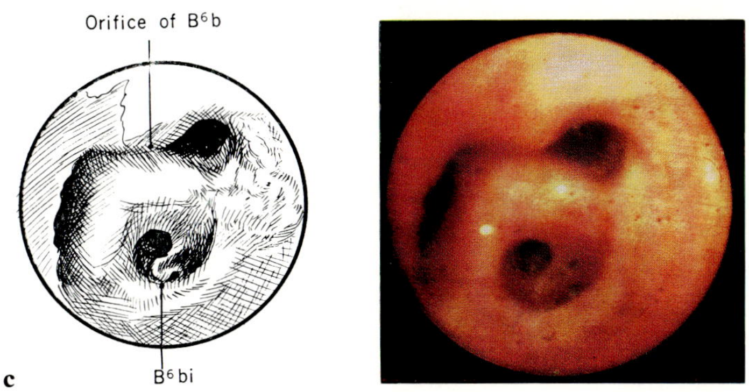


417 c

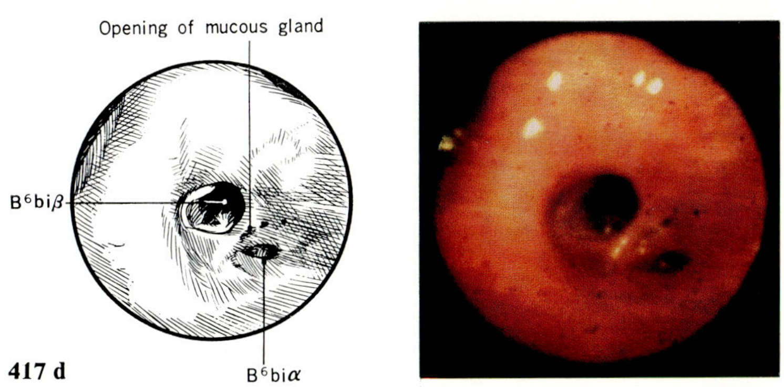


417 d

**Fig. 417 Fiberscopic findings:**

**a.** Inflammatory changes are seen at the entrances of B$^6$ and the basal bronchi. Especially intense is the swelling at the orifice of B$^6$, which is filled with thin purulent sputum.

**b.** When the thin suppurative sputum is removed, the orifices of B$^6$ and B$^6$a+c come into view. Reddening and swelling are prominent, especially the septum between B$^6$b and B$^6$a+c.

**c.** In the three smaller branch bronchi in B$^6$b (B$^6$bi, ii, iii), redness and swelling are similarly marked.

**d.** A bit farther into B$^6$bi, at the bifurcation into $\alpha$ and $\beta$ the opening of a mucous gland is visible.

These bronchoscopic findings are typical of suppurative disease.

## Case 55 Bronchiectasis (55, male)

**Chief complaint :** Bloody sputum.
**Case history :** Patient has had recurrent bloody sputum for the last 7 years.

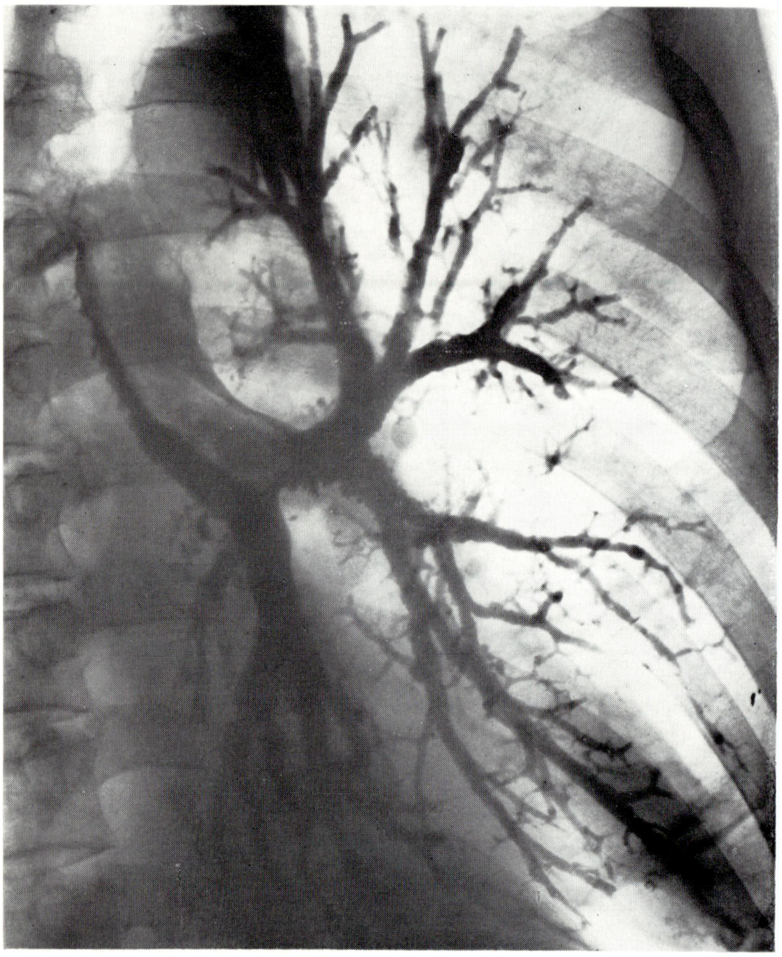

**Fig. 418 Bronchogram :** Abnormally coalesced bronchi are located in the left lower lobe, and ectasis is observed at $B^8$, $B^9$ and $B^{10}$. These findings led to a diagnosis of bronchiectasis.

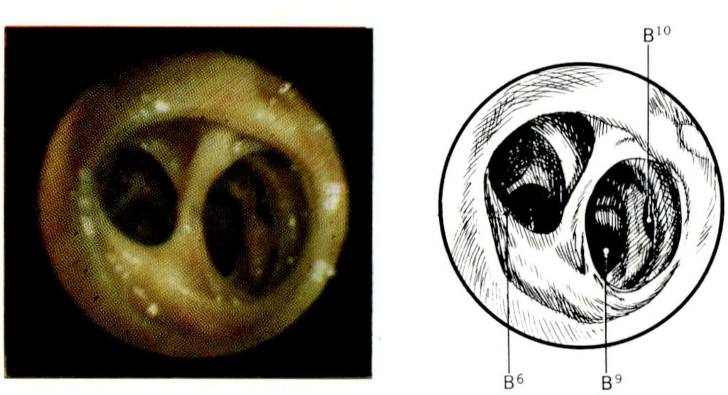


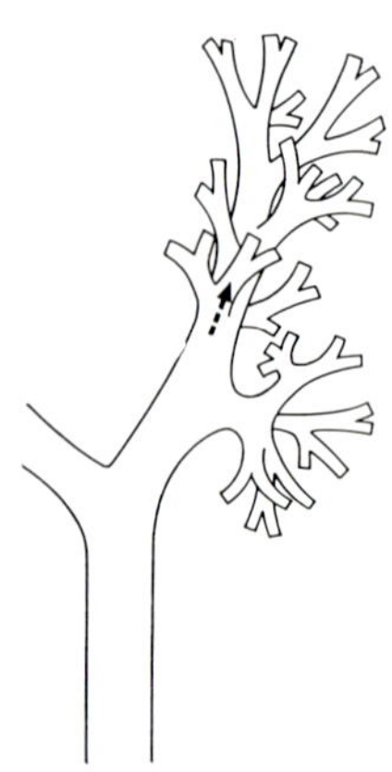

**Fig. 419 Fiberscopic findings :** The mucosa of $B^8$, $B^9$ and $B^{10}$ trifurcations is markedly swollen. This is indicative of the presence of inflammation.

## Case 56 Bronchiectasis (46, male)

**Chief complaint :** Bloody sputum.

**Case history :** The patient had bloody sputum since a year ago, and suspecting lung cancer, came to our hospital.

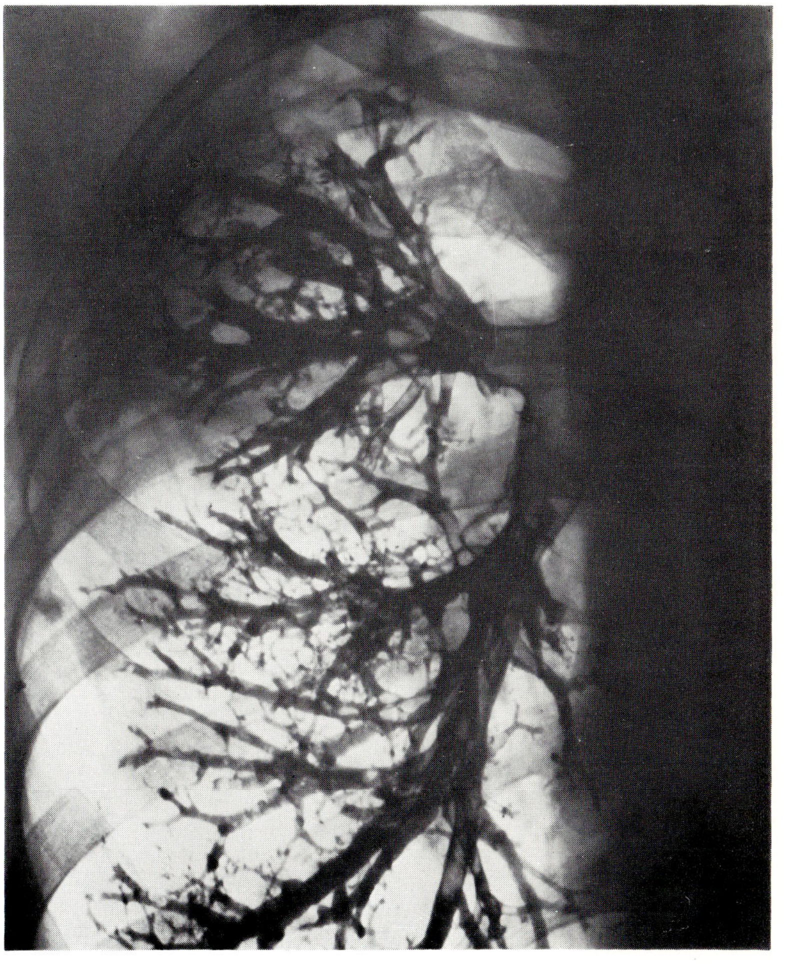

**Fig. 420 Bronchogram :** Moderate bronchiectasis is demonstrated in the peripheral branches of the right $B^1$, $B^2$ and $B^3$.

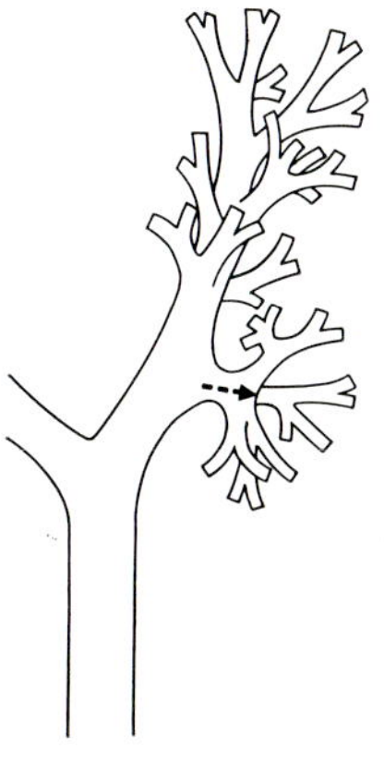

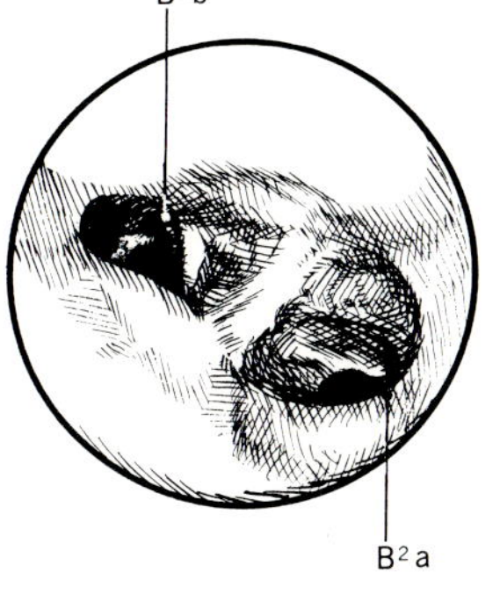


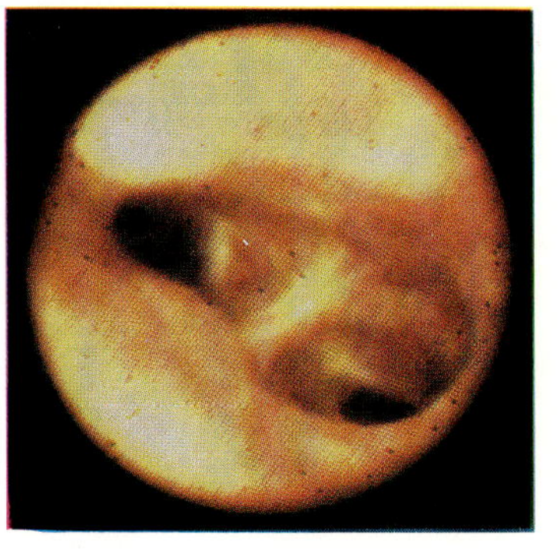

**Fig. 421 Fiberscopic findings :** The entrance to both $B^2a$ and $B^2b$ is atrophic. Atrophic cartilage rings are visible in the subsegmental bronchi. Further peripherally, the bronchi appear to be ectatic. These findings are characteristic of post-inflammatory bronchiectasis.

# III. Foreign Body in a Bronchus

## Case 57 Foreign Body in a Bronchus (67, female)

**Case history :** Thirteen years ago a fish bone (sea bream) was inhaled accidentally into a bronchus. Since then the patient has had a slight fever or sputum with blood streaks on occasions, and this had continued for three years. About 10 years ago, the patient was hospitalized in a certain college hospital and rigid bronchoscopy was performed. A foreign body, apparently a fish bone, and granulation tissue reaction were localized. They were unable to remove the fish bone. The bloody sputum continued but no further attempts were made to remove the bone. During the past year the bloody sputum became much worse. The patient visited our hospital for removal of the fish bone.

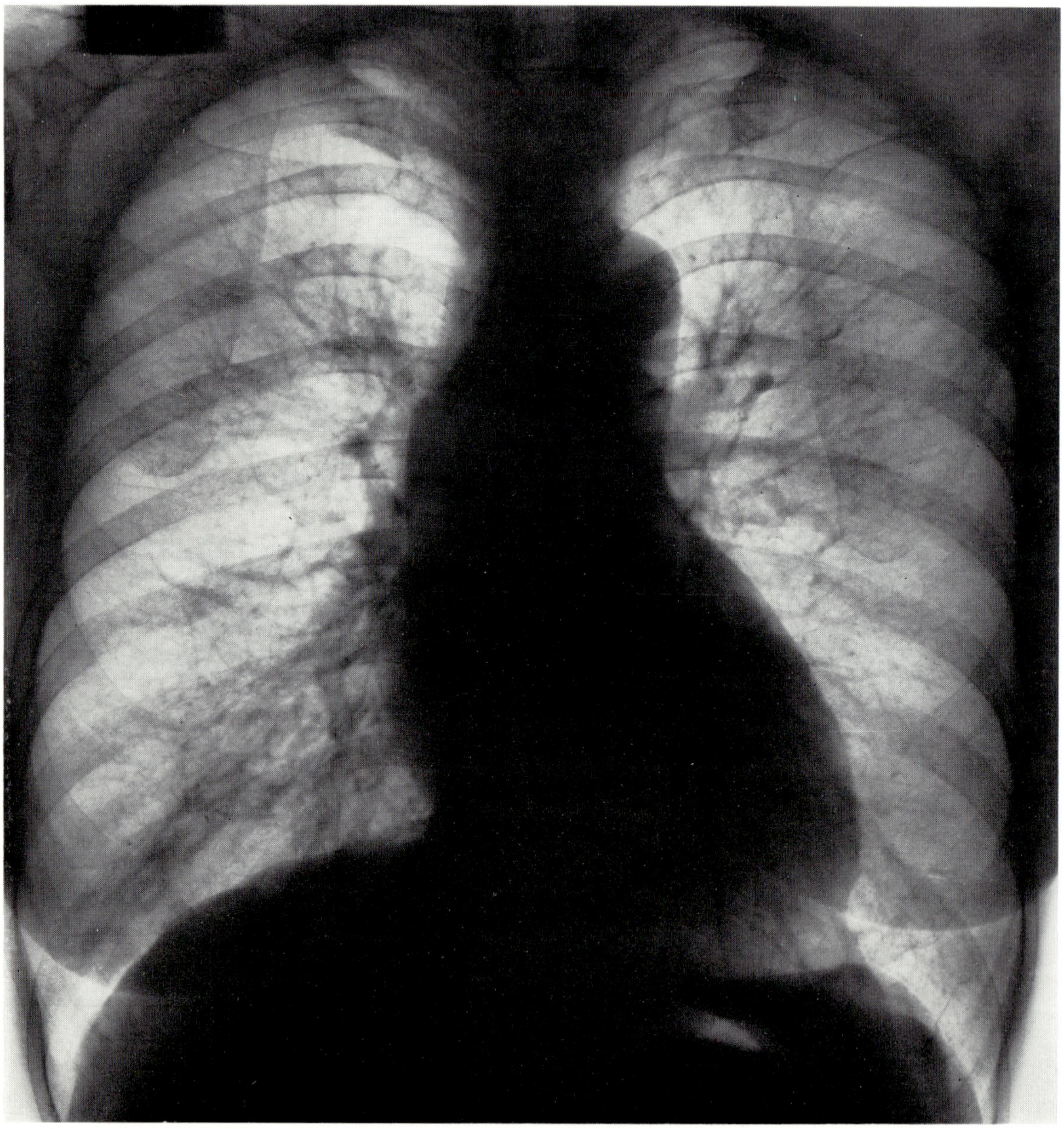

**Fig. 422 Chest X-ray, frontal :** Engorgement of vascular shadow is noted in the right lower lung field. Pneumonia is considered to be present.

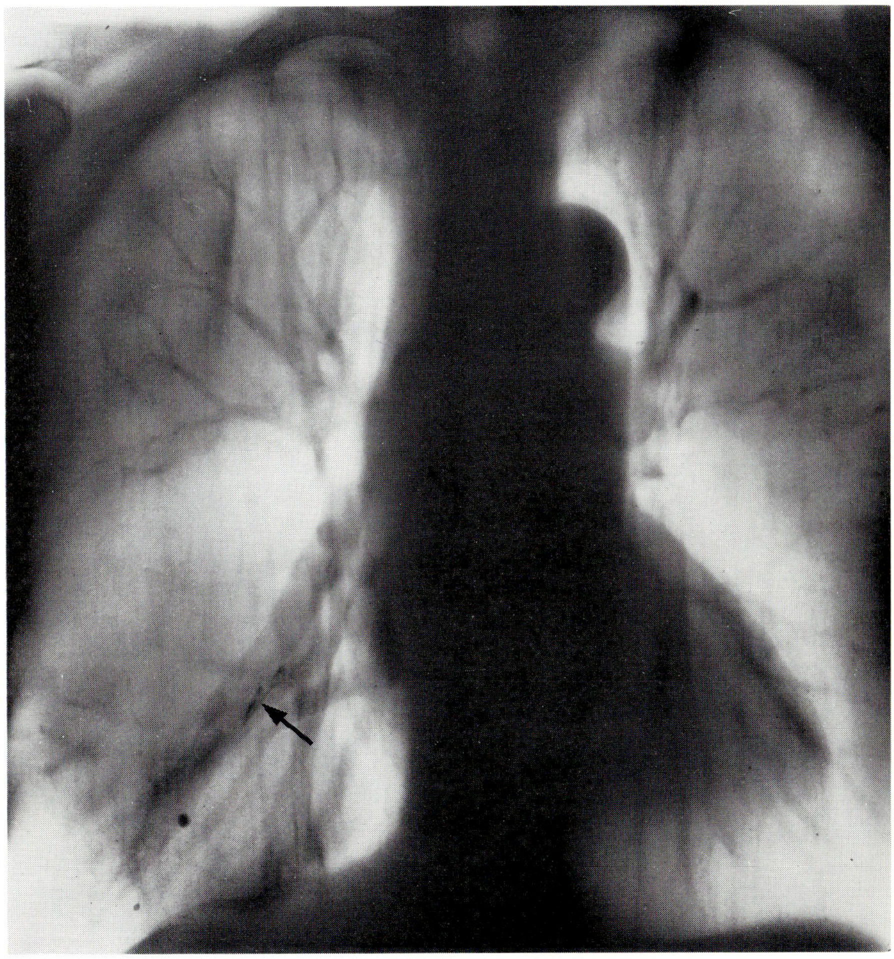

**Fig. 423 Tomogram:** A sharp fish bone (arrow) is present in the wall a of peripheral subsegmental bronchus of $B^8$. An airbronchogram is visible in the periphery of the bronchus.

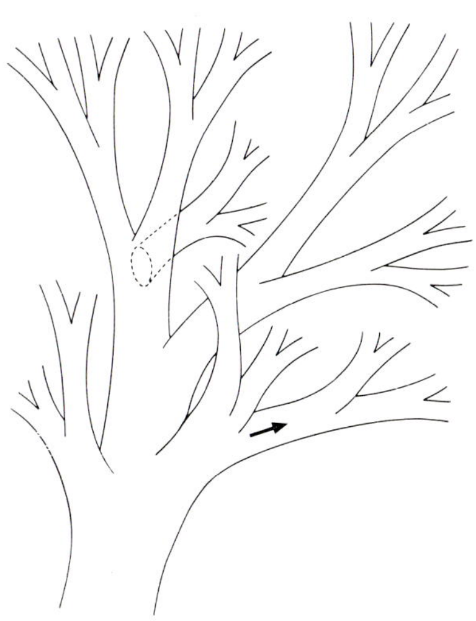

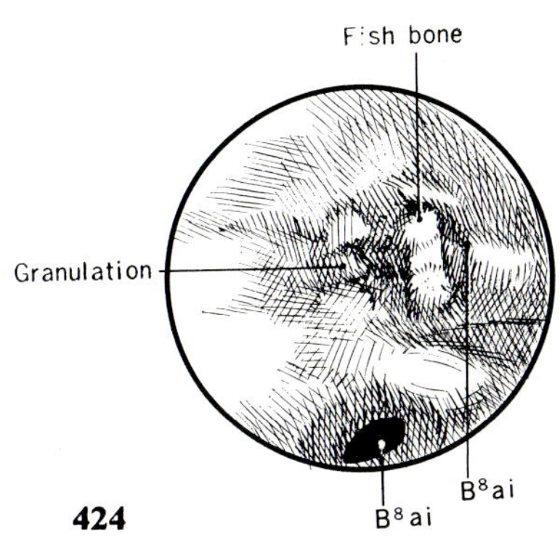


424

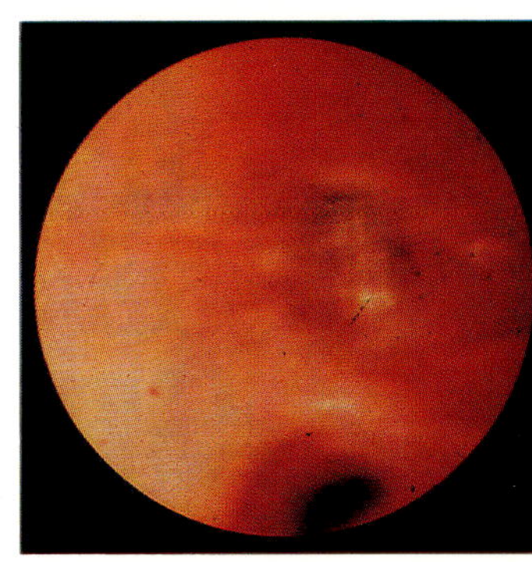

425

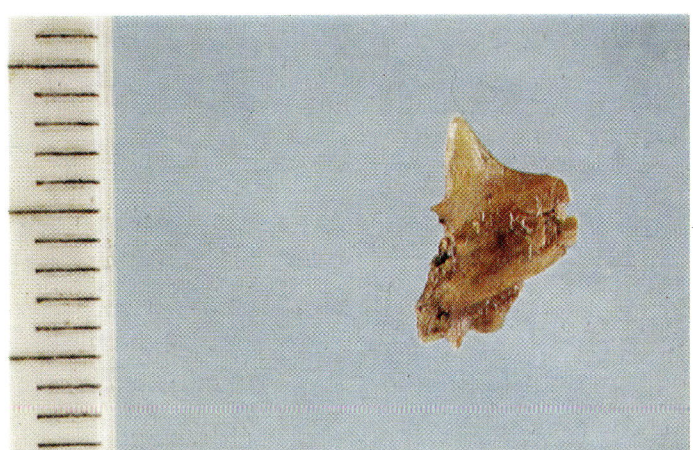

**Fig. 424 Fiberscopic findings:** The fish bone is stuck in the granulation tissue in $B^8$aii which bled readily. The lower part is free from the bronchial wall but the upper end has become so firmly entrenched in the wall that it could not be removed by mere pulling. A biopsy forceps inserted through a 5 mm flexible bronchofiberscope was successful in removing the bone by grasping the free edge of it.

**Fig. 425 Macroscopic findings:** The fish bone measured 8 mm in length and part of it was misshaped due to corrosion.

## Case 58 Foreign Body (26, male) (Courtesy of Dr. M. Amo, National Sanatorium Matsudo Hospital)

**Case history :** During the dental operation 10 days ago, a tip of small drill was dropped into a bronchus. The chest X-ray was taken at the nearby clinic, which indicated the location of the drill at the right peripheral bronchus. Rigid bronchoscopy, immediately performed, was not successful. The patient was transferred to the National Sanatorium Hospital at Matsudo near Tokyo and underwent bronchofiberscopy. The drill was successfully taken out under X-ray TV fluoroscopy.

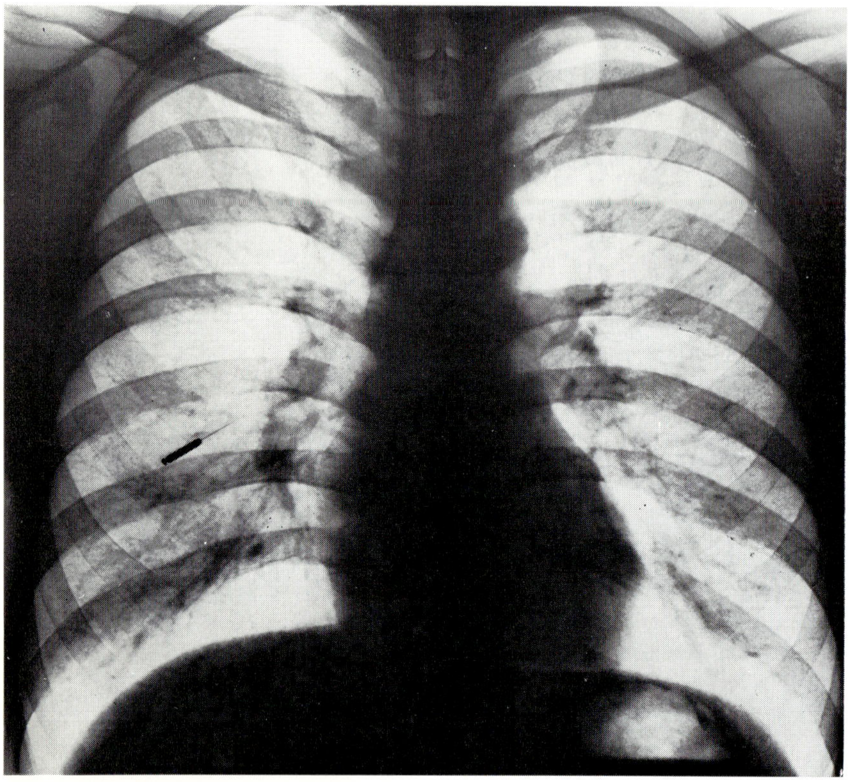

**Fig. 426 Chest X-ray, frontal :** A small drill is clearly observed in the periphery of $B^6b$. In order for the location to be determined exactly, a lateral photograph is essential.

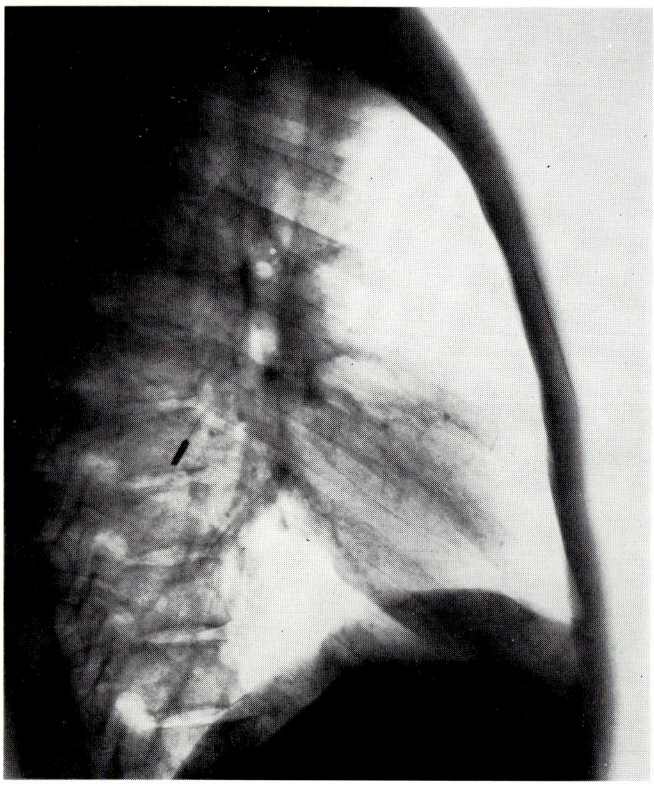

**Fig. 427 Chest X-ray, lateral :** This reveals the small drill to be in the peripheral bronchus of $B^6bii$.

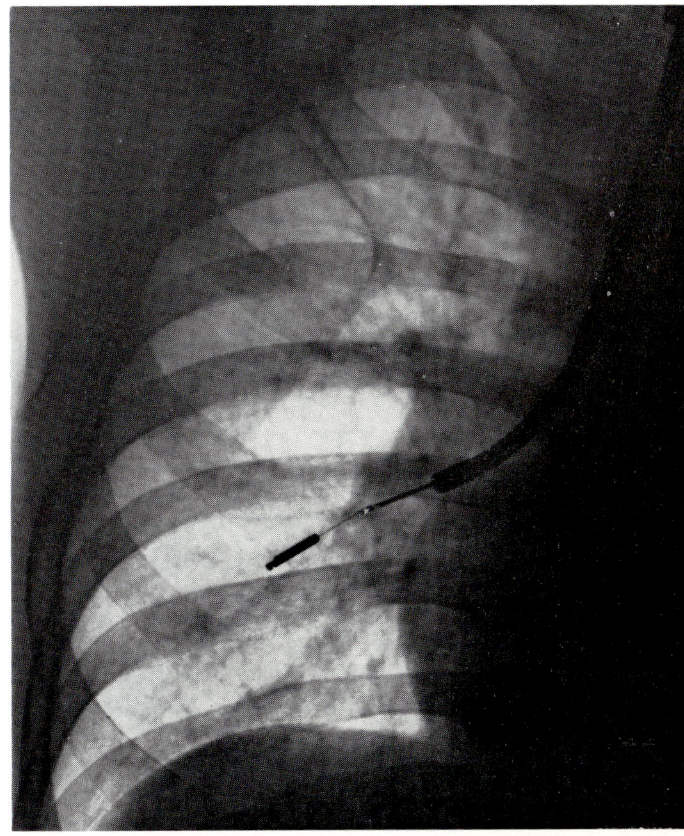

**Fig. 428 Bronchofiberscopic X-ray film, frontal:** Flexible bronchofiberscopy was performed under local anesthesia. When the 5 mm fiberscope was inserted into the right $B^6b$, a slightly glittering body was discovered in the direction of $B^6bii$. Under X-ray fluoroscopy, the tip of the fiberscope and the pointed end of the drill were found to be in good contact. This relative position did not change even when the patient's body was rotated slightly for further confirmation. A biopsy forceps for the 5 mm scope was introduced and the glittering body was firmly grasped and removed under X-ray vision.

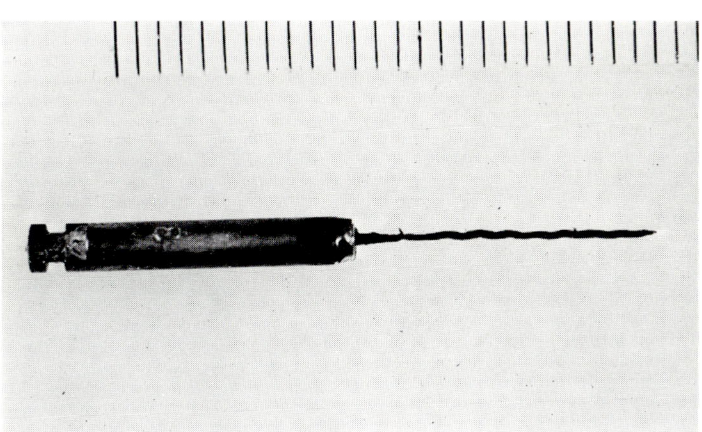

**Fig. 430** The small dental drill which was removed.

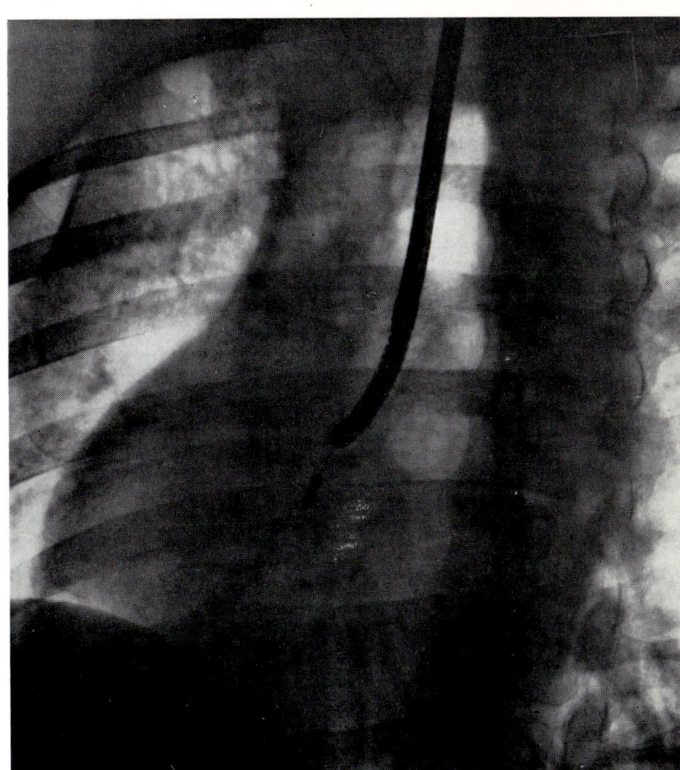

**Fig. 429 Bronchofiberscopic X-ray film, oblique:** Notice the drill securely held by the biopsy forceps.

## COMMENT:

The flexible bronchofiberscope exercises its great power in removing such a foreign body. The rule is to confirm the precise location of the foreign body by means of the X-ray TV, and then under its direct vision the foreign body should be extracted by using the biopsy forceps through the bronchofiberscope.

# References


ABRAMS, L. D.: A pleural biopsy punch. Lancet, 1 : 30, 1958.

ABRAMS, W. B. et al.: Current concept of tuberculosis, pleurisy with effusion as derived from pleural biopsy studies. Dis. Chest, 38 : 60, 1960.

AGLIOZZO, C. M. et al.: Scalene lymph nodes in necropsies of malignant tumors. Analysis of one hundred sixty-six cases. Cancer, 20 : 2148, 1967.

ANACKER, H.: Lungenkrebs und Bronchographie. Georg Thieme Verlag, Stuttgart, 1955.

ANDERSON, R. W.: Bronchoscopy. In : Davis-Christopher ; Textbook of Surgery. p. 1773, W. B. Saunders Company, Philadelphia, 1972.

BAIRD, J. L.: British Patent Specification No. 20, 969/27, 1927.

BAIRD, J. L.: British patent 285, 738, February 15, 1928.

BAIRD, J. L.: An Improved Method of and Means Producing Optical Images. British Patent Specification, 20 969, 1968.

BERQUO, G. and CARDOSO, P.. Anesthesia for bronchoscopy and bronchography. Anesth. & Analg., 39 : 523, 1960.

BLADY, J. V.: Aspiration biopsy of tumors in obscure or difficult locations under roentgenoscopic guidance. Am. J. Roentgenol., 42 515, 1939.

BLUTH, I.: Laminagraphic studies of the vascular patterns in cancer of the lung with special reference to the "circumscribed" variety. Am. J. Roentgenol., 98 : 397, 1966.

BORRIE, J.: Lung Cancer, Surgery and Survival. Appleton-Century-Crofts, New York, 1965.

BOYDEN, A.: Segmental Anatomy of the Lungs. McGraw-Hill, New York, 1955.

CAHAN, W. G. et al.: Radical pneumonectomy. J Thorac. Surg., 22 : 449, 1951.

CAHAN, W. G. Radical lobectomy. J. Thorac. Cardiovasc. Surg., 39 : 555, 1960.

CARLENS, E.: Mediastinoscopy : A method for inspection and tissue biopsy in the superior mediastinum. Dis. Chest., 36 : 343, 1959.

CARLENS, E.: "Some aspects of mediastinoscopy." Rev. Méd. Internat. Photo Cinéma Télévision, 1 : 86, 1926.

COCCHI, U. und SCHINZ, H. R. et al.: Differentialdiagnose der Erkrankungen von Lunge, Pleura, Mediastinum und Zwerchfell, Lehrbuch der Röntgendiagnostik. Band III. Innere Organe, Teil I., Georg Thieme Verlag, Sturttgart, 1952.

CONNAR, R. G.: Prescalene and deep cervical lymph node biopsy. Surg. Gynec. Obstet., 101 : 732, 1955.

CRAVER, L. P. et al.: Aspiration biopsy of tumors of lung. J. Thorac. Surg., 8 : 436, 1939

CRUZE, K. et al.: Prescalene node biopsy. Ann. Surg., 148 : 895, 1958.

DAMELS, A. C.: A method of biopsy useful in diagnosing certain intrathoracic disease. Dis. Chest, 16 : 360, 1949.

DAVIES, D. F.: A review of detection methods for the early diagnosis of lung cancer. J. Chron. Dis., 19 : 819, 1966.

DREVVATEN, T. and FRIMANN-DAHL, J.: Peripheral carcinomas : A radiological and pathological study. Brit. J. Radiol., 34 : 180, 1961.

EINHORN, M.: A new oesophagoscope. Med. Record, 61 : 159, 1902.

ESGNRRA, A., WETMORE, J. and RICKERT, R. R.: Transbrochial lung biopsy ; Laboratory evalution of a biopsy instrument capable of obtaining specimens suitable for histologic studies. Am. Rev. Resp. Dis., 102 : 808, 1970.

FARBER, S.M., ROSENTHAL, M., ALSTON, E.F., BENIOFF, M.A. and MCGRATH, A. K.: Cytologic Diagnosis of Lung Cancer. Charles C Thomas, Springfield, Illinois, 1950.

FENNESSY, J. J.: A technique for the selective catheterization of segmental bronchi using arterial catheters. Am. J. Roentgenol., Rad. Therapy & Nuclear Med., 96 : 963, 1952.

FRY, W. A. and MANALO-ESTRELLA, P.: The techinical details of bronchial brushing. J. Thorac. Cardiovasc. Surg., 60 : 636, 1970.

FUKUMA, S.: Bronchoscopic examination in pulmonary cancer (in Japanese). Jap. J. Clin. Med., 24 : 465, 1966.

GLEDHILL, E. Y. et al.: Needle aspiration in the diagnosis of lung cancer—Report of experience with seventy five aspirations. Amer. J. Clin. Path., 19 : 235, 1949.

GORDON, W.: Lymphatic spread in the surgical treatment of lung cancer. Amer. J. Surg., 104 : 866, 1962.

GRILLO, I. A.: Pulmonary Endoscopy : From KILLIAN to IKEDA ; An Historical Appraisal. J. Jap. Broncho-esophago. Soc., 22 : 107, 1971.

GRZYBOWSKI, S. and COY, P.: Early diagnosis of carcinoma of the lung ; Simultaneous screening with chest X-ray and sputum cytology. Cancer, 25 : 113, 1970.

HANSELL, C. W.: U. S. Patent 1, 751, 584, 1930.

HARRISON, B. and ACKERMAN, L. V.: The importance of epidermoid carcinoma in situ in the histogenesis of carcinoma of the lung. Ann. Surg., 136 : 44, 1952.

HARKEN D. E. et al.: A simple cervicomediastinal exploration for tissue diagnosis. New Eng. Med. J., 251 : 1041, 1954.

HERBUT, P. et al.: Bronchogenic carcinoma ; Diagnosis by cytologic study of bronchoscopically removed secretion. JAMA, 130 : 1006, 1946.

HIGGINS, G. A. et al.: Prescalene fat pad biopsy. J. Thorac. Cardiovasc. Surg., 38 : 402, 1959.

HINSON, K. F. W.: The Spread of Carcinoma of the Lung. In : Carcinoma of the Lung (J. R. BIGNALL, Ed.). E. & S. Livingstone., Edinburgh, p. 130, 1958.

HOLINGER, P. and ANDREWS, A. H.: Bronchial obstruction, Signs, symptoms and diagnosis. Amer. J. Surg., 54 : 193, 1941.

HOLMAN, C. W. and OKINAKA, A.: Occult carcinoma of the lung. J. Thorac. Cardiovasc. Surg., 47 : 466, 1964.

HORNYKIEWYTSCH, TH and STENDER, H. ST.: Normale und pathologisch veränderte Lungengefässe in Schichtbild. Fortschr. Röentgenstr., 79, 1953 ; 80, 81, 1954.

HUERZELER, D.: Zur Frueherkennung des Bronchuskarzinoms. Schweiz. med. Wschr., 100: 1879, 1970.

IKEDA, S.: Bronchogram; Lung cancer (in Japanese). Clinics of Respiratory Organs, 12: 869, 1957.

IKEDA, S.: Periphenal bronchogram of lung cancer (in Japanese). Jap. J. Clin. Med., 24: 451, 1966.

IKEDA, S.: Recording of the endoscopic picture (in Japanese). J. Jap. med. Instr., 37: 291, 1967.

IKEDA, S., YANAI, N. and ISHIKAWA, S.: Flexible Bronchofiberscope. Keio J. Med., 17: 1, 1968.

IKEDA, S., YANAI, N. and ISHIKAWA, S.: Flexible bronchofiberscope (in Japanese). J. Jap. Broncho-esophago. Soc., 19: 54, 1968.

IKEDA, S.: Bronchoscopy, Flexible bronchofiberscopy. In: Atlas of Lung Cancer (S. ISHIKAWA, Ed.) (in Japanese). p. 206, Nakayama-Shoten, Tokyo, 1968.

IKEDA, S.: Bronchofiberscope. In: Japanese Bronchoesophagology (Japan Bronchoesophagolgical Society, Ed.) (in Japanese). p, 145, Igaku Shoin Ltd., Tokyo, 1968.

IKEDA, S. et al.: Endoscopy; Bronchoscopy (in Japanese). Gendai Iryo, 1: 6, 1969.

IKEDA, S.: Clinical application of flexible bronchofiberscope (in Japanese). Lung and Heart, 16: 12. 1969.

IKEDA, S. et al.: Bronchofiberscopic diagnosis (in Japanese). Internal Med., 24: 2, 1969.

IKEDA, S.: New flexible bronchofiberscope (in Japanese). J. Jap. Broncho-esophago. Soc., 20: 167, 1969.

IKEDA, S. et al.: Development of flexible bronchofiberscope (in Japanese). Surg. Diag. & Treatm., 11: 391, 1969.

IKEDA, S. et al.: Diagnosis of lung cancer using flexible bronchofiberscope (in Japanese). Diagn. & Treatm., 57: 1789, 1969.

IKEDA, S.: Diagnosis of Lung Cancer. In: Gendai Gekagaku Taikei 30 (S. ISHIKAWA, Ed.) (in Japanese). p. 75, Nakayama-Shoten, Tokyo, 1969.

IKEDA, S. and TAKASHU, Y.: Eodoscopic color television (in Japanese). Medicina, 6: 1090, 1969.

IKEDA, S.: Flexible Bronchofiberscope. Ann. Otol., 79: 916, 1970.

IKEDA, S. et al.: Flexible Bronchofiberscope. Jap. J. Clin. Oncol., 1: 55, 1971.

IKEDA, S.: Endoscopic diagnosis of lung cancer (in Japanese). Internal Med., 28: 651, 1971.

IKEDA, S. et al.: Early lung cancer (in Japanese). J. Clin. Surg., 27: 31, 1972.

IOANNOU, J.: Atlas D'endoscopie Bronchologique, Aspects Normaux et Pathologiques. Masson, Paris, 1967.

ISHIKAWA, S. and IKEDA, S.: Diagnosis of early lung cancer (in Japanese). Jap. J. Cancer Clin., 11 (Suppl.): 225, 1965.

JACKMAN, R. J., GOOD, C. A., CLAGETT, O. T. and WOOLNER, L. B.: Survival rates in peripheral bronchogenic carcinomas up to four centimeters in diameter presenting as solitary pulmonary nodules. J. Thorac. Cardiovasc. Surg., 57: 1, 1969.

JACKSON, C.: Foreign bodies in the trachea, bronchi and esophagus. Laryngoscope, 15: 527, 1905.

JACKSON, C. and JACKSON, C.L.: Peroral pulmonary drainage —natural and therapeutic, with especial reference to the "tussive squeeze". Amer. J. Med. Sci., 186: 849, 1933.

JACKSON, C. and JACKSON, C. L.: Bronchoscopy, Esophagoscopy and Gastroscopy: Third Edition. W. B. Saunders Company, Philadelphia, 1934.

JACKSON, C. and JACKSON, C. L.: Bronchoesophagology. W. B. Saunders Company, Philadelphia, 1950.

JACKSON, C.L. and HUBER, J.F.: Correlated applied anatomy of the bronchial tree and lungs with a system of nomenclature. Dis. Chest, 9: 319, 1943.

JOSEPHS, B. N. et al.: Prescalene lymph node biopsy. Arch. Surg., 76: 93, 1958.

KAPANY, N. S.: Fiber Optics Principles and Applications. Academic Press, New York, London, 1967.

KAPUR, K. K. et al.: Scalene node biopsy in pulmonary diseases. Report of 110 cases. Dis. Chest, 52: 195, 1967.

KASSAY, D.: Clinical Applications of Bronchology. McGraw-Hill Book Company, New York, 1960.

KILLIAN, G.: Meeting of the Society of Physicians of Freiburg. Dec. 17, 1897, München. Med. Wschr., 45: 378, 1898.

KLASSEN, K. P. et al.: Biopsy of diffuse plumonary lesions. Arch. Surg., 59: 694, 1949.

KOPPENSTEIN, E. et al.: Beitrag zur Punktionsdiagnostik der Brustorgane. Fortschr. Röntgenstr., 85: 563, 1956.

KOVACS, S.: Method of Ventilation during Bronchoscopy. Anesthesiology, 18: 335, 1957.

KOVÄTS, F. Jr. and ZSEBÖK, Z.: Röntgenanatomische Grundlagen der Lungenutersuchungen. Akadémiai Kiado, Budapest, 1959.

LAMM, H.: Z. Instrumentenk., 50: 579, 1930.

LEES, A. W. et al.: Scalene node biopsy in bronchial carcinoma. Amer. Rev. Resp. Dis., 86: 648, 1962.

LEMOINE, J. M. and FABRE, CH.: L'examen bronchoscopique aprés les hémoplysies. J. Fr. Méd. Chir. Thor., 25: 621, 1971.

MASSEN, W.: Die Mediastinoskopie (Biopsie nach Carlens), eine neue diagnostische Methode bei Thoraxerkrankungen. Dtsch. Med. Wschr., 87: 2004, 1902.

MESTITS, P. et al.: Pleural biopsy in the diagnosis of pleural effusion. Lancet, 2: 1349, 1958.

MILLER, W. S.: The lymphatics of the lung. Anat. Anz., 12: 110, 1896.

MIYAJI, T. et al.: Morphological study of bronchogenic carcinoma in Japan. Gann, 46: 523, 1955.

MORGAN, S. W. et al.: A critical reappraisal of scalene fat pad biopsy. J. Thorac. Cardiovasc. Surg., 43: 548, 1962.

MUENDNICH, K. and HOFLEHNER, G.: Die Narkose-Beatmungs-bronchoscopie. Anesthetist, 21: 121, 1953.

MÜNZ, J.: Die Bronchotomographie mit besonderer Berücksichtigung der postoperativen Zustände. VEB Georg Thieme, Leipzig, 1963.

NAGAISHI, C.: Fuctional Anatomy and Histology of the Lung. Igaku Shoin Ltd., Tokyo, 1972.

NAKATSUBO, H. and KAWASHIMA, T.: History of glass fibers and fiberscope (in Japanese). J. Jap. Med. Instr., 37: 273, 1967.

NARABAYASHI, K. and IKEDA, S.: Bronchography and bronchoscopy in pulmonary cancer (in Japanese). Diagn. & Treatm., 54: 422, 1966.

NOHL, H. C.: The value of scalene node biopsy in intrathoracic disease. Brit. J. Tuberc., 52: 286, 1958.

ONUIGBO, W. I. B.: Contralateral cervical node metastases in lung cancer. Thorax, 17: 201, 1962.

ONUIGBO, W. I. B.: Surgical significance of mediastinal metastases in lung cancer. Am. J. Surg., 106: 929, 1963.

ONUIGBO, W. I. B.: Amons-block formalin-fixation method for investigating cancer metastasis, Z. Krebsforsch., 65: 209, 1963.

OSWALD, N. C., HINSON, K. F. W., CANTI, G. and MILLER, A. B.: The diagnosis of primary lung cancer with special reference to sputum cytology. Thorax, 26: 623, 1971.

OVERHORT, R. H. et al.: The neccessity for exploration in silent lung cancer. New York State J. Med., 51: 1915, 1951.

OVERHOLT, R. H. et al.: Surgical treatment of lung cancer found on X-ray survey. New Eng. Med. J. 252: 429, 1955.

PALUMBO, L. T. et al.: Evaluation of scalene node biopsy. Surgery, 53: 639, 1963.

PALVA, T.: On the technique of mediastinoscopy. Rev. Méd. Internat. Photo Cinéma Télévision, 1: 84, 1962.

PAPANICOLAOU, G. N. and TRAUT, H. F.: Diagnosis of uterine cancer by the vaginal smear. The Commonwealth Fund, New York, 1943.

PINKERS, L. H. et al.: Does a carcinomatous scalene node contraindicate pulmonary resection? Dis. Chest, 38: 516, 1960.

PRIMER G.: Früherkennung des Bronchialkarzinoms bei chronischen Bronchitikern. Prax. Pneumol., 26: 209, 1972.

QUARZ, W.: Die periphere Bronchosopie mit Hilfe Flexibler Bronchoskope. Endoscopy, 3: 171, 1971.

RADNER, S.: Suprasternal node biopsy in lymphspreading intrathoracic disease. Acta Med. Scand., 152: 413, 1955.

RATH, G. S., SCHAFF, J. T. and SNIDER, G. L.: Flexible fiberoptic bronchoscopy; Techniques and review of 100 bronchoscopies. Chest, 63: 689, 1973.

RENZ, L.E., SMIDDY, J.W. and RAUSCHER, C.R. et al.: Bronchoscopy in respiratory failure. JAMA, 219: 619, 1972.

Di RIENZO, S.: Radiologic Exploration for the Bronchus. Blackwell Scientific Publications, Oxford, 1949.

RIGLER, L. G.: Emphysema; An early roentgen sign of bronchogenic carcinoma. Radiology, 49: 578, 1947.

RIGLER, L. G.: The roentgen signs of carcinoma of the lung. Am. J. Roentgenol., 74: 415, 1955.

RIGLER, L. G.: Planigraphy in the differential diagnosis of the pulmonary nodule. Radiology, 65: 692, 1955.

RIGLER, L. G.: The Chest; A Handbook of Roentgen Diagnosis. Second Edition. Year Book Medical Publishers, Chicago, 1956.

RIGLER, L. G.: A roentgen study of the evolution of carcinoma of the lung, J. Thorac. Surg., 34: 283, 1957.

RIGLER, L. G.: The earliest roentgenographic sign of carcinoma of the lung. JAMA, 195: 655, 1966.

RINK, H.: Der Lungenkrebs, Klinik, Praxis, Problematik. F. K. Schattauer Verlag, Stuttgart, 1965.

ROUVIÉRE, H.: Anatomie des lymphatiques d l'homme, Masson et Cie, Éditeurs, Paris, 1932.

SAFAR, P.: Ventilating Bronchoscopy. Anesthesiology, 19: 406, 1958.

SENOO, T.: Metastasis of 400 necropsy cases of bronchogenic cacinoma; Statistical and morphological studies. Med. J. Osaka Univ., 7: 515, 1956.

SEPPÄLA, A. J.: Endoscopic aspects of bronchogenic carcinoma. Acta Oto-Laryng., 49: 81, 1950.

SHARP, G. S.: The diagnosis of primary carcinoma of the lung by aspiration. Am. J. Cancer, 15: 863, 1931.

SHEFTS, L. M. et al.: Scalene node biopsy. Am. Rev. Tuberc., 68: 505, 1953.

SHIELDS, T. W. et al.: Preoperative evaluation of patients with clinically resectable bronchogenic carcinoma. Arch. Surg., 76: 707, 1958.

SMIDDY, J. F., RUTH, W.E. and KERBY, G.R., et al.: Flexible fiberoptic bronchoscope. Ann. Intern. Med., 75: 971, 1971.

STRADLING, P: Diagnostic Broncnoscopy; An Introduction. E. & S. Livingstone, Edinburgh, 1968.

STÜTZ, E. und VIETEN, H.: Die Bronchographie. Georg Thieme, Stuttgart, 1955.

TAHIR, A. H.: Ventilation during bronchofiberscopy. Ann. Thorac. Surg., 14: 680, 1972.

TAJIMA, M., IKEDA, S. and TSUBOI, E.: Cytologic diagnosis and biopsy in pulmonary cancer (in Japanese). Surg. Diagn. Treatm., 7: 16, 1965.

TILDON, T.T.: An evaluation of bronchoscopy as a diagnostic and prognostic aid in lung cancer. J. Nation. Med. Assoc., Tuskegee, 54: 198, 1962.

TSUBOI, E.: Atlas of Transbronchial Biopsy. Igaku Shoin Ltd., Tokyo, 1970.

TSUBOI, E., IKEDA, S., TAJIMA, M., SHIMOSATO, Y. and ISHIKAWA, S.: Transbronchial biopsy smear for diagnosis of peripheral pulmonary carcinomas. Cancer, 20: 687, 1967.

VALAITIS, J., MCGREW, E. A., CHOMET, B., CORRELL, N. and HEAD, J.: Bronchogenic carcinoma in situ in asymptomatic high-risk population of smokers. J. Thorac. Cardiovasc. Surg., 57: 325, 1969.

VERSTEEGH, R. M. and SWIERENGA, J.: Bronchoscopic evaluation of the operability of pulmonary carcinoma. Acta Oto-Laryng., Utrecht, 56: 603, 1963.

VOZNESENSKII, A. N. and SHESTERINA, M. V.: K diagnostike bronkho-legochnykh opukholei. Probl. tbk., Moskva, 49: 14, 1971.

WALLACE, F. J.: Fiber optic endoscopy. J. Urology, 90: 324, 1963.

WANNER, A., AMIKAN, B. and SACKNER, M. A.: A technique for bedside bronchofiberscopy. Chest, 61: 287, 1972.

WANNER, A., ZIGHELLIOIM, A. and SACKNER, M. A.: Nasopharyngeal airway; A facilitated access to the trachea. Ann. Intern. Med., 75: 593, 1971.

WESSEL, T., JACOBSEN, C. D. and ÖVREBERG, K.: The diagnostic value of bronchoscopy. Acta Tuberc. Pneum. Scand., 43: 17, 1963.

WETZER, K.: Die Zytologie als ein Bestandteil der bronchologisch-pneumologischen Diagnostik. Z. Erkr. Atm., 136: 361, 1972.

WILSON, J.A.S.: The flexible fiberoptic bronchoscope. Ann. Thorac. Surg., 14: 686, 1972.

WILT, K. E. et al.: The role of bronchography in the diagnosis of bronchogenic carcinoma. Dis. Chest, 35: 517, 1959.

WOLFSON, R. J.: The diagnosis of bronchogenic carcinoma. Ann. Oto-Rhino-Laryng., 70: 677, 1961.

WOOLNER, L. B., DAVID, E., FONTANA, R. S., ANDERSEN, H. A. and BERNATZ, P. E.: In situ and early invasive bronchogenic carcinoma; Report of 28 cases with postoperative survival data. J. Thorac. Cardiovasc. Surg., 60: 275, 1970.

ZOLLNER, F.: Gustav Killian, Father of Bronchoscopy. Arch. Otolaryng., 82: 656, 1965.

# Index